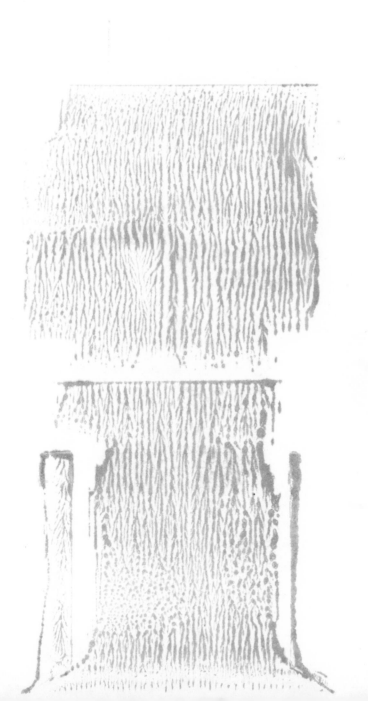

NUTRITION AND HEALTH ENCYCLOPEDIA

David F. Tver
and
Percy Russell, Ph.D.

VNR VAN NOSTRAND REINHOLD COMPANY
————————————————————— NEW YORK

Copyright © 1981 by Van Nostrand Reinhold Company Inc.
Library of Congress Catalog Card Number: 80-19933
ISBN: 0-442-24859-8

Manufactured in the United States of America

Van Nostrand Reinhold Company Inc.
135 West 50th Street, New York, N.Y. 10020
Published simultaneously in Canada by Van Nostrand Reinhold Ltd.

15 14 13 12 11 10 9 8 7 6 5 4

Library of Congress Cataloging in Publication Data
Tver, David F
    Nutrition and health encyclopedia.
    1. Nutrition. 2. Health. I. Russell,
Percy, 1926–   joint author. II. Title.
OP141.T88   613.2   80-19933
ISBN 0-442-24859-8

Preface

One of the most important health objectives today is an understanding of the part nutrition plays in the preservation of good health. The subject of nutrition is broad and encompassing, and covers many sciences—from molecular biology, physiology, and chemistry to the general field of medicine. It involves various nutritional diseases and diseases of the nervous system, the understanding both of bodily functions and of the structure of the body itself. It covers drugs, toxins, chemicals, food additives, all food man eats and their content and function.

Nutrition is still a growing science. There are many controversial areas to be researched and issues to be resolved. The subject of vitamins and their particular functions in the human body are being studied and debated. The effects of cholesterol, polyunsaturated fats, starches, sugar, food additives, and many other related subjects are still being evaluated. The effects and functions of minerals and trace elements are not entirely clear. The general subject of dieting is confusing; from carbohydrate to high-protein diets, the public is being subjected to claims and counterclaims which may or may not be valid. Diseases related to nutrition are being clarified and better understood.

From the growing, to the processing, packaging, storing, and distribution of food, nutrition is involved. Nutrition science has advanced in many directions with no clearly defined boundaries or limits. It is because of this great diversity in the field of nutrition that it was felt a comprehensive nutrition encyclopedia was needed to cover all the areas relating to nutrition. In the area of physiology, the composition and structure of the body is included; carbohydrates, fats, proteins, lipids, water and electrolytes, minerals and trace elements, fat- and water-soluble vitamins are among a few of the subjects covered.

For the food entries, a description of most of the various foods is given, with their caloric value, and food tables are included with the nutritional values. Cereals, starches, pulses, nuts, seeds, vegetables, meats, fish, eggs, milk and milk products, oils and fats, herbs, spices, beverages, and food toxins are examined and described.

Nutritional diseases are reviewed, obesity, protein-energy, malnutrition, rickets, ostemalacea, scurvy, beri-beri, gout, hyperlipemia, diabetes mellitus, and nutritional disorders of the nervous system are included. Diseases of the kidneys and urinary tract, gastrointestinal tract, liver, biliary tract, and pancreas are included.

The subjects of adsorption and metabolism are covered, including catabolic reactions, ketosis, amino acids, glucose, urea, acetyl coenzyme A, and many related functions. The various body chemicals are described and their structures and formulas given. Food additives are detailed, their functions and reliability are assessed. This and much more is included.

HOW TO USE THIS BOOK

The definitions have been made concise but all necessary detail has been included, and where a more thorough analysis was necessary, definitions have been given in greater depth. Every definition is complete with its own tables, formulas, and structures, or other pertinent information related to it. The book can be used by either the layman or the science-oriented individual. It is cross-referenced to aid those without a scientific background in gaining a full understanding of the context. For those with a scientific background, there are formulas and other more technical information. Entries in italics that are not scientific names are cross-referenced, and the asterisk (*) specifies that a diagram of the chemical structure exists with the definition or explanation.

It is believed that the Nutrition and Health Encyclopedia is one of the most comprehensive of its kind and should be an invaluable reference guide to anyone interested or involved in nutrition.

A

abalone (*Haliotis*). A red or pink mollusk or shellfish found in the Pacific Ocean off the coast of California. The muscle of the shell is the edible part of the abalone and has a clamlike flavor. Fresh, 100 gm = 98 calories; canned, 100 gm = 80 calories.

absorption. Products of digestion pass through the lining of the intestines (the intestinal mucosa) into the blood and lymph system. This process is known as absorption. Water, some simple sugars (*monosaccharides*), and many inorganic ions are absorbed in their original form. *Carbohydrates* must be converted into simple sugars, fats into *fatty acids* and *glycerol,* and *proteins* into *amino acids* during digestion to make them absorbable and therefore available to the body for building tissue and to provide a source of energy. Although limited amounts of water, *alcohol,* simple salts, and *glucose* are absorbed through the stomach (gastric mucosa), the small intestine is by far the most important organ for absorption. The most active absorptive area in the small intestine is the lower part of the duodenum and the first part of the jejenum. See *digestive system* and *active transport.*

acerala. Cherries or berries from the Caribbean Islands, a rich source of *ascorbic acid** (vitamin C), sometimes used in "natural vitamin" formulations.

acetic acid. Mol. Wt. 60. CH_3COOH. Most widely used of the organic acids. Vinegar, for example, is an aqueous solution of 4 to 5 percent acetic acid, plus flavor and colors imparted to vinegars by the constituents of the alcoholic solutions from which they are made. Ethyl alcohol (*ethanol**) in the presence of certain bacteria and air is oxidized to acetic acid. CH_3CH_2OH (ethyl alcohol) + O_2 (oxygen) = CH_3OHO (acetic acid) + H_{20} (water). Various forms of acetic acid are important intermediates in the biochemistry of all living systems. The active form of acetic acid is *acetyl coenzyme A *.* See *acetyl choline ** also.

acetoacetic acid. Mol. Wt. 102. One of the ketone bodies found in the blood and urine during *metabolic acidosis.* See *metabolic acidosis.*

1

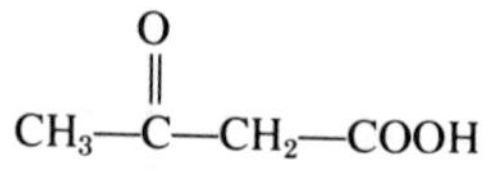

$$CH_3-\overset{\overset{\displaystyle O}{\|}}{C}-CH_2-COOH$$

Acetoacetic acid

acetohexamine (Dymelor). A hypoglycemic agent reported to lower the blood sugar level and to reduce *glycosuria* in certain diabetics. The drug acts by stimulating the release of *insulin* from the *pancreas*. The insulin appears to exercise its main effect by promoting the uptake of glucose from the bloodstream and storage as liver and muscle *glycogen**.

acetone. Mol. Wt. 58. One of the ketone bodies formed during metabolic acidosis. It arises from the nonenzymic decarboxylation of *acetoacetic acid**. It is of clinical significance because acetone or sweet breath indicates metabolic acidosis.

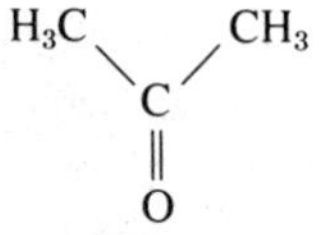

$$\underset{\underset{\displaystyle O}{\|}}{\overset{H_3C\diagdown \quad \diagup CH_3}{C}}$$

Acetone

acetone bodies. *Acetone**, *acetoacetic acid**, and *beta-hydroxybutyric acid**. Called ketone bodies and are in the blood and urine of individuals with metabolic acidosis or ketosis. See *ketone bodies*.

acetone peroxide. A chemical agent used to improve flour by bleaching in addition to aging it. An oxidizing agent solid at room temperature and normally used at levels of 5 to 120 parts per million (ppm), depending upon the flour.

acetylcholine. Mol. Wt. 182. A metabolism fundamental to the mechanism of nerve-impulse transmission. An impulse reaching a nerve ending in the normal cycle liberates acetylcholine, which then stimulates a receptor. To enable the receptor to receive further impulses, the enzyme cholinesterase breaks down

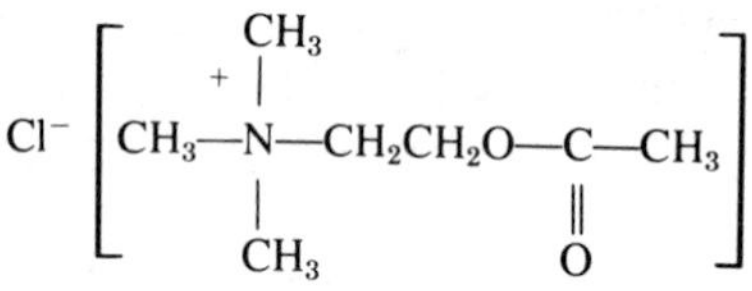

$$Cl^- \left[CH_3-\overset{\overset{\displaystyle CH_3}{\overset{\displaystyle +}{|}}}{\underset{\underset{\displaystyle CH_3}{|}}{N}}-CH_2CH_2O-\overset{\overset{\displaystyle }{}}{\underset{\underset{\displaystyle O}{\|}}{C}}-CH_3 \right]$$

Acetylcholine chloride

acetylcholine into *acetic acid** and *choline**. Other enzymes resynthesize these into more acetylcholine. Botulinus and Dinoflagellate toxins inhibit the synthesis or the release of acetylcholine.

acetyl-coenzyme A. A combination of an acetyl group with *coenzyme A**. Previously known as active acetate, it is a key material in metabolism. See *acetic acid** and *coenzyme A**.

acetylsalicylic acid. See *aspirin.*

achalasia (cardiospasm). A disturbance of normal peristalsis of the esophagus causes foods to stick at the junction of the esophagus and stomach. This area lacks normal ability to "open up" when a *bolus* of food arrives. Chief symptom is difficulty in swallowing food into the stomach.

achylia gastrica. A condition in which the secretion of gastric juice is diminished or absent.

achlorhydria. Absence of hydrochloric acid in the gastric secretions.

acid. An acid may be defined as a compound that has hydrogen ions that are released in water solutions. Acids are essentially ionized hydrogen donors. In solution, acids provide H-ions (H^+) or protons. The pH of a solution is a measure of acidity, neutrality, or alkalinity. A pH of 7.0 is neutral, a value below pH 7 is in the acid region of hydrogen-ion concentration, and above pH 7 is the alkaline or basic region.

acids and bases (alkaline substances). Chemical entities with opposite behavior. Acid solutions are sour to the taste, like *vinegar;* base or alkaline solutions feel soapy, like lye. When combined equally, acids and bases neutralize one another and produce a salt solution. The products of metabolism are largely acidic. Most foods as they are eaten are neutral, neither acid or base. However, as the food materials are broken down by enzyme action in the digestive tract and by combustion in the cells, their comparative neutrality is changed and they exhibit reactions dependent on the products formed. Thus, carbohydrate *catabolism* (metabolic breakdown) forms such acids as *lactic acid** and *pyruvic acid** which ordinarily are broken down further by oxidation to give carbon dioxide, water and energy. Fats are split into fatty acids and glycerol and under normal conditions are also oxidized to carbon dioxide, water, and energy. Proteins in hydrolysis yield amino acids which are incorporated into body proteins or after transmission can be converted into carbon dioxide and water in the process of oxidation.

acid ash residue. The preponderance in a food of inorganic (fixed) acid radicals, chiefly chloride, sulfate, and phosphate, which form acid irons (anions) in the body. The value is computed and expressed as the amount of 0.1 N alkali which would be required for neutralization.

acid–base balance. The maintenance of acid-base balance is a function of normal metabolism. The blood is slightly alkaline, varying only within narrow limits, regardless of the amount of acid products formed in metabolism. This equilibrium is maintained by a series of *buffers* (see *buffers*) in the blood and the tissue fluids. Buffers have a tendency to resist changes in hydrogen-ion concentrations (and hence pH) when treated with acids or bases. Chemically, buffers are combinations of a weak acid or base and a salt of this acid or base. The principal buffers in humans are the bicarbonate-carbonic acid system, the phosphate buffer system, the hemoglobin-oxyhemoglobin system and the proteins (see *acids and bases*).

acid-forming foods. Foods that have an acid ash residue exceeding the alkaline ash residue. Examples are meat, fish, poultry, eggs, cereals, and some nuts. Certain fruits such as cranberries and some varieties of prunes and plums, although they have a predominantly alkaline residue, are acid-forming because the organic acids are not metabolized by the body. Pure starches, sugars and fats, which produce carbonic acid during metabolism, are not included as acid forming since *carbonic acid* is readily excreted by the lungs as carbon dioxide (CO_2) without affecting the alkaline reserve. ·

acidemia. When human blood decreases from pH 7.4, it is more acidic; the condition is called acidemia. Normally the body tends towards acidemia because of the accumulation of carbon dioxide and the acid waste products of metabolism. Acidemia also occurs in starvation and diabetes. The acid products are buffered by the buffer systems present in the blood and tissue fluids, and there is an increase in rate and depth of breathing which removes CO_2 from the blood, thus removing *carbonic acid*. Later the kidney excretes highly acid urine, and there is a return towards normal.

acidity or alkalinity food controls. Substances added to food to control acidity or alkalinity include acids, alkalies, buffers, and neutralizing agents. (See *acids and bases* and *buffers*.) Fruit flavors used in various products differ in their level of acidity. Thus "fruit" acids may be added to increase flavor intensity. The same "fruit" acids are sometimes added to processed cheese to improve texture and impart tartness. Additives in this group are also used to give an acid or tart taste to soft drinks, to facilitate heat processes of canned vegetables without discoloration, and to compensate for insufficient acid in fruit when making jellies and jams. These additives also facilitate peeling of tubers and fruits, neutralize part of the natural acids as when making tomato soup, and help control the texture of candy.

acidophilus milk. See *milk, fermented milk sources*.

acidosis. A term to indicate a blood pH value below the normal value of 7.4. A condition in which the body's *alkaline reserve* is lowered due to abnormal loss of alkaline salts or abnormal accumulation of acids. Acidosis may be caused by an accumulation of organic acids (see *metabolic acidosis*) as in diabetic acidosis, or by excess loss of bicarbonates (as in renal disease), or in respiratory disorders that interfere with adequate release of carbon dioxide from the lungs and thereby cause an accumulation of *carbonic acid* in the blood (*respiratory acidosis*).

acini. Groups of secretory cells in glands such as the salivary glands, the pancreas, and the liver. These organized clusters of cells are called acini because their shape resembles that of a bunch of grapes. Secretions of enzymes from the acini of the pancreas, for example, feed into ducts that empty into the small intestine to promote digestion.

acne. Seen most commonly in the skin of the face, neck, and chest. The characteristic sign is the blackhead or comedo, with the skin surrounding the central blackened area often slightly raised or reddened. Sometimes the central area is white and called a whitehead. The blackhead is a plugging of the opening of a hair follicle. This plug consists of a mixture of sebum, the normal oily secretion of the sebaceous glands (microscopic glands connected to the shaft containing the root of the hair), and of keratin, the normally present outermost layer of the skin. The sebum produced by these glands serves to lubricate the hair and give it its oily sheen. There is no known cure for acne, nor is there any known way of preventing this common problem.

acne rosacea. Involves excessive flushing of the blood vessels of the nose and cheeks. A nervous reflex may be a factor in such excessive flushing. Drinking alcohol may encourage the reflex, but it is not essential. With long-continued abnormal flushing the blood vessels become more apparent, and nose size may increase.

acorn squash. A fall and winter vegetable that belongs to the gourd family. It has a dark-green rind, yellow-orange flesh, and many seeds. Acorn squash can grow as large as 8 inches long and 5 inches across. Its flavor is on the sweet side. An excellent source of *carotene* * (vitamin A activity); fair source of *ascorbic acid* * (vitamin C), *riboflavin* *, and iron. Raw, 100 gm = 44 calories.

acrolein. Mol. Wt. 56. A substance formed from the glycerol of fat when heated to high temperature. The acrid odor of overheated fat is due to acrolein.

$$
\begin{array}{ccc}
\text{H} & \text{H} & \text{H} \\
| & | & | \\
\text{H---C} & \!\!=\!\!\text{C---C} & \!\!=\!\!\text{O}
\end{array}
$$

Acrolein

acromegaly. A chronic progressive disease due to increased secretion of the growth-stimulating hormone from the *pituitary gland*. In most instances a benign tumor of the pituitary is the cause of the trouble. Acromegaly is characterized by enlargement of the hands and feet, cartilaginous part of bones, soft tissues of the body, and such structures as the heart, spleen, and liver. The frontal bones and jaw become prominent, the nose widens, the teeth become spaced, the lower eyelids are baggy, the tongue markedly enlarged.

ACTH. See *adrenocorticotropin* (adrenocorticotropic hormone).

activators. Substances that bring about or increase the activity of enzymes.

active site. That portion of an enzyme surface where combination with the substrate takes place and the chemical or molecular changes in the substrate occur.

active transport. By active transport nutrients and other substances are concentrated within the cell from a lower concentration outside the cell. Active transport is in contradistinction to simple diffusion where the material, such as water and some salts, pass freely through the membrane in either direction, and to facilitated diffusion where the rate of transfer is increased by enzymes or carriers in the membrane. Both simple diffusion and facilitated diffusion are passive diffusions since the processes are in the direction of equilibrium, i.e., concentrations on both sides of the membrane are equal. Active transport requires energy, and the major source of the energy is *adenosine triphosphate* (ATP). The details of how the chemical energy is coupled to the active transport of nutrients across membranes is not clearly understood. Amino acids are actively transported into the intestinal mucosa. Sodium is actively transported in the opposite direction, i.e., sodium ions are pumped out of the cell, which in turn is coupled to the active transport of *glucose* * and *galactose* *. Calcium is an example of facilitated diffusion in the intestines in which *vitamin D* * plays a major role. The transport of *cobalamin** (vitamin B_{12}) is also facilitated and needs a specific factor, a mucoprotein called intrinsic factor, in order to be absorbed. See *absorption*.

acute. A condition or disease of short duration. The opposite of chronic.

addictive. A substance leading to the habituation of use, usually of a drug, the deprivation of which leads to withdrawal symptoms and an impulse to take the drug again.

Addison's disease. A rare metabolic disorder in which there is adrenal insufficiency of the hormones of the *adrenal cortex*, either because of infection such as tuberculosis, or a tumor, or general wasting or *atrophy* following removal of the *pituitary gland* in the treatment of *cancer*. A person with Addison's disease is unable to store sodium chloride and excretes it in the urine in excessive quantities, while there is decreased ability to excrete potassium, and the percentage of potassium in the blood rises sharply. With sodium loss, water excretion increases and severe dehydration follows, which can result in a crisis.

additives. See *food additives*.

adequate. An amount sufficient to meet a specific requirement. The term "adequate diet" is often incorrectly used in reference to an individual diet which provides the dietary allowances of nutrients as recommended by the Food and Nutrition Board of the National Research Council.

adenine. A *purine* base. See *adenosine triphosphate*.

adenohypophysis. See *pituitary gland*.

adenosine. See *adenosine triphosphate*.

adenosine diphosphate (ADP). See *adenosine triphosphate*.

adenosine monophosphate (AMP). See *adenosine triphosphate*.

adenosine triphosphate (ATP). Mol. Wt. 507. The adenosine nucleotides, AMP, ADP, and ATP, are the most important compounds in terms of energy balance and metabolism. The oxidation of foodstuffs leads through a system called the *terminal respiratory chain* where electrons are donated to oxygen, and water is formed. The process is called *oxidative phosphorylation*, because coupled to the oxidation of foodstuffs is the phosphorylation of ADP to form

ATP. These reactions take place in the *mitochondria*. ATP is the principal form of chemical energy in the body. It is used in many biosynthetic processes which require energy. The activation of glucose, amino acids and fatty acids all require the formation of phosphate intermediates, and ATP is the source of the phosphate and the chemical energy. The result of these reactions is the formation of AMP or ADP, depending upon the reaction, which can be used to form more ATP by oxidative phosphorylation.

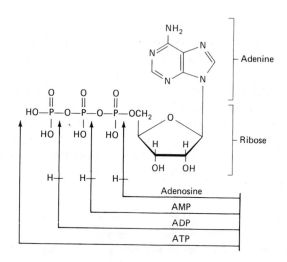

Adenosine triphosphate

S-adenosylmethionine. Mol. Wt. 434. A derivative of *adenosine triphosphate* (ATP) involved in the transfer of methyl groups ($-CH_3$) in the formation of lecithin (phosphatydyl choline). Other compounds involved in one carbon transfers are the vitamins *cobalamin* * (vitamin B_{12}) and *folacin*.

S-adenosylmethionine

ADH. See *antidiuretic hormone* (vasopressin).

adipic acid (hexanedioic acid). Mol. Wt. 146. Used in bottled drinks and throat lozenges, because this additive has little tendency to pick up moisture, and is frequently used to supply tartness to powdered products, such as gelatin desserts and fruit-flavored drinks. Adipic acid is occasionally added to edible oils to prevent them from going rancid.

$$HOOC \cdot CH_2CH_2CH_2CH_2COOH.$$

adipose. Animal fat. Commonly used in describing the part of the body where neutral fat is stored, which is the adipose tissue.

adipose tissue. A fatty connective tissue which is found under the skin and in many other regions of the body. It serves as a padding and insulation around and between organs. It insulates the body by reducing heat loss and serves as a food reserve.

ADP. Adenosine diphosphate. See *adenosine triphosphate**.

adrenal cortex. The outer layer of the adrenal glands. See *adrenal glands*.

adrenal glands. The two adrenal glands are located one above each kidney (suprarenal). Each adrenal gland actually functions as two separate glands, producing different hormones from its two parts, the medulla, the inner portion, and the cortex, the outer portion. The adrenal medulla is a physiologically separate organ from the cortex. The medulla produces *epinephrine**, the "fright or flight hormone," and *norepinephrine**. The hormones of the medulla, epinephrine and norepinephrine, are important in preparing the body for action against external danger or fright. Epinephrine (sometimes called adrenaline) dilates blood vessels so that more blood can flow through them and increase the amount of work done by the heart. Both epinephrine and norepinephrine elevate the blood glucose level by stimulation of the breakdown of the glycogen store in the liver. Dilation of the tiny coronary arteries in the heart is also engendered by both hormones. Epinephrine and norepinephrine are both modified forms of a single amino acid *phenylalanine*. The medulla is stimulated to release epinephrine by the sympathetic branch of the autonomic nervous system in order to give the body the extra energy it needs in emergencies by causing the release of glucose from liver *glycogen**. The cortex, the outer part of the adrenal glands, produces a series of adrenocortical hormones including *hydrocortisone**. The adrenocortical hormones influence the salt and *water balance* of the body, the metabolism of foods, and the ability of the body to handle stress. The cortex of the adrenal glands requires stimulation by a hormone produced by the pituitary gland, adrenocorticotropin.

adrenaline. See *epinephrine*.

adrenocorticotropic hormone (adrenocorticotropin, ACTH). A hormone liberated by the anterior *pituitary gland,* which stimulates the cortex of the *adrenal glands*. The basophilic cells of the hypophyseal pituitary anterior lobe secrete adrenocorticotropin, often referred to as adrenocorticotropic hormone (ACTH). ACTH is a polypeptide with 39 amino acids. ACTH acts upon the *adrenal gland* cortices. When there is too little ACTH, the cortical layers atrophy. Hyperplasia occur when excessive quantities of ACTH are given. Under the influence of ACTH all the adrenal cortical hormones are secreted. In addition, ACTH has a direct lipolytic action. Fat is mobilized and the fatty acid level in the blood increases due to *lipolysis*.

aerobic. Living or functioning in air or free oxygen.

aflatoxins. Mol. Wt. 312. Several closely related toxic compounds produced by certain molds which cause liver injury in poultry. Some may be carcinogenic.

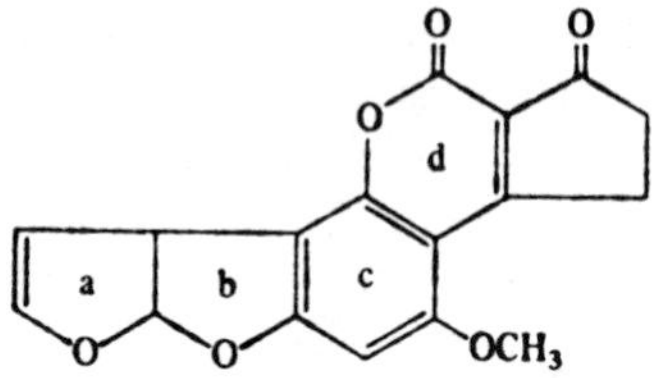

All aflatoxins contain the same tetracyclic ring
systems shown above, a b c d.

agar. A vegetable gelatin made from various kinds of algae or seaweed, used as a jellying agent in home cooking. Used in the Orient in the preparation of soups and jellies as a thickening agent. Also used in the commercial manufacture of jams, jellies, ice creams, and mayonnaise. It is used in medicine and is essential in microbiology where it is used as a solid support on which bacteria are grown in culture.

agglutination. Clumping of cells or other particles, as in the blood when there is a mixture or transfusion involving incompatible bloods.

agglutinin. The substance, or antibody, in the blood serum which causes the clumping or *agglutination* of cells.

agglutinogen. The substance, or antigen, in the red blood cells which is affected by the conflicting agglutinin of another person.

alanine. Mol. Wt. 89. One of the amino acids found in proteins. It is the amino acid derivative of *pyruvic acid**. See *amino acid*.

$$CH_3—CH—COOH$$
$$|$$
$$NH_2$$

Alanine

albacore (*Thunnis germo*). A type of tuna fish. Albacore has true white meat of all tuna and is used for the finest canned tuna. Canned tuna labeled "all white meat, solid pack," is albacore. Excellent source of protein; small amounts of calcium, phosphorus, and iron. Fresh, raw, 100 gm = 177 calories; canned and packed in oil, ½ cup = 194 calories.

albinism. An inborn error of the metabolism of the essential amino acid *tyrosine* that results in the failure to produce the pigment *melanin*.

albino. An animal or human being with *albinism*.

albuminoids. The simple proteins characteristic of the skeletal structure of animals (also called scleroproteins) and also of the external protective tissues such as the skin, hair, etc. Example is collagen, which when boiled with water yields gelatin. See *protein*.

albumins. Simple proteins soluble in pure water and coagulable when heated. Examples are egg albumin (in egg whites), serum albumin (blood), leucosin (wheat), legumelin (peas). See *serum albumins*.

albuminuria. The presence of albumin in the urine. It is an indication of renal dysfunction.

***Alcaligenes*.** A species of bacteria which usually produces an alkaline reaction in the medium of growth. *A. viscolactis* (viscosus) causes ropiness of milk, and *A. metalcaligenes* gives a slimy growth on cottage cheese. These organisms come from manure, feeds, soils, water and dust.

alcohol. A class of organic compound that contains the hydroxyl (–OH) group. A general term often applied to ethyl alcohol (ethanol). Alcohol in its pure form is a transparent, colorless liquid, volatile, and very flammable. It is distilled from a great variety of fruits and grains that contain either natural sugar or substances that can be transformed into sugar. By the addition of natural or artificial yeast strains and mineral compounds, the sugar is changed by the process of fermentation into alcohol and other by-products which are used commercially. This is the alcohol commonly known as grain or wine alcohol. Its technical name is ethyl alcohol or *ethanol**. It is found in beer, whiskies, wines, brandies, liqueurs, and rum. Alcohol should not be regarded as a single substance. *Methyl* or wood alcohol, which is very different from the grain or ethyl alcohol we drink, is the poisonous alcohol most frequently encountered.

aldosterone. Mol. Wt. 360. One of the three major hormones of the *adrenal glands* (cortex) concerned mainly with the level of sodium ions (Na^+) in the body and the *water balance*. The hormone cannot actually increase the amount of Na^+ in the body, it can only prevent excessive loss. It does this by acting directly on the filtering system of the kidneys. The aldosterone modifies the membranes involved in filtration so that Na^+ does not pass into the urine. At the same time, potassium ions (K^+) tend to be excreted in increased quantities. The amount of Na^+ in the body is important both for the activity of certain enzymes and for the normal functioning of the nervous system. See *water balance*.

Aldosterone

ale. Ale is fermented malt beverage; *beer* is its brother. Ale, like beer, is brewed from malt, cereals, and hops, but the method of brewing ale is different from that of brewing beer. Ale is "top fermented," that is, during fermentation at a higher temperature, its *yeast* rises to the top. The result is a brew with a more pronounced hop flavor than that found in beer. Porter and stout are two well-known varieties of ale, both sweeter and darker than the others. Porter has less hop flavor than stout, which has a full hop flavor with a slightly burnt taste. 1 cup = 84 calories. See *beer* and *yeast*.

alewife (*Pomolobus pseudoharengus*). An inexpensive edible fish belonging to the herring family. Alewives grow to about 10 inches in length and to about a half pound in weight. The fish is rather bony, but the flavor is pleasant and less oily than that of shad. They can be cooked like fresh herring. Fresh, raw, 100 gm = 127 calories; canned, fish and liquid, 100 gm calories.

alfalfa (_Medicago sativa_). A leguminous plant chiefly used for animal forage, prized by health-food devotees as a rich source of vitamins, usually consumed in the form of alfalfa tablets. Alfalfa sprouts are rich in _ascorbic acid.*_

alginate or **propylene glycol alginate.** As a food additive it acts as a thickening and stabilizing agent. The most important commercial source of algin is giant kelp. Algin solutions can be converted to gels by adding calcium. These chemically set gels are extremely stable, and help prevent jelling in pastries from oozing over the oven. Industry uses algin to help maintain the desired texture in ice cream, candy, cheese, pressure-dispensed whipped cream, yogurt, canned frostings, and many other factory-made goods.

alimentary canal. See _digestive system._

alkalemia. As human blood increases above pH 7.4, the blood becomes more alkaline and the condition is called alkalemia. Alkalemia is less common than acidemia, but can occur from loss of acid from the stomach in vomiting or the intake of too much alkaline medicine, for example, in the treatment of gastric or duodenal ulcer. To compensate for alkalemia, buffer mechanisms come into action in the opposite direction and respiration is depressed so that carbon dioxide is retained and the H-ion concentration rises again with the resulting increase in _carbonic acid._ The kidney secretes an alkaline urine and body conditions return towards normal, pH 7.4.

alkali. One of a group of compounds that form salts when united with acids, and soaps when combined with fatty acids. The chemical opposite of an acid. A base or substance capable of neutralizing acids. See _acids and bases._

alkaline ash residue. The preponderance in a food of the elements sodium, potassium, calcium, and magnesium, yield basic or alkaline reactions with water, the cations in the body. The alkaline value is computed and expressed as the amount of O.1 N acid which would be required for neutralization.

alkaline-phosphatase test. An enzyme test performed on blood; used as a screening test in bone disease, prostate cancer, and for diagnosis in obstructive jaundice.

alkaline reserve. The amount of alkaline or basic material available in the body to neutralize acids.

alkaline tide. The slight change in blood pH towards the alkaline side following a meal. A consequence of the production of hydrochloric acid in the stomach.

alkaloid. An organic nitrogenous base. Many alkaloids are of great medical importance, such as morphine, strychnine, atropine, cocaine, quinine. They occur in the animal and vegetable kingdoms, and some have been synthesized.

alkalosis. A condition in which there are excess alkaline substances in the body fluids. Can be caused by excessive vomiting or improper use of a gastric-suction apparatus and by hyperventilation when an individual breathes too rapidly. Symptoms include shallow respiration, a tingling sensation of the fingers, toes, and lips, muscular cramps, tetany convulsions. The physiological opposite of *acidosis*. See *alkalemia*.

allele (allelomorphs). Genes which are assigned to the same functions and are located in the same position in matching chromsomes.

allergen. Any substance capable of inducing an *allergy*.

allergy. A special type of inflammatory response in various parts of the body to a foreign substance in the environment. Allergic reactions may take several forms, depending upon which part of the body is affected, but all involve the immunological system. The parts of the body most likely to show allergic responses are the lungs, nose, eyes, skin, middle ear, and the stomach and intestines. Depending on the site, allergic reactions can result in asthma, hay fever, conjunctivitis, eczema, hives, sinusitis and any combination of abdominal pain, nausea, vomiting, or diarrhea. Substances that provoke an allergic reaction are known as *allergens*. An individual who is allergic to grass, for example, produces antibodies that are distributed throughout the body but cause symptoms only where and when they come in contact with their allergen. Allergic symptoms arise from the interaction of an allergen with an *antibody* made by the allergic individual. The meeting of allergen and antibody sets in process a reaction that releases various substances, which cause the dilation (opening up) of small vessels and the leaking of fluids through these vessels into the surrounding tissues, resulting in swelling, spasm of the mouth muscles, spasm in air passages, and an outpouring of mucous secretions. The particular resulting symptoms depend upon where the antibody and allergen meet.

almond (*Prunus Amygdalus*). The word covers the tree and nut, the seed or kernel of a subgenus which includes the peach tree. The almond closely resembles the peach in its blossom and young unripe fruit, although the almond tree grows larger. The almond tree bears a leathery fruit which upon maturing, splits open and exposes the nut in its shell. The pitted shell is light tan in color. The nut is covered with a medium-brown skin and is white inside. Basically there are two kinds of almonds, sweet and bitter. Almonds provide some protein, iron, calcium, phosphorus, and B vitamins. They are also high in fat. Raw, 100 gm = 598 calories; roasted and salted, 100 gm = 627 calories.

alopecia. Loss of hair from part of the body that is normally hairy. A symptom of *retinol* * (vitamin A) toxicity.

alpha (α) ketoglutaric acid. See *ketoglutaric acid.*

alpha (α) tocopherol. See *tocopherols.*

aluminum (Al). Element No. 13. Atom. Wt. 27. A light silver-colored metal. The amount of aluminum ingested in the average human diet ranges widely from about 10 mg to more than 100 mg daily. This element is found in many plant and animal foods. Despite this wide intake and distribution, no clear function in human nutrition has been established. The total aluminum content of the human body is from 50 to 150 mg.

aluminum hydroxide. Mol. Wt. 78. $Al(OH)_3$. A basic substance used in antiacids. See *antacid.*

ameba. A one-celled animal organism. A naked rhizopod or other ameboid protozoan.

amebic dysentary (amebiasis). Disease primarily caused by *ameba* affecting the colon, but may affect other organs, especially the liver. Severe amebiasis is characterized by diarrhea with blood and/or pus and mucus in the watery discharges. Infection generally takes place following the drinking of water contaminated with sewage containing amebae. Complications of amebic infections are hepatitis, abscess of the liver, abscess of the lung, and perforation of the bowel.

ameboid movement. The method of locomotion for amoeba which involves the formation and contraction of cellular extensions sometimes referred to as pseudopodia (false feet). Many f the cells in the human body, especially the *white blood cells,* have ability to move about by ameboid movement.

ameloblasts. Special epithelial cells surrounding tooth buds in gum tissue, which form cup-shaped organs for producing the enamel structure of the developing teeth. Insufficient vitamin A (*retinol**) causes faulty production of ame-loblasts and therefore impairs the soundness of tooth structure.

amenorrhea. The word means absence of menstruation. The term is used to cover the absence of regular monthly periods at any time between the onset of puberty and menopause. Usually classified as primary amenorrhea, in which the menses have never occurred, and secondary amenorrhea in which there is an absence of menstrual periods in women who have formerly had normal men-strual cycles.

amination. The addition of an amino group (NH_2) to an organic compound to produce an *amine*. See *transamination*.

amine. An organic compound with basic properties containing an amino group—NH_2.

amino acids. Amino acids are the simplest structural unit of the proteins. They have the same relation to proteins that letters have to words. At least 22 dif-ferent letters make up the amino alphabet, and combinations of these amino acids produce a great variety of proteins. There are eight essential or indispens-able amino acids for man, *tryptophan**, *threonine**, *methionine**, *isoleucine**, *lysine**, *valine**, and *phenylalaine**. The body is unable to produce these and must get them from food. The other amino acids may be synthesized in the body. The amino acids in a protein determine its chemical characteristics, and the essential amino acids determine its nutritive or *biological value* (BV). All amino acids contain carbon, hydrogen, oxygen, and nitrogen. Three amino acids have sulfur, and two contain iodine. A unique feature of the amino acids is the arrangement of its asymmetric carbon, which can exist in two patterns. One pattern is the mirror image of the other (L-form and D-form), like the left and right hand. Nature makes only the L-form of amino acids in all proteins, the pattern found in all foods. In general, the body can use only the L-form. Some bacterial nonprotein products contain the D-forms of amino acids. For ex-ample, some antibiotics and cell walls of some bacteria contain D-amino acid forms. Two naturally occurring amino acids, L-*ornithine** and L-*citrulline**, do not occur in proteins. The structures of the amino acids are given under the name of the individual amino acid.

amino-acid metabolism. The metabolism of the amino acids follows several directions. The amino acid can be degraded and oxidized as a source of energy, incorporated into proteins, or used in the synthesis of nitrogen-containing com-pounds. The diagram on p. 17 summarizes and simplifies the various meta-bolic paths amino acids take.

Amino Acid Classification

Classification	Essential Amino Acids	Nonessential Amino Acids
Neutral—one amino and one carboxyl group Aliphatic	threonine valine leucine isoleucine	glycine alanine serine
Aromatic—contains benzene ring	phenylalanine	tyrosine
Heterocyclic	tryptophan histidine (children)	proline hydroxyproline
Sulfur-containing	methionine	cysteine
Basic—two amino and one carboxyl group	lysine	arginine hydroxylysine
Acid—one amino and two carboxyl groups		aspartic acid glutamic acid

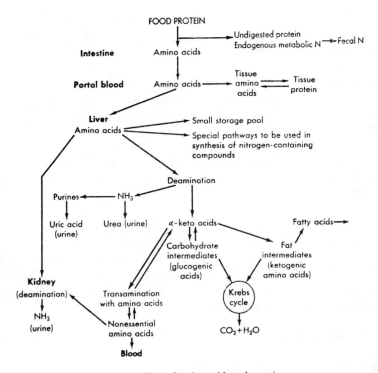

The metabolism of amino acids and protein.

In terms of their metabolism, amino acids are classified as *glucogenic* (resulting in a net increase in *glucose* production), *ketogenic* (resulting in a production of *ketone bodies*) or both. The metabolic classification is only of importance in that it indicates the pathway a given amino acid may take. Most of the amino acids are glucogenic. Only leucine is wholly ketogenic. The table below shows the metabolic fates of the carbon skeletons of the common amino acids.

Carbon Skeleton Ultimately Converted to Amphibolic Intermediates Forming:

Glycogen ("Glycogenic" Amino Acids)		Fat ("Ketogenic" Amino Acids)	Both Glycogen and Fat ("Glycogenic" and "Ketogenic" Amino Acids)
L-alanine	L-hydroxypoline	L-leucine	L-isoleucine
L-arginine	L-methionine		L-lysine
L-aspartate	L-proline		L-phenylalanine
L-cystine	L-serine		L-tyrosine
L-glutamate	L-threonine		L-tryptophan
L-glycine	L-valine		
L-histidine			

The diagram on p. 19 shows the metabolic pathways central to the *Kreb's* (*tricarboxylic acid*) *cycle.**

amino acids oxidase. The catalyst for oxidative deamination of amino acids. The reaction occurs primarily in the liver and kidneys. The enzyme uses flavin mononucleotide* (FMN) as a cofactor, which is a derivative of the B-vitamin *riboflavin.* *

amino sugars. Sugars that contain an amino group (NH_2). An important example of their occurrence is in antibiotics such as the mycin drugs and in mucopolysaccharides.

ammoniated glycyrrhizin. A toxic agent having a variety of physiological effects; it raises blood pressure, alleviates stomach ulcers and reduces the toxicity of strychnine, carbolic acid, and diptheria toxin. Food companies use it in licorice flavoring and as a compound of root beer and wintergreen flavoring in beverages (50 ppm), candy (5 to 60 ppm), and baked goods (5 ppm). Glycyrrhizin is one of the sweetest natural substances known.

amoeba. see *ameba.*

AMP (adenosine monophosphate). See *adenosine triphosphate* (ATP).

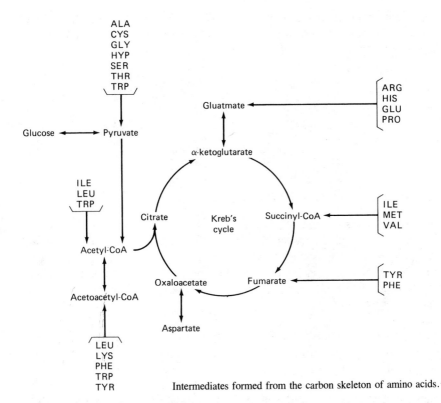

Intermediates formed from the carbon skeleton of amino acids.

amphetamine sulfate (benzidrine sulfate). Mol. Wt. 369. A synthetic drug that stimulates the central nervous system, reduces appetite and reduces nasal congestion. Amphetamines are addictive.

Amphetamine sulfate

amphoteric. A single compound having properties of both an acid and a base, and therefore able to function as either. *Amino acids* have this dual chemical nature because of their structure; they contain both an acid (carboxyl, COOH) group and a base (amino, NH_2) group, as do *proteins*. See *zwitterion*.

amygdalin (vitamin B$_{17}$, laetrile). Mol. Wt. 457. The active principle of laetrile or vitamin B$_{17}$ is shown below. It occurs in almond seed extracts and has been controversial in the treatment of cancer.

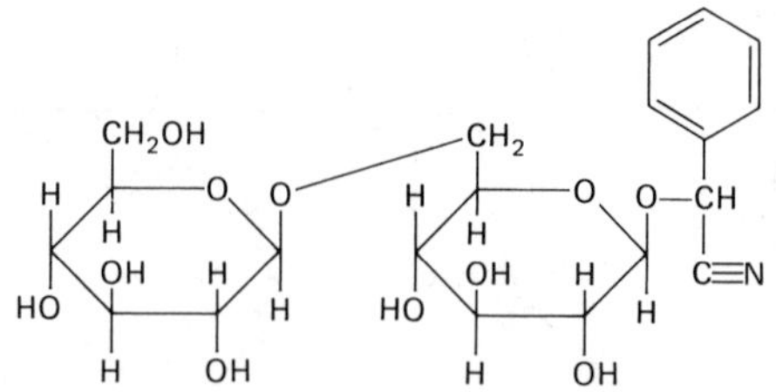

Amygdalin (vitamin B$_{17}$, laetrile)

amylase. A classification of enzymes that digest starch, e.g., *ptyalin* in the *saliva*. To distinguish between the different enzymes, the starch splitting enzyme found in saliva is called salivary amylase and the one secreted by the pancreas is known as pancreatic amylase. The amylases that hydrolyze the starches are classified in various ways depending on how and where they act on the *starch* * molecules.

amylopectin. The branched-chain, insoluble form of *starch* from plants which stains violet red with iodine and forms a paste with hot water. The animal equivalent of amylopectin is *gylcogen* *. See *starch*.

amylose. The straight chain of linked *glucose*, a soluble form of starch which stains blue with iodine. Potato starch is an example of amylose. See *starch*.

anabolism. The opposite of catabolism. Anabolism includes all chemical changes that build new substances in growth or maintenance. *Metabolism* = anabolism + *catabolism*. Constructive processes that build up the body substances—the synthesis in living organisms of more complex substances from simpler ones, are anabolic processes. Anabolism uses energy made available from certain catabolic processes, for example, the oxidation of fat to carbon dioxide + water + energy.

anaerobe. A microorganism living or functioning in the absence of air or free oxygen. The opposite of an aerobe. A strict anaerobe is an organism which cannot survive in the presence of oxygen. Organisms that can live under either aerobic or anaerobic conditions are called *facultative* organisms. Most *yeasts* are facultative.

analgesia. Absence of sensitivity to pain.

analgesics. One of the largest groups of pain killers. Narcotics such as morphine and codeine sulfate are derivatives of opium and all three may cause addiction. *Aspirin* acts as an analgesic and as an antipyretic. As an *analgesic,* it relieves headache and muscular pain. Aspirin normally is used in 0.324-gm tablets. Often it is combined with other analgesics such as *phenacetin** and *caffeine** (APC). In large and continued doses, aspirin produces gastric irritation.

anaphase. The stage in cell division at which the newly formed duplicated chromosomes separate and go to opposite sides of the dividing cell.

analphylaxis. An extreme hypersensitivity induced as a result of the presence of an *antigen* to which the animal or individual has been sensitized by injection. It is an extreme reaction of the immunological system.

anastomosis. A communication between two vessels either naturally or surgically.

androgens (androgenic hormones). One of a class of steroid hormones that produces secondary male characteristics. They are derivatives of cholesterol. The opposite of the female hormones, the *estrogens.* See *testosterone**.

anemia. A condition in which the total quantity of *hemoglobin* in the circulating blood is less than normal. This deficiency in circulating hemoglobin may be due to a decreased number of red blood cells per unit volume of blood or to a deficient hemoglobin content in the erythrocytes. The various anemias may be classified in the following simplified fashion on an etiologic basis.

I. Anemia caused by blood loss: (A) Anemia of chronic blood loss; B) Acute posthemorrhagic anemia.
II. Anemias caused by excessive destruction of erythrocytes: (A) Acute *hemolysis:* (1) Due to immune bodies, as in erythroblastosis or hypersplenism, (2) due to toxic reactions to bacteria toxins or chemicals (drugs). (B) Chronic hemolysisis as in, (1) congenital disorders such as sickle-cell anemia, Mediterranean anemia, congenital hemolytic *jaundice,* (2) acquired disorders such as paroxysmal nocturnal hemoglobinuria.
III. Anemias due to impaired production of erythrocytes: (A) Caused by deficiency of substances essential for erythropoesis, (1) iron, (2) *cobalamin** (vitamin B_{12}), (3) *folacin**, (4) *protein,* (5) *ascorbic acid** (vitamin C), (6) trace minerals, (7) other vitamins. (B) Caused by congenital defects in *erythropoesis,* (1) congenital hemolytic disease, (2) formation of abnormal *hemoglobins.* (C) Caused by acquired impairment

of erythropoesis, (1) infection, (2) chronic disease, (3) replacement or infiltration of the bone marrow, (4) inhibition or destruction of the marrow by noxious chemicals, drugs or irradiation, (5) hormonal disorders.

anemias, iron deficiency. A group consisting of a number of chronic anemias which are characterized by small pale *erythrocytes*. The basic cause is depletion of iron stores due to a discrepancy between iron intake and iron requirements. In adults, chronic blood loss is the most common cause for iron deficiency anemia. It may be physiologic, as in excessive or prolonged menstruation, or pathologic, as in occult intestinal blood loss due to ulcerations, parasites, or maligancy. Disorders of the gastrointestinal tract such as *achlorhydria*, or chronic diarrhea may also lead to iron deficiency anemia because of impaired iron absorption. The symptoms of iron deficiency anemia are similar to those of other types and include easy fatigability, pallor, dyspnea on exertion, and a constant feeling of tiredness. The skin, mucous membranes, and nails are pale in proportion to the reduction in the circulating hemoglobin. Nails may be brittle, individual blood cells are pale (hypochromic) and smaller than normal (microcytic).

anemia, nutritional. The anemias that result from a deficency of iron, proteins, certain vitamins, *cobalamin** (vitamin B_{12}), *folacin,* and *ascorbic acid** (vitamin C), copper, and other heavy metals are frequently termed nutritional anemias. The deficiency may be caused also by chronic blood loss or hemmorrhage, inadequate ingestion, defective absorption, imperfect utilization, or injury to the bone marrow. The vast majority of the cases of hypochromic or nutritional anemia seen in the United States are related to iron deficiency. For many years, diet has been recognized as a remedial agent in overcoming nutritional anemia.

anemia, pernicious. An *anemia* caused by the lack of *vitamin B^{12}* (extrinsic factor)*. A failure to absorb vitamin B^{12} due to a failure of the gastric mucosa (stomach lining) to excrete mucoproteins, called intrinsic factor, required for absorption. Pernicious anemia is characterized by giant red cells (*macrocytes*) and each red cell appears to be overloaded with hemoglobin (hyperchromic) while the total number of red blood cells is decreased (anemia). Numbness in the fingers and toes is common. The disease generally occurs in males between the ages of 40 and 65 years. Treatment and maintenance usually involves intermuscular injection of a vitamin B^{12} derivative, cyanocobalamin, and the prognosis is excellent. Vitamin B^{12} deficiency is sometimes found in strict vegetarians of long standing, since vitamin B^{12} does not occur in plants. Rarely are individuals such strict vegetarians or vegans that dairy products, eggs, or fish are not eaten at some time. Vitamin B^{12} deficiency has been reported in infants born of mothers who were strict vegetarians. The administration of microgram quantities of cyanocobalamin daily by mouth is sufficient to overcome vitamin B^{12} deficiencies when there is normal production of intrinsic factor. Vitamin B^{12} is required to remove methyl groups ($-CH^3$) from folic acid (folacin). Unmethylated folacin is required for the production of red blood cells. See *folate deficiency* and *folacin*.

angina. Spasmodic choking or suffocating pain; also used for the disease or condition producing the pain.

angina pectoris. Similar to myocardial infarction in that it results from an inadequate oxygen supply to the myocardium. The difference is that myocardial infarction is a result of a rather sudden blockage of a coronary artery, whereas angina pectoris is a more gradual process in which the coronary vessels cannot bring sufficient blood supply (or oxygen) to the myocardium because they are occluded by atherosclerotic plaques and their walls have lost their elasticity.

angiocardiogram. A special type of x-ray examination using radio-opaque dye to aid in visualizing heart and large blood vessels leading to and from the heart. The dye is injected through a catheter into an artery. Immediately after the dye is injected, X-rays are taken in rapid sequence. The dye is radio opaque, i.e., it does not allow X-rays to pass through, and its passage through the heart can be visualized. This type of examination is done for congenital heart diseases or other structural defects of the heart, its valves, or the large blood vessels.

angioneurotic edema. Patches of circumscribed swelling of the skin, mucous membranes, and sometimes, viscera. Giant hives.

angitis. Inflammation of a vessel such as a blood vessel, lumpy vessel, or bile duct.

angiotensin (vasopressin). A polypeptide hormone that acts as a pressor substance (elevates the blood pressure). Angiotensin is produced in the body by interaction of the enzyme renin, produced in the kidneys by the *renal cortex,* and a serum globulin fraction, angiotensinogen, produced by the liver. Angiotensin also has an effect on *water balance* since it stimulates the secretion of *antidiuretic hormone* (ADH) by the adrenal glands.

Ångstrom (Å). A linear unit of measure equivalent to 1/100,000,000 of a centimeter. The measure is named after a Swedish physicist.

anions. An ion carrying a negative charge. Since unlike forms of electricity attract each other, it is attracted by, and travels to, the anode or positive pole. The anions include all the nonmetals, the acid radicals, and the *hydroxyl* ion (OH^-).

anise (*Pimpinella anisum*). A culinary herb belonging to the parsley family, growing to a height of 2 feet, with feathery leaves and tiny grayish brown fruits which are dried for use. The plants and fruits have a distinctive licorice flavor. The dried fruits are called aniseed.

annatto. A yellowish-red vegetable dye made from the pulp around the seeds of a small tropical tree, **Bixa orellana.** The tree is a native of the Caribbean. Annatto is widely used in coloring cheese, especially Cheddar, and to a lesser extent, butter.

anodyne. Relieving pain. A medicine that eases pain.

anorexia. Lack or loss of appetite for food.

anorexigenic. Producing anorexia or diminishing the appetite.

anosmia. Lack or loss of sense of smell.

antagonist. A substance that counteracts the action of another substance. The antagonist prevents the normal action because its molecular structure is so like that of the first substance that it almost fits into the first substances's position in a metabolic process. It gets in the way and prevents the reaction from taking place.

anterior. Situated toward the front.

antacid. A substance that counteracts or neutralizes acidity. *Aluminum hydroxide* and *magnesium trisilicate* tablets act on the gastrointestinal system relieving excess acidity in the stomach and the consequent pain of gastritis and peptic ulcer. The combination of the two drugs provides relief without causing constipation. The tablets should be chewed and swallowed with a small amount of water; unless some fluid is taken the drug preparation may only coat the esophagus and not reach the stomach.

antibiotics. Substances that are "against life." They are chemical substances produced by certain living cells, such as bacteria yeasts and molds, that are antagonistic or damaging to other living cells, such as disease-producing bacteria. Antibiotics may kill living cells or prevent them from growing and multiplying. *Penicillin* is an example of an antibiotic that damages certain bacteria that cause disease in man.

antibodies. Specific serum proteins or *immunoglobulins* formed in more complex organisms, including man, in response to the intrusion of antigens, substances alien to the body. Each antibody binds itself specifically to an appropriate site (antigenic determinant) on the antigen. Antibodies are involved principally in resisting infection.

anticaking agent. Keeps salts and powders free flowing. They are used in such products as table salts, garlic and onion salts and powders, powdered sugar, and malted-milk powders.

anticoagulant. An agent that prevents coagulation. In blood chemistry, anticoagulants prevent the clotting of blood. Examples of anticoagulants are *dicumarol** and *heparin*. The mechanisms of anticoagulants vary since different anticoagulants interfere with the blood-clotting mechanism at different stages of the process.

antidiuretic hormone (ADH, vasopressin). A hormone secreted by the pituitary gland, which acts upon the distal renal tubule, causing the reabsorption of water. The result is diminished urinary output; hence the term antidiuretic hormone (ADH). The posterior *pituitary gland* secrets ADH in response to body stress. The ADH mechanism is the body's primary water-conserving mechanism and is therefore essential to life. See *water balance*.

antigens. Substances foreign to the body that lead to the formation of specific antibodies. Most antigens contain several antigenic determinants. Chemically, antigens may belong to the proteins, the polysaccharides or to other classes of substances.

antihemorrhagic. Preventing *hemorrhage* (bleeding).

antihistamine. A drug that counteracts the effects of histamine in a mucous membrane. It is of value in the treatment of certain allergic conditions such as hay fever, nettle rash, and certain forms of eczema.

antimetabolite. A chemical compound that resembles a substance occurring naturally and prevents its metabolism. Generally, the antimetabolite replaces metabolites in enzyme reactions. Certain antimetabolites are used for medicinal purposes, e.g., dicumarol in the treatment of blood clots. *Dicumarol* * is an antimetabolite of *vitamin K* and is also an *antivitamin*.

antineuritic. Counteracting *neuritis*. Often applied to thiamine, because it counteracts the neuritis resulting from B-complex deficiency (avitaminosis).

antioxidant. A substance that prevents or delays oxidation. A substance capable of chemically protecting other substances against oxidation. One of the most common groups of additives used to prevent change in color or flavor caused by oxygen in the air. For example, some fruits and vegetables containing certain enzymes (such as apples, apricots, bananas, cherries, peaches, pears and potatoes), darken when exposed to air after being cut, bruised, or allowed to overmature. Antioxidants also are used to prevent rancid taste and odor from developing in fats and oils during storage, and in commercial cake mixes. The vitamins *ascorbic acid* * (vitamin C) and the *tocopherols* * (vitamin E) act in the body as water soluble and fat soluble antioxidants, respectively.

antimyotic agents. A preservative used to prevent or control the spoilage organisms such as mold, bacteria and yeast. Otherwise, foods such as bread become moldy quickly, especially in warm weather. One mold that sometimes appears in bread lacking antimyotics is called ''rope,'' making the bread inedible. Rope is caused by certain bacteria not destroyed during baking. Other antimyotics are used in cheese, including *scorbic acid* *, sodium and potassium sorbates.

antipyresis. The application of remedies against fever. See *antipyretic*.

antipyretic. Reducing temperature in fever but not affecting normal body temperature.

antirachitic. Preventive, curative, or corrective of rickets. *Vitamin D* * has antirachitic activity.

antiscorbutic. Prevents or cures *scurvy*. *Ascorbic acid* * (vitamin C) has antiscorbutic activity.

antivitamins. An antimetabolite against a vitamin which it replaces or competes with metabolically. For example, deoxypyridoxine is an antimetabolite to *pyridoxine* * (vitamin B_6); oxythiamine and pyrithiamine are antivitamins to *thiamine* * (vitamin B_1); and *dicourmarol* * is an antimetabolite to *vitamin K* *. On p. 27 some of the antivitamins are listed.

Riboflavin (B_2) antivitamins:	isoriboflavin; galactoflavin
Pyridoxine (B_6) antivitamins:	deoxypyridoxine (isoniazid, a drug used in the treatment of tuberculosis, also has an antagonistic effect on vitamin B_6).
Niacin antivitamin:	3-acetylpyridine: pyridine-3-sulfonic acid.
Pantothenic acid antivitamin:	omega-methylpantothenic acid, raw egg white which contains a substance called avidin.
Folic acid antivitamin:	methotrexate or aminopterin, used as a drug in the treatment of cancer.
Vitamin K antivitamin:	dicoumarol which is really not an antivitamin but an antimetabolite, a small but often substantial difference.

anus. Opening at the posterior end of the digestive tract, through which indigestible solid wastes are expelled.

anxiety. Apprehension, tension, or uneasiness that stems from the anticipation of danger, the source of which is largely unknown or unrecognized; it is primarily of intrapsychic origin, in distinction to fear, which is the emotional response to a consciously recognized and usually external threat or danger.

aortosclerosis. Hardening of the walls of the aorta. See *arteriosclerosis*.

A.P. See *As Purchased*.

aphasia. A defect in or the loss of the power of speech.

aphrodisiac. Something which excites sexual activity (usually a drug.)

aplastic anemia. Since blood cells are manufactured in the bone marrow, anemia may result when the marrow is damaged and becomes sluggish or fails to function at all. In this type of anemia, not only are red blood cells reduced in numbers, so too are the white cells. Resistance to infection is reduced, blood platelet count drops as well, and there may be bleeding.

apoenzyme. The protein portion of an enzyme to which the *prosthetic* group or *coenzyme* is attached.

apoferritin. Protein base in intestinal mucosa cells, which will bind with iron (from food) to form ferritin, the storage form of iron. Apoferritin is the iron-free protein.

appendicitis. The vermiform appendix is a narrow, shallow, blind tube, about three inches long, that looks much like an earthworm. It is located at the juncture of the large and small intestines. It serves no known purpose. Appendicitis is an inflammation of the appendix. Appendicitis cannot be caused by swallowing seeds.

appetite. Similar to hunger but a less physiologically related activity. The desire for a specific food is related to appetite, whereas when one is hungry, any one of a variety of foods may satisfy. Food intake is regulated by the *hypothalamus,* and many centers in the brainstem and spinal cord are involved in the actual process of eating, e.g., salivation, chewing, swallowing. Appetite is very complex and not well understood.

apple (*Malus*). Apples come in many varieties, with an estimated 6500 or more horticultural forms, and in many shapes and forms. In shape it can be round like a McIntosh or egg-shaped like the Delicious. In size, it can vary from a 2-inch crabapple to a 6-inch Rome Beauty. The flesh may be white as a Cortland, yellow as a Golden Delicious, crisp as a Northern Spy, mellow as a Baldwin, sweet as a Grimes, or tart as a new Winesap. The skin is thin and glossy and ranges in color from bright or russet red, to yellow, to green. Fresh apples are a good supplement to the diet, since they contain carbohydrates and *carotene* * (vitamin A activity) and *ascorbic acid* * (vitamin C). Apples contain cellulose to maintain body regularity and, when eaten raw, help clean the teeth.

  1 apple, medium, fresh = 75 calories
  Applesauce, unsweetened, ½ cup = 50 calories
  Applesauce, sweetened, ½ cup = 92 calories
  Apple juice, 1 cup = 126 calories
  Apple butter, 100 gm = 186 calories

apricot (*Prunus armeniaca*). Oval stone fruit of a golden yellow color which grows on a small tree belonging to the peach family. Excellent source of vitamin A, high in natural sugars. Three medium apricots = 54 calories.

arachidonic acid. Mol. Wt. 304. Has four double bonds and 20 carbon atoms, used to be included as an *essential fatty acid,* but since it is found in nature only in animal foods, and since it can be readily made in the body from *linoleic* *acid**, it is not actually essential in the diet. Arachidonic acid is a precursor to the *prostaglandins **.

$$CH_3(CH_2)_4(CH\!\!=\!\!CHCH_2)_4(CH_2)_2COOH$$

areolar tissue. A fibrous connective tissue which forms the *subcutaneous* layer of tissue. It fills many of the small spaces in the body, and helps hold organs in place.

arginine. Mol. Wt. 174. One of the nonessential *amino acids* found in proteins. It is the member of the *urea cycle* from which urea is formed by action of the enzyme arginase. See *amino acids* and *urea cycle*.

$$\underset{\textstyle NH_2}{H_2N-\overset{\textstyle \overset{NH}{\|}}{C}-NH-CH_2-CH_2-CH_2-\underset{|}{CH}-COOH}$$

ariboflavinosis. A disease resulting from the deficiency of *riboflavin **. It is characterized by lesions of the tongue and at angles of the mouth, dermatitis, and ocular changes.

aromatic compounds. Chemical compounds containing characteristic ring structures of atoms related to benzene; known for their stability and characteristic behavior. Some are known or believed to be carcinogenic.

arrector muscles. The follicles contain hairs and narrow pits which slant obliquely upward. Connected with each follicle are small bundles of involuntary muscle fibers called the arrector muscles. They arise from the papillary layer of the corium and are inserted into the hair follicle, below the entrance of the duct of a sebaceous gland.

arrowroot (*Maranta arvndinacea*). The starch obtained from the tubers of several kinds of tropical plants. The roots are peeled, washed, and pulped to produce a white fluid. This is made into a powder which is then milled into a recognized form. Arrowroot is an excellent thickening agent and can be used in lieu of flour or cornstarch. It is neutral in flavor and produces soups, sauces, pie fillings, and puddings, that are clear and sparkling, with none of the heaviness of other starches. Arrowroot is easily digested.

arteriogram. An x-ray test after injecting a radio opaque "dye"; for the diagnosis of brain tumors. See *angiogram*.

arteriosclerosis. One of the most common changes within the brain tissue itself is that known as arteriosclerosis, or "hardening of the arteries." There is primarily a loss of elasticity in the arteries feeding the brain tissue, producing profound somatic and resulting psychological reactions. Most everyone who reaches old age suffers to some extent from an arteriosclerotic involvement. The anatomical changes in the arteries supplying blood to the brain result in major pathological changes within the brain itself. These are primarily the result of: the decreased amount of oxygen available to the brain cells; waste products of the brain cells are not as readily removed and tend to accumulate; a decreased amount of sugar is furnished to the brain as fuel; and hemorrhages, either minor or major, may result with the attendant destruction of the brain tissue involved and the consequent loss of function.

artery. A blood vessel that carries blood away from the heart.

arthritis. The term arthritis is used to cover all inflammatory diseases of the joints. Research has shown there are approximately 100 different types of arthritis, but all are capable of producing disability. The exact cause of arthritis is not well known, but there are some definitely established predisposing factors: infection, the most common being streptococcus, staphylococcus, and pneumococcus; trauma; overweight, and/or poor posture; prolonged physical stress and strain; emotional disturbances; metabolic disorders (e.g., gout); and heredity.

artichoke (*Cynara scolymus*). Globe or common artichokes are the leafy buds from a plant resembling the thistle. The artichokes cultivated in the United States are grown mainly in the midcoastal regions of California. Artichokes may be eaten in many ways. One way is to eat them with the fingers; pulling off the leaves one at a time and dipping them into a sauce. Eventually a core of thin light-colored leaves is reached; this covers the choke and the heart. Artichokes contain small amounts of vitamins and minerals. Fresh, 1 cooked = 50 to 60 calories; canned or frozen, about ½ cup = about 40 calories; caloric values vary greatly.

articular cartilage. Covers the joint surfaces at the ends of a long bone. The cartilage provides a smooth contact surface in joint formation and gives some resilience for shock absorption.

ascariasis (roundworm infection). Usually contracted from eggs reaching the mouth by way of fingers that have been in contact with contaminated soil. The worm inhabits the small bowel. Mild roundworm infection may not bother most people who have it. If the worm migrates to various parts of the body it may cause serious effects. Ordinarily, symptoms of infection with these worms are nondescript abdominal complaints and anemias.

ascites. Accumulation of fluid in the abdominal cavity.

ascorbic acid (vitamin C). Mol. Wt. 176. Both the reduced form of ascorbic acid and the oxidized form (dehydroascorbic acid) have equal vitamin activity. This level of oxidation should not be confused with oxidations (catalyzed by heavy metals and heat) that inactivate vitamin C by changing the structure irreversibly. Ascorbic acid is related chemically to the sugars. One of its functions in the body is to maintain the connective tissues. In the absence of ascorbic acid, the structure of the connective tissue becomes weakened. The linings of blood vessels, as well as the sheath of connective tissue about them, become weakened so that bleeding occurs. Ascorbic acid serves as a cofactor or a coenzyme in several metabolic systems. It also takes part as a cofactor in a number of reactions involving amino acids, such as *tyrosine*,* and *tryptophan**. It is involved in: the hydroxylation of proline to hydroxyproline; the synthesis of collagen, an important component of connective tissue; the hydroxylation of tryptophan to 5-hydroxytryptophan, a precursor in the biosynthesis of *serotonin;* the conversion of 3,4-dihydroxyphenylethylamine to *norephinephrine*;* and hydroxylation of p-hydroxyphenlypyruvate to homogenistic acid in the catabolic pathway of *tyrosine**. It has been shown that ascorbic acid lowers the blood cholesterol of people with artherosclerosis. It also influences the formation of hemoglobin, the absorption of iron from the intestine and deposition of iron in liver tissue. Ascorbic acid is found in many parts of the body. Since ascorbic acid is water soluble, it is readily absorbed from the gastrointestinal tract into the bloodstream within a few hours after it is ingested and taken up by the tissues. Studies using radioactive ascorbic acid show that it is rapidly taken from the serum and transported to the adrenal glands, kidneys, and liver. Transfer to such tissues as the eyes, muscles, testes, and brain is more gradual. Ascorbic acid also functions in protecting the body against infection and bacterial toxins. Tissues that have higher metabolic activity contain the highest concentrations of ascorbic acid.

The Food and Nutrition Board of the United States recommends a daily allowance of 60 mg per day for adult males, and 55 mg for females. Practically all vitamin C comes from fruits and vegetables which may be eaten raw or cooked, whether cooked fresh produce, frozen or canned. Foods rich in vitamin

dehydro-ascorbic acid

Ascorbic acid

C are citrus fruits, liver, tomatoes, and most vegetables. Fruits, except citrus fruits, generally have a lower vitamin C content than vegetables. Vitamin C is not destroyed by heat but by the oxidation that heat accelerates. Since this vitamin is susceptible to oxidation, the cooking of vegetables, if done to the point of palatability (whether by steaming, boiling or pressure cooking), preserves only about half of the ascorbic acid. Freezing, canning, and dehydration also cause about the same degree of destruction. Citrus fruits and juices, and tomato juice perhaps are the most convenient sources of ascorbic acid.

The following table gives the ascorbic acid content of some foods:

Food	Range (mg ascorbic acid/100 gm edible portion)
Bananas	10–30
Black currants, fresh	90–300
Black currant syrup	60
Broccoli and brussel sprouts	70–100
Cabbage and lettuce	10–60
Canned fruit, various	1–25
Citrus fruits, fresh or juice	25–60
Eggs	trace
Fresh meat	trace
Green leafy vegetables, tropical, raw	50–220
Guava	200
Mango	10–50
Melon	1–45
Papaya	30–120
Pineapple	25
Potato, boiled	5–15
Potato chips	10–30
Potato, raw	10–30
Roots and pulses, fresh	10–30
Rose hips, fresh	70–460
Rose hip syrup	150–200
Soft fruits—strawberries, raspberries	25–60
Stone fruits—apples, pears, plums	5–10
Sweet potato	20–30
Tomato, fresh or juice	20–25

ascorbyl palmitate. Formed by combining *ascorbic acid* * (vitamin C) with palmitic acid (a *fatty acid*). This additive functions as an *antioxidant* in shortening in the same fashion as ascorbic acid. It readily reacts with oxygen, preventing the latter from reacting with unsaturated fats and causing rancidity. Also used as a source of vitamin C in vitamin pills and fortified foods.

asepsis. Absence of infectious material; freedom from infection.

ash (chemical analysis). Mineral matter is ascertained by completely burning the combustible portion and weighing the noncombustible residue.

asparagine (Asn). Mol. Wt. 132. One of the amino acids found in proteins. Formed from aspartic acid by the addition of ammonia to the free carboxylic acid group to from an amide group.

$$\underset{\text{H}_2\text{NC}-\text{CH}_2-\text{CH}-\text{COOH}}{\overset{\text{O} \qquad \text{NH}_2}{\overset{\|}{} \qquad \overset{|}{}}}$$

asparagus (*Asparagus offinicinalis*). A member of the lily-of-the-valley family. The name comes from a greek word meaning "stalk" or "shoot." Especially prized is the variety of asparagus that yields very thick, white, fleshy stalks that are very tender. These asparagus are grown in little individual mounds and cut when only the green tip shows, so that the stalks are still white. A good source of *carotene* * (vitamin A activity), fair for vitamin B, and *ascorbic acid* * (vitamin C) and iron. gm Raw, $100 = 26$ calories; Cooked, canned or frozen, 100 gm = 21 calories.

aspartic acid (Asp). Mol. Wt. 133. One of the nonessential amino acids found in proteins. Aspartic acid contains two carboxylic acid groups and is classified as an acidic amino acid. It can be synthesized in the body from *oxalacetic acid* *. See *amino acid*.

$$\underset{\text{NH}_2}{\overset{}{\text{HOOC}-\text{CH}_2-\text{CH}-\text{COOH}}}$$

Aspergillus flavus. A mold found on corn, peanuts and certain grains when improperly dried and stored; source of *aflatoxin* *.

aspirin (acetylsalicylic acid). Mol. Wt. 180. Aspirin acts as an analgesic and an *antipyretic*. As an analgesic, it relieves headache and muscular pain. Aspirin normally is used in 0.324 gm tablets, often being combined with other analgesics such as *phenacetin* * and *caffeine* * (APC). In large and continued doses, aspirin produces gastritis (gastric irritation), and a ringing in the ears.

Aspirin

As Purchased (A.P.). Refers to food as offered for sale on the retail market. In tables that give nutritive value for food "as purchased," the nutrient content is stated in terms of the weight of the food before inedible portions, usually discarded, are removed.

asthma. A respiratory problem whose chief feature is labored or difficult breathing. Often accompaned by a characteristic wheezing or whistling sound. The whistling or wheezing sounds of asthma is loudest when breathing air out. The symptoms of asthma are caused by changes in the respiratory system, the system of passageways that carries air from the mouth into the lungs. In asthma, the small air passageways are the ones which are chiefly affected. The muscles in these passages go into spasms, narrowing the width of the tubes and thus making the passage of air in and out of the lungs more difficult. In addition to muscle spasm there is an outpouring of mucus into the small air passages, further obstructing the flow of air. Finally, the mucosa become inflamed and swollen thus narrowing the air passageway even further, much as an accumulation of rust on the inner surface of a pipe would partially obstruct the flow of water through the pipe. All these changes, the spasms, the swelling, and the outpouring of mucus, occur together, affecting to a greater or lesser degree almost all of the air passages. The resistance to the flow of air, particularly during expiration, or breathing out, is significantly increased, and the individual must work harder to move air in and out of the lungs, which results in a whistling sound. Asthma is considered to be the result of an allergy.

astigmatism. A defect in vision in which the lens of the eye is curved differently in one direction than in the other (like the sides of a football), so that it is impossible to see all of an object in focus at once.

asthenia. Without strength. Weakness.

atherosclerosis. Term derived from two Greek words: athere meaning "porridge" or "mush," and skleros meaning "hard." A chronic, usually progressive vascular disease characterized by thickening, induration, and loss of elasticity of arterial walls, followed by secondary degenerative changes. The changes may be generalized or more prominent in certain organs or locations—heart, kidneys, lungs, brain, and extremities. The cause of the disease has been variously attributed to abnormal fat transport or metabolism, dietary habits, disorders of blood flow and blood clotting, hormonal disturbances, and mechanical factors. Heredity also appears to be a factor in individual susceptibility. Long-standing hypertension and diabetes are predisposing factors. The onset usually takes place gradually during the early adult years; progressive symptoms and specific secondary illness are usually observed in the fifth and sixth decades of life. See *arteriosclerosis*.

atonic. Lack of normal tone or vigor of an organ or part.

atrophy. A wasting away or reduction in size of a cell, organ, or part of the body.

auditory nerve. The eighth cranial nerve. It consists of two branches; one of these is concerned with hearing; the other is distributed to the vestibule and semicircular canals of the internal ear and is concerned with the sense of balance. Disturbance of the former causes deafness, the latter, giddiness.

Aureomycin. Mol. Wt. 479. A proprietary brand of chlortetracycline an antibiotic. It generally is prepared as a hydrochloride.

Aureomycin

auscultation. The act of listening for sounds in the body in order to determine the condition of the organs and also for the detection of pregnancy.

autonomic nervous system. A system of motor nerves, intimately connected with *cerebrospinal nervous system,* having centers in the medulla, midbrain, hypothalamus and cerebral cortex, yet it is to some extent set apart both anatomically and functionally. The autonomic system acts upon the glands and smooth muscles of the viscera and blood vessels. The autonomic nervous system is divided into two subdivisions, the *sympathetics* and *parasympathetics,* which have somewhat antagonistic effects. The sympathetic system is mainly concerned with mobilizing the resources of the body for use in work or in emergencies. The parasympathetic division is mainly concerned with conserving and storing the bodily resources. Both divisions of the autonomic nervous system act with less precision and more diffuseness than the cerebrospinal system, sometimes referred to as the voluntary nervous system. The diagram on p. 36 is a schematic representation of the autonomic nervous system. The light lines represent nerve pathways for the sympathetic impulses. The heavy lines are nerve pathways for parasympathetic impulses. The circles are ganglia.

autosome. Any one of the chromosomes other than the sex chromosomes.

autotrophic. Capable of manufacturing organic nutrients from carbon dioxide (CO_2). Bacteria with such capacity are called autotrophs.

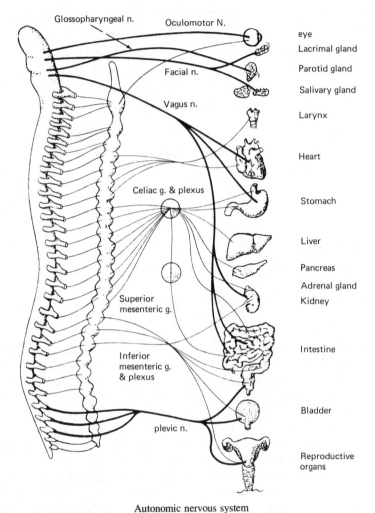

SPINAL   SYMPATHETIC   NERVES (N. or n.)   ORGANS
CORD   TRUNK   AND GANGLIA (g.)

Glossopharyngeal n.

Oculomotor N.

Facial n.

Vagus n.

Celiac g. & plexus

Superior
mesenteric g.

Inferior
mesenteric g.
& plexus

plevic n.

eye
Lacrimal gland
Parotid gland
Salivary gland
Larynx
Heart
Stomach
Liver
Pancreas
Adrenal gland
Kidney
Intestine
Bladder
Reproductive
organs

Autonomic nervous system

avidin. A protein isolated from egg white that can combine with *biotin* *, a B vitamin, causing the vitamin to be unavailable to the body. Cooking renders avidin inactive.

avitaminosis. A condition or clinical symptom due to the lack or the deficiency of a vitamin in the diet, or to lack of absorption or utilization of it. The avitaminoses are given under the vitamin listings.

avocado (*Persea Americana*). A fruit native to Central or South America, also called an alligator pear. In the United States it grows along the southern coast from California to Florida, especially in the Rio Grande Valley. The fruit may vary from the small round bell variety, which is shiny green, to the pear-shaped, slightly russet-coated fruit; the fruit may weigh from 5 to 6 ounces, to 2 to 3 pounds. Avocados have a coarse shell-like skin or a smooth thin skin, depending upon the variety. The flesh is yellowish green and fairly firm, with a single large seed, round or conical. Avocados have fair amounts of *thiamine**, *riboflavin** and *ascorbic acid** (vitamin C). Unlike most fruits, they have a high fat content which varies from less than 5 percent to more than 20 percent. Raw 100 gm = 167 calories.

axon. A fiber of a nerve cell that conducts impulses away from the cell body and can release, but cannot itself be stimulated by, transmitter substance. See *neuron*.

azodicarbonamide. Mol. Wt. 66. A dough conditioning agent employed by the baking industry. Dough conditioning replaces months of storage as the standard way of aging flour. Natural and chemical aging have identical chemical affects on flour; both produce more manageable dough and lighter, more voluminous loaves of bread. Azodicarbonamide does not bleach flour, so it must be used with a bleach such as benzoyl peroxide. When azodicarbonamide reacts with flour the additive is rapidly and completely converted to a second compound, biurea. In the same chemical reaction the protein (gluten) of flour is oxidized, accounting for the changes in the dough's properties. The nutritive value of vitamins and amino acids in bread is not affected by azodicarbonamide or biurea.

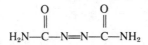

B

bacillary dysentery. A common form of dysentery caused by different strains of dysentery bacillus, resulting from poor sanitation. Attacks come on abruptly, with fever, nausea, vomiting, abdominal pain, and cramps and diarrhea. Blood and mucus are present in the watery stools in severe cases. Untreated, it is a self-limited disease, as a rule clearing up in a week or 10 days, but may become chronic and debilitating and progress to a chronic colitis. Treatment aimed at maintaining salt and water balance is very important.

bacon. The cured and smoked fat and lean meat from the side of the pig, after the spareribs have been removed. Canadian-style bacon, which resembles ham rather than ordinary streaky bacon, is the eye muscle that runs along the pig's back. The word, bacon, originally French, meant pork and cured pork products.

Bacon, raw, 100 gm = 665 calories
Bacon, cooked, broiled or fried, drained, 100 gm = 611 calories
Salt pork, raw, 100 gm = 739 calories
Canadian-style bacon, raw, 100 gm = 277 calories

bacteria. Very small one-celled microorganisms, the smallest living things with self-contained metabolic processes. There are many families and strains; some require oxygen in order to multiply and are called aerobic bacteria. The anaerobic will not grow if oxygen is present. Some strains are hemolytic (destructive to red blood cells). Bacteria have different shapes: the cocci are spherical, streptococci grow in chains and are known as "step germs." There are bacilli, rod shape; spiral cork screw shaped (spirilla), and common shaped, vibrios. Bacteria are widely distributed in the air, water, soil, animal, and plant tissues. Some bacteria have useful functions such as decay of dead matter, fermentation of fruit and vegetable juices; they can also produce disease or cause harmful spoilage of foods.

bacterial toxins. Food poisoning is caused by the ingestion of bacteria toxins that have been produced in food by the growth of specific kinds of bacteria. The powerful toxin is ingested directly, and symptoms of food poisoning therefore develop rapidly, usually within 1 to 6 hours after the food is eaten. See *food poisoning*.

bacteriophage. A virus that attacks bacteria.

Baker's yeast (*Sacchromyces cerevisiae*). A microorganism, one of the fungi. Baker's yeast has replaced brewer's yeast in baking. It is composed of strains specially selected for both their flavor and their ability to produce a great deal of carbon dioxide and little alcohol. See *yeast* and *brewer's yeast*.

baking powder. A leavening agent used in batters and doughs to make them rise and become light and porous during baking. In mixtures it produces carbon dioxide,, one of the three leavening gases (the other two are air and water vapor or steam). Today, commercial baking powders contain at least three ingredients: (1) Baking soda, also known as sodium bicarbonate or bicarbonate of soda, and in less-refined form, saleratus. (2) An acid salt that produces carbon dioxide, the leavening agent, and may be a tartrate compound, a phosphate compound, or sulfate and phosphate combinations. (3) Starch which is used as a stabilizer to keep the powder from caking and reacting in the can. There are three different kinds of baking powders, named according to the type of acid salt used in the formula. The common names sometimes found in recipes are: (1) Tartrate which contains cream of tartar and tartaric acid. This type releases most of its gas quickly in the batter or dough at room temperature. (2) Phosphate which contains calcium acid phosphate, and may also be combined with sodium acid pyrophosphate. This type of powder releases two thirds of its gas at room temperature and the remainder when heat is applied. (3) Double-acting or SAS phosphate in which the acids are sodium aluminum sulfate (SAS) and calcium acid phosphate. This type releases a small portion of gas when the ingredients are combined at room temperature, but the greater amount is released in the oven. Baking can be delayed a few minutes.

baking soda (bicarbonate of soda). Mol. Wt. 84. The chemical formula of this product is $NaHCO_3$. Its home use lies mostly in baking where it is used to leaven cakes containing acid ingredients such as butter, milk, vinegar, molasses, and fruit juices. It is also used along with cream of tartar or baking powder when the amount of acid in the ingredients being combined varies a great deal, as it does when such things as chocolate, brown sugar, honey, sour cream, apples, etc., are used together. The acid in the ingredients combines with the baking soda to produce a gas which leavens the dough.

balance. In nutrition, the term balance refers to the relationship between nutrient intaken and subsequently excreted by the body. When the intake and output are the same, the condition is described as balance, or equilibrium. When the intake exceeds the output, the balance is positive and retention of the nutrient has occurred. A negative balance describes the state in which the intake is less than the output, and the body stores have been used. The balance study has been a useful tool for measuring protein and mineral metabolism, although the balance is greatly affected by other dietary components and by body stores. See *energy balance, nitrogen balance,* and *water balance.*

balm or Lemon balm (*Melissa afficinalis*). A hardy perennial reaching a height of from 1½ to 2 feet. It has broad, dark green leaves, with a faint lemon flavor, and flowers growing in pale yellow clusters. Leaves and tender springs lend a subtle flavor to lemonade, teas, meats, sauces, stuffings, soups, and salads. Industrially, balm is used in making perfume and liqueurs.

bamboo shoot (*Bambusa, Arundinaria,* and *Dendrocalamus*). The inner white part of the young shoot of the tropical bamboo plant. The shoot is prepared by stripping off the tight tough, overlapping sheaths of the plant. The shoots are then cut into strips and are ready for cooking. Bamboo shoots are a basic ingredient in Chinese, Japanese, and other oriental cooking. 100 gm = 27 calories.

banana (*Musa paradisiaca*). Bananas are seedless fruit grown on a plant that resembles the palm, each plant bearing a single bunch of fruit. The plant is first cousin to the tough, fibrous Manila hemp plant. Bananas are harvested green, and their food value and flavor are the result of carefully controlled conditions and temperatures during ripening, when their starch is converted to sugar. The skin of the partly ripened fruit is usually yellow, but there are also red-skinned varieties. Bananas provide *ascorbic acid* * (vitamin C) with good quantities of vitamin A and some vitamin B_1. They are low in protein and fat. 1 medium banana = 85 calories.

barbital (diethylbarbituric acid). Mol. Wt. 184. A habit-forming white powder, the basis of many sedatives, such as barbiturates, which depress the central nervous system.

Barbital

barbiturates. Drugs derived from barbituric acid; one of the most extensive series of sedative, hypnotic, and anesthetic drugs presently in use. Among the better known barbiturates are barbitone, hexobarbitone and phenobarbitone.

barley (*Hordeum*). A hardy cereal grass related to wheat, which it resembles. It comes in a number of varieties and seldom grows higher than 3 feet. Barley is high in nutritive value. It is an essential ingredient in the brewing of beer and in the distillation of Scotch whisky. Barley is high in carbohydrates with moderate amounts of protein, calcium, and phosphorus, and small amounts of B vitamins. Pearl barley, raw, 100 gm = 349 calories; Scotch barley, raw, 100 gm = 113 calories.

basal metabolism. The minimum metabolic activity necessary for maintenance of life and vital processes is called the basal metabolism. It is measured as the heat production or energy expenditure of an individual at rest and after a 12-hour fast. This is determined from the oxygen consumption measured over a short period of time. A value of 4.8 calories per liter of oxygen consumed yields the heat production for the period of measurement. The measurement is called the basal metabolic rate or BMR and is normally around 1200 to 1800 calories (5000 to 7600 KJ) per day. The BMR may also be expressed as percent above or below normal value for an age and sex. Normal values have a range of 20 plus or minus. The basal rate is greatly influenced by secretions of the thyroid gland. A list of the factors that influence the BMR is given below. See *energy balance* and Appendix 10.

A. Factors excluded in all basal tests on normal controls:
1. Muscular movements during test
2. Recent muscular exertion (within ½ to 1 hour)
3. Food within 12 or 14 hours
4. Strong emotions, noises, discomforts
5. Extremes of environmental temperature
6. Diseases

B. Factors taken into account in interpretation of determinations of basal metabolism.

1. Age
2. Sex
3. Weight and height
4. Surface area
5. Undernutrition or overnutrition
6. Athletic training
7. Climate
8. Altitude
9. Sleep
10. Body temperature

C. Additional factors which may or may not be of importance.

1. Occupation
2. Race
3. Previous diet
4. Vigorous exercise or emotion on day before test
5. Novelty of situation
6. Time of year

base. A base may be defined as a substance that combines with acids to form neutral salts. It may also be defined as a substance that increases the concentration of hydroxyl ions, or conversely decreases the concentration of hydrogen ions when dissolved in water. The solution has a pH greater than 7. See *acids, acids and bases*.

base pairings. The specific linkage of two nucleotides in the structures of deoxyribonucleic acid (DNA) and ribonucleic acid (RNA). Nucleotides contain nitrogen base derivatives of either *purines* * or *pyrimidines* *. Pairings are either the pyrimidine base thymine in DNA or uracil in RNA with the purine base adenine and the pyrimidine base cytosine, a purine base guanine. In DNA, there are 2 purine nucleotides, adenine and guanine, and 2 pyrimidine nucleotides, cytosine and thiamine. In the DNA chain, adenine always forms *hydrogen bonds* to thiamine, and guanine always forms hydrogen bonds to cytosine. This rule of base pairings is fundamental; along with the amino acid sequence it determines the intracellular double-standard structure of DNA, the replication of DNA, and the translation of the nucleotide sequence of DNA or of messenger-RNA into the amino acid sequence of protein. See *deoxyribonucleic acid* *

basic foods. The seven basic food groups established by the U.S. Department of Agriculture are: (1) Green and yellow vegetables; (2) citrus fruits, tomatoes, and salad greens; (3) other fruits and vegetables; (4) milk, including all its recognized forms except butter; (5) meats, fish, poultry, eggs; (6) nuts and mature legumes, including peanut butter; and (7) butter and fortified margarine.

basil, sweet (*Ocimum basilicum*). There are five or six varieties of basil, which belong to the mint family, all differing in height, color, and taste. The basil most often used in the United States is sweet basil and Dwarf basil. All basil varieties have a unique fragrance and taste that add zest and flavor in cooking. The word basil comes from the Greek basilikon meaning "royal" or "king." Sweet basil is a culinary seasoning, useful in almost any dish that can be herbed and is especially pleasant in seafoods, salads, potatoes, vegetable soups, dishes that contain tomatoes. Basil may be used fresh or dried.

bass (*Micropterus*). The name covers more than a dozen species of spiny-rayed North American food and game fish that belong to at least half-a-dozen different fish families. Some bass are freshwater fish; others, saltwater fish. The most common freshwater varieties include white or silver bass, and yellow bass. The best-known saltwater basses are common sea bass, and striped bass. Bass is a good source of protein and phosphorus. Raw, 100 gm = 104 calories.

beach plum (*Prunus maritima*). A member of the prune tree family. Beach plums grow wild. Although highly prized for jams and jellies, the plums are seldom cultivated. The fruit is small and dark purple blue when ripe, with a thick tough skin and bullet hard seed. The flavor is a combination of grape, plum and cherry on the bitter and sour side. They are used mostly cooked. See *plum*.

bean. Beans are the seed or seeds of many plants, both trailing vines and erect bushes. They belong to the group of foods called legumes, which also includes peas, lentils, and peanuts. When cooked for a short time in a small amount of water, they are a fair source of *carotene** (vitamin A) and *ascorbic acid* (vitamin C).

Green beans, raw, 100 gm = 32 calories
Green beans, boiled and drained, 100 gm = 25 calories
Wax beans, raw, 100 gm = 27 calories
Wax beans, boiled and drained, 100 gm = 22 calories

beef. Beef is the flesh of an adult animal of the Bovidae family of ruminants. Practically all the beef eaten comes from steers, heifers, and cows. High quality beef comes from animals that generally weigh from 900 to 1300 pounds each, and range in age from 1 to 3 years. The better known breeds of cattle are the Shorthorn and Hereford, Aberdeen, Angus, the Brahman and Santa Gertrudis. Beef is an excellent source of high-quality protein, and provides good amounts of iron and *niacin**. 100 gm of cooked, boneless, lean beef, supplies the following percentages of the recommended daily allowances for a 25-year-old man: 30 percent protein, 27 percent iron, 10 percent *riboflavin**, 22 percent *niacin**, and 4 percent *thiamine**. 100 gm of raw beef, choice grade, gives the following calories:

Chuck (82% lean, 18% fat) = 257 calories
Flank steak (100% lean) = 144 calories
Hamburger (lean) = 179 calories
Porterhouse steak (63% lean, 37% fat) = 390 calories
Rib roast (64% lean, 36% fat) = 401 calories
Round (89% lean, 11% fat) = 197 calories
Rump (75% lean, 11% fat) = 303 calories
Sirloin steak (73% lean, 27% fat) = 313 calories

100 gm of variety meat, raw, gives the following calories:
Brains = 125 calories
Heart, lean = 108 calories
Kidney = 130 calories
Liver = 140 calories
Tongue = 231 calories
Tripe, fresh = 231 calories

Cured beef, 100 gm gives the following calories:
Beef, corned, boneless, uncooked, medium fat = 293 calories
Beef, corned, boneless, cooked, medium fat = 372 calories
Beef, canned corned, boneless, medium fat = 216 calories
Beef, dried, chipped = 203 calories
Beef, dried, uncooked = 203 calories
Canned corned beef hash, with potato = 181 calories

beer. A foamy, fermented beverage brewed from a malted cereal, with hops
added. Beer is brewed from a variety of grains, such as wheat, millet, barley
and rice. Today's American beer is brewed from barley, which has been germinated in water and dried, cereal adjuncts such as corn or rye, and hops, the
dried cones of the hop vine. In addition, cultured yeast is needed for the fermentation which creates beer's characteristic sparkle. Also needed is pure filtered water which by volume makes up about nine-tenths of the finished beer.
There are many varieties of beer, including ale, porter and stout. The most popular American beer is lager. The word lager comes from the German and means
"to store," and that is what lager beer is, beer stored for various periods of
time to age or mellow. The nutrient content of beer is as follows: For 355 ml
(12 fluid oz); water content, 92 percent; caloric content, 150 cal; *protein,* 1 gm;
carbohydrate, 18 gm; *thiamin* *, 0.01 mg; *riboflavin* *, 0.11 mg; and *niacin* *,
2.2 mg.

beet (*Beta*). The enlarged red root of a plant which is first cousin to *chard.*
Beet greens, the tops of the plants are also edible, and some varieties are purposely grown for this. Beets are also grown for sugar. Beets have small

amounts of vitamins and minerals. Beet greens are an excellent source of *carotine* * (vitamin A activity) and calcium.

Greens, cooked, boiled and drained, 100 gm = 18 calories
Beets, cooked, boiled, and drained, 100 gm = 32 calories
Canned beets, 100 gm = 34 calories

benign. Not malignant; not having a tendency to recur; having a favorable outcome.

benzoyl peroxide. Mol. Wt. 232. As a food additive it is an important flour bleach which doesn't "age" flour, but is used in conjunction with "aging" agents, (*azodicarbonamide* *, *potassium bromide*). Benzoyl peroxide is a powder that bleaches flour within 24 hours after being mixed with it. As the bleach does its work, most of it decomposes to benzoic acid which remains in the flour after baking. The benzoic acid residue is not hazardous.

Benzoyl peroxide

bergamot. The name is used for three very different plants. (1) A native American herb, (*Monarda*) which belongs to the mint family. The leaves have a pleasant lemon scent. There are several varieties of the herb bergamot, the best-known one is the *Monarda didyma,* commonly known in the Eastern states as "Oswego tea," from the tribe of Indians that used it extensively. (2) A pear, one of the oldest to be cultivated in the British Isles. The bergamot pear is a winter pear, with several varieties. (3) A tree of the citrus family cultivated in Italy for the essential oils of the rind of its small, pear-shaped orange. These oils are only used commercially, chiefly in perfumes or as a flavoring.

beri-beri. A nutritional disease of the peripheral nerves caused by a deficiency of *thiamine* * (vitamin B_1). It is characterized by pain (neuritis) and paralysis of the extremities, cardiovascular changes, and edema. Beri-beri is common in the Orient where diet consists largely of milled rice with little protein. See *thiamine.*

berry. The word describes not only the fruits that have berry as part of their names, but also cherries, tomatoes, and even the hips of roses, for the definition says that berries are any kind of small, pulpy fruit, no matter what its structure may be. In cookery there are certain fruits thought of as strictly berries, such as barberries, bilberries, blackberries, blueberries, cloudberries. cranberries, currants, elderberries, gooseberries, loganberries, mulberries, raspberries, rowanberries, and strawberries.

beta (β) carotene. See *carotene**.

betaine. Mol. Wt. 118. A methyl donor (—CH_3) that derives from *choline** and functions to synthesize the essential amino acid *methionine** from homocysteine.

$$CH_3-\overset{\overset{\displaystyle CH_3}{\overset{+}{|}}}{\underset{\underset{\displaystyle CH_3}{|}}{N}}-CH_2-CO\overset{-}{O}H$$

Betaine

beta (β) lipoproteins. Low-density lipoproteins (LDL), carrying in addition to other lipids about two-thirds or more of the total plasma cholesterol, formed in the liver from endogenous fat sources. See *lipoproteins*.

bicarbonate. (HCO_3^-) One of the main buffer systems of the human body. Bicarbonate is formed by the CO_2 dissolved in water to form carbonic acid (H_2CO_3). The salts of that acid, sodium bicarbonate ($NaHCO_3$), and potassium bicarbonate ($KHCO_3$) with carbonic acid form the *buffer* system. (Also see *acids and bases* and *buffers*). The pKa of the bicarbonate buffer system is 6.3.

bile. An alkaline viscous yellow to green bitter fluid (pH 8–8.6) which is secreted continuously by the liver at a rate of 0.5–1 liter per day. It is stored and concentrated in the gall bladder, which contracts when fat enters the duodenum and forces bile into the intestine along with the pancreative juice. The mechanism for this is a hormone called *cholecystokinin* which is secreted by the duodenal wall when fat enters it. Bile is composed of water, *bile pigments**, *bile salts**, *cholesterol** and electrolytes. The bile salts are largely concerned in the digestion and absorption of fats. They assist in the emulsification of fat globules by the reduction of surface tension. They react with insoluble fatty compounds such as stearic acid, cholesterol and the fat-soluble vitamins to produce *micelles* which are soluble in water and can be absorbed. After absorption the bile salts are reabsorbed in the blood stream and carried to the liver where they stimulate further bile secretions. Bile pigments are the waste products of hemoglobin breakdown. Bile is essential for the absorption of *vitamin*

$K*$ and other fat-soluble vitamins. It also stimulates intestinal motility and neutralizes the acid *chyme,* creating a favorable hydrogen ion concentration for
pancreatic and intestinal enzyme activity, just as salts help to keep cholesterol
in solution.

bile pigments. Derived from the heme of hemoglobin contained in red blood
cells broken down in the liver. The bacterial action on these pigments give the
characteristic brown color to feces. The major bile pigments are bilirubin, Mol.
Wt. 585, and biliverdin, Mol. Wt. 585. The structures are:

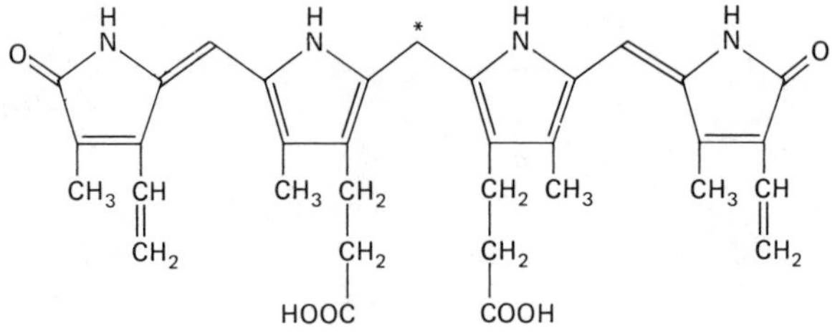

Bilirubin

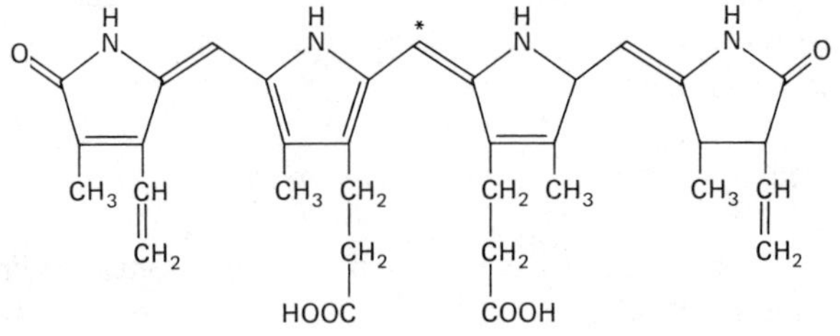

Biliverdin

Bilrubin and biliverdin are red and green, respectively, but become brown
when oxidized by intestinal bacteria. The position with the asterisk (*) indicates
the difference between these two structures.

bile salts. Act as emulsifying agents causing large fat droplets to be broken up
into many smaller droplets. Also aids in the absorption of fats by the small intestine. The bile salts are themselves absorbed through the wall of the large intestine and returned to the liver for reuse. The bile salts are derivatives of
cholesterol. They derive from the conjugated derivates of the bile acids, *cholic
acid*, *chenodeoxycholic acid*, *deoxycholic acid** and *lithocholic** as major
bile salts. The bile acids conjugate with *glycine** and *taurine** The salts of
these conjugated bile acids are the bile salts. As an example, the structure of a
bile salt, cholyltaurine (taurocholic acid) is given.

Cholyltaurine (Taurocholyic Acid)

The bile salts are water soluble and are power emulsifiers.

biliary system. Bile is formed in the liver. It is then transported by the hepatic duct from the liver to a point where the hepatic and cystic ducts join to form the common bile duct. The common bile duct unites with the pancreatic duct before entering the small intestine. The opening of the common bile duct is guarded by the sphincter of Oddi. When this sphincter is closed the bile formed by the liver flows down the hepatic duct and then through the cystic duct to reach the gallbladder.

bilirubin. A red pigment in bile. See *bile pigments*.

binary fission. Reproduction by the division of a cell into two essentially equal parts by a nonmitotic process.

biochemical analysis. Biochemical assessments of nutritional status are made primarily in blood and urine. For certain nutrients the blood is said to reflect the adequacy, the urine serves as an indicator of adequacy or inadequacy with respect to these nutrients. Biochemical tests are designed to measure specific nutrients in relation to specific body functions. Biochemical methods are applied to the blood in evaluating contents of *protein, enzymes,* and several vitamins. They also serve to determine hemoglobin level as an assessment of anemia. Biochemical tests of the urine are used to evaluate body contents of certain vitamins.

bioflavin. A substance once known as *vitamin P,* found mainly in the pulp and connective tissue of citrus fruits. Some vitamin distributors add it to vitamin combinations and claim it is useful to help build resistance to infection and colds and beneficial in cases of hypertension. However, there is no clinical evidence of its need.

biogenesis. Origin of living organisms from other living organisms.

biological catalyst. See *enzyme.*

biological function. The role played by a chemical compound or a system of chemical compounds in living organisms.

biological magnification. Increasing concentration of relatively stable chemicals as they are passed up a food chain from initial consumers to top predators.

biological value (BV). The biological value of a food protein is the efficiency with which that protein furnishes the proper proportions and amounts of the essential or indispensible amino acids needed for the synthesis of body proteins in man or animals. The more nearly a protein supplies the tissues with the necessary proportion and amounts of these indispensible amino acids, the higher is its biological value. Egg protein has the highest biological value and is the standard by which other proteins are measured. The BV is one of several values used to measure the quality of a protein and represents a value obtained under controlled, experimental conditions. The methods for conducting these measurements are not fully standardized, nor is there full agreement concerning the way to express the result. The BV is defined as:

$$BV = \frac{\text{Nitrogen retained}}{\text{Nitrogen absorbed}} \times 100$$

$$= \frac{(\text{dietary N}) - (\text{F-Fm}) + (\text{U-Ue})}{(\text{dietary N}) + (\text{F-Fm})} \times 100$$

Where F equals the fecal nitrogen during the testing of a protein; Fm equals the fecal nitrogen on a protein-free diet (endogenous fecal nitrogen); U equals urinary nitrogen excreted during the testing of a protein; and Ue equal urinary nitrogen excreted on a protein-free diet (endogenous urinary nitrogen excretion). The BV of proteins in food are as follows:

Beef	75
Casein	75
Corn	72
Eggs	100
Fish	75
Milk	93
Rice	86
Wheat flour	44

A protein with a BV of 70 or greater is capable of supporting growth (maintaining a positive nitrogen balance) if sufficient calories are also taken.

The protein to be tested for a BV is fed to the animal as (1) the only source of nitrogen, and (2) at a level just below a predetermined level required for nitrogen balance. The BV makes no allowances for the losses of nitrogen in the digestive process. See *net protein utilization* (NPU); *net dietary protein value* (NDpV); *Net dietary protein calories percent* (NDpCal%); and *chemical score.*

biopsy. The removal of a sample of living cells from a living patient for the purpose of diagnosis, or the prognosis of a disease, or of confirmation of normal conditions. The specimen is sent to a specially trained pathologist who examines the cells and determines the type of growth they represent.

biosynthesis. The chemical synthesis of materials in living plants or animals. *Enzymes* usually are the catalysts for biosynthetic reactions.

biotic. Pertaining to life.

biotin. Mol. Wt. 244. A water-soluble vitamin, belonging to the vitamin B-complex group. This vitamin plays an important role as a *coenzyme* for biochemical reactions, in which *carbon dioxide* (CO_2) is incorporated into metabolites. Biotin even in very small amounts appears to function as a coenzyme mainly in carboxylation and deamination reactions. Biotin serves as a coenzyme with active acetate in reactions that transfer carbon dioxide from one compound and fix it onto another. It also serves as a coenzyme in reactions which split off the amino group from certain amino acids, (*aspartic acid* *, *serine* *, *threonine* *). It has been demonstrated that biotin aids in the synthesis of saturated fatty acids. Biotin has been found necessary also in conversion of *ornithine* * into *citrulline* *, an important step in *urea* formation, for protein synthesis, *oxidation phosphorylation,* and carbohydrate metabolism. The factor is required for purine metabolism, and in the presence of carbon dioxide, for conversion of pyruvate to oxalacetate and then to aspartate. It is closely interrelated with *folacin* *, *pantothenic acid* *, and *cobalamin* * (Vitamin B_{12}) in metabolic processes. The human requirement for biotin has not been established in quantitative terms, since the amount needed for metabolism is so

Biotin

small. This coenzyme occurs in many natural foods, and is apparently synthesized by intestinal bacteria. Examples of excellent food sources of biotin include egg yolk, liver, kidney, tomatoes, and yeast.

Below are the biotin sources in some food.

Micrograms (μgm) Per 100 Grams of Food.			
Bananas	4	Milk	5
Beans, dried, lima	10	Molasses	9
Beef	4	Mushrooms	16
Carrots	2	Onions, dry	4
Cauliflower	17	Oysters	9
Cheese	2	Peas, fresh	2
Chicken	5–10	Peas, dried	18
Chocolate	32	Peanuts, roasted	39
Corn	6	Pork, bacon	7
Eggs, whole fresh	25	Pork, muscle	2–5
Filberts	16	Salmon	5
Grapefruit	3	Spinach	2
Halibut	8	Strawberries	4
Hazel nuts	14	Tomatoes	2
Liver, beef	100	Wheat, whole	5

birch beer. The sap of the Sweet Birch, also called Black Birch or Cherry Birch, can be fermented into a mild or potent beer. Birches are tapped like maples and their sap is delightful to drink, faintly sweet and tasting of wintergreen.

blackberry (Rubus). An oblong, conical fruit composed of many small fruits called druplets. Blackberries are also called brambles, since they are the fruit of various brambles. Ripe blackberries are purple-black in color, although they are red when they are unripe. Berries contribute to the vitamin and mineral content of the diet. Iron content is fair and the *ascorbic acid* * (vitamin C) content is fair to good, depending upon the amount eaten. Fresh, raw, 100 gm = 58 calories; canned, light syrup, 100 gm = 72 calories; canned, heavy syrup, 100 gm = 91 calories.

blackstrap molasses. See *sucrose* and *molasses*.

bladder. A vesicle, blister, or hollow structure, normal or pathological, which contains watery fluid. Gall bladders and urinary bladders are examples of normal bladders. A tube or ureter, leads from each kidney to the urinary bladder. The bladder empties through the urethra, a tube leading to an external opening called the meatus. The bladder which functions as a collecting and temporary storage point for urine, expands to accommodate increasing amounts. With the accumulation of about half a pint, reflex contractions lead to a desire to urinate. The contraction stimulates pressure receptors in the muscles of the bladder wall, from which nervous impulses go to the brain. When it is convenient to urinate, the brain sends out signals which cause the bladder's external sphincter to relax. Under the *urinary bladder* * is a diagram of the urinary bladder and its relationship to that system.

bleaching and maturing agents. Bleaching and maturing agents are used in flour milling and bread baking. Freshly milled wheat flour has a yellowish color and lacks the qualities needed for an elastic stable dough. When flour is stored and allowed to age for several months, it gradually becomes white due to ox-idation and "matures" to make it satisfactory for baking. Natural aging is costly so the flour millers speed up the bleaching and aging (which modifies the gluten characteristics of the flour) by adding oxidizing and/or bleaching chemi-cals such as *benzoyl peroxides* *, the calcium and ammonium phosphates, and chlorine dioxide.

blood. A tissue consisting of cells suspended in a fluid called plasma in the ap-proximate proportion of 45 parts of corpuscles to 55 parts of plasma. Its spe-cific gravity is 1.005, and its reaction is faintly alkaline (pH 7.4). The majority of the corpuscles in blood are red blood cells (erythrocytes), but white blood cells (leucocytes) and platelets are also found. All the oxygen and part of the carbon dioxide are carried by the red blood cells, but everything else travels in the plasma. If the blood plasma or whole blood is allowed to stand outside the body, clotting occurs and a protein called fibrin is deposited leaving a fluid called serum. Plasma is in fact, serum plus 0.3–0.5 gm per 100 ml of fibrin-ogen, the substance from which fibrin is formed. The blood corpuscles are heavier than the plasma which has a specific gravity of 1.028. Blood constitutes 5–10 percent of the total body weight.

A reduction in blood volume leads to a fall in the capillary blood pressure as a result of which fluid is transferred from the tissues and so restores the blood volume but dilutes the blood. The motor functions of blood are all carried out when blood circulates normally through the blood vessels. These functions are: (1) To carry oxygen from the lungs to tissue cells and carbon dioxide from the cells to the lungs. (2) To carry food materials absorbed from the digestive to the tissue cells and to remove waste products for the elimination by excretory organs, the kidneys, intestines, and skin. (3) To carry hormones which help regulate body functions from ductless (endocrine) glands to the tissues of the body. (4) To help regulate and equalize body temperature. Body cells generate large amounts of heat, and the circulating blood absorbs this heat. (5) To pro-tect the body against infection. (6) To maintain the fluid balance of the body.

The average man has a blood volume of 5–6 liters, the average woman 4–5 liters. See Appendix 7 for the normal constituents of human blood.

blood-brain barrier. A general term that loosely describes the fact that the number of substances in the blood that transfer into brain cells is limited relative to transfer into other cells. It is a complex phenomenon involving several concepts. The major source of energy for the brain is glucose which can pass the "barrier," other sugars cannot. Since the brain depends on glucose, hypoglycemic (low blood sugar) states can bring on convulsions, as in *insulin shock*. The brain can adapt to the utilization of ketone bodies as a source of energy under a prolonged state of *metabolic acidosis* or *ketosis*. Amino acids vary greatly in their ability to be actively taken up (active transport) by the brain cells. *Glutamine* * is the amino acid taken up to the greatest extent by the brain. *Tyrosine* * is readily taken up and *glutamic acid* *, *lysine* * and *leucine* * exchange rapidly between the brain cells and blood but with no net uptake. The blood-brain barrier mechanisms, anatomically and biochemically are complex and not well understood.

blood cells, red (erythrocytes). Human red blood cells are discs about 7.5 thousandths of a milliliter (ml) or 7.5 microns in diameter. There are about 5.5 million in every milliliter of whole blood from men, and nearly 5 million per milliter from women. There are about 25 billion red blood cells in the whole body and they are constantly being destroyed and replaced at a rate of about 9000 million an hour. The normal red cell lasts approximately 120 days before it is destroyed. Red blood cells are flexible and withstand much bending, squeezing and deformation as they are pushed through the narrow capillaries. They consist of an intricate, spongy network of protein-filled spaces (sinusoids) in the red marrow. The development of a mature red cell takes about a week, during which the endothelial cell enlarges, dividing, forms hemoglobin and finally loses its nucleus. This process is called maturation.

blood cells, white (leucocytes). There are several different kinds of white blood cells, the main ones being the polymorphonuclear leucocytes, the monocyte, and the lymphocyte. There are normally 5,000–10,000 white cells per. milliter of blood but the number varies during the day. There is a rapid turnover with constant destruction and replacement, they live for 7 to 14 days. There is usually a rise in white blood cells (leucocytosis) after meals, severe exercise or other forms of stress, such as infection. About 70 to 75 percent of the leucocytes are polymorphonuclear, less than 5 percent are monooytes, and the rest are lymphocytes. Their function is primarily one of protection. They can ingest and destroy foreign particles, such as bacteria, in the blood and tissues. This function is called *phagocytosis* and the white cells performing it are phagocytes.

White cells are capable of ameboid movement and thus can pass through the walls of capillaries into surrounding tissues. This ability to enter tissue makes them very useful in fighting infection. An area of infection is characterized by a great increase in white cells which gather about the site to destroy bacteria. Below is a diagram of blood cells:

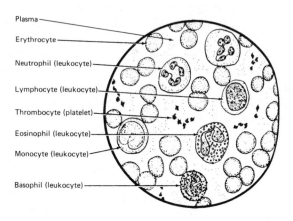

Plasma
Erythrocyte
Neutrophil (leukocyte)
Lymphocyte (leukocyte)
Thrombocyte (platelet)
Eosinophil (leukocyte)
Monocyte (leukocyte)
Basophil (leukocyte)

blood count. A laboratory test performed on a drop of blood which measures the number and characteristics of the red blood cells, white blood cells, and platelets. The measurement of these cells is then compared with standards for the normal individual. The red blood count is done in several parts, including the hematocrit, the hemoglobin, and the blood smear. The hematocrit measures the proportion of red cells in a unit of blood. The blood smear measures a number of things including the number of white cells per cubic centimeter (cc) of blood and the differential white count (the proportion of the various kinds of white cells present).

blood cyscrasis. An abnormal or pathologic condition of the blood, especially one that involves some imbalance in its elements. There are two general types, those present at birth (congenital), and those acquired after birth. Most are a result of the body's inability to produce blood elements that are primarily concerned with the formation of blood clots. The person who has such a condition maintains most normal physiological functions, but if there is any damage to the blood vessels, there is a tendency to bleed freely, for the blood will not clot normally. One of the best-known examples present at birth is *hemophilia*.

blood plasma. Proteins. Plasma contains 7–8 gm percent of protein which is made up of *fibrinogen* and *prothrombin* in small amounts, *albumin* 4–5 gm percent, and globulin 2–3 gm percent. Fibrinogen and prothrombin are concerned with the clotting of blood. Albumin is a protein of low molecular weight, 68,000, and small particle size, which is responsible for 80 percent of the osmotic pressure exerted by the blood. Globulin is a mixture of proteins of much larger size, which are of little importance osmotically, but are intimately concerned with the defense mechanism of the body, the antibodies. The plasma proteins are constantly changing because of new formation, especially in the liver, and utilization in the tissues. The plasma proteins are completely renewed about once a week.

Salts. The following electrolytes are found in solution in blood plasma; sodium (330 mg percent), *potassium* (20 mg percent), *chloride* (360 mg percent), calcium 10 mg percent), *bicarbonate* (165 mg percent) and smaller quantities of phosphate, sulphate, and organic radicals.

Other constituents. Plasma also contains glucose (100 mg percent), ura (30–40 mg percent), cholesterol (200 mg percent), uric acid (3 mg percent), small quantities of lactic acid, amino acids, fatty acids, and traces of many other substances.

blood platelets. A minute particle of protoplasm (the basic material of cells) which is much smaller than the red blood cell. The normal platelet count is 180,000 to 350,000 per milliliter of blood. One of the functions of the platelets is to maintain the texture of the smallest blood vessels (capillaries) in proper condition. In the absence of platelets, red cells often leak out from the capillaries, and tiny bleeding points may be seen.

blood pressure. The force that blood exerts on the walls of vessels through which it flows. All parts of the blood vascular system are under pressure, but the term blood pressure usually refers to arterial pressure. Pressure on the arteries is highest when the ventricles contract during systole (systolic pressure). Pressure is lowest when the ventricles relax during diastole (diastolic pressure). The brachial artery in the upper arm is the artery generally used for blood-pressure measurement. Blood pressure is measured in terms of millimeters (mm) of mercury (Hg). A pressure of 120/80 (120 over 80) means a systolic pressure of 120 mm Hg and diastolic pressure of 80 mm Hg. A systolic pressure above 140 mm Hg indicates hypertension. The blood pressure may temporarily rise or fall under various states or conditions. The following represent some normal changes.

Musculary activity. May increase systolic pressure 60 to 80 mm Hg.

Sleep. Systolic pressure falls during quiet sleep, rises slowly before awakening, and may become high during dream periods.

Emotion. Increases systolic pressure.

Weight. An increase in body weight after age 60 is generally accompanied by a rise in blood pressure.

Sex. Blood pressures in women are usually 8 to 10 mm Hg lower than in men.

blood sugar. The normal functioning of all the cells in the body depends upon an adequate supply of *glucose* * in the blood which reaches them and the amount present (the blood sugar level) varies from 70 to 100 mg per 100 ml in the fasting state. The blood sugar level is controlled partly by dietary intake, and mainly by hormones of the pancreas (*insulin* and *glucagon*), the pituitary, and adrenal glands. Glucose is a *monosaccharide* of low molecular weight and diffuses rapidly out of the blood into the tissues because of the differences in concentration and an enzyme-facilitated uptake by the cells. The blood sugar level usually remains relatively constant even in a fasting state, although it is constantly being removed and used by the cells of the various tissues. The glucose needed to maintain the blood sugar level is obtained primarily by absorption from the intestine during *digestion.* If this is inadequate, breakdown of the liver *glycogen* * provides a further supply through the influence of the hormone glucagon. The level of the blood sugar (glucose) at any moment depends upon the balance between the uptake and utilization by the tissues, its absorption from the intestines and the mobilization of glycogen in the liver. The following four hormones control these functions: (1) anterior pituitary hormone; (2) *pancreas* (insulin and glucagon); (3) adrenal medulla (*epinephrine* *); (4) adrenal cortex (*cortisone* *).

blood types. All human blood may be divided into four main types or groups; O, A, B, AB. This system of typing is used to prevent incompatible blood transfusion, which causes serious reactions and sometimes death. Certain types of blood are incompatible or not suited to each other if combined. Two bloods are said to be incompatible when the plasma or serum of one blood causes clumping of the cells of the other. Two bloods are said to be compatible and safe for transfusion if the cells of each can be suspended in the *plasma* or *serum* of the other without clumping. Blood typing and cross-matching are done by a trained laboratory technician. The blood type A, B, AB or O is determined by the presence of different mucopolysaccharides on the membrane surface of red blood cells. Red cells in type A blood are clumped (agglutinated) by anti-A serum (see diagram p. 57), those in type B blood are agglutinated by anti-B serum. Type AB blood cells are clumped by both serums and type O blood is not agglutinated by either serum. Blood serum is defined as the watery part of the blood that remains after the clot has been removed.

blood type (RH factor). In addition to blood groupings and cross-matching for compatibility, the RH factor must be considered. The RH factor is carried in

Anti-B Serum   Anti-A Serum

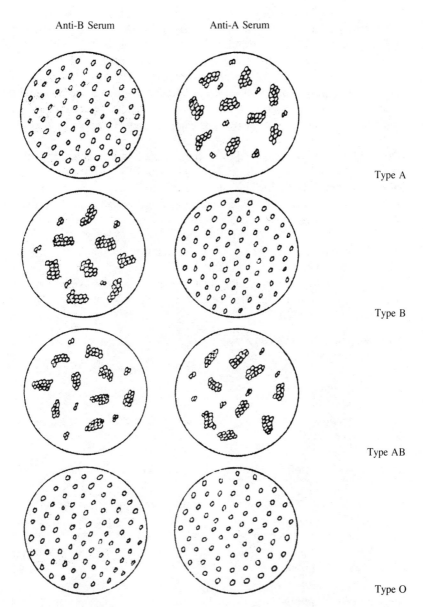

Type A

Type B

Type AB

Type O

red cells, and about 85 percent of all individuals have this factor and therefore are RH positive. Individuals who do not have the RH factor are RH negative. As a general rule, RH negative blood can be given to anyone, provided it is compatible in the ABO typing system, but RH positive blood should not be given to an RH negative individual.

blood vessels. The blood vessels are the closed system of tubes through which the blood flows. The *arteries* and *arterioles* are distributors. The capillaries are the vessels through which all exchange of fluid, oxygen, and carbon dioxide takes place between the blood and tissue cells. The venules and veins are collectors, carrying blood back to the head. The capillaries are the smallest of these vessels but are of greatest importance functionally in the circulatory system. The diagrams on p. 59 show the major arteries and veins in man.

blueberry (*Vaccinium*). The edible berry of a plant of the same name. Blueberries belong to the Vaccinium genus, and there are many varieties, ranging in color from purplish-blue to blue-black. Bilberries and whortleberries are blueberry varieties. Blueberries have fair amounts of *ascorbic acid* * (vitamin C) and iron. Fresh, 100 gm = 62 calories.

bluefish (*Pomatomus saltatrix*). A vivacious fish, bluish above and silvery below, an important food source along the Atlantic Coast. Bluefish get to be as large as 10 pounds, but those sold in fish markets usually weigh from 3 to 6 pounds. Bluefish are meaty fish, delicate in flavor. A good source of protein and phosphorus.

  Baked, 100 gm = 159 calories
  Fried, 100 gm = 205 calories

bologna. A mildly seasoned sausage made of finely ground beef, pork or veal. The meat is packed into a casing and smoked. Good source of protein and fat with small amounts of *thiamine* *, *riboflavin* *, and *niacin* *. All meat, 100 gm = 277 calories.

BMR (basal metabolic rate). See *energy balance, basal metabolism.*

bonito (*Thunnus*). Any of various medium sized *tuna*. A relative of the *mackerel,* and kingfish, which lives in both the Atlantic and the Pacific. A saltwater fish caught commercially on a large scale. More of it is canned in flakes and chunks than is sold fresh. Caloric value: Fresh, raw, 100 gm = 168 calories; canned drained, and oil removed, 100 gm = 198 calories.

body cavities. The organs of the body are located in certain cavities, the major ones of which are the dorsal cavity (toward the back part of the body) and the ventral cavity (toward the front part of the body). The dorsal cavity has a cranial area which contains the brain, and a vertebral area which contains the spinal cord. These areas are continuous. The ventral cavity has a thoracic cavity and an abdomino-pelvic cavity. These areas are separated by the diaphragm.

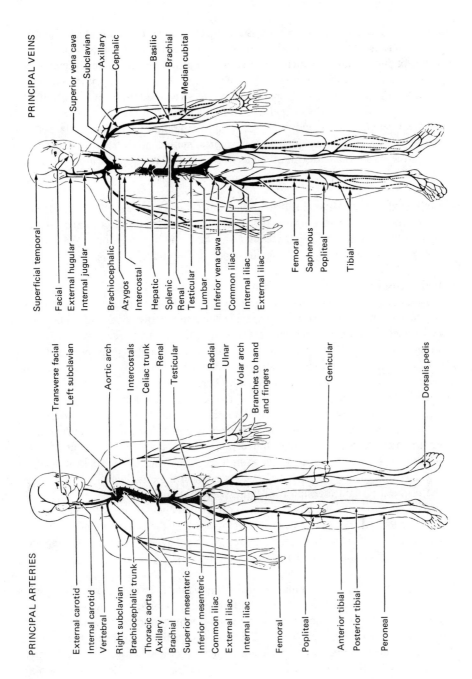

PRINCIPAL VEINS

Superficial temporal
Facial
External hugular
Internal jugular
Brachiocephalic
Azygos
Intercostal
Hepatic
Splenic
Renal
Testicular
Lumbar
Inferior vena cava
Common iliac
Internal iliac
External iliac

Superior vena cava
Subclavian
Axillary
Cephalic
Basilic
Brachial
Median cubital

Femoral
Saphenous
Popliteal
Tibial

PRINCIPAL ARTERIES

External carotid
Internal carotid
Vertebral
Right subclavian
Brachiocephalic trunk
Thoracic aorta
Axillary
Brachial
Superior mesenteric
Inferior mesenteric
Common iliac
External iliac
Internal iliac
Femoral
Popliteal
Anterior tibial
Posterior tibial
Peroneal

Transverse facial
Left subclavian
Aortic arch
Intercostals
Celiac trunk
Renal
Testicular
Radial
Ulnar
Volar arch
Branches to hand and fingers

Genicular

Dorsalis pedis

59

body fat. The amount of body fat is an objective measure of the state of nutrition. There are several methods of making the evaluation. Measurement of the width of the fat layer, which lies directly beneath the skin, is one method. It takes into account the fact that subcutaneous tissue is a repository for fat. Fat-layer width can therefore be estimated by measuring skinfold thickness with a pincerlike device called a caliper. Skinfold thickness can then be translated into terms of percentage of body fat. The caliper is applied in designated areas of the body, which are considered to be representative of overall fat thickness. The three-headed extensor muscle along the back of the upper arm is one such area.

body regulators. Mineral salts and vitamins act as body regulators by promoting oxidative processes, normal functioning of nerves and muscles, and vitality of tissues, and are of assistance in many other bodily functions. Water also serves as an important regulating substance in the body.

body temperature. Warm-blooded animals maintain an about constant body temperature even though their environment may undergo relatively gross temperature changes. Basically, two mechanisms are involved in heat regulation: (1) A metabolic or chemical process which produces heat breakdown of foods in the body, and (2) physical processes, which eliminate losses. The metabolic processes involve to a large extent the oxidation of foods which results in the production of heat. When more food is consumed than is required for caloric needs, the maintenance of the body temperature and physical activity, the excess food is converted into fat and stored as such. The losses of body heat, takes place as follows: (1) About 70 percent is normally lost to the surrounding environment through radiation, convection, and conduction; (2) About 25 percent through evaporation of water from the external surface of the skin and internal surface of the lungs; (3) About 3 percent of the total heat is used to bring the inspired air and ingested cold foods to body temperature; (4) About 1 to 2 percent is lost with the excreta. The normal body temperature for humans is 37°C or 98.6°F, no matter what the temperature of the environment. It should be recognized that the body temperatures given are average values and temperatures may vary slightly under normal conditions.

boiling point. The temperature at which the vapor pressure of a liquid equals the atmospheric pressure. At the boiling point, bubbles of vapor rise continually and break on the surface. The boiling temperature of pure water at sea level (barometer 30 inches) is 212°F (100°C). At high altitudes, the boiling point of water is lower because the atmospheric pressure is lower. At 5,000 feet above sea level, for example, the boiling point of water is 203°F, at 10,000 feet, 194°F.

bolus. The mixture of food particles and saliva that results from mastication (the chewing process).

bomb calorimeter. An apparatus for measuring calories stored in foods or any organic material. The apparatus is carefully designed for measuring all the heat produced by the complete oxidation of an accurately measured amount of any food. The apparatus is insulated thoroughly against loss of heat, and the amount of heat produced is measured by the change in temperature of a measured amount of water. In an experiment, a weighed portion of the food whose calorie value is to be determined is placed in the bomb; after the bomb is charged with pure oxygen it is submerged in water. An electrical circuit causes combustion to take place. The heat given off into the water is measured by a thermometer calibrated to 100° Centigrade or Celsius (^{0}C). The rise in temperature of the water and the total heat capacity of the water bath and bomb are determined; it is then possible to determine the energy released by food. Below is a diagram of a bomb calorimeter with bomb in position. (A) Platinum dish holding weighed food sample. (B) Bomb filled with pure oxygen enclosing food sample. (C) Container holding water of known weight in which the bomb is submerged. (D) Outer double-walled insulating jacket. (E) Fuse, which is ignited by an electric current. (F) Motor-driven water stirrer. (G) Thermometer calibrated to 1/1000°C. (H) Electric wires to send current through food.

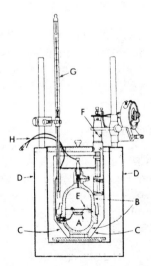

bonds. The chemical forces that hold atoms together in molecules.

bone. Living tissue containing blood vessels and nerves within the hard bone structure. The living cells that form bones are osteocytes. Bone cells have the ability to select calcium and other minerals from blood and tissue fluid and to deposit the calcium phosphate and calcium carbonate in the connective tissue fibers between cells. Periosteum, the membrane covering bone surfaces, carries blood vessels and nerves to the bone cells. Two kinds of bone are formed by the bone cells, compact and cancellous. Compact bone is hard and dense, while cancellous bone has a porous structure. The combination of compact and cancellous bone cells produces maximum strength with minimum weight. Bone contains 99 percent of the body's total metabolic calcium pool. Several vitamins are involved in bone development and maintenance. *Vitamin D* * has a direct effect on the mobilization of calcium to and from bone. A vitamin D deficiency in a child results in the nutritional disease *rickets,* and the adult counterpart *osteomalacia. Retinol* * (vitamin A) is also required for proper bone development which stops if a retinol deficiency is continued. *Ascorbic acid* * (vitamin C) is also required for a normal skeleton since abnormal *collagen* is formed and this leads to an impaired calcium deposition (calcification).

bone marrow. Two kinds of marrow, yellow and red, are found in the marrow cavities of bones. Red bone marrow is active blood cell manufacturing material, producing red blood cells and many of the white blood cells. Deposits of red bone marrow in the adult are in cancellous proteins of some bones, the skull, ribs, and sternum, for example. Yellow bone marrow is mostly fat and is found in marrow cavities of mature long bones.

boron (B). Element number 5. Atomic wt. 11. Minute traces of boron are found in body tissue, but no clues to its purpose have been discovered. Boron has been found to be essential for plant nutrition and growth, but experiments in animals have not demonstrated any evidence of deficiency after boron deprivation.

botulinus poisoning or botulism. Poisoning due to the ingestion of a toxic substance found preformed in food. Botulism is caused by the ingestion of a potent toxin secreted by different strains of *Clostridium botulinum,* an anaerobic, spore-forming organism which is widely distributed in soils. The bacterium grows readily under anaerobic conditions in improperly sterilized preserved foods which have a near-neutral or slightly alkaline reaction. The toxin of *Cl. botulinum* is one of the most potent poisons known. The ingestion of even minute quantities will result in a severe syndrome which may be fatal within 2 to 10 days. The entire human population could be eliminated by 200 g. (7 oz.) of the toxin. Symptoms include headache, nausea, prostration, oculomotor abnormalities, blindness, progressive difficulty in swallowing and talking, ascending paralysis and death. Treatment is primarily supportive in addition to the administration of polyvalent botulinus antitoxin. Inadequately processed home canned foods are most often the cause of botulism, preserved meats and fishes also are causes. In general, the low- and medium-acid canned foods are most often incriminated. Of the canned foods, those most often responsible for botulism have been string beans, sweet corn, beets, asparagus, spinach, and chard. Meats, fish and seafood, and milk products also have been responsible for outbreaks of botulism. Sausage and ham are also often involved. The name botulism is derived from the Latin word for sausage, botulus, because the first recognized European outbreaks were caused by spoiled sausages. See *food poisoning*.

bradycardia. Abnormal slowness of the heartbeat and pulse.

brain. The brain, a mass of nervous tissue, is the highest level of the nervous system. It coordinates activities of the entire body; carries on the learning, thinking, and reasoning processes; and directs the voluntary movements of the body. The brain may be divided into three parts; the cerebrum, cerebellum, and the brainstem, the last consisting of the forebrain, midbrain, pons, and medulla. The midbrain serves as a connective pathway between the right and left halves of the cerebrum and also between the cerebellum and the rest of the brain.

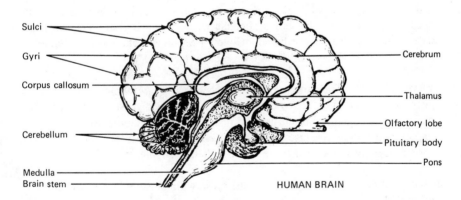

Sulci
Gyri
Corpus callosum
Cerebellum
Medulla
Brain stem

Cerebrum
Thalamus
Olfactory lobe
Pituitary body
Pons

HUMAN BRAIN

bran. The outer layers of food grains, obtained during flour-making are called by this name. Bran contains carbohydrates, vitamins, and minerals. It adds bulk to the diet and has a laxative effect. Bran is used as a breakfast food and as an ingredient in baking. Pure bran is dark brown in color and sold in the shape of flour, small strips, curls, and buds. Pure bran is often combined with another cereal such as wheat, and then pressed into flakes or little strips. The percentage of bran in these combinations is generally 40 percent. Nutritive values: Bran cereal is a good source of carbohydrates, has fair amounts of calcium and phosphorus. Flakes, 40 percent bran, 100 g. = 303 calories. See *cereal grains* and *wheat*.

brandy. This colorless, spirituous liquid is obtained by the evaporation, by distillation, of most of the watery portion of wine. The alcohol content is usually 50 to 60 percent. The wine can be made from grapes and other fruits, although the word brandy implies the use of grapes. The word itself comes from the middle English "brandywine" or "brandwine" which means burnt wine, or wine distilled by high heat.

Brazil nut (*Bertholletia excelsa*). Botanically speaking, Brazil nuts are not nuts at all, but the edible seeds of the rough-barked giant tree of the Amazon forest of South America. The fruit is globular, 4 to 6 inches in diameter, hard-walled and contains 8 to 24 seeds, arranged like the sections of an orange. These seeds are white and are known as Brazil nuts. The shell of the individual nut is triangular, dark brown, and very rough. The kernals are white with a rich flavor and are quite oily. Brazil nuts provide some protein, iron, and *thiamine**. Because of their high fat content, they are high in calories. Four average, or 3 large nuts = 97 calories.

bread. A food made from flour or meal, liquid, and shortening. Leavening agents are usually added, and the dough or meal is shaped, allowed to rise and baked. Breads are usually named after the meal or flours from which they are made, e.g., corn bread, rye bread, whole wheat bread. The nutritive value of various breads is given on the table on pp. 66–67.

brewer's yeast. The fungi *Saccharomyces cerevisiae* which will ferment sugars to alcohol under anaerobic conditions. Brewer's yeast is a concentrated source of high quality protein and of many of the B-vitamins except *cobalamin** (vitamin B_{12}). Because it is also a good source of iron and phosphorus, it is sometimes prescribed for those needing dietary supplements. See *yeast*.

brine. A strong salt solution used in the preservation of fish, meats, vegetables, and in pickling.

broccoli (*Brassica oleracea*). A dark-green vegetable, that is closely related to cauliflower, cabbage and Brussel sprouts. Broccoli has tight small heads called curds, which sit like buds on a thick stem. Both heads and stems are eaten. One of the richest vegetable sources of *ascorbic acid** (vitamin C), if vegetable is cooked quickly in a small amount of water. Excellent source of *carotene** (vitamin A) *riboflavin**, *iron* and *calcium*. Raw, 100 g. = 32 calories.

bromelain. A proteolytic enzyme from pineapple that digests proteins. See *papain*.

brominated vegetable oil (BVo). Chemically BVo is vegetable oil (olive, sesame, corn, or cottonseed) whose density has been increased to that of water by being combined with bromine. Flavoring oils are dissolved in BVo, which is then added to carbonated or noncarbonated fruit-flavor drinks. The lighter-than-water oils are dispersed throughout the drink by BVo, without which they would float to the surface and form a ring at the neck of the bottle. BVo also makes the soft drink slightly cloudy, giving the illusion of thickness or "body."

bronchi. The trachea divides to form the two bronchi. One bronchus enters each lung and these divide into many small air passages called bronchioles or bronchial tubes which lead air into the final air spaces within the lungs (See *respiratory system*).

bronchitis. An inflammation of the bronchii, the passageways of the lungs. It is usually an extension of colds or upper respiratory infection and has many of the same symptoms as pneumonia, cough, fever, and labored breathing. Asthmatic bronchitis is a loose term for the wheezing and cough which occur in allergic individuals who have symptoms, particularly in response to infection. Bronchiolitis is a viral inflammation of the smallest air passageways (bronchioles), usually occurring in infants. Its symptoms and signs are fever, cough, and labored breathing. Bronchitis, upper respiratory infection, laryngitis, and pneumonia may coexist in any given illness. An infection often involves several parts of the respiratory tree to varying degrees.

brucellosis. Milk from infected cows or goats may transmit the coccobacilli that cause brucellosis (undulant fever), transmitted through cuts or scratches in the skin of persons.

Brunner's glands. Mucus-secreting glands in the duodenum which provide mucus to protect the mucosa from irritation and erosion by the strongly acid gastric juices entering from the stomach. Emotional tension and stress inhibit these mucus secretions, a large factor in duodenal ulcer formation.

brussel sprouts (*Brassica oleracea*). A member of the cabbage family, looking like miniature cabbages. The plant, instead of making one large cabbage head, produces a number of rows of small heads where the leaves are attached. By pulling away the lower leaves, the little heads are given room to develop.

Food, Approximate Measure, and Weight (in grams)			Water	Food Energy	Protein	Fat
Breads:						
Boston brown bread, slice 3 by ¾ in.	1 slice	48	45	100	3	1
Cracked-wheat bread:						
Loaf, 1 lb.	1 loaf	454	35	1,190	40	10
Slice, 18 slices per loaf.	1 slice	25	35	65	2	1
French or vienna bread:						
Enriched, 1 lb. loaf	1 loaf	454	31	1,315	41	14
Unenriched, 1 lb. loaf.	1 loaf	454	31	1,315	41	14
Italian bread:						
Enriched, 1 lb. loaf	1 loaf	454	32	1,250	41	4
Unenriched, 1 lb. loaf.	1 loaf	454	32	1,250	41	4
Raisin bread:						
Loaf, 1 lb.	1 loaf	454	35	1,190	30	13
Slice, 18 slices per loaf.	1 slice	25	35	65	2	1
Rye bread:						
American, light (⅓ rye, ⅔ wheat):						
Loaf, 1 lb.	1 loaf	454	36	1,100	41	5
Slice, 18 slices per loaf.	1 slice	25	36	60	2	Trace
Pumpernickel, loaf, 1 lb.	1 loaf	454	34	1,115	41	5
White bread, enriched: *						
Soft-crumb type:						
Loaf, 1 lb.	1 loaf	454	36	1,225	39	15
Slice, 18 slices per loaf.	1 slice	25	36	70	2	1
Slice, toasted	1 slice	22	25	70	2	1
Slice, 22 slices per loaf.	1 slice	20	36	55	2	1
Slice, toasted	1 slice	17	25	55	2	1
Loaf, 1½ lbs.	1 loaf	680	36	1,835	59	22
Slice, 24 slices per loaf.	1 slice	28	36	75	2	1
Slice, toasted	1 slice	24	25	75	2	1
Slice, 28 slices per loaf.	1 slice	24	36	65	2	1
Slice, toasted	1 slice	21	25	65	2	1
Firm-crumb type:						
Loaf, 1 lb.	1 loaf	454	35	1,245	41	17
Slice, 20 slices per loaf.	1 slice	23	35	65	2	1
Slice, toasted	1 slice	20	24	65	2	1
Loaf, 2 lbs.	1 loaf	907	35	2,495	82	34
Slice, 34 slices per loaf.	1 slice	27	35	75	2	1
Slice, toasted	1 slice	23	35	75	2	1
Whole-wheat bread, soft-crumb type:						
Loaf, 1 lb.	1 loaf	454	36	1,095	41	12
Slice, 16 slices per loaf.	1 slice	28	36	65	3	1
Slice, toasted	1 slice	24	24	65	3	1
Whole-wheat bread, firm-crumb type:						
Loaf, 1 lb.	1 loaf	454	36	1,100	48	14
Slice, 18 slices per loaf.	1 slice	25	36	60	3	1
Slice, toasted	1 slice	21	24	60	3	1

* Values for iron, thiamin, riboflavin, and niacin per pound of unenriched white bread would be as follows:

	Iron Milligrams	Thiamine Milligrams	Riboflavin Milligrams	Niacin Milligrams
Soft crumb	3.2	.31	.39	5.0
Firm crumb	3.2	.32	.59	4.1

| | Fatty Acids | | | | | | | | | |
| | | Unsaturated | | | | | | | | |
Satu-rated (total)	Oleic	Lin-oleic	Carbo-hy-drate	Cal-cium	Iron	Vita-min A Value	Thia-mine	Ribo-flavin	Niacin	Ascor-bic Acid
			22	43	.9	0	.05	.03	.6	0
2	5	2	236	399	5.0	Trace	.53	.41	5.9	Trace
			13	22	.3	Trace	.03	.02	.3	Trace
3	8	2	251	195	10.0	Trace	1.27	1.00	11.3	Trace
3	8	2	251	195	3.2	Trace	.36	.36	3.6	Trace
Trace	1	2	256	77	10.0	0	1.32	.91	11.8	0
Trace	1	2	256	77	3.2	0	.41	.27	3.6	0
3	8	2	243	322	5.9	Trace	.23	.41	3.2	Trace
			13	18	.3	Trace	.01	.02	.2	Trace
			236	340	7.3	0	.82	.32	6.4	0
			13	19	.4	0	.05	.02	.4	0
			241	381	10.9	0	1.04	.64	5.4	0
3	8	2	229	381	11.3	Trace	1.13	.95	10.9	Trace
			13	21	.6	Trace	.06	.05	.6	Trace
			13	21	.6	Trace	.06	.05	.6	Trace
			10	17	.5	Trace	.05	.04	.5	Trace
			10	17	.5	Trace	.05	.04	.5	Trace
•5	12	3	343	571	17.0	Trace	1.70	1.43	16.3	Trace
			14	24	.7	Trace	.07	.06	.7	Trace
			14	24	.7	Trace	.07	.06	.7	Trace
			12	20	.6	Trace	.06	.05	.6	Trace
			12	20	.6	Trace	.06	.05	.6	Trace
4	10	2	228	435	11.3	Trace	1.22	.91	10.9	Trace
			12	22	.6	Trace				
			12	22	.6	Trace	.06	.05	.6	Trace
8	20	4	455	871	22.7	Trace	2.45	1.81	21.8	Trace
			14	26	.7	Trace	.07	.05	.6	Trace
			14	26	.7	Trace	.07	.05	.6	Trace
2	6	2	224	381	13.6	Trace	1.36	.45	12.7	Trace
			14	24	.8	Trace	.09	.03	.8	Trace
			14	24	.8	Trace	.09	.03	.8	Trace
3	6	3	216	449	13.6	Trace	1.18	0.54	12.7	Trace
			12	25	.8	Trace	.06	.03	.7	Trace
			12	25	.8	Trace	.06	.03	.7	Trace

Brussel sprouts are high in *carotene* * (vitamin A activity) and *ascorbic acid* * (vitamin C), and contain fair amounts of iron. Raw, 100 gm = 45 calories.

BSP test. Bromsulphthalein, a chemical measure of liver function. An injection is given, and some time later a blood specimen is taken for analysis.

buckwheat (Fagopyrum esculentum). The triangular seeds of this plant are used as a cereal although botanically speaking, it is an herb. It is not a member of the family of cereal grasses to which wheat belongs. High in carbohydrates, with small amounts of vitamins and minerals. Dark flour, 100 gm = 333 calories; light flour, 100 gm = 347 calories; whole-kernel, 100 gm = 335 calories.

buffer. A substance that can help a solution resist or counteract changes in free acid or alkali concentration. There are many buffers in the body. The word buffer comes from a Middle English root meaning "to protect from blows." In chemistry, a buffer is a combination of a weak acid and its salt, or a weak base and its salt, which protects a solution against wide variations in its pH (hydrogen ion or proton concentration) even when strong bases or acids are added to it. A solution containing such a protective mixture is called a buffer solution. A buffer protects the acid-base balance of a solution by rapidly offsetting changes in its ionized hydrogen concentration. It works by protecting against either added acid or base. Blood contains many buffer systems which include the *protein, hemoglobin, bicarbonate* and *phosphate* buffer systems which maintain a pH of the blood and body fluids at pH value of 7.4. See *acids and bases*.

bulgur. A cracked wheat that retains the bran and germ.

bulk. Fruits, vegetables, and cereals such as bran, in addition to being good sources of carbohydrate and minor sources of protein also provide bulk. Fruits and vegetables also contain fiber which is undigestible and nonabsorbable. As it travels through the intestines, it stimulates inactivity which is helpful in formation and maintenance of normal bowel habits.

bursa. A sac or saclike structure filled with fluid that acts as a cushion and prevents friction between two moving parts.

bursitis. Bursa is a small fluid-filled sac that permits one part of a joint to move easily over another part or over another structure. Bursae act to facilitate the gliding of muscles or tendons over bony or ligamentous surfaces. They are found throughout the body. In bursitis, a bursa becomes inflamed as the result of injury, gout, acute or chronic infection.

butter. An edible animal fat, obtained from milk and cream which have been made solid by churning. Butter can be made from fresh or slightly acid milk; it can be salted or it can be sweet, that is nonsalted. Butter is high in fat with moderate amounts of *carotene* * (vitamin A). Whipped butter contains ⅓ less calories than regular butter. Sweet or salted, 1 tablespoon = 100 calories. (One pat is ½ tablespoon). See *milk products*. The table on p. 70 gives the nutritive content of butter.

butternut (*Juglans cinerea*). A native North America nut, also known as a white walnut, used primarily in cakes and cookies. Butternuts are very difficult to shell, but do not need blanching. They grow in small clusters inside spongy, hair-covered husks. Butternuts contain some protein and iron and are high in fat. 100 gm = 629 calories.

butternut squash (*Cucurbita*). A winter squash, smooth and hard shelled, long and slender, with seeds contained in a small hollow in the base. The squash gets its name from its color which, for most of the year, is light brown or dark yellow. The flesh is almost orange. Its flavor is sweet, it mashes smoothly and is comparatively quick cooking. Butternut squash is an excellent source of *carotene* * (vitamin A) and also provides fair amounts of *ascorbic acid* * (vitamin C), iron and *riboflavin* *. Raw, 100 gm = 171 calories. See *Squash*.

butylated hydroxanisole (BHA), butylated hydroxytoluene (BHT). Used in many vegetable oils and in almost every processed food that contains fat or oil. These additives may increase slightly the shelf life of food by preventing polyunsaturated oil from oxidizing and becoming rancid; they may also protect

Butylated hydroxanisole. The —C(CH₃)₃ group may be in any one of the Positions marked (X).

Butylated hydroxytoluene

Food, Approximate Measure, and Weight (in grams)		gm	Water Per Cent	Food Energy Calories	Protein gm	Fat gm	Fatty Acids			Carbohydrate gm	Calcium mg	Iron mg	Vitamin A Value I.U.
							Saturated (total) gm	Unsaturated					
								Oleic gm	Linoleic gm				
Regular, 4 sticks per pound:													
Stick	½ cup	113	16	810	1	92	51	30	3	1	23	0	[21]3,750
Tablespoon (approx. ⅛ stick)	1 tbsp.	14	16	100	Trace	12	6	4	Trace	Trace	3	0	[21]470
Pat (1-in sq. ⅓-in high; 90 per lb)	1 pat	5	16	35	Trace	4	2	1	Trace	Trace	1	0	[21]170
Whipped, 6 sticks or 2, 8-oz containers per pound:													
Stick	½ cup	76	16	540	1	61	34	20	2	Trace	15	0	[21]2,500
Tablespoon (approx. ⅛ stick)	1 tbsp.	9	16	65	Trace	8	4	3	Trace	Trace	2	0	[21]310
Pat (1¼-in sq. ⅓-in high; 120 per lb)	1 pat	4	16	25	Trace	3	2	1	Trace	Trace	1	0	[21]130

the fat-soluble vitamins, *retinol** (vitamin A) and *tocopherol** (vitamin E). Manufacturers add BHA and BHT to breakfast cereal packaging, chewing gum, convenience foods, vegetable oil, shortening, potato flakes, enriched rice, potato chips, candy, and many other oil-containing products. The total concentration of antioxidants ranges from as low as 0.0001 percent in gelatin desserts to 0.1 percent in chewing gum. The usual concentration is about 0.01 percent.

butyric acid. Mol. Wt. 88. A saturated fatty acid that occurs as a glyceride to the extent of about 5 to 6 percent in butter and in very small amounts in a few other fats. Butyric acid is a mobile liquid, mixing in all proportions with water, alcohol, and ether; boiling without decomposition and readily volatile with steam.

$$CH_3CH_2CH_2COOH.$$

C

cabbage (*Brassica*). The word "cabbage" itself is an anglicized version of the colloquial French word caboche, which means "head." Cabbage comes in many varieties, some with loose heads, some with firm ones, and others with flat, conical, or eggshaped heads. Some cabbages are white, some green, some red; some have plain leaves and some curly ones. Raw cabbage is a very good source of *ascorbic acid* * (vitamin C) and some *carotene* * (vitamin A activity). Celery cabbage has a smaller amount. Cabbage also contains the goitogenic agents *thiourea* * and *thiocyanates* *. During the cooking process, there may be some vitamin loss. Raw, 100 gm = 24 calories; Cooked, 100 gm = 20 calories; Celery, raw 100 gm = 14 calories.

cabbage palm (*Oreodoxa*). The name given to several kinds of palm trees, which have edible parts. One of these is *O. oleracea,* which is cut down for food when about 3 years old. The parts eaten are the tender central leaves, used as greens, and especially the terminal bud and the tender inside of the thick stem, the "hearts of palm." The taste of these is bland and delicate.

cacao (*Theobroma cacao*). When taken from the pod, the cacao or cocoa beans are covered with a limey or fruity pulp which is removed by means of a fermentation process. The pulp-covered seeds are placed in piles, in pits, or in a "sweating box," where the beans are covered with banana or plantain leaves. During the 3 to 13 days of fermentation the beans are stirred and turned to aerate them and to keep down the temperature. The fermentation has the purpose of removing the adhering pulp from the bean; killing the embryo in the seed; and giving aroma, flavor, and color to the bean.

cactus pear. Prickly pear is another name for this fruit of one of a group of plants known as succulents. There are a number of edible varieties, with a water content that averages 85 percent and a high sugar content. The two most common ones are the *Fiscus-indica* and the Tuna. The *Fiscus-indica* has an oval fruit and is about 1½ to 3 inches in diameter, with a yellowish skin and pink or reddish pulp. The fruit of the *Tuna* is pearshape or roundish, and measures about 1 to 1½ inches in diameter. Cactus pears have a mild sweet flavor and are usually eaten raw. Raw, 100 gm = 42 calories.

cadmium (Cd). Element No. 48. Atom Wt. 112. Cadmium inactivates certain enzymes. It is also believed to be a micronutrient, but in large quantities it is a poison. Cadmium can be absorbed from drinking water that has not run sufficiently through galvanized pipes. Traces of cadmium are present in body tissues and their existence has been known for some time. It wasn't until 1960 that cadmium was isolated as a definite component of a metal containing protein. The protein metallothionein, found in the renal cortex of the horse, contains cadmium, zinc, and sulfur. The significance of this cadmium-containing protein is not yet clear, but it points to the possibility that the mineral functions in some basic biologic system.

caffeine. Mol. Wt. 194. An example of a mildly addicting cortical stimulant present in coffee, tea, cocoa, and cola drinks. The effect on the user depends on the tolerance he may or may not have for the drug. Tolerance is increased by habitual usage. Small doses of caffeine seem to improve performance in tasks such as typing. Doses that exceed individual tolerance levels can result in indigestion, nervousness, and inability to sleep.

Caffeine

Calciferol. Vitamin D_2, produces by irradiating *ergosterol* * from yeast. (See *vitamin D*).

calcification. Process by which organic tissue becomes hardened by a deposit of calcium salts.

calcitonin. A thyroid hromone concerned with the metabolism of calcium in the body. Calcitonin works in collaboration with a hormone from the parathyroid gland. The major effect of calcitonin on calcium metabolism is to increase the deposition and to prevent the removal of the mineral matter from the bones. Calcitonin is antagonistic to the activity of the hormone from the *parathyroid gland,* parathromone. Together the two hormones maintain a steady balance of Ca^{++} in the blood. Alone calcitonin tends to decrease the blood Ca^{++} level. Calcitonin production is regulated by feedback through Ca^{++}. Vitamin D is also involved in this regulatory system since it is needed for the transport of Ca^{++} through the blood. Calcitonin is a polypeptide consisting of a single chain of 32 amino acids. The sequence of these amino acids has been established and the substance has been synthesized.

calcium (Ca). Element No. 20. Atom Wt. 40. Of all the minerals in the human body, calcium is present in the largest amounts. It comprises about 1.4 to 2.0 percent of the total body weight. About 90 percent of the body calcium is in the skeletal tissue (bones and teeth) as deposits of the calcium salts dahllite or apatite. The remaining, which occurs in the plasma and other body fluids performs highly important metabolic tasks. It occurs in three forms: (1) nondiffusible, (2) diffusible, or (3) diffusible, but a constituent of an organic complex. From 10 to 30 percent of the calcium in an average diet is absorbed through the intestine. The physiologic function of 99 percent of the calcium in the body is to build and maintain skeletal tissue, and in tooth formation. The remaining 1 percent of the body's calcium performs several vital physiological functions. In blood clotting, calcium ions are required for bonding between fibrin molecules and to give stability to the fibrin threads. Calcium is also required for conversion of prothrombin to thrombin. Thrombin is an enzyme necessary for blood clotting. *Vitamin K* is also involved in these clotting reactions. Diary products supply the bulk of dietary calcium. One quart of milk contains about 1 gm of calcium, and cheese contains a comparable amount. Secondary sources are egg yolks, green leafy vegetables, legumes, nuts, and whole grains. Calcium in the body is usually associated with phosphorus, which is 0.8 to 1.1 percent of the body weight. A male person who weighs 154 pounds will have 2.3 to 3.1 pounds of calcium and 1.2 to 1.7 pounds of phosphorus in his body, about 99 percent of the calcium and 80 to 90 percent of the phosphorus are in the bones and teeth. The rest is in the soft tissue and body fluids and is important to their normal functioning. Phosphorus is an essential part of every living cell and occurs primarily as phosphate (PO_4^{-3}), and takes part in the chemical reaction with protein, fats, and carbohydrates to give the body energy and vital materials for growth and repair. It is one of the buffers in the blood and helps the blood neutralize acid and alkali. Both calcium and phosphorus are essential for the work of the muscle and for the normal response of nerves to stimulations. The calcium and phosphorus and other minerals in food are dissolved as the food is digested. Then they are absorbed from the gastrointestinal tract into the bloodstream. The blood carries them to different parts of the body where they are used for growth and upkeep. *Vitamin D* is essential for the absorption of calcium from the gastrointestinal tract. Egg yolk, butter, fortified margarine, and certain fish oils are the chief sources. Too much vitamin D can be dangerous in that it overloads the blood and tissues with calcium. Two hormones secreted by the parathyroid gland, *calcitonin* and *parathromone* have an important part in the body's use of calcium. The parathormone and calcitonin in the presence of vitamin D keep the amount of calcium in the blood at a normal level of about 10 mg per 100 ml of blood serum. The amount of calcium absorbed by the body is affected by the body's need for it, the amount supplied by the diet, the kind of food that supplies it, and the speed with which the food passes through the gastrointestinal tract.

calcium propionate. The calcium salt of proprionic acid is a chemical used to prevent growth of mold and certain bacteria in bread and rolls and also provides a calcium supplement to the diet. The sodium salt, sodium propionate, is preferred in pies and cakes because calcium alters the action of chemical leavening agents. Propionic acid occurs naturally in many foods and acts as a natural preservative in Swiss cheese. Propionate is also formed and used as a source of energy when the body metabolizes certain fats and amino acids. Propionates inhibit the growth of, but do not kill germs. See *proprionic acid* for structure.

calcium test. A chemical test on blood; used as a screening test and also for the diagnosis of bone disease and certain parathyroid, kidney, and pancreatic diseases.

calcium to phosphorus ratio (Ca : P ratio). Since calcium and phosphorus are intimately related in metabolism, two ratios between them are significant. (1) The dietary calcium to phosphorus ratio affects absorption of these minerals; a 1 : 1 ratio is ideal for growth, pregnancy, and lactation periods. Otherwise, for adults a 1 : 1½ ratio of calcium to phosphorus is required. (2) The serum calcium to phosphorus ratio is the solubility product of two minerals in the serum. An increase in one mineral causes a decrease in the other to maintain a constant product of the two. The normal serum level of calcium is 10 mg per 100 ml; of phosphorus, 4 mg per 100 ml in adults.

calculus. Any abnormal accretion within the body of material which forms a "stone." Calculi are usually composed of mineral salts. The most commonly formed renal calculi are composed of calcium salts. See *tartar*.

caloric. Pertaining to heat or energy; used in reference to the caloric value of a food, meaning the heat or energy that can be obtained as muscular work and heat when the body uses or metabolizes that food. See *calorie*.

caloric equivalent. The number of calories produced per liter of oxygen (O_2) for each of the foodstuffs, fat, carbohydrates, and protein is the caloric equivalent. The values for the three foodstuffs are almost the same (within 10 percent). Therefore, by determining the amount of oxygen utilized and multiplying it by the caloric equivalent, the number of calories produced can be determined. This is the basis for *indirect calorimetry* measurements. The caloric equivalent value is 4.8 calories/liter of O_2. See *indirect calorimetry* and *energy balance*.

caloric requirements. The amount of energy required to maintain life is the sum total of calories needed to satisfy requirements for basal metabolism, the specific dynamic action of food, as well as for growth, repair, and physical activity. Even minor physical activity adds to caloric requirements above the basal requirement or BMR. The act of walking on level ground at 2.5 mph requires an expenditure of about 180 calories per hour for an average adult; walking uphill on a 5 percent grade requires 270 calories per hour, and on a 15 percent grade 490 calories. See *energy balance*.

calorie. The commonly used standard for measurement of the energy value of substances is the calorie. The same term is used to express the body's energy requirement. The unit used in nutritional work is the large calorie (Cal) or the kilocalorie (kcal) and is the amount of heat required to raise the temperature of 1 kg of water 1° Centigrade. The small calorie (cal) or gram calories is one-thousandth of the value of the large unit and is used when minute amounts of heat are to be considered. 3500 calories equal 1 pound of body fat. The relationship between calorie input and energy output is called "calorie balance." Another unit of energy measurement is the joule, a unit used in some other scientific fields. To convert calories to joules the factor used is 1 calorie equals 4.184 joules. Calories are derived from the metabolism of carbohydrates, protein and fat. Proteins and carbohydrates contain 4 calories per gram, fat has nine. The difference is in the concentration of calories. Proteins and carbohydrates contain more water and fiber, ounce for ounce than fat does. All calories are alike, and four protein calories are precisely equal to four fat calories. So there is really no such thing as a "fattening food."

calorie measurements (values). The original work in establishing calorie values was done with the *bomb calorimeter* using weighed amounts of pure fat, pure carbohydrate, and pure protein. From data thus derived it was possible to arrive at average daily values for a specified weight of each. It was soon discovered that certain corrections were necessary when calculating energy values for human diets because some foods are not completely absorbed, and some are not completely oxidized to carbon dioxide and water, as in the calorimeter. Extensive experimentation showed the following rounded figures were suitable for practical use in calculating values of the usually mixed diets eaten; 1 gram of pure carbohydrate yields 4 calories; 1 gram of pure fat yields 9 calories; 1 gram of pure protein yields, 4 calories.

calorimeter. An instrument for measuring the heat change in any system, and the *bomb calorimeter* used to measure the calorie (energy) value of foods. See *bomb calorimeter*.

calorimetry. The measurement of heat loss. An instrument for measuring heat output of the body or the energy value of foods is called a calorimeter. See *direct calorimetry* and *indirect calorimetry*.

canker sores. More technically called aphthous or aphthous stomatitis, which are small ulcers inside the cheeks or on the sides of the tongue. Unlike fever blisters, canker sores develop only on the wet, pink tissue known as mucosa. A blister usually forms first, without notice, then breaks to form the open sore or canker; a small, oval, light-yellow ulcer ringed by red. The acute pain begins. Usually only one sore, appears, but there can be many. They are caused by bacteria (rather than viruses, as are fever blisters). They appear to come during times of emotional stress. Allergies and otherwise small injuries, such as a bruise while brushing the teeth too hard, seems to produce them also.

cantaloupe (*Cucumis melo cantalupenis*). A variety of muskmelon, with a sweet and fragrant taste. The cantaloupe was named for a castle in Italy. Cantaloupe is an excellent source of *carotene**** (vitamin A) and *ascorbic acid*** (vitamin C) ½ melon, 5 inches in diameter = 37 calories.

capers (*Capparis*). The unopened flowers of the caper bush. During the flowering season, the buds are picked before the petals can expand and preserved in vinegar and salt. Capers add liveliness to white and other sauces, to salads and creamed dishes, and as condiments, to appetizers, meats, and seafood.

capillaries. Small microscopic vessels forming networks in all tissues lying between the arterial and venous systems. Somewhat larger than a red cell, thin walled, permitting oxygen, nutrients and other substances to diffuse through their walls to reach the living tissues.

capillary fluid shift mechanism. The process which controls the movement of water and small molecules in solution (electrolytes, nutrients) between the blood in the capillary and the surrounding interstitial area.

caproic acid. Mol. Wt. 116. A *saturated fatty acid* occurring in cow and goat butter and coconut fat.

$$CH_3CH_2CH_2CH_2CH_2COOH.$$

caprylic acid. Mol. Wt. 148. A *saturated fatty acid* occurring in coconut oil, goat, and cow butter, and human fat.

$$CH_3CH_2CH_2CH_2CH_2CH_2COOH.$$

caramelize. The word "caramel" has two meanings. It describes a candy with a chewy consistency and it is also a culinary term that refers to burnt sugar by itself or thinned with water. To caramelize is to heat sugar or foods containing sugar until a brown color and characteristic flavor develop.

caraway (*Carum carvi*). An oval-shaped brown seed named after the ancient district of Caria in Asia Minor. The caraway plant grows to a height of about 2 feet, with feathery green leaves and yellow-white flowers that resemble Queen Anne's Lace. Fresh young leaves add flavor to soups, salads, cheeses, vegetables, and meat. The roots may be steamed and eaten as a vegetable. Caraway seeds are used to season soups, meats, vegetables, breads such as rye, cakes, and pasteries. Oil extracted from the seed provides the distinctive flavor of the liqueur kümmel.

carbohydrates. Class name is suggested by the fact that they are made up of the elements carbon, hydrogen, oxygen, with the hydrogen and oxygen present in the same 2 : 1 proportion as in water, hence the name hydrate. Carbohydrates are subdivided into three groups, according to the relative complexity and size of their molecules. The more complex carbohydrates must all be broken down by the digestion into the simple sugars before they can be absorbed and used by the body. Carbohydrates are classified as simple sugars or *monosaccharides* (one sugar group per molecule); *disaccharides* (two simple sugars per molecule); *oligosaccharides* (several simple sugars per molecule); and *polysaccharides* (many simple sugar groups per molecule). Carbohydrates supply about 20 percent of the energy needed to act and move, perform work, live. Among the carbohydrates are *sugars, starches,* and *celluloses*. All green plants form carbohydrates. Carbohydrates are important in nutrition, some make food sweet. Some carbohydrates serve as food for bacteria that cause tooth decay. The body needs carbohydrates in order to use fat efficiently. Some carbohydrates are relatively small molecules. Others, larger and more complex, such as glycogen, consist of many of the smaller monosaccharide molecules chemically linked in long chains. The chains of the largest molecules may contain more than 1000 units. They may be straight as in potato starch, or branched as in *glycogen* and *amylopectin*. Some contain only one kind of unit, others several different kinds. Less complex carbohydrates are *lactose* or milk sugar which is a disaccharide complex of one *glucose** and one *galactose** molecule. Cane sugar or *sucrose** is also a disaccharide complex of one *glucose* and one *fructose** molecule. Carbohydrates made up of long chains of monosaccharides are known as *polysaccharides*. Among them are *glycogen* (animal starch), *starch, cellulose, plant gums,* and *mucilages,* and other structural and storage carbohydrates. Glucose is the commonest of the *monosaccharides*. Although carbohydrates function in nutrition primarily as a source of energy, there is no definite nutritional requirement for carbohydrates. Starch which consists of glucose units is the only polysaccharide that man can use efficiently. Potatoes and cereal grains, the most important sources of carbohydrates, are rich in starch. Rice, wheat, sorghum, corn (maize) millet, and rye contain 70 percent starch. Potatoes and other tubers and roots are also rich in starch. Beans and the seeds of many other legumes are high in protein, and also contain 40 percent or more of their dry matter as starch. Digestable starches are about 97 percent absorbed by the digestive tract under ordinary circumstances. A constant amount of glucose is necessary for the proper functioning of the central nervous system. Its regulatory center, the brain, contains no stored supply of glucose and is therefore, especially dependent upon a minute-to-minute supply of glucose from the blood. Sustained and profound hypoglycemic shock may cause irreversible brain damage. In all nerve tissue carbohydrate is indispensible for functional integrity.

carbohydrate, available. This term, available carbohydrate, represents the portion of the carbohydrate of foods which is available to the human body for glycogen formation. It includes starch, dextrins, glycogen, *maltose**, *sucrose**, *lactose**, as well as the monosaccharides *glucose**, *fructose**, *galactose**, *mannose**, and pentoses.

carbohydrate combustion. The average value for the heat of combustion of carbohydrates ordinarily accepted is 4.1 calories per gram; the caloric value of the oxygen needed to oxidize glucose is 4.047 calories per liter and varies slightly depending on the carbohydrate. If the organism were burning only glucose, the heat production could be computed by determining the liters of oxygen consumed and multiplying by the factor 5.047.

carbohydrate digestion. Starches are complex forms of sugars. When starch is eaten a digestive enzyme in the saliva of the mouth, salivary amylase, mixes the starch and begins the digestive process. As the food is swallowed, this step continues in the stomach process, where starch is converted to oligosaccharides and sugars. In the small intestine digestive enzymes from the pancreas, pancreatic amylases, and from the walls of the intestine itself complete the process. The final products are *monosaccharides*. A similar transformation takes place when sugar replaces starch in the ripening of fruit. *Cellulose,* the carbohydrate that forms the cell walls of vegetables and fruits of all plants is not digested by humans or mammals. Cellulose is important in the mechanics of the digestive process, however, because it provides fiber bulk and thus aids in discarding residues of digestion.

carbohydrate, indigestible. Substances which make up the cell-wall structure of plants, consisting of varying amounts of cellulose, hemicellulose, lignin, pectin substances, gums, mucin, etc., which cannot be hydrolyzed by enzymes of the human gastrointestinal tract. They are not available for glycogen formation.

carbohydrate metabolism. The metabolism of carbohydrates proceeds in the liver and other body tissues. Glucose is carried in the bloodstream to the liver. In the presence of the enzyme hexokinase and a high-energy phosphate com-

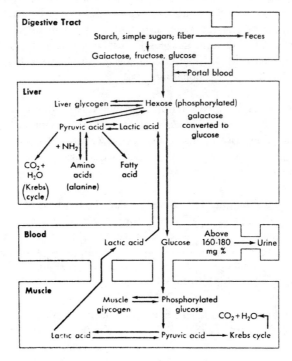

Pathways of carbohydrate metabolism.

plex, *adenosine triphosphate* * (ATP), glucose is phosphorylated to glucose-6-phosphate, then to glucose-1-phosphate, and finally to glycogen. The high energy compound *uridine triphosphate* * (UTP) is involved in the latter reactions. This polysaccharide glycogen is found in muscle tissue as well as in the liver, the heart, brain, and other tissues. The liver glycogen acts as an energy reserve for the other tissues. For carbohydrate metabolism to proceed normally, several B vitamins, as well as the minerals, magnesium, and phosphorus are required. *Niacin* *, *riboflavin* *, *thiamine* *, *pyridoxine* * and *pantothenic acid* * function as coenzymes, and magnesium and phosphorus, as cofactors in the chemical reactions involved in the metabolism of carbohydrates. When energy is required glycogen is broken down to glucose and oxidized. Hormones are involved in this breakdown process, notably epinephrine or glucagon. The hormones initiate the formation of the "second messenger" *cyclic 3',* *5'-adenosine monophosphate* * (C-AMP) which in turn initiates the breakdown of glycogen* to glucose-1-phosphate. The diagram traces the major metabolic pathways of carbohydrates in man.

carbohydrate oxidation. The process in which oxygen unites with carbohydrates to form carbon dioxide, water and heat, and chemical energy, ultimately through the *terminal respiratory chain*. Heat represents the energy available for the maintenance of body temperature. Chemical energy, mainly in the form of ATP is used for synthetic, mechanical, electrical, and physical work.

carbohydrate storage. Carbohydrate is stored in the liver and other cells as the polysaccharide, *glycogen* *. In the liver, glycogen is not only stored as fuel for other tissues, but also serves two other important functions. First, it exerts a protective action by being present as glycogen and by participating in specific detoxifying metabolic pathways. Second, carbohydrate has a regulatory influence on protein and fat metabolism. The presence of sufficient carbohydrates for energy demands prevents the oxidation of too much protein for this purpose. This protein-sparing effect of carbohydrate allows a major portion of protein to be used for its basic structural purposes of tissue building. The amount of carbohydrate present also determines how much fat will be broken down.

carbon (C). Element No. 6. Atom Wt. 12. This chemical element is present in all substances designated as organic. These include proteins, carbohydrates, and fats. When a compound containing carbon combines with oxygen in the body, energy is liberated and carbon dioxide is formed. Compounds that do not contain carbon are classed as inorganic. Carbon has several chemical features that make it unique as a foundation for life. Its four *valances* and tetrahedral structure allow a wide variety of compounds to be formed with a carbon backbone and the compounds themselves can be stereospecific. Living reactions involving carbon are stereospecifically selected. For example, all proteins contain only L-amino acid forms. Biochemical reactions then differ from chemical reactions by the specificity that the structure of carbon allows.

carbonic acid. Mol. Wt. 53.

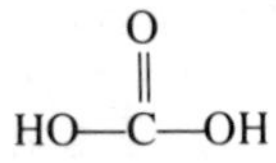

$$\underset{\text{HO-C-OH}}{\overset{\overset{\textstyle O}{\|}}{}}$$

Carbonic acid is a part of the important *bicarbonate buffer* system in the body. Carbonic acid is formed when carbon dioxide dissolves in water.

$$CO_2 + H_2O \rightleftharpoons H_2CO_3$$

Acid drives the reaction to the left and CO_2 is formed. *Base* drives the reaction to the right and *bicarbonate* salts (HCO_3^-) are formed. The exchanges are important in respiration at the cellular level; in hemoglobin chemistry, and in the lungs.

carbonyl group. Carbon-oxygen groups found in acetones and ketones. $\geq C = O$ this group is found in all monosaccharides (sugars).

carboxylation. Reaction which involves the addition of carbon dioxide (CO_2) to an organic compound is called a carboxylation. The reactions are often referred to as CO_2 fixation in plants. The vitamin *biotin* * is often involved in CO_2 fixation reaction. For example, biotin is a coenzyme for the reaction of methyl malonyltranscarboxylase that forms methylmalonyl coenzyme A, an intermediate in fatty acid synthesis that requires CO_2 fixation. *Vitamin K* * is also involved in the carboxylation of a terminal glutamic acid residue in the formation of normal *prothrombin*.

carboxyl group. The acid group of organic compounds. The structure —COOH dissociates a hydrogen ion (proton, H^+) in aqueous solution and it is therefore

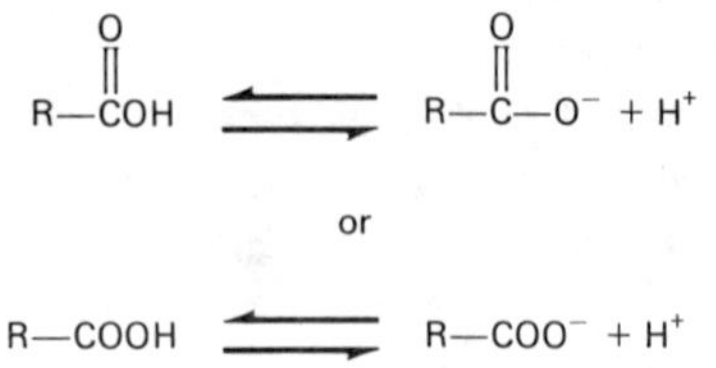

$$R-\overset{\overset{\textstyle O}{\|}}{C}OH \rightleftharpoons R-\overset{\overset{\textstyle O}{\|}}{C}-O^- + H^+$$

or

$$R-COOH \rightleftharpoons R-COO^- + H^+$$

Carboxyl group

an acid. Carboxyl group are weak acids because there is a great tendency to associate with a proton, i.e., the reaction tends towards the left.

carboxylic acid. An organic compound containing a *carboxyl* group.

carboxypeptidase. A digestive enzyme formed initially in an inactive state called procarboxypeptidase. Carboxypeptidase is quite different from other proteolytic digestive enzymes. It hydrolyzes only peptide bonds that are adjacent to the free carboxylic acid end of the peptide chain. Each molecule of the enzyme contains an atom of zinc, which is involved in the active site of the enzyme. When the *zinc* atom is removed all enzyme action is lost.

carcinogen. Means cancer-producing. Carcinogenic agents are substances which can cause the development of cancer cells. Over 400 different carcinogens have been identified.

carcinoma. A form of cancer consisting of malignant growth originating in the epithelial tissue and tending to spread to other tissues.

cardamom (*Elettaria cardamomum*). A plant growing to a height of 8 to 12 feet, the seeds of which are used as a flavoring, grow in groups within a pod that resembles a capsule. The capsules are sun-dried and marketed whole. Cardamom is said to be the world's second most precious spice, the costliest one being saffron. Cardamom seeds are brown, and they have an aromatic odor and a warm, spicy taste. They are used in curries and in such meats as frankfurters and sausages, in pickling-spice blends, and in baked foods.

cardiac muscle. A specialized form of muscle in which the individual muscle cells are joined together by bridges of protoplasm forming a network (syncytium). It has intrinsic rhythmical properties and if any part of the cardiac muscle contracts the wave of contraction spreads throughout the muscle as a whole. Conditions which affect the cardiac muscle include: (1) The length of the muscle when it contracts (degree of diastolic filling). (2) The neuro-humoral background, a general term for the degree of activity exerted by the autonomic nervous system and the level of hormones such as *epinepherine* and *norepinepherine* circulating in the blood. (3) The concentration of electrolytes such as *potassium* and *calcium* in the blood circulating through the heart. The metabolism of cardiac muscle is essentially the same as that of skeletal muscle but it has far less reserves and is unable to contract in the absence of oxygen (anaerobically) for more than a few seconds. See *skeletal muscle* and *smooth muscle*.

cardiac output. The amount of blood pumped by the left venticle into the aorta in 1 minute. An average person has a cardiac output of 5.6 l per minute with an average pulse of 66 per minute. Stroke volume is output of left venticle during one contraction.

cardiovascular system. This system, which maintains the heart and all blood vessels is a closed system, transporting blood to all parts of the body. Blood flowing through the circuit brings heat, oxygen, food, and other chemical elements to tissue cells and removes carbon dioxide and other waste products resulting from cell activity.

cardoon (*Cynara cardunuculus*). A thistlelike, silver-green, prickly plant closely related to the artichoke but which looks more like an outsize stalk of celery. Cardoons are grown from the leafy midribs of the plant, which are fleshy and tender. The flavor is delicate and resembles that of the related artichoke and the oyster plant. See *artichoke*.

carnitine. A growth factor in the mealworm. In animals it forms esters with fatty acids that allow passage through the membrane of mitochondria.

$$\overset{\displaystyle CH_3}{\underset{\displaystyle CH_3}{CH_3\!-\!\overset{+}{N}\!-\!CH_2\!-\!\underset{\displaystyle OH}{CH}\!-\!CH_2COOH}}$$

carob (*Ceratonia siliqua*). The carob tree is native to the Mediterranean region. Known since biblical times as St. John's bread, the powder made from the seed pods tastes something like chocolate. Carob is popular as a health food, and as a chocolate substitute in candy because of its low fat content. Carob has 180 calories and 1.4 gm of fat per 100 gm (3.5 ounces) compared to 528 calories and 35 gm of fat for the same amount of sweet chocolate.

carotene (*provitamin A*). Mol. Wt. 537. A group of yellow-red plant pigments which yield vitamin A upon oxidative scission. A yellow pigment occurring in many fruits and vegetables, as well as in animal fat. Important in a good diet because the digestive tract converts it to *retinol* * (vitamin A), in animals. Food manufacturers add carotene to margarine, nondairy coffee whiteners, shortenings, butter, milk, cake mix, dessert topping, and other products either as artificial coloring, as a nutritional supplement or both. Retinol is obtained from fish oil and requires no conversion. The average adult should consume 5000 international units of vitamin A. Carotene in food has about one-sixth the activity of retinol. Carotene is the most abundant form in green leafy and yellow vegetables. Because of inefficient conversion of carotene to retinol in the body, six

Carotene

molecules of β-carotene are considered equivalent to one molecule of vitamin A in man; approximately two-thirds of the vitamin A activity of the average diet is provided by carotene. The most common form of carotene is beta (β)-carotene. Other forms exist, but they are not so active as β-carotene. The other carotenes differ from β-carotene in the position of the methyl (—CH₃) groups in the ionone ring. The retinol requirement is easily satisfied by beef liver, chard, kale, spinach, and other greens, beans, broccoli, carrots, yellow squash, apricots, and sweet potatoes.

carotenoid. (1) Pertaining to a number of compounds related to carotene. They are primarily yellow pigments. (2) Any of a group of red, orange, and yellow accessory pigments of plants.

carotenoid pigments. The carotenoid pigments are related to retinol. Plant precursors contribute to vitamin A value of a food, and in a popular manner, frequently are referred to as the vitamin itself. Of the plant precursors, β-carotene is the most important since it has the highest vitamin A activity and occurs most plentifully in foods. In human beings the biologic activity of the carotenes is less than that of retinol, due in part to the extremely variable availability of some of them and the low efficiency of conversion. Beta-carotene is a dark-red crystalline compound. The carotenoid pigments are comparatively heat stable compounds but are labile on exposure to radiation and oxidation, especially when in liquid form and when associated with free radicals or peroxides.

carotin. A ruby-red crystal-like parent substance of vitamin A occurring naturally in green vegetables, carrots, and yellow turnips. After absorption it is converted by the liver into retinol. It is also an organic pigment found in certain chloroplasts.

carrageenin. A substance obtained from Irish moss. The active chemical is the carbohydrate carrageenin. Food manufacturers use carrageenin because of the unique way it reacts with milk protein. A weak gel that forms in the milk prevents cocoa particles from settling in chocolate milk and prevents butterfat from separating out of evaporated milk. The seaweed derivatives have similar stabilizing effects in canned milk drinks, instant breakfasts, and infant formula. Manufacturers use carrageenin to add ''body'' to soft drinks, to thicken ice cream, jelly, sour cream, and syrup, to stabilize the foam in beer, and to prevent oil from separating out of frozen whipped topping. It is used as the gelling component of gelatin-type desserts and milk puddings. Carrageenin gel has no nutrient value. Companies that manufacture canned infant formula use carrageenin to prolong the shelf life of their product.

carrots (*Daucus carota*). Carrots have been cultivated for over 2000 years. They are one of the best sources of vitamin A, which is necessary for good eye health and good bone formation. Carrots also contain small amounts of vitamins and minerals. Raw, 100 gm = 42 calories.

cartilage tissue. A tough, resilient connective tissue found at the ends of the bones, between bones, and in the nose, throat, and ears. It contains large quantities of the protein *collagen*.

casaba. Any or several large winter melons, globular in shape with pointed stem ends and round furrowed rinds. When ripe, the flesh is creamy white, soft and juicy, but almost without fragrance. It has a distinctive, mild cucumberlike flavor. The rind is yellow and although wrinkled, it is not netted. 100 gm = 27 calories.

casein. The principal protein of milk, the basis of cheese. A phosphoprotein. Casein is a nutritious protein, because it contains adequate amounts of all the essential amino acids. Food manufacturers add casein to ice cream, ice milk, frozen custard, and sherbert to improve their texture; in nondairy coffee creamers, casein adds body and acts as a whitener.

cashew (*Anacardium occidentale*). A sweet, plump, white kidney-shaped nut, the edible seed of a tropical evergreen tree related to the sumac, native to tropical America and found widely in India and equatorial Africa. Cashews contain some protein, iron, and various B vitamins. They are high in fat content. 100 gm = 561 calories.

cassava. See *Maniac*.

catabolism. Refers to processes by which nutrients, reserve tissue material, and cellular substances are broken down into chemically simpler compounds with the liberation of energy. In catabolism energy nutrients are oxidized gradually, ultimately yielding carbon dioxide and water plus some nitrogen compounds, from protein catabolism. Part of the energy released by catabolism, is converted to chemical energy (*adenosine triphosphate* *), and the remainder is usually converted to heat. See *anabolism*. (Anabolism + catabolism = *metabolism*). See *oxidative phosphorylation* and *kreb's cycle*.

catalase. An enzyme usually obtained from animal organs but can be prepared from a mold grown in an aerated, agitated culture or from *Micrococcus lysodeikticus*. It is used to neutralize excess hydrogen peroxide in processes involving the combined action of mild heat and the peroxide as applied to milk and other foods. The reaction catalaze catalyzes is as follows: $H_2O_2 \longrightarrow H_2O + HO_2$. In animal cells catalase is found in organelles called peroxisomes.

catalyst. A substance which regulates the speed at which a chemical reaction occurs without affecting the end point of the reaction and without being used up as a result of the reaction. Biochemical catalysts are called enzymes.

cataracts. Opaque spots that form on the lens and impair vision. Spreading throughout the lens over a period of time, they keep light rays from getting through to the retina. Cataracts may result from injuries to the eyes, exposure to great heat or radiation, or inherited factors.

catecholamines. Derivatives of *catechol* * in which the amine ($-NH_2$) group is attached to a side chain. Catecholamines of biological interest are *epinephrine* * (adrenaline) and *norepinephrine* * (noradrenaline).

catecholamine test. A chemical test on blood or urine; used for diagnosis in tumors of the adrenal gland.

catfish. A freshwater fish that derives its name from its barbels, or feelers, which resemble a cat's whiskers. Catfish live in streams. The best eating, is the channel cat, which weighs from 5 to 10 pounds. The smaller bullhead is the most common. The channel cat is usually baked; the bullhead is fried. Raw, freshwater, 100 gm = 103 calories.

cauliflower (*Brassica oleraccea*). The word cauliflower is a combination of the Latin caulis, meaning "stalk," and floris, "flower." A member of the cabbage family. Cauliflower is a good source of *ascorbic acid* * (vitamin C); a fair source of iron. Raw, 100 gm = 27 calories; Cooked, 100 gm = 31 calories.

caustic. Burning or corrosive; capable of destroying living tissue.

caviar. A fish roe which has been sieved, lightly pressed, and treated with salt. It may come from any of the following fish, among others; beluga (a member of the sturgeon family), sterlet, sturgeon, salmon, carp, herring, whitefish, or cod.

cayenne. The hot, pungent red pepper known as cayenne is prepared by grinding the dried ripe fruit of several species of the Capsicum plant, chiefly *Capsicum frutescens* and *C. annum*. Cayenne is an ingredient of sausage seasonings and curry powders.

cecum (caecum). The first portion of the large intestine. It is about 7 cm long and 8 cm wide. It lies between the ileum and colon. See *digestive system.*

celeriac (*Apium*). A dark, turnip-rooted European variety of celery which also goes by the names of celery root or celery knob. Only the root is eaten. It is eaten hot, or used as a cold salad and as a flavoring for soups and stews. Celeriac is seldom eaten raw. Raw, 100 gm = 40 calories.

celery (*Apium graveolens*). A stalk vegetable which is a cultivated version of a white-flowered herb that grew wild in both Europe and Asia. The leaves, stalk, and root of cultivated celery are all edible. Raw, 100 gm = 17 calories.

celiac disease. A disease characterized by fatty diarrhea (steatorrhea) and caused by intolerance to glutin; similar to nontropical sprue.

cellibiose. Mol. Wt. 343. The basic disaccharide unit of the plant polysaccharide cellulose. Cellibiose is composed of two glucose molecules but is not digestible, while *maltose* * is digestible. The difference between cellibiose and maltose is in the configuration of the linkage between the glucose molecules.

Cellibiose

cells. The basic functioning unit in the composition of the human body. The human body is composed of millions of cells varying in shape and size, microscopic in size, the largest being only about 1/1000 of an inch. A group of cells is called a tissue when the cells associate and coordinate to perform particular functions. The interior of cells are composed of a substance called *protoplasm*.

A typical cell is made up of a cell membrane and two main parts, the nucleus and the *cytoplasm,* which are types of protoplasm. The nucleus contains the genetic determinants *chromosomes* and controls all activities of the cell, including growth and reproduction. The cytoplasm is the matter surrounding the nucleus and is responsible for most of the work done by the cell. The cytoplasm contains formed elements such as *lysosomes, mitochondria* and the *endoplasmic reticulum.* The cell membrane encloses the protoplasm and permits the passage of fluid and specific materials into and out of the cell. This specific permeability of the cell membrane is an important structural feature of the cell. It is through the cell membrane that all materials essential to metabolism are received and all products of metabolism are disposed of. The bloodstream and tissue fluid which constantly circulate around the cell transport the materials to and from the cells. The diagram on p. 90 is a schematic representation of a "typical cell" cell. It is a composite of several animal cell types.

cellulose. Mol. Wt. 20,000–400,000. A plant polysaccharide of glucose consisting of β $1\rightarrow4$ linkages that are not digestible by animal enzymes. Ruminants such as cattle depend upon intestinal bacteria to digest the cellulose in the fodder. *Cellibiose** is considered the disaccharide building block.

cellulose, methyl. A methyl ester of *cellulose* which swells in water to produce a colloidal solution; used as a thickening agent, an emulsifier, and as a noncaloric source of bulk.

central nervous system. The central nervous system (CNS) consists of the brain and spinal cord. These are delicate structures that are protected by two coverings, bones and special membranes. The brain is encased by the bones of the skull that form the cranium; the spinal cord by the vertebrae. The membranes enclosing both brain and spinal cord are the meninges.

cephalins. A class of phospholipids found in tissues, especially brain and nerve tissue.

Cephalins

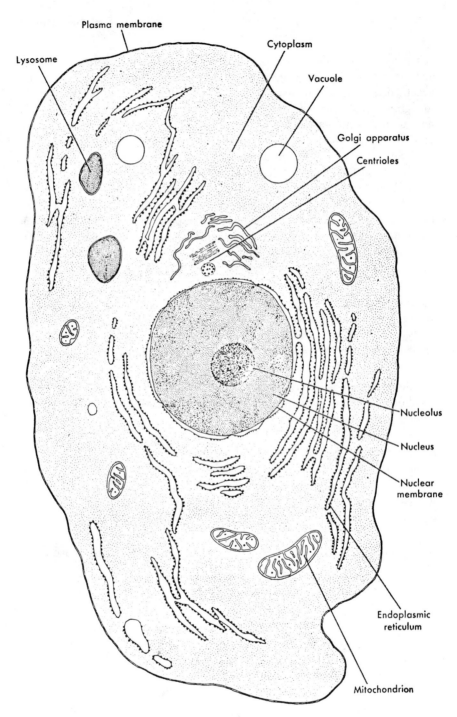

Plasma membrane

Lysosome

Cytoplasm

Vacuole

Golgi apparatus

Centrioles

Nucleolus

Nucleus

Nuclear
membrane

Endoplasmic
reticulum

Mitochondrion

Diagram of a ''typical'' animal cell.

cereal. An edible seed, also called grain, of the grass family. The word "cereal" goes back to Ceres, the Roman goddess of grain. Rice, wheat, and corn are the mainstays of nutritious diets, followed by rye, barley, millet, and oats. The common grains have a roughly similar composition. They contain from 7 to 14 percent protein, and 75 percent carbohydrates. The proteins are of low biologic value but when supplemented with simultaneously consumed proteins of a better quality they are capable of supplying man's protein requirements. The vitamin and mineral constituents of grains are held mostly in the outer layers of the kernel or in the embryo (germ). Since much of this is lost in the process of milling, phosphorus remains the major mineral contribution of most grains. Today's enrichment of flour restores *thiamine*, riboflavin*, niacin** and iron to the grain.

cereal grains. Cereal grains are the seeds of domesticated grasses. The principal cereals are *wheat, rice, corn, millets, oats* and *rye.* All cereals can be ground into flour but only wheat and rye bake into *bread.* Wheat is basically the choice in temperate or dry climates. Rice is the cereal of choice for most damp tropical climates. Corn is grown widely and considered essentially a poor person's food, having the merit of being hardy, and easily cultivated. Millets grow in hot climates in poor soil with limited water supply. Oats is chiefly grown for cattle fodder. Barley is mainly used for brewing, but is also eaten by man and cattle. Whole grains of all cereals have a similar chemical constitution

Nutritive Value of the Main Whole Cereal Grains
(Values per 100 gm)

	Energy		Protein	Limiting Amino Acid	Fat	Calcium	Iron	Thiamine	Nicotinic Acid	Riboflavin	Carotene	Ascorbic Acid
	MJ	kcal	g		g	mg	mg	mg	mg	mg	μg	mg
Wheat (whole meal)	1·40	334	12·2	lysine	2·3	30	3·5	0·40	5·0	0·17	Trace	0•
Rice (husked)	1·49	357	7·5	lysine	1·8	15	2·8	0·25	4·0	0·12	Trace	0
Maize (whole meal)	1·49	356	9·5	tryptophan	4·3	12	5·0	0·33	1·5	0·13	Up to 800	0
Millet Sorghum)	1·44	343	10·1	lysine	3·3	30	6·2	0·40	3·5	0·12	Trace	0
Oats (rolled)	1·61	385	13·0	lysine	7·5	60	3·8	0·50	1·3	0·14	Trace	0
Rye	1·34	319	11·0	lysine	1·9	50	3·5	0·27	1·2	0·10	Trace	0

and nutritive value. They provide energy and also some protein. They contain appreciable amounts of calcium and iron, but the value of these minerals is partly discounted by the presence of *phytic acid* which may interfere with their absorption. Whole cereals are totally devoid of *ascorbic acid* * (*vitamin C,*) and practically devoid of *carotene* * (vitamin A activity). Whole cereal grains contain useful amounts of the water-soluble B groups of vitamins, except for *cobalamin* * (vitamin B_{12}). Listed on p. 91 are the nutritive values of the cereal grains.

cerebellum. The second largest part of the brain, located above the medulla at the back of the cranial cavity covered dorsally by the cerebral hemispheres.

cerebral cortex. The outer layer of the cerebrum, consisting of cells known collectively as "gray matter" where the principal brain centers are located; these are the motor, sensory, visual, auditory, olfactory, and association centers. See *brain.*

cerebral hemisphere. Two cerebral hemispheres fill the major part of the skull, each hemisphere being largely responsible for the sensation and movement of the opposite half of the body, although certain automatic processes, such as swallowing, breathing, and some trunk movements are doubly controlled from both hemispheres. The cerebral hemispheres consist of an outer layer of nerve cells or gray matter, called the cortex, surrounding a complex network of nerve fibers or white matter. The two cerebral hemispheres are each divided for descriptive purposes into four lobes; (a) frontal, (b) parietal, (c) occipital, and (d) temporal.

(a) Frontal lobes: The frontal lobe extends forward and contains nerve cells which transmit impulses to the brainstem and spinal cord and on to all the voluntary muscles of the body. Much of the frontal lobe is concerned with emotional expression and experience but its functions are not well understood. The production of words, phrases, and sentences in correct order and balance depends on the activity of this part of the brain.

(b) Parietal lobes: The parietal lobes are the middle part of the cerebral hemispheres behind the fissure of Rolando. They are mainly concerned with the reception of a response to nerve impulses from sensory nerve endings all over the body. The detailed appreciation, assessment, integration, and judgment of sensation depend on the parietal lobes.

(c) Occipital lobes: The posterior parts of the cerebral hemispheres form the occipital lobes which contain the nervous structure necessary for vision. The neuronal equipment necessary for the recognition of light, shade, shape, and color is localized at the back and the more forwardly placed structures are responsible for the appreciation and interpretation of visual patterns.

(d) Temporal lobes: The cerebral hemispheres jut out to form the temporal lobes, which are their lower parts. The lobes are especially concerned with hearing but their other functions are not understood, although they seem to be concerned with memory to some extent.

cerebral thrombosis. Formation of a clot in the brain artery eventually leading to occlusion of the artery. The result is a stroke or a cerebral vascular accident.

cerebrospinal. Pertaining to the brain and spinal cord.

cerebrospinal fluid (CSF). The cerebrospinal fluid fills ventricles of the brain and the subarachnoid space which surrounds the brain and spinal cord. The central nervous system is suspended in this collection of fluid and its chief function is to protect the delicate nervous tissue from jarring and injury. It is possible that the cerebrospinal fluid may also be of value for the transfer of biologically important protective substances to various parts of the central nervous system. The cerebrospinal fluid is formed, both by filtration and active secretion by the choroid plexuses which lies in the lateral ventricles of the brain. It is a clear, colorless, alkaline fluid which is slightly modified blood plasma free of protein. At any one time an adult has about 135 ml of this fluid circulating, although over 500 ml is produced daily. If anything interferes with its circulation or its reabsorption, the fluid accumulates. Hydrocephalus (water on the brain) is an abnormal accumulation of cerebrospinal fluid.

cerebrum. The dorsal anterior part of the vertebrate brain consisting of two hemispheres; or the largest region of the human brain, considered to be the seat of emotions, intelligence, and other nervous activities.

ceroid pigment. Ceroid pigment, also called old-age pigment, is believed to result from the oxidation and peroxidation of polyunsaturated fats, with the formation of insoluble long-chained polymers. The ceroid pigments appear as brown spots on skin surfaces. Ceroid pigment is found also in human atheromatous aortas and coronary arteries. Under some circumstances it may interfere with the normal process of dissolving blood clots.

ceruloplasmin. A blue copper-containing enzyme. It is an alpha globulin of blood plasma. It catalyzes the oxidation of *ascorbic acid, amines* and *phenols*.

chard (*Beta vulgaris cicia*). This vegetable is a variety of beet, of which the leaves and stalk, not the root, are eaten. Chard, also called Swiss Chard, has all the attributes of the green leafy vegetables. It is an excellent source of *caro-*

*tene** (vitamin A), a very good source of iron, and a good source of *ascorbic acid** (vitamin C). Raw, 100 gm = 25 calories.

chayote (*Sechium edule*). The gourdlike fruit of a trailing vine of tropical America, which is eaten as a vegetable, chayote has a deeply ribbed, greenish-white rind and one soft seed. It is extremely bland squash and its main virtues are that it is low in starch and that it keeps its shape even when overcooked. Peeled or unpeeled, it can be boiled, fried, baked, stuffed, or combined with other foods such as meats and vegetables. 100 gm = 28 calories. See *Squash*.

cheese. See *milk products*.

chelate. A chemical compound capable of incorporating a metallic ion into its molecular structure and thus removing it as an available ion in solution. Desterrioxamine is a chelating agent developed for the treatment of *hemochromatosis* and *hemosiderosis* diseases in which excess iron is stored in body tissues. The desterrioxamine removes iron from the tissue and transports it to excretion sites.

chelation. The formation of a bond between a metal ion and two or more polar groupings of a single molecule.

chemical additives. Synthetic substances added to foods to improve their flavor, color, and texture or keeping quality. See *food additives*.

Chemical Score. The Chemical Score is a value which quantifies the quality of proteins. In this regard, the Chemical Score is similar to the *biological value* (BV), and the *net protein utilization* (NPU) value. The BV and NPU are based upon animal test systems for value determination. The Chemical Score is based upon the amino acid analysis. Specifically, the Chemical Score is a measure of the percent concentration of the *essential amino acids* in a protein relative to the percent concentration of the essential amino acids in eggs. The amino acid with the lowest percent concentration relative to its concentration in eggs is

Protein	Chemical Score	NPU	BV
Egg	100	94	100
Beef	67	80	75
Cow's milk	60	75	95
Rice	53	59	86
Corn	49	52	72
Wheat	53	48	44

taken as the Chemical Score. Because of the lower relative cost and convenience, most biological values of proteins are determined as Chemical Scores. The relative agreements between the Chemical Scores, BV, and NPU are generally good. Listed on p. 94 are comparisons of the Chemical Score, the BV and the NPU of some foods.

chemogenic disorders. Chemogenic disorders are those resulting from the effects of various chemical agents upon the brain tissue. This includes reactions resulting from poison taken into the body (such as alcohol, morphine, carbon monoxide, etc.), poisons resulting from internal physiological malfunctioning (such as endocrine disturbances), and the toxic effects of various disease processes (such as encephalitis). Severe reactions to the continued use of alcohol are usually classified among the chemogenic disorders, although it is the combined effect of the oral intake of alcohol which produces certain physiological results and unconscious needs that explain the total behavior.

chenodeoxycholic acid. Mol. Wt. 393. A bile acid derivative of cholesterol that occurs in bile as a conjugate of *glycine* or *taurine*. See *bile salts*.

Chenodeoxycholic acid

cherry (*Prunus*). The small, smooth, long stemmed, round-stoned fruit of a tree that has a birchlike bark and pink or white flowers. Cherries are divided into two groups; sweet and sour. Sweet cherries are the larger of the two, heart-shaped, and firm, yet tender. Sour cherries are rounder, softer-textured fruit. Fresh cherries, both sweet and sour, contain small amounts of vitamins and minerals. Canned and frozen cherries are similar in food value except that those processed with sugar contain more calories.

Fresh, sweet, 100 gm = 70 calories
Fresh, sour, 100 gm = 58 calories
Canned in light syrup, sweet, 100 gm = 65 calories
Canned in light syrup, sour, 100 gm = 74 calories
Maraschino, 100 gm = 116 calories

cherry liqueur. A number of well-known European liqueurs and brandies are made from special strains of cherries cultivated for the purpose. The best known ones are Kirsch, a strong colorless spirit, made in France, Switzerland, and Germany; Cherry Heering, a rich, red cordial made in Denmark; and cherry brandy made in Holland and England.

chervil (*Anthriscus cerefolium*). A delicate herb used to flavor soups, salads, and stews. Chervil is an annual, and grows to a height of 2 feet. In appearance, it resembles a delicate parsley with lacy leaves. The flowers are tiny and white. Chervil may be used fresh or dried.

chestnut (*Castanea*). The edible nut of a tree of the same name. Chestnuts are peeled (both the hard brown outer shell and the thin bitter brown inner peel), and are eaten in a variety of ways. They may be boiled or roasted. Chestnuts provide some protein, iron, and B vitamins, but their main contribution is calories. Fresh, 100 gm = 194 calories. Dried, 100 gm = 377 calories.

chicken (*Gallus gallus*). An excellent source of high-quality protein, very good to excellent for *niacin* *, and a fair source of iron. Broiler-fryers are lower in fat and calories than most other meats. The light meat of chicken has a lower fat content and is higher in niacin than the dark meat; however, it is lower in iron.

Light meat without skin, raw, 100 gm = 117 calories
Light meat without skin, cooked, roasted, 100 gm = 166 calories
Dark meat without skin, raw, 100 gm = 130 calories
Dark meat without skin, cooked, roasted, 100 gm = 176 calories

chick-pea (*Cicer arietinum*). The chick-pea, also known as garbanzo bean, Spanish bean, or ceci pea, is a branching, bushy annual, which is well adapted to arid and semiarid regions. The sparse foliage is poisonous, eliminating any use of the plants as forage. Large green pods produce one or two edible seeds, or peas, that wrinkle as they dry and are described as looking like "ram heads." Peas vary in size and color (white, red, and black) in the different varieties. Good source of protein, *iron* and *thiamine* *. Dry, 100 gm = 360 calories.

chicory (*Cichorium intybus*). A salad green which is a member of the endive family, with finely cut, feathery leaves that have dark green edges and almost white centers. Some varieties of chicory are cultivated for their roots which are roasted, then ground and added to certain coffees as stretchers. An excellent source of *carotene* * (vitamin A). Raw, 100 gm = 20 calories.

chili (*Capsicum frutescens*). A tropical American plant from whose small elongated pods or peppers we get *cayenne* (red) *pepper* and hot pepper sauce. Chili powder is a blend of dried ground chili pepper pods, which may or may not contain other powdered herbs and spices.

chitterlings. The intestines of young pigs that have been emptied, turned inside out, and scraped clean while still warm. They are then soaked for 24 hours in cold salted water, and washed at least six times before being cut up into 2-inch lengths. Chitterlings are eaten either boiled or deep fried.

chive (*Allium schoenoprasum*). A member of the onion family, it grows in clumps of slender, green, tubular leaves. Chives may be used to flavor any food in which a mild onion flavor is desired.

chloride ion (Cl⁻). The major anion of the extracellular fluid occurring for the most part in combination with sodium. Less than 15 percent of the total body chloride is located intracellularly. Chloride in blood easily transfers between the blood fluid and erythrocytes in what is commonly known as the chloride shift, a primary homeostatic mechanism for the control of blood pH. Although chloride is generally considered with sodium, with which it functions in maintenance of *extracellular fluid* pH and osmolarity, the chloride ion also functions as an activator for amylases and obviously is essential for the formation of gastric *hydrochloric acid* *

chlorine (Cl). Element No. 17. Atomic Wt. 35. A common water purifier and bleach, which is an essential nutrient that comes into the diet automatically as long as the *chloride ion* (Cl⁻) with sodium in the salt is added to foods. Chloride ions have a special function in forming the *hydrochloric acid* present in gastric juice. This acid is necessary for proper absorption of the *colalamin* * (vitamin B$_{12}$) and iron, and it supresses growth of microorganisms that enter the stomach with food and drink. Chloride ion is also involved in the acid-base economy of the body. One of the best agents for aging flour is chlorine gas, which at a level of 400 ppm, instantly ages the flour and bleaches it white. It affects the flour by causing changes in the protein fraction of flour. In addition chlorine reacts to limited extent with the small amounts of unsaturated oil that is present in white flour.

chlorine dioxide (ClO$_2$). A bleaching and maturing agent which works by releasing oxygen which causes changes in the protein fraction of flour and bleaches the yellow pigments. Fourteen parts per million of chlorine dioxide has an immediate bleaching and maturing effect and is the normal amount used to treat flour. Chlorine dioxide and other bleaching agents reduce the *tocopherol* * (vitamin E) content of flour.

chlorpropamide. A hypoglycemic agent. Reported to lower the blood sugar level and to reduce *glycosuria* in certain diabetics. The drug acts by stimulating the release of *insulin* from the pancreas. The insulin appears to increase its main effect on the liver by promoting a decrease in the output of glucose from the liver into the bloodstream.

$$CH_3CH_2CH_2—NH\overset{\overset{\displaystyle O}{\|}}{C}—NH—\overset{\overset{\displaystyle O}{\|}}{\underset{\underset{\displaystyle O}{\|}}{S}}—\!\!\!\left\langle\bigcirc\right\rangle\!\!\!—Cl$$

Chlorpropamide

chocolate. Chocolate and *cocoa,* are made from the beans of the *cacao* tree, a perennial evergreen tree of the cola family. Chocolate is a mixture of roasted cocoa, cocoa butter (also obtained from the cacao bean), and very fine sugar. The word comes from the Mexican Indian choco, "foam," and atl, "water." Chocolate, apart from its palatability, has a considerable stimulating effect on the heart and the general musculature of the body. Chocolate contains an appreciable amount of fat and carbohydrates. It is a good source of quick energy.

> Unsweetened, 100 gm = 505 calories
> Semisweet, 100 gm = 507 calories
> Sweet, 100 gm = 528 calories
> Milk chocolate, 100 gm = 520 calories

chokecherry (*Prunus virginiana* and *Prunus demissa*). A small, wild cherry grows on a large shrub, and is a native of North America. The flowers are white, and the fruit turns from red to black as it matures. Chokecherries have a puckery taste, and they are best used for jams and jellies. See *cherry.*

cholecalciferol (vitamin D_3). The first crystalline *vitamin D* * was obtained in 1931 and was synthesized shortly thereafter. Soon it became evident that there are at least 10 natural substances which exert vitamin D-like activity in varying degrees, but only 2 of these are of practical importance from the standpoint of their occurrence in foods; ergocalciferol (vitamin D_2) which is found in yeast, and cholecalciferol (vitamin D_3). See *vitamin D.*

cholecystitis. An inflammation of the gallbladder, usually resulting from a low-grade chronic infection. The infectious process produces changes in the gallbladder mucosa which affect its absorptive powers. Normally, the cholesterol which is insoluble in water, is kept in solution by action of the *bile salts* * and especially the *bile acids* *. However, when mucosa changes occur in cholecystitis, the absorptive powers of the gallbladder may be altered, affecting the solubility ratios of the bile ingredients. Excess water may be absorbed, or excess bile acids may be absorbed.

cholecystokinin. A hormone produced in the wall of the duodenum in the presence of fat, which stimulates the contraction of the gallbladder, with the emission of *bile*. Bile is necessary to emulsify fat before digestion.

cholesterol. Mol. Wt. 387. A fatlike pearly substance which crystalizes in the form of circular crystals. When stored in the intima (lining) of the arteries it begins to irritate, and over a period of time sets up an inflammatory reaction which may damage the arterial lining and lead to narrowing of the artery due to atheroma (see *arteriosclerosis*). Found in all animal fats and oils, brain, whole milk, yolk of eggs, liver, kidneys, adrenal glands, and pancreas. When taken with food it combines with bile salts to get through bowel membrane and then combines with protein to form a lipoprotein with the cell. From the cell it circulates through the blood, and through the entire body. Derivatives of cholesterol (dehydrocholesterol) form *vitamin D* and the steroid hormones.

Listed below is the cholesterol content of some common foods.

Cholesterol

Food	Mg Cholesterol Per 100 gm of Food
Butter	110
Cheese, cheddar	100
Chicken	60
Egg	550
Liver	300
Lobster, Oyster	200
Margarine (All vegetable fat)	0
Meat, Fish	70
Sweetbreads	250
Whole milk	10

cholic acid. See *bile salts*.

choline. Mol. St. 121. A trimethyl amino ethanol which occurs in biological tissues in the free form and as a component of lecithin, acetylcholine, and certain of the phospholipids, *plasmalogens,* and *sphingomyelins*. Choline is important as a source of labile methyl groups. A choline deficiency has never been demonstrated in man, and it is not known if a dietary supply is required in addition to that formed by biosynthesis. Choline has many important functions in the body, as a constituent of several phospholipids (primarily *lecithin*). As a constituent of acetylcholine, choline plays a role in normal functioning of nerves. It is estimated that an average mixed diet for adults in the United States contains 500 to 900 mg per day of choline, or about 0.1 to 0.18 percent of the diet. Choline is present in all foods in which phospholipids occur liberally, as in egg yolk, whole grains, *legumes,* meats of all types, and wheat germ. Fresh egg yolk contains about 1.5 percent choline, beef liver 0.6 percent, legumes such as soybeans, peas, and beans, contain from 0.2 to 0.35 percent; vegetables and milk have moderate choline activity.

$$CH_3-\overset{\overset{\displaystyle CH_3}{|}}{\underset{\underset{\displaystyle CH_3}{|}}{N^+}}-CH_2-CH_2OH$$

Choline

chondroitin and chondroitin sulfates. Polysaccharides containing D-*glucuronic acid* * and acetyl *glactosamine* *. Their general structure is similar, but they differ in the content and location of sulfate ester groups in the molecule. Chondroitin contains only a small number of sulfate ester groups. Chondroitin sulfates have a high viscosity and a capability for binding water, and in connective tissue apparently play a role similar to that of *hyaluronic acid* *. In addition, these compounds are distinguished by the ion-binding capacity of the sulfate groups. Chondroitin is a component of the cell coat, and chondroitin 4-sulfate is the principal organic component of the ground substance of cartilage and bone.

chorionic gonadotropin. A biological test on blood or urine; for the diagnosis of pregnancy. Human chorionic gonadotropin (HCG) has been used to control appetite, but scientific evidence of its effectiveness is negative.

chromatin. A complex structure that contains in addition to *deoxyribonucleic acid** (DNA), large amounts of histone and nonhistone proteins and small amounts of *ribonucleic acid** (RNA). It is packaged as distinct bodies called chromosomes in the nucleus. The total chromosomal DNA of any cell is its genome.

chromium (Cr). Element No. 24. Atomic Wt. 52. Chromium activates insulin action. Insulin plays a vital role in carbohydrate or glucose utilization during a state of well-being and even more in diabetes, in which there is a disarrangement of carbohydrate or glucose metabolism. Chromium has a variety of functions including the stimulation of the synthesis of fatty acids and cholesterol in the liver; an involvement in insulin metabolism; and a role as a part of several other enzymes including one of the protein-digesting enzymes in the intestine. The human body contains only a small amount of chromium, less than 6 mg, with a decline in age. A typical daily intake ranges between 50 and 130 mg. Only a small amount of that ingested is absorbed (1 to 5 percent). The biologically active form is quite nontoxic and is rapidly excreted. Good food sources of chromium are fats such as corn oils and meats, black pepper, thymes, brewer's yeast, mushrooms, beef liver, and bread. Refined sugar increases chromium excretion.

chromosomes. Filamentous or rod-shaped bodies in the cell nucleus which contains the hereditary units, the genes.

chronic. Of long duration; denoting a disease or condition of long duration. The opposite of acute.

chyle. The milk like contents of the lacteals and lymphatic vessels of the intestine. It consists principally of absorbed fats. Chyle is carried from the intestine by the lymphatic vessels to the cisterna chyli. The cisterna chyli (the cistern or receptacle of the chyle) is a dilated sac at the origin of the lymphatic vessels. The cisterna chyli lies in the abdomen between the second lumbar vertebra and the aorta. It receives the lymph from the intestinal trunk, the right and left lumbar lymphatic trunk, and two descending lymphatic trunks. The chyle after passing through the cisterna cyli, is carried upward to the chest through the thoracic duct and empties into the venous blood at the point where the subclavian vein joins the left internal jugular vein.

chylomicron. Particles of emulsified lipoproteins containing primarily triglycerides from dietary fat and very little protein. Very small (micro-) globules of fat in varying sizes are transported after digestion and absorption. *Chyle is a* product of digestion of fats absorbed into the lymphatic circulation and from there into the thoracic duct. See *lipids*.

chyme. The thick, grayish, semiliquid mass into which food is converted by gastric (stomach) digestion. In this form it passes into the small intestine.

chymotrypsin. One of the proteolytic enzymes of the *pancreatic juice*. A digestive enzyme, occurs initially in an inactive *zyomgen* state called chymotrypsinogen. Chymotrypsin continues the hydralytic action begun by pepsin, and together they break molecules into smaller and smaller peptide fragments. It hydrolyses proteins at the amino acids *phenylalanine* * and *tyrosine* * linkages.

chytothorax. Effusion of chyle (fat) from the thoracic duct into the thoracic cavity.

cider. Cider is the juice of apples that have been ground to a pulp and pressed to extract their juice. Cider may be "sweet" or "hard," that is, nonfermented or fermented. Sweet, bottled, 100 gm = 47 calories.

cider vinegar. a mild, yellow-brown vinegar, made from hard (fermented) cider. Vinegar results from the oxidation of *ethanol* * to *acetic acid* *.

cinnamon (*Cinnamomum*). A reddish-brown spice which comes from the dried bark of the shrublike evergreen trees which belong to the laurel group. It is one of the very few spices not obtained from the seeds, flowers, or fruits of a plant. The kinds of cinnamon most commonly used are cassia and Ceylon cinnamon. Cinnamon is sold both ground and whole in sticks.

cirrhosis (digestive diseases). Means scarring of the liver that interferes with its normal function and with blood flow through the liver. The most common cause of the scarring is repeated injury to the liver from drinking large amounts of alcoholic beverages; but other known causes include poor nutrition, hepatitis, rare metabolic disease, in which large amounts of iron or copper are deposited in the liver, and possibly, the long continued effects of irritating or toxic drugs. The treatment for cirrhosis involves first, the complete abstinence from alcohol and other agents known to damage the liver. Additional important measures include eating a well-balanced, nutritious diet and getting plenty of rest.

***cis-* and *trans-*isomerism.** Any fatty acid which contains a double carbon bond (ethylene linkage) can exist in either of two geometrically isomeric forms. For example, the trans-isomers of the natural *unsaturated fatty acid, oleice acid* is elaidic acid. They are structurally related as follows:

$$CH_3(CH_2)_7 \diagdown \diagup H$$
$$C$$
$$\|$$
$$C$$
$$HOOC(CH_2)_7 \diagup \diagdown H$$

Oleic acid
(*Cis*-form)

$$CH_3(CH_2)_7 \diagdown \diagup H$$
$$C$$
$$\|$$
$$C$$
$$H \diagup \diagdown (CH_2)_7 COOH$$

Elaidic acid
(*Trans*-form)

Oleic acid is an oily substance, elaidic is a solid. This is known as *cis* and *trans* isomerism. When two carbon atoms are held together by the double bond, there is no freedom of rotation for these groups about the axis of the bond. The natural unsaturated fatty acids exist in the *cis*-form, with their molecules bent back at each double bond. *Trans*-isomers of polyunsaturated acids do not have essential fatty acid activity and lack the ability possessed by *cis*-isomers of lowering the level of lipoproteins in plasma.

cistron. The genetic unit of biochemical function; the sequence of nucleotide pairs in *deoxyribonucleic acid* * (DNA) that specify the amino acid sequence of a single peptide chain.

citric acid. Mol. Wt. 192. An important intermediate in the citric acid or tricarboxylic acid or *Kreb's cycle* *, the pathway by which foodstuffs are oxidized. Citric acid is a metabolic product of living systems. Most citric acid is produced by fermentation. *Aspergillus niger* is the principal mold used in citric acid production. Most citric acid is made from molasses, with beet molasses preferred over cane. In the food industry, citric acid is added to flavoring extracts, soft drinks, and candies. It has been added to fish to adjust the pH to about 5.9 to aid in its preservation. A large portion of citric acid produced is used for medicinal purposes. Citric acid is an important food additive because it is a strong acid, inexpensive, has a tart flavor, and serves as an antioxidant. The food industry uses it on ice cream, sherbet, fruit juice drinks, carbonated beverages, jellies, preserves, canned fruits, and vegetables, cheeses, candies, and chewing gum. In soft-centered candy, citric acid has the added function of solubilizing the sugar. Manufacturers use citric acid as an antioxidant in instant

$$H_2C-COOH$$
$$|$$
$$HO-C-COOH$$
$$|$$
$$H_2C-COOH$$

Citric acid

potatoes, wheat chips and potato sticks. Citric acid prevents spoilage by trapping (chelating) metal ions which might otherwise promote reactions that spoil or discolor the food. Humans produce their own citric acid as in the citric acid cycle (*Kreb's cycle* *).

citric acid cycle. The common final oxidative pathway for the intermediate compounds of carbohydrate, fat, and protein catabolism. It is also known as the tricarboxylic acid cycle or the *Kreb's cycle. Citric acid* is an intermediate in the cycle. See *Kreb's cycle.*

citron (*Citrus media*). The oldest of the citrus fruits; it grows on a small thorny tree whose flowers are purple and white. The citron resembles a lemon, and grows to a length of 6 to 9 inches. It has a greenish-yellow, tough and warty, fragrant peel, and a scanty, acid pulp. The fruit is grown for its peel, which is used in baking, and it is a most important ingredient of fruitcakes. The peel is first treated with brine, to remove the bitter oil, to bring out the flavor, and to prevent spoilage. Then it is candied in sugar and glucose. Caloric value: 100 gm = 314 calories.

citrovorum factor (CF). A biologically active form of *folacin* *. This bacterial vitamin factor was first described in 1948 as required for the growth of *Leuconostoc citrovorum,* a microorganism used in the dairy industry. It was isolated in the pure state from horse liver in 1952 and the chemical structure has been determined.

citrulline. Mol. Wt. 175. One of two naturally occurring L-amino acids that do not occur in proteins, *ornithine* * being the other. Both of these amino acids are a part of the urea cycle which leads to urea formation. See *urea cycle.*

$$\underset{\text{Citrulline}}{H_2N-\overset{\overset{\displaystyle O}{\|}}{C}-CH_2CH_2CH_2\overset{\overset{\displaystyle NH_2}{|}}{CH}-COOH}$$

clarifying agents. Clarifying agents remove all particles of mineral elements such as iron and copper from liquids. Vinegar for example, may turn "cloudy" unless a clarifying agent is added to settle out traces of minerals.

clone. A group of cells or organisms derived asexually from a single ancestor and hence genetically identical.

clove. (*Eugenia aromatica*) The dried, unopened flower bud of the evergreen clove tree, which belongs to the myrtle family. The name originated from the fact that the flower buds resembled small nails, and in French, the word for nail is clou, in Latin, clavus. Cloves are sold whole or ground, and are one of the most useful spices. They are used in gingerbreads, spicecakes, fruitcakes, chili sauce, and pickles. They are good to flavor cooked beets and meat loaves.

coacervates. Minute droplets of organic material suspended in water.

coagulated proteins or derived proteins. Insoluble products which result from (1) the action of heat on protein solutions, or (2) the action of alcohol in the protein. Examples are cooked egg albumin, or egg albumin precipitated by means of alcohol.

coagulation. The change from a fluid state to thickened jelly, curd, or clot.

coagulation time test. A blood-clotting test used for diagnosis of individuals having a tendency to hemorrhage, and also as a guide to treatment in those receiving anticoagulant drugs.

coal tar dyes. Coal, when heated in the absence of air, is converted to coke, coal gas, and coal tar. The coal tar, a viscous black liquid, is a mixture of many organic compounds. The synthetic substances made by chemists from coal tar are known as coal tar dyes, and are used widely by the food, fabric, and cosmetic industries. Over 95 percent of these dyes are used in foods, particularly beverages, candy, ice cream, dessert powder, baked goods and sausages. Levels used range from approximate 10 parts to 500 parts per million, the lower levels being used in liquid foods, (beverages, gelatin desserts), the higher levels in solid foods (pet food, breakfast cereals). Coal tar dyes frequently provide the only color in factory-made foods. The presence of coloring in food generally indicates an absence of natural and often nutritous ingredients whose colors the synthetic dye seeks to imitate.

cobalamin (extrinsic factor, vitamin B₁₂). Mol. Wt. 1355. Cobalamin is a generic name for the various forms of vitamin B_{12}. Cyanocobalamin is one of the most active forms.
Cobalamin has two forms that function as coenzymes in two separate set of reactions. In one set of reactions, cyancobalamin reacts with a *folacin* derivative, N^5 methyl (CH_3) tetrahydrofolic acid to yield a CH_3-vitamin B_{12} derivative and free tetrahydrofolic acid. The CH_3-vitamin B_{12} can then react with homocysteine to form the *essential amino acid* methionine. This last reaction is important in the symptoms of vitamin B_{12} deficiency, *pernicious anemia*. In another set of reactions, an adenosine derivative of cobalamin called coenzyme B_{12} serves in a reaction which converts methyl malonyl-coenzyme A, a fatty acid synthesis intermediate, into succinyl-coenzyme A, an intermedi-

Vitamin B$_{12}$ (cyanocobalamin).   Coenzyme B$_{12}$

ate of the Kreb's cycle. Coenzyme B$_{12}$ is also required for the synthesis of the nucleic acids. A lack of cobalamin (vitamin B$_{12}$) results in a nutritional disease called pernicious anemia, a rare disease that results from the failure of the intestinal mucosa to produce a mucoprotein required for cobalamin absorption. The mucoprotein was called intrinsic factor. The same symptoms of pernicious anemia became evident on a cobalamin free diet. Hence, cobalamin was called the extrinsic factor in the disease. It was found that one of the symptoms, the macrocytic anemia, could be alleviated by high doses of *folacin* * even in the absence of cobalamin, but the neurological and other symptoms remained. It became clear that red blood cell synthesis requires methyl (—CH$_3$) free folacin, and canocobalamin is required to remove the CH$_3$ group. The reactions involving these two vitamins then are closely interwoven. A deficiency of cobalamin then results in a deficiency in another vitamin, the folacin derivative tetrahydrofolic acid.

Cobalamin occurs only in animal food sources. Therefore, strict vegetarianism for a long term (years) may result in an *avitaminosis,* and in the case of a pregnant female, an avitaminosis in the infant. Recovery is rapid and the levels of cobalamin required for good health are in the few micrograms (μg) range. Cobalamin is stable to heat but is inactivated by *acids* or *alkalies*. Good sources of cobalamin are any animal tissues and foods derived from milk. See *water soluble vitamin* chart and *pernicious anemia*. Daily needs are met by the average diet supplying 3–5 μg, vitamin B_{12}; major sources are liver, kidney, and muscle meats.

Vitamin B_{12} Food Sources	Micrograms per 100 gm Edible Portion
Beans, green	0–0.2
Beef, kidney	18–55
Beef, liver	31–120
Beef, round	3.4–4.5
Beets	0–0.1
Bread	0–0.3
Bread, whole wheat	0.2–0.4
Carrots	0–0.1
Cheese, American	0.6
Cheese, cream	0.2
Cheese, Swiss	0.9
Corn, yellow	0–0
Egg, whole	0.3
Haddock	0.6
Ham	0.9–1.6
Milk, evaporated	0.1–0.3
Milk, powder, skim	2.5–4.0
Milk, powder, whole	1–2.6
Milk, whole	0.3–0.5
Oats	0.3
Peas	0–0.1
Scallops	0.7
Sole, fresh, filet	1.3
Soybean meal	0.2
Wheat	0.1

cobalt (Co). Element No. 27. Atom. Wt. 59. Cobalt stimulates the production of red blood cells in many aimals. A most important function of cobalt is as a metallic component in several enzyme systems which convert enzymes into forms probably necessary in cell metabolism. Cobalt, obtained by man through animal materials in his diet is found in liver, kidneys, and bones. A diet containing a moderate amount of meat probably supplies the small amount needed. There is no evidence that humans must ever be concerned about their intake of inorganic cobalt. Cobalt is an important part of *cobalamin* * (vitamin B_{12}).

cobamide. Refers to *cobalamin* * (vitamin B_{12}) containing coenzymes.

cocarboxylase. Another name for the coenzyme derivative of thiamin, thiamin pyrophosphate. See *thiamine* *

cocci (bacteria). Cocci are characterized by formation of pus (pyogenic bacteria). Primary members of this group are staphylococci, streptococci, and diplococci.

cochlea. Part of the inner ear; a spirally coiled tube of two-and-a-half turns, resmbling a snail's shell.

cocoa. The word comes from the Mexican Indian cacahuatl and describes a beverage and dessert flavoring made from the beans of the cacao tree which grows only in tropical climates. The cacao or coca bean is the source of *chocolate*. Cocoa differs from chocolate in fat and sugar content. After the beans are cleaned, dried, roasted, and ground, some of the fat, or cocoa butter is removed. It is then ground again to form the powder known as cocoa. In Dutch process cocoa, cocoa is treated with an alkali which gives it a darker color and a richer flavor. Instant cocoa is a mixture of cocoa, sugar, flavoring, and an emulsifier, to be added to hot or cold water or milk for use as a beverage.

cocoa beans. See *cacao* and *cocoa*.

cocoa butter. The fat removed from caco beans during their conversion into chocolate and cocoa. It is used primarily in making candy and pharmaceutical products. Cocoa butter is whitish-yellow and smells of cocoa.

coconut. The fruit of a palm (*Cocus nucifera*), native to Malaya, which has been transplanted to all parts of the tropical and subtropical world. The fruit is 12 to 18 inches in length and 6 to 8 inches in diameter. It takes about a year to mature. The outer covering is smooth, the husk fibrous, and a woody brown shell encases a layer of firm white meat with a milky fluid at its center. Caloric value: Fresh, 100 gm = 346 calories; varied, shredded, 100 gm = 548 calories.

cod (*Gradus morrhua*). A soft-finned saltwater fish averaging from 3 to 4 feet in length and 7 to 10 pounds in weight. The cod is brownish on the upper body and sides and creamy below, with small brown and yellow spots. The roe sometimes constitutes a full half of the weight of the female fish. The flesh is firm and white. Cod is a lean fish, a good source of protein, some iron, calcium, and B vitamins. Fresh, raw, 100 gm = 78 calories; dried, salted, 100 gm = 130 calories.

cod liver oil. Intended for use for medicinal purposes, derived from the fresh liver of the cod. Cod liver oil is the most important of the fish liver oils. The better qualities are valued for their content of *retinol* * (vitamin A), and *vitamin D* *, and are used as medicinal oils and for animal feeding. The lower grades (cod oils) are used in the leather industry. See *vitamin D*.

coenocytic. Having more than one nucleus in a single mass of cytoplasm.

coenzyme. A nonprotein organic substance that works with or is bound to the protein part of an *enzyme*, which part is called an apoenzyme. The complete enzyme is called a holoenzyme. Many enzymes do not work unless the coenzyme is attached. Coenzymes are often necessary for the enzyme to function as a biological catalyst. Most of the vitamins, the water-soluble vitamins, in particular, function as coenzymes in some chemically modified form. For example, *thiamine* * functions as a coenzyme thiamin pyrophosphate; *niacin* * functions as the coenzyme *nicotinamide adenine dinucleotide* * (NAD); *riboflavin* * functions as the coenzyme *flavin adenine dinucleoitde* *; and *pyridoxine* * (vitamin B$_6$) functions as the coenzyme *pyridoxal* or pyridoxamine phosphate.

coenzyme A (CoA). A complex nucleotide containing *panthothenic acid.* Coenzyme A combines with acetyl groups to yield active acetate, acetyl coenzyme A, which can enter the *Krebs cycle* * for oxidation or serve as an intermediate in fatty acid synthesis and cholesterol synthesis. Coenzyme A is a central biochemical intermediate in many *anabolic* and *catabolic* reactions. Acid derivatives with CoA, such as acetyl—CoA or amino acid—CoA or Acyl—CoA are high-energy compounds and are capable of doing synthetic work. In order to form these CoA derivatives, energy must be put into the reaction. That source of chemical energy is usually *adenosine triphosphate* (ATP) or a nucleoside triphosphate equivalent. The pantotheine portion, shown in the structure below is also the active portion of the complex enzyme *fatty acid synthase.*

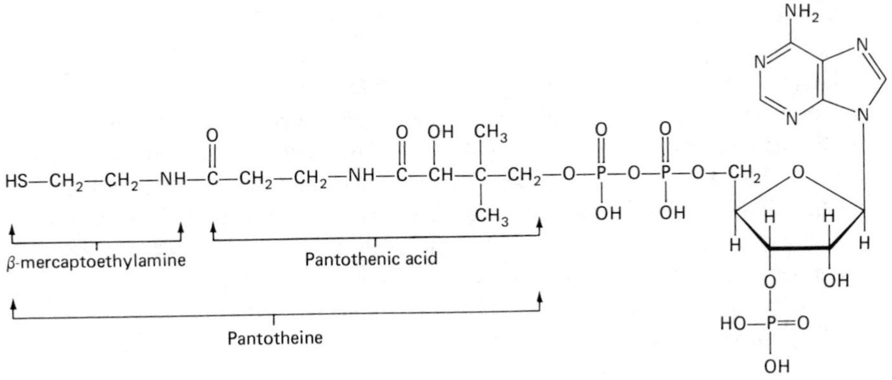

Coenzyme A (CoA)

coenzyme B$_{12}$. See *cobalamin* *

cofactor. A substance required for enzyme activity, such as a coenzyme.

coffee (*Coffea*). A beverage brewed from roasted and ground coffee beans. The beans themselves, whole or ground, are also known as coffee. The two chief methods of curing coffee are: (1) The dry method, in which the berries or "cherries" are spread out and air-dried in the sun or artificially; and (2) The wet, or "washed coffee" method in which the berries, after removal of the outer skin, are soaked in water. The removal of pulpy material is accomplished primarily by pectinolytic bacteria, mostly coliforms, although pectinolytic bacilli and fungi may be present. This is followed by an acid fermentation by lactic acid bacteria such as *Leuconostoc mesenteroides, Lactobacillus brevis and plantarum,* and *Streptococcos faecalis.* The acids produced may be degraded by oxidizing organisms. After the pulp and its residues have been washed away, the beans are dried and hulled.

cola or **kola**. The word covers a tree, a nut, and a complex syrup used for making a carbonated beverage. The cola tree (*Cola nitida*) produces fruit containing numerous seeds. These brownish bitter seeds are the cola nuts from which the cola extract is obtained. Containing a small amount of caffeine, the cola nut is a mild stimulant. In the United States the extract of the cola nut is widely used in the drug and beverage industries.

colchicine. An alkaloid drug used in the treatment of gout. It interferes in the metabolic pathway of *uric acid* *.

colectomy. The removal of the diseased portion of the *colon*.

colitis. Inflammation of the colon.

collagen. A protein, the main organic constitutent of connective tissue and of the organic substance of bones. Collagen in the native state is insoluble in water and changes into gelatin by boiling. *Proline* * and *glycine* * are the major amino acids of collagen. A protein that forms the chief constituent of the connective tissue, tendon, bone, and skin. *Ascorbic acid* * (vitamin C) is required for a reaction that adds a hydroxyl group onto proline and lysine residues in procollagen to yield the hydroxyproline and γ-hydroxylysine residues required for normal collagen. The synthesis or normal collagen is vital for proper wound healing. In ascorbic acid deficiency wound healing is greatly diminished. See *ascorbic acid* * and *scurvy*.

collard (*Brassica olercea*). Collards are a member of the cabbage family and most closely related to kale. Their leaves are smooth, tall, and broad, but they do not form a head as cabbage does. The usual method of cooking them is to boil them with a piece of bacon or salt pork. The resulting juice is known as "pot likker" and is eaten with corn bread. Collards can also be cooked like spinach, chard, cabbage, or kale. Excellent source of *carotene* * (vitamin A), *iron, calcium,* and *ascorbic acid* * (vitamin C); fair source of *thiamine* *, *riboflavin* *, and *niacin* *. Raw, 100 gm = 45 calories

colloid. (1) A two-phase system in which particles of one phase ranging in size from 1 to 100 millimicrons are dispersed in the second phase. Dispersion of particles less than 11 μm is usually considered a solution and above 100 μm it is a suspension. (2) A gelatinous material secreted by cuboidal epithelial cells, arranged in hollow spheres one cell thick, as in the thyroid. Proteins dissolved in water are examples of colloidal solutions.

colon. The large intestine. The colon extends from the ileocecal sphincter in the right iliac fossa, around the outer portion of the abdominal cavity to end at the anus. When food enters or leaves the stomach there is a reflex discharge of intestinal contents from the lower *ileum* into the colon through the ileocecal sphincter. This is called the gastrocolic reflex. There is also a passive filling of the colon from the ileum about 4 or 5 hours after the ingestion of food. Normally about 350 gm of fecal matter pass into the colon daily. Water is absorbed by the colon and the feces become formed or semisolid in the next 36 hours.

color additives. Food colors can be synthetic or natural origin but more than 90 percent of the colors now in use are synthetic. Sometimes these are called coal-tar colors because originally they were made from chemicals obtained from coal tars. Synthetic colors are often used in soft drinks, candy, or confectionary products, frozen desserts, gelatin desserts and puddings, maraschino cherries, meat casings, prepared mixes, and some dairy and bakery products. There are actually thousands of synthetic coloring agents. Some colors added to foods are substances found in carrots and are a source of *carotene* * (vitamin A), often used to color dairy products as well as margarine.

colostrum. Milk secreted during the first week of lacation.

combustion. The combination of substances with oxygen accompanied by the liberation of energy.

complete protein. A protein that contains the essential amino acids in quantities sufficient for maintenance of the body and for a normal rate of growth.

Such proteins are said to have a high biological value (BV). Egg, milk, cheese, and meat are complete protein foods. See *biological value.*

condensed milk. See *milk.*

congenital. Existing at or before birth with reference to certain physical or mental traits.

conjugated proteins. Proteins with some nonprotein substance attached to their structure. Protein molecules may be conjugated with fat such as the lipoproteins in the blood, or carbohydrates, such as the glycoproteins, which are found in the mucus secreted into the *digestive* system. Other important conjugated proteins are formed by linkage with phosphoric acid (phosphorproteins); with the lipid *lecithin* * (*fibrin* in clotted blood, vitellin in egg yolk); with an iron-containing compound (*heme*) to form the oxygen-carrying substance hemoglobin in the blood.

conjugation. Process of genetic recombination between two organisms (e.g., bacteria, algae) through a cytoplasmic bridge between them.

conjunctivitis. An inflammation of the conjunctiva, the membrane lining the inner eyelid and whites of the eyes. Its characteristics are redness, discharge, discomfort (itching and/or burning), and sensitivity to light. The conjunctiva can be inflammed as a result of exposure to chemicals, bacteria, viruses or allergens, and is a common feature of *retinol* * (vitamin A) deficiency. The well-known pinkeye is an example of conjunctivitis caused by bacteria. Viruses are common causes of conjunctivitis. The watery slightly reddened eyes seen in many colds result from an attack on the conjunctiva by the cold viruses. Conjuctivitis associated with retinol (vitamin A) deficiency is marked by dryness. One virus, *herpes simplex,* is notoriously dangerous when it affects the cornea of the eye.

contact dermatitis (allergic eczema). An inflammation of the skin resulting from exposure to, or contact with some substance in a person's environment. The substance may be animal, mineral, or vegetable in origin and must be a substance to which the person has developed a sensitivity.

contracture. A condition in which there is fixed resistance to the stretching of a muscle. It results from fibrosis of the tissues surrounding a joint or from disorders of the muscle fibers.

Coomb's test. An antibody test on blood; used in selecting blood suitable for transfusion, and in the diagnosis of certain anemias.

copper (Cu). Element No. 29. Atomic Wt. 64. The human body contains 1.5–2.5 mg per Cu/kg fat-free body weight. The mineral is distributed in all body tissues, but liver, brain, heart, and kidney contain the highest amounts. In blood, copper appears to be about equally divided between plasma and erythrocytes; plasma contains about 110 μg/100 ml. Symptoms of copper deficiency include anemia, hypopigmentation, and changes in the texture of hair, abnormalities in bone structure, failure of myelination, and central nervous system defects. Copper occurs along with other mineral elements in the most natural foods. The richest sources are organ meats, crustaceans, shellfish, nuts, dried legumes, and cocoa. Human milk contains an adequate amount. Only 30 percent of the copper consumed is absorbed. This occurs in the stomach and upper intestine in an acid medium. From the intestine copper moves into the bloodstream. About 93 percent of the serum copper is bound tightly to *ceruloplasmin* and is released from it only when this protein is catabolized. Ceruloplasmin is considered the molecular link in copper and iron metabolism and has been shown to be directly involved in hemoglobin biosynthesis. About 7 percent of the serum copper is loosely bound to albumin and amino acids, and is transported to the various body tissues in these forms. The liver is the main organ for copper storage. The liver also synthesizes ceruloplasmin and prepares the mineral for biliary excretion.

copper, dietary sources. (Micrograms per 100-gm edible portion)

Almonds	1210	Halibut	230
Apples	120	Kale	328
Asparagus	141	Liver, beef	2450
Avocado	690	Lobster	730
Bananas	200	Mackerel	230
Beans, dry	960	Mushrooms	1790
Beans, lima, dry	915	Oats	738
Beef, round	80	Oranges	80
Bread, white	205	Oysters	3623
Cabbage	50	Peas, dried	802
Carrots	80	Pecans	1360
Cheese, American	180	Pork chops	310
Chicken, dark meat	410	Prunes, dried	291
Chicken, white meat	270	Rye, whole	656
Chocolate, bitter	2670	Shrimp	430
Cocoa	3340	Spinach	197
Corn	449	Sweet potatoes	184
Eggs	253	Turkey, dark meat	200
Flour, whole wheat	435	Turkey, white meat	150
Flour, white	170	Walnuts	1000
		Wheat	787

corn or **maize (Zea mays).** One of the *cereal grains*. It originated in the Americas and is now grown worldwide. It is a hardy crop, more resistant to drought and predation by birds than most cereal grains. The nutrient value is similar to the other cereal grains and information is under cereal grains. Corn has more *retinol* * (vitamin A) activity than most of the cereals and while it appears to contain adequate amounts of *niacin* * it appears to be in a bound form and unavailable for absorption. Consequently, in those poor societies or economic groups that depend on corn as a major source of food, the nutritional disease due to a niacin deficiency, pellagra, is widespread, as it was among the poor in the southern United States several decades ago. Interestingly enough, pellagra was once thought to be a heritable disease associated with other "traits" of the poor, such as laziness and slowness of wit. The Mexican Indians who are poor, and who depend on corn as a major source of food never develop pellagra. It is believed that their customary treatment of corn flour with slaked-lime (an alkali) in the preparation of tortillas, releases the bound niacin in corn and the tryptophan, which has some niacin activity, and so niacin deficiencies never develop.

Fresh, 1 small ear = 85 calories
Canned, whole kernel, 100 gm = 66 calories
Canned, cream-style, 100 gm = 82 calories
Frozen, kernels on the cob, cooked and drained, 100 gm = 94 calories
Frozen, kernels cut from cob, cooked and drained, 100 gm = 70 calories

cornmeal. Corn, coarsely ground. In "new process" cornmeal, the corn is ground after the hull and germ of the kernel is removed. In "old process" cornmeal, the whole grain is ground into meal. Although old process cornmeal is richer in *carotene* * (vitamin A activity), new process cornmeal keeps better because it has a lower fat content. Enriched, cooked, 100 gm = 46 to 50 calories.

corn oil. The fruits *corn* (kernels), a large number of which are united with a fleshy stalk to form the "cob", are commercially divided into (1) bran (testa + pericarp) (2) hominy (endosperm), (3) germ (scufellum). Oil is obtained only from the germ which is commercially separated from the endosperm by various processes (steaming, rolling, and sifting) before pressing. It is also obtained as a by-product in starch making. Corn oil is a golden yellow liquid, giving a small deposite of "stearine" in cold weather, and a very strong tenacious test and smell, characteristic of the original fruit. The theory that the *polyunsaturated fatty acids* contained in vegetable oils are "essential" to human metabolism and that they tend to combat the onset of thrombosis has made vegetable and seed oils' high content of polyunsaturated acids highly recommended as substitutes for butter and for use in the diet generally. In the same class are safflower and sunflower oils. They are also used for salad purposes and in margarine.

cornstarch. A starch obtained from the *endosperm* portion of the kernel. It is used as a thickener in sauces, gravies, and puddings. It is also the basis of laundry starch.

corn syrup. A sweet, thick solution made by digesting cornstarch with acids or enzymes. It contains *dextrose* (glucose*), *maltose*, and *dextrin*. Food manufacturers use corn syrup to sweeten and thicken foods and beverages. In some foods, such as candy, icings, and fillings, it retards crystallization of sugar, and prevents the loss of moisture from cakes, cookies, and whipped foods. There are two kinds, light and dark. Light corn syrup has been clarified and decolorized. Dark syrup has a stronger flavor.

coronary arteries. The heart gets its blood supply from the right and left coronary arteries. These arteries branch off from the aorta just above the heart, then subdivide into many smaller branches within the heart muscle. If any part of the heart muscle is deprived of its blood supply through interruption of blood flow through the coronary arteries and their branches, the muscle tissue deprived of blood cannot function and will die. This is called myocardial infarction. Blood from the heart tissue is returned by coronary veins to the right atrium.

coronary heart disease. Although the heart muscle itself may be normal, the circulation to it is reduced or cut off by narrowing or blocking of branches of the coronary arteries. There is a constant changing pattern of the circulation in the complex branching distribution of the coronary arteries, some of which become thickened and blocked with clots or fatty deposits, which narrow the caliber. In some a clot in the artery may become partially dissolved and nature then attempts to open up new channels to replace those which have degenerated. The following factors are known to increase the risk of coronary heart disease, but are not necessarily "abnormalities" per se and are not readily amenable to preventive intervention: (1) Maleness, (2) Increasing age, (3) A family history of premature vascular disease, (4) Endomorphic body build, (5) Certain behavior patterns and personality traits. The following factors are known to increase the risk of coronary heart disease: (1) *Hyperlipemias*, (2) *Hypertension*, (3) *Diabetes mellitus*, (4) *Obesity*, (5) *Hyperuricemia* and *gout*. (6) Certain electrocardiographic abnormalities. The following factors, which are primarily due to culture and environment, are known to increase the risk of coronary heart disease: (1) Cigarette smoking, (2) Dietary habits (high intake of saturated fats, etc.), (3) Lack of physical exercise, (4) Occupational hazards.

coronary occlusion. Obstruction or narrowing of one of the coronary arteries which hinders blood flow to some part of the heart muscle.

cortex. Outer layer of an organ, e.g., adrenal cortex and cerebral cortex. In plants, it is the tissue beneath the epidermis.

corticorophin. A hormone of the anterior *pituitary gland* that specifically stimulates the adrenal cortex.

cortisol (hydrocortisone) and cortisone. Cortisol and cortisone belong to a class of steroid hormones synthesized in the cortex of the adrenal glands, known as glucocorticoids. They have a primary effect on carbohydrate, protein, and lipid metabolism. Increased concentrations of cortisol or cortisone may cause a stimulation of appetite and a negative calcium balance (antagonistic to *vitamin D* * effects). The production and liberation of cortisol and cortisone are under the control of *adrenocorticotropin* (ACTH). Four of the cortical hormones including cortisol and cortisone affect carbohydrate, protein, and fat metabolism in many ways antagonistic to *insulin*. They elevate blood glucose and increase production of glucose from protein, and they slow the growth of connective tissue cells and the formation of complex polysaccharides in these tissues. Injections of cortisone give relief from pain and crippling effects in some cases of rheumatoid arthritis. Cortisone is addictive in some individuals.

Cortisol (hydrocortisone) and cortisone

Cortisol   Cortisone

coumarin. A compound found in sweet clover. A derivative of coumarin, dicumarol is a antivitamin of vitamin K and is used clinically to prevent blood clotting. See *dicumarol*.

cranberry (Vaccinium). A bright red berry of a plant, of the heath family, *Ericacae*. Cranberries are high in ascorbic acid (vitamin C). Raw, 100 gm = 46 calories; sauce, 100 gm = 146 calories; juice, 100 gm = 65 calories.

cream. The rich, fatty part of whole milk which rises to the top and which can be separated from the milk. The longer sweet cream stands, the thicker it will be. There are different kinds of cream, regulated by their butterfat content. Cream can be sweet or sour. 18 percent butterfat content, 1 tablespoon $=$ 30 calories. See *milk*.

cream of tartar (sodium acid tartrate). Mol. Wt. 172. The common name for potassium acid *tartrate* *, an acid salt that is used in angelcake to stabilize the eggwhite foam, to whiten the color, and to increase the tenderness of the cake. It is also used as an acid ingredient in the tartrate baking powder.

$$
\begin{array}{c}
\overset{-}{C}O\overset{+}{O}\,Na \\
| \\
H—C—OH \\
| \\
HO—C—H \\
| \\
COOH
\end{array}
$$

creatine. Mol. Wt. 131. A nitrogenous constituent of muscle which in phosphorylated form is essential for muscle contraction. See *phosphocreatine*.

$$
\begin{array}{c}
HN \qquad NH_2 \\
\diagdown \;/ \\
C \\
| \\
H_3C—N—CH_2—COOH
\end{array}
$$

creatinine. Mol. Wt. 131. A nitrogen-containing substance derived creatine catabolism and present in urine. It is the end product of creatine. Creatinine is excreted at a relatively constant rate. The rate varies roughly in proportion to the muscle mass. Because of the relatively constant excretion rate it is often used as an index of kidney function since a kidney malfunction will sometimes show decreased creatinine excretion rates.

Creatinine

cretinism. A glandular disease, cretinism is easily recognizable within the first 4 months of an infant's life. It is due to insufficient secretion of the *thyroid gland*. Two types of cretinism have been identified, sporadic and endemic. The child may be born with a rudimentary thyroid gland, or the thyroid gland may be absent. In either case the child is not able to furnish his body with sufficient *thyroxin**. Cretinism manifests itself in early infancy and is recognized by symptoms such as small stature (dwarfism) accompanied by short, thick legs; disproportionally large head; short, broad hands and fingers with square ends; dry and coarse or scaly skin, with an edematous appearance; coarse and scant hair; peg-shaped and chalky teeth, with delayed dentition; half-shut eyes and swollen eyelids; low *basal metabolic rate* (BMR), and little perspiration; short and thick neck; delayed sexual development; hoarseness and strident voice. In personality these infants and later these children tend to be restive and stubborn; they lack spontaneity. They are not troublesome in behavior, usually being placid and taciturn rather than quarrelsome and aggressive. In intelligence, cretins range from the idiot level through the moron level and some reach the borderline normal classification.

crossing over. A process during meiosis in which the homologous chromosomes undergo synapses and exchange segments.

cryptoxanthin. The yellow pigment of corn. Three provitamin A carotenoids are known as carotenes (alpha-, beta-, and gamma-carotene), and a fourth is cryptoxanthin.

cucumber (*Cucumis sativus*). The succulent fruit of a rough-stemmed trailing vine belonging to the gourd family. Cucumbers come in a number of varieties, from thick, stubby little fruit 3 to 4 inches long, to greenhouse giants. The most popular cucumbers have a smooth dark-green rind. Pickles, called gherkins are made from small cucumbers. They are soaked in brine, treated with boiling vinegar, and flavored with dill or with spices. Caloric value: 1, raw 7½ x 2 inches = 25 calories.

cumin (*Cuminum cyminum*). The cumin plant, source of the aromatic cuminseed, is a delicate member of the parsley family, an annual which rarely grows more than 5 to 6 inches high. The seed is tiny and oval, with a strong, warm and slightly bitter taste. Since cuminseed resembles caraway seed in flavor as well as looks its uses are much the same.

curd. Semisolid mass formed when milk comes in contact with an acid, such as the acid secretion in the stomach or with an enzyme. See *milk products*.

curing agents. Originally used to preserve meat. Salt and certain other curing compounds are still important in curing ham, bacon, and many other meats such as frankfurters and bologna. But curing agents also are used to modify the flavor and stabilize or add color. The most controversial curing agents are *sodium nitrates* and *nitrites*.

currant (*Ribes* and *Vitis*). The name is applied to two totally different fruits. One, a fresh currant, is a berry of the genus *Ribes*, a member of the gooseberry family; the other, a dry currant, is a dried grape of the genus *Vitis*. Currants are sweet tart berries which come in red, white, or black varieties. Red currants are the best known and most frequently used. Red currants are eaten fresh as a fruit, as well as cooked in jams and jellies. White currants are used in salads and fruit cups, and black currants are used primarily in jams, jellies, and beverages. Small amounts of *carotene* * (vitamin A) and *ascorbic acid* * (vitamin C). Raw, 100 gm = 54 calories.

Cushing Syndrome (hyperadrenalism). A result of an increased production of hormones from the adrenal cortex. It may be caused by a tumor or other disease of the adrenal gland, or it may result from overstimulation of the adrenal glands by the pituitary gland. See *cortisol* and *cortisone* *

custard apple (*Annona reticulata*). Aside from the common custard apple, the name covers several fruits of tropical and subtropical America, such as the cherimoya and the sweetsop, or sugar apple, all of which have a sweet soft pulp. The do not taste like apples. The outside of the true custard apple looks scaly, rather like an artichoke. The fruit is 4 to 6 inches in length, heart-shaped, and the pulp is cream-colored. All custard apples have a bland taste, with the pulp eaten as is, either directly from the fruit or spooned into a serving dish. Raw, 100 gm = 101 calories.

cyanocobalamin (cobalamin, vitamin B_{12}). See *cobalamin* *

cyanogens. Hydrogen cyanide (HCN) is a constituent of a large number of edible plants. Cyanogens or the cyanogenic glucosides which on hydrolysis in the human intestine yields cyanide, are found in such garden variety foodstuffs as lima beans, sweet potatoes, yams, sugar cane, peas, cherries, plums, and apricots. The initial symptoms of acute cyanogen poisoning have been described as numbness in fingertips and toes and giddiness or lightheadedness. Small, nonfatal doses often produce headache sensations of tightness in both throat and chest, perceptible heart beating (palpitations), and general weakness. Full recovery is usual as the body processes eliminate the offending chemical.

cyclamate, sodium salt. The sodium or calcium salts of cyclohexylsufamic acid. It is water soluble, with a sweet taste (30 times that of sucrose). Used as noncaloric sweetener. The use of cyclamate as sweeteners was banned in the U.S. as a health hazard, because it was shown to produce cancer in mice under certain conditions.

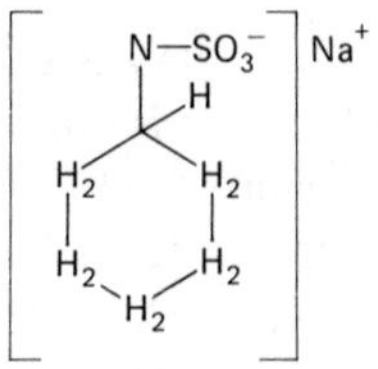

Cyclamate

cyclic AMP (c-AMP). Mol. Wt. 329. A compound produced by ATP through the action of an enzyme, adenylate cyclase, which is stimulated by a vast number of hormones, including *epinephrine, catecholamines, glucagon, luteinizing hormone* (LH), *vasopressin, parathyroid hormone, prostaglandins,* and *thyrocalcitonin* as well as other biologically active agents such as *histamine* and *serotonin*. It is believed that c-AMP mediates the effects of hormones and other active agents, and plays a regulatory role in cellular metabolism by stimulating the phosphorylation of enzymes and controls the rate of a number of cellular reactions as varied as the synthesis and activity of proteins, *glycogenolysis, lipolysis,* steroidogenesis, and *active transport*. Because of the role that c-AMP plays it is often referred to as the "second messenger". Hormones then are the primary messengers.

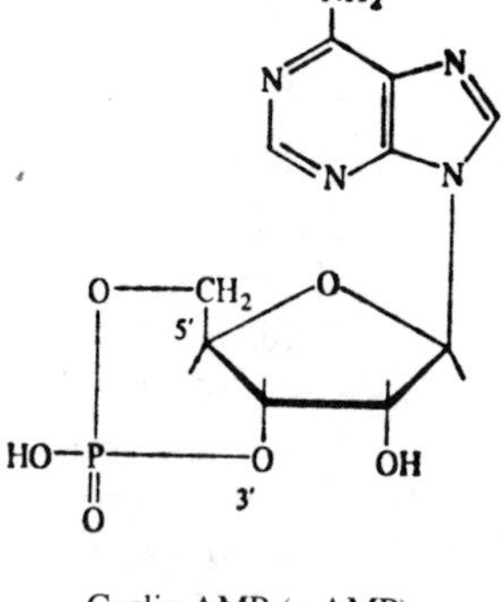

Cyclic AMP (c-AMP)

cyst. A sac or saclike structure, usually abnormal, containing liquid or semisolid matter and often caused by blockage of a passage.

cysteine (Cys). Mol. Wt. 121. An *amino acid* and one of two principal sources of sulphur in the diet of man. The other source is *methionine* *. The body can make cysteine from methionine but not vice versa, so that methionine is an *essential amino acid*. *Cystine* * is formed when two molecules of cysteine are reduced and lined by an – S—S– bond. Cystine is present in the keratin of hair and in insulin, in each of which it forms about 12 percent of the whole protein molecule.

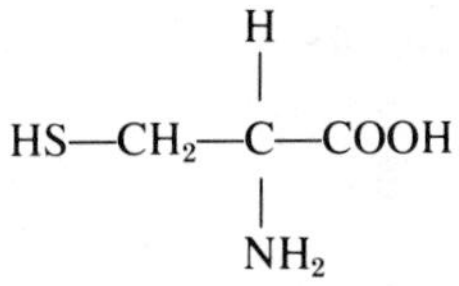

$$\begin{array}{c} H \\ | \\ HS\!-\!CH_2\!-\!C\!-\!COOH \\ | \\ NH_2 \end{array}$$

Cysteine

cysticerosis. Infestation of the body with a form of tapeworm called cysticerus, which is sometimes present in raw beef. Beef should be cooked at least to the rare done stage (140°F) to avoid danger.

cystine (Cys-Cys). Mol. Wt. 240. Cystine is the oxidative condensation product of two molecules of the amino acid *cysteine* *. Cystine as a separate compound has no major important function. However, the condensation of two cysteine residues within protein chains to form cystine residues is very important to the structure and conformation of a large number of proteins and enzymes. Some examples are chymotrypsin and insulin, both of which require peptide chains held together by cystine residues for their biologic activity.

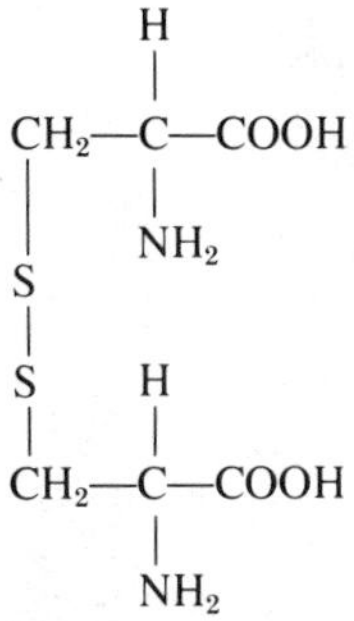

$$\begin{array}{c} H \\ | \\ CH_2\!-\!C\!-\!COOH \\ | \quad\; | \\ | \quad\; NH_2 \\ S \\ | \\ S \quad\; H \\ | \quad\; | \\ CH_2\!-\!C\!-\!COOH \\ | \\ NH_2 \end{array}$$

Cystine (Cys-Cys)

cystinuria (cystine stones). Cystinuria is an inborn error of metabolism characterized by faulty absorption of the amino acids cystine, ornithine, arginine, and lysine in the intestinal tract, slightly retarded growth, and the appearance of the four amino acids in the urine, due to defective tubular reabsorption. Of these cystine is the least soluble. It will precipitate when there is increased concentration in the urine and form stones.

cystitis. An inflammation of the bladder and one of the most common disorders of the urinary tract. It is rarely a primary disease and is often a symptom of some other disturbance in either the urinary tract or the genital tract.

cytochromes. Respiratory enzymes consisting of a number of hemochromogens which are similar to the *heme* in *hemoglobin*. The iron-containing heme proteins of the electron transport system or terminal respiratory chain that are alternately oxidized and reduced in biological oxidation. It is the electron transport system in cells that uses oxygen to form water in an oxidative phosphorylation processes. See *terminal respiratory chain* and *oxidative phosphorylation*.

cytokinesis. The division of the cytoplasm during mitosis or meiosis.

cytoplasm. Contains a variety of structures, organelles, organized living material, and inclusions, lifeless and often temporary material, such as pigment granules, secretory granules, and nutrients such as protein and carbohydrate particles. Materials which will be utilized by the cell in its life processes or excreted. The material within the cell, with the exception of nucleus.

cytosol. The liquid portion of the *cytoplasm* after the organelles and other formed elements have been removed, usually by high speed centrifugation. It is essential a colloidal suspension of the soluble proteins of the cell.

cytosine. One of the *pyrimidine* nitrogenous bases found in the *nucleic acids*. See *pyrimidines*.

D

D. A symbol to denote a configuration about an asymmetric carbon relative to D-gyceraldehyde. The mirror image is the L-configuration. All naturally occurring asymmetric carbons are either all L- or all D-. For example, all *amino acids* found in proteins have the L-configuration.

damson (*Prunus*). A variety of *plum* tree and its fruit, which, like all plums, belongs to the great rose family. The word "damson" is derived from Damascus, capital of Syria, where the plums were cultivated before the time of Christ. Damson plums are small, firm, oval purple plums. There is a variety with yellow flesh. These are spicier and more acid than ordinary plums. Damson plums are not eaten raw, but are used for cooking and are made into pies, compotes, jams, and preserves. Caloric value:1 plum = 10 to 15 calories; jam, 1 tablespoon = 55 calories.

dandelion (*Tarasacum officinale*). A familiar weed of the *chicory* family. The name comes from the French dent de lion or "lion's tooth," which the sharply indented leaves of the plant are said to resemble. Wild or cultivated, dandelion leaves are eaten as a vegetable, raw or cooked. They have a somewhat bitter flavor. The roots can be eaten as vegetables or roasted and ground and made into a root coffee. Dandelion greens are an excellent source of *carotene** (vitamin A activity), very good for iron, and good for calcium. Raw, 100 gm = 45 calories; cooked, 100 gm = 33 calories.

dasheen (*Colocasia*). A starchy root vegetable with large and small tubers side by side on one plant. It is a variety of *taro* and in southern and tropical climates is used as a substitute for potatoes. The larger tubers (corms) weigh up to 6 pounds; the smaller tubers (cormels) are egg size. Both have brown fibrous skins. When peeled and cooked, the flesh becomes cream-colored, mealy, and nutty-flavored. Dasheens have more carbohydrates and proteins than potatoes. Raw, 100 gm = 98 calories.

date (*Phoenix dactylifera*). The fruit of the date palm. The date itself, is a one-seeded berry and grows in thick clusters. Unripe, it is green; ripe, yellow or red, with thick and very sweet flesh. Depending upon the variety, dates can be soft, or hard and dry. Dates are ripened off the tree and dried before shipping. Dates are a good source of iron and sugar, as well as protein. Pitted, 100 gm = 274 calories.

deamination. Removal of an amino group ($—NH_2$) from an amino acid or other organic compound. Usually the first step in the *catabolism* of amino acids is a deamination which is accomplished by transfer of the amino group (*transamination*) to another compound. All amino acids are ultimately catabolized in man to carbon dioxide, water, urea, and energy. After removal of the nitrogen (deamination) to form an *alpha keto acid,* the nonnitrogenous fraction of the amino acid molecule has one of several uses, depending on the need: (1) Some circulate directly to the tissues to form tissue protein by recombining with amino groups to reform the amino acid; (2) the alpha-keto acid is metabolized to carbon dioxide, water, urea, and energy at that time; or (3) converted to fat or carbohydrate and stored to be metabolized at a later time; or (4) incorporated into other compounds.

debilitated. Weak; lacking strength. See *anorexia.*

decalcification. The withdrawal of calcium from the bones where it has been deposited. It may be caused by an inadequate supply of calcium in the diet so that calcium has to be taken from the bones to help meet the body's needs. It may be caused by an imbalance in some of the hormone activity in the body. *Parahormone, calcitonin,* and *vitamin D* are involved in calcium metabolism.

decarboxylation. The removal of carbon dioxide from an amino acid. It is necessary for the formation in the body of at least three vital physiological regulators (hormones or similar compounds) from the amino acids, *histidine* * to form *histamine* *, *tryptophan* * to *serotonin* * and *tyrosine* to form *epinephrine* *, as well as for the oxidation of amino acids for energy. The vitamin *pyridoxine* *, as the coenzyme pyridoxal phosphate, is involved in the decarboxylation reactions of the amino acids, with the exception of the decarboxylation of histidine. *Thiamine* * as the coenzyme thiamine pyrophosphate is involved in the oxidative decarboxylation of *pyruvate* * and *α-ketoglutarate* *.

deficiency disease. A disease resulting from an inadequate dietary intake of something required nutritionally; most commonly refers to diseases resulting from dietary deficiencies of vitamins or trace elements.

deglutition. The act of swallowing is termed deglutition. After food has been grasped and divided by the anterior teeth, it is ground into fine particles by the posterior dentition. At the same time it is tossed about by the tongue and thoroughly mixed well with saliva. Saliva makes it possible to swallow the mass of food called *bolus*. In the first stage food is ground and rolled into a bolus which has been thoroughly soaked with saliva. The tongue then directs the bolus to the back of the mouth and forces it to enter the pharynx. In the second stage, the bolus passes through the pharynx to enter the esophagus. In the third stage, the food traverses the esophagus to enter the stomach.

dehydrated foods. Products from which most of the water has been removed in order to improve their stability during storage. See *lyophilize*.

dehydration. (1) Removal of water from food or tissue; or the condition that results from undue loss of water. (2) Dehydration also refers to excessive loss of water or losses without replacement. Common causes of dehydration in man are *diarrhea* and *vomiting* (emesis).

dehydrocholesterol (7-dehydrocholecalciferol). The cholesterol derivative in the skin that is converted to vitamin D_3. See *vitamin D* *

dehydrogenase. A class of enzymes which facilitates the transfer of hydrogen from one compound to another. The vitamins *niacin* *, as the coenzymes *nicotinamide adenine dinucleotide* * (NAD) and *nicotinamide adenine dinucleotide phosphate* * (NADP), and *riboflavin* *, as the coenzyme *flavin mononucleotide* * (FMN) and *flavin adenine dinucleotide* * (FAD), serve in many dehydrogenase reactions.

denature. (1) Denature may refer to the alcohol *ethanol* * when a poison is added to make it unsuitable for consumption. It is referred to as denatured alcohol. *Methanol* * or wood alcohol does not have to be denatured since it is a poison. (2) Denature or the process of denaturation most frequently refers to proteins when they lose the natural physical, chemical, or biological characteristics by any means. Proteins are denatured by heat. The *coagulation* of egg white when boiled is an example of denaturation. That is to say, the physical properties of the protein have changed from soluble to insoluble. Enzymes when denatured lose their catalytic activity, and yet may remain soluble protein. Proteins may be denatured by a wide variety of substances or conditions including heat, acid, alkali, organic solvents, and mechanically agitation are only a few. Most cooking or preparation for meals causes denaturation of proteins which only alters its internal structure and has no effect on the quality of protein in general. One clear exception is dry heat, such as occurs in the formation of "puffed wheat" and "puffed rice" type cereals. Dry heat tends to destroy the *essential amino acid lysine* *.

deoxycholic acid. Mol. Wt. 393. One of the *bile acids* that forms *bile salts* in *bile*. The bile salt is conjugated with taurine or glycine to form deoxycholyltaurine (taurodeoxycholate) and deoxycholylglycine (glycodeoxycholate). The bile salts are powerful emulsifiers. See *bile salts*.

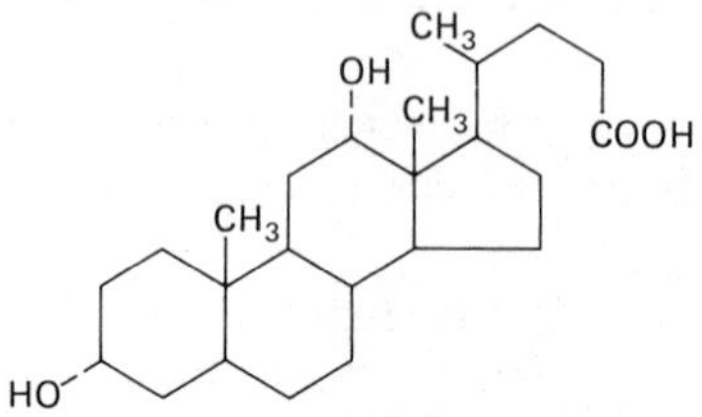

Deoxycholic acid

11-deoxycorticosterone. Mol. Wt. 330. A steroid hormone produced by the cortex of the adrenal glands. It is a precursor to the more powerful hormones *aldosterone* * and *corticosterone* *. The 11-deoxycorticosterone has about 4 percent of the activity of aldosterone in its influence on salt and *water balance*. See *aldosterone* *.

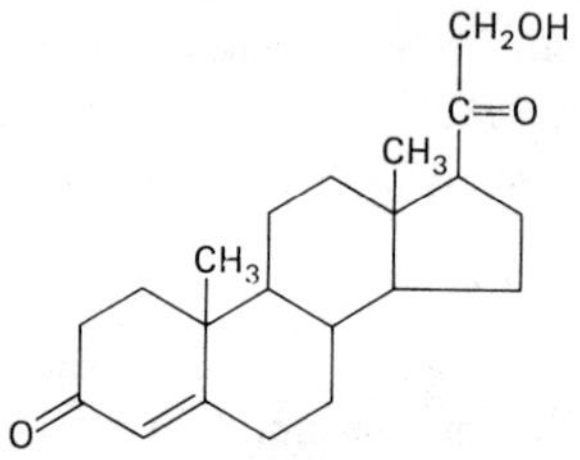

11-deoxycorticosterone

deoxypyridoxine. Mol. Wt. 154. An antivitamin (antimetabolite). A compound similar in structure to pyridoxine that is antagonistic to the action of *pyridoxine* * (vitamin B_6) See *pyridoxine* *.

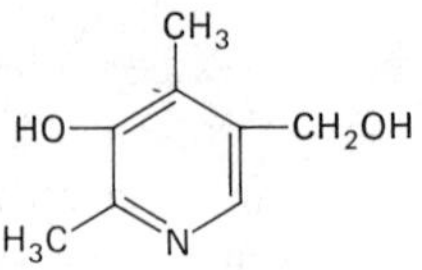

Deoxypyridoxine

Deoxyribonucleic acid (DNA). Found in the nucleus of living cells and functions in the transfer of genetic characteristics. The primary genetic material of the cell consists of long chains of nucleic acid called DNA or deoxyribonucleic acid. These chains contain genes. DNA is organized into larger units called *chromosomes* which contain protein and other substances, which are microscopically visible components of cell nuclei. It has been established that DNA molecules consist of a pair of polymeric chains of alternate units of a particular

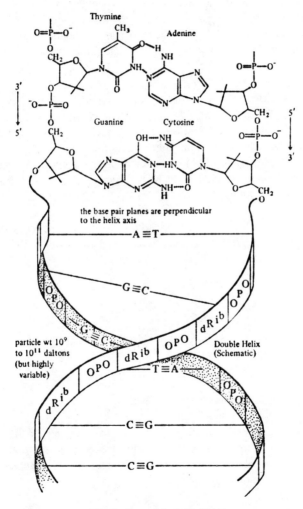

Deoxyribonucleic Acid (DNA)

sugar (deoxyribose) and a phosphate group. Attached to each sugar is any one of four nitrogenous bases, two *purines* and two *pyrimidines*. The arrangement of these bases along the strand is the key factor that gives each DNA molecule its identity. The strands of DNA are complementary strands in that each base specifically pairs with one another. Adenine and thymine are one specific pairing, and guanine and cystosine are the other specific pairing. The two complementary strands entwine naturally to form a double helix. DNA is the hereditary material of the cell, and there exists a biochemical process by which the DNA in a cell can be replicated and passed to successive generations. The position of a particular amino acid in the polypeptide chain is given in each case by the sequence of three nucleotides (a triplet code). The sequence of deoxyribonucleotides in DNA fixes the sequence of ribonucleotides in *messenger ribonucleic acid* (m-RNA) which in turn determines the sequence of amino acids in proteins.

deoxyribonucleotides. Building blocks of *deoxyribonucleic acids** (DNA), each consisting of a sugar *deoxyribose*, a phosphate group and a nitrogenous bases, the deoxyribonucleotides. There are four different deoxyribonucleotides, all containing deoxribose and phosphate and differing in the bases, deoxyadenosine monophosphate (dAMP); deoxythymidine monophosphate (dTMP); deoxycystosine monophosphate (dCMP); deoxyguanosine monophosphate (dGMP).

2-deoxyribose. Mol. Wt. 134. A five-carbon sugar with one less oxygen atom than the parent sugar, ribose. It occurs as a constituent of DNA. See *deoxyribonucleic acid** and *ribose**.

2-deoxyribose

derived proteins. See *coagulated proteins*.

dermatan sulfate. Contains largely L-iduronic acid in place of the acid sugar D-glucuronic acid. Dermatan sulfate generally occurs in tissues that are rich in collagen. Its biological role appears to be different from the *chondroitin sulfates* and it is present mainly in the skin.

dermatitis. An inflammatory, recurring skin reaction, caused by contact with an irritating agent that is ingested or found in the environment. Dermatitis is usually associated with hereditary allergic tendencies and may be aggravated by emotional stress and fatigue. A primary symptom of dermatitis is *eczema,* a type of skin eruption characterized by tiny blisters that weep and crust. Chronic forms are characterized by scaling, flaking and eventual thickening and color changes of the skin. Itching is almost always present. Deficiency of any of the B-vitamins can cause dermatitis. A protein deficiency can cause chronic eczema.

desiccate. To dry.

detoxication. Reduction of the toxic properties of a substance.

dewberry. Closely related to the blackberry, dewberries differ from blackberries by growing on trailing rather than upright vines. There are many different species. Berries contain a fair amount of iron and *ascorbic acid* * (vitamin C) Raw, 100 gm = 58 calories.

dextran. A polysaccharide, made by *Leuconostoc mesenteroides* from a molasses or refined sucrose medium dextran may serve as a stabilizer for sugar syrups, ice cream, or confections. Dextrans are characterized by $\beta 1 \rightarrow 2$ glycosidic linkages as contrasted with the $\alpha 1 \rightarrow 4$ linkages in *starch* *.

dextrin. Formed from starch by the action of certain enzymes, acids, or heat. The term dextrin designates a group rather than an individual substance. Malt diastase, acting for some time upon starch in fairly concentrated solutions, yields usually about one part of dextrin to four of *maltose* *. Dextrins thus formed by partial hydrolysis of starches are sometimes called hydrolytic dextrins. Commercial dextrin, the principal constituent of British gum is obtained by heating starch either alone or with a small amount of a dilute or a weak acid. The dextrins formed essentially by dry heating are sometimes called torrefaction dextrins. The dextrins are much more soluble than the starches. The dextrin molecules while very large and complex are smaller in size than the starch molecules from which they are derived.

dextrose. *See glucose* *. Food manufacturers use dextrose primarily as a sweetener, but it serves additional functions in certain foods. Dextrose (and other sugars) turn brown when heated and contribute to the color of bread crust and toast. The same browning reaction accounts for the brown color of caramel. In soft drinks, dextrose contributes "body." Only three-fourths as sweet as table sugar and may be used in place of table sugar.

diabetes mellitus. A group of diseases in which the body cannot oxidize *glucose* * properly because of a lack of *insulin* or its improper function. A disturbance of metabolism, not fully understood, in which the body behaves as if it were partially or entirely deficient in insulin. In diabetis mellitus the blood sugar (glucose) is abnormally high and there is no apparent secretion of insulin in response to a carbohydrate meal. There is also increased breakdown of liver *glycogen**, defective storage of glucose as glycogen in muscle, and therefore a defective utilization of glucose in the tissues for energy. Although the cause and cure of this disease are not known, heredity is a predisposing factor. With proper medical attention the disease can be controlled often by diet, insulin, and exercise. Common symptoms include polydipsia (extreme thirst), polyphagia (constant hunger), and polyuria (excessive urine), which may cause bed wetting and "accidents" in the day. Complications include *ketosis* or diabetic *acidosis*. The extreme of an uncompensated diabetic condition may result in a diabetic coma. Acidosis from diabetes often causes the face to flush, the lips to become red, the breath to have a characteristic sweet odor due to the presence of *acetone**, the respiration to increase and to become labored and dehydration to occur. Hypoglycemia which can be caused by too much insulin is characterized by irritability, hunger, weakness, double vision, and tremors and pyogenic infections. An extreme of insulin administration may result in insulin shock. The condition of hypoglycemia in an individual is often considered as an indication of a predisposition for diabetes. The condition of diabetes leads to an alteration from normal glucose and fat metabolism.

dialysis. A sensitive method for separating lower molecular weight components from macromolecules. A thin membrane in the form of a tube is filled with the solution containing the molecules to be separated. The pore size of the membrane allows the diffusion of small molecules such as salts or amino acids; larger molecules such as *proteins* or *nucleic acids* cannot pass through the pores and so remain inside the dialysis tube. Dialysis is a convenient method of exchanging solvents in the isolation of enzymes or other macromolecules.

diarrhea. A medical term for liquid stools, the color of the stools varying from light brown to green. Flecks of blood, mucus, or partially digested food may appear in the bowel movement. Most diarrhea results from viral infections of the intestines and stomach, (*gastroenteritis*). The inflamed and irritated intestine affected by an infection is less able to absorb food and liquids. It leaks fluid, is overactive, and tends to pass its contents through and out of the body more rapidly than normal. Bacteria can also cause diarrhea. Salmonellosis and Shigellosis are among the more common types of bacterial infections. These can be transmitted from humans and from animals as well. Because there is no cure for virus diseases and therefore for most cases of diarrhea, doctors concern themselves mainly in treating the effects of diarrhea, which include dehydration, rather than the ailment itself.

diastase. The first enzyme to be discovered. It converts starch into sugars. "Diastases" is a general term for enzymes that hydrolyze starches.

diastole. Relaxation of the heart muscle especially that of the ventricle, during which the lumen becomes filled with blood.

diastolic blood pressure. Minimum arterial pressure when left ventricle relaxes after contracting. Average, 75 mm of mercury; normal range 60–90 mm of mercury.

diastolic hypertension. Results from an excessive constriction or narrowing of the arterioles throughout the body. The greater the degree of arteriolar narrowing, the greater is the diastolic blood pressure elevation.

diathermy. The generation of heat produced by the resistance of the body tissues to the passage of high-frequency electric impulses.

Diazepam (Valium). A minor tranquilizer useful in treating anxiety states, fatigue, nausea, and ataxia. Valium has addictive qualities.

dicoumarin. An anticlotting factor first isolated from sweet clover. It is an *antivitamin,* structural related to *vitamin K*.

dicumarol. Mol. Wt. 336. An antivitamin. The registered name of dicoumarin, a coumarin derivative isolated originally from spoiled sweet clover and later made synthetically. It is used clinically as an *anticoagulant* in thrombotic states, and acts to depress the factors concerned with the formation of thrombin because of its *antivitamin K* activity.

Dicumarol

Diencephalon. Lying centrally within the brain between the cerebrum and the pons are the diencephalon and midbrain, covered at the sides by the cerebral hemispheres. The diencephalon lies to either side of the narrow midline third ventricle. Adjacent to the third ventricle the thalamic portion of the diencephalon is subdivided into an epithalamus, thalamus, hypothalamus, and subthalamus. See *brain.*

diet (general definition). Any combination of foods that constitutes a regular proportion of basic foodstuffs and alcohol over a specified period of time. Usually, even though the individual foods may vary from day to day, the ratios of the basic foodstuffs does not vary. For example, the relative proportions of fats, protein, and carbohydrates has not changed radically over the last 80 years. However, within the carbohydrates there has been a radical change in type, in that starch has been largely supplanted by table sugar (*sucrose* *). The average American diet is approximately 55 percent fat, 35 percent carbohydrate, and 10 percent protein. Below are some variations of diets and the purposes for which such diets are prescribed.

Caloric, high: A diet which has caloric value above the total energy requirements and is often prescribed to gain weight.

Caloric, low: A diet which has a caloric value below the total energy requirement and is often prescribed to lose weight.

Cholesterol, low: A combination of foods in which the dietary intake of total cholesterol is restricted. The dietary prescription should include the permissible amounts of fat and cholesterol.

Fat, modified: A combination prescribed to meet a specified level of fat in the diet, or specified amounts of ratios of fatty acids. When used for regulation of abnormal serum lipids or in the treatment of individuals with vascular disease, fat-modified diets may be combined with a low cholesterol diet.

Fiber, high: A normal diet including an additional serving of foods high in indigestible carbohydrate fiber and unrestricted amounts of connective tissue.

Fiber, low: A diet which contains a minimum of indigestible carbohydrates (fiber) and no tough connective tissue.

Galactose-free: A diet which has been made almost free of galactose by the elimination of milk and milk products; or those containing complex forms of galactose, as for example peas, lima beans, and beets which contain raffinose and stachhose as complex forms of galactose.

Ketogenic: A diet in which the ratio of fatty acid (ketogenic) value to glucose (antiketogenic) value equals two or more, i.e., is sufficiently high to produce ketosis. Such a diet generally provides small amounts of carbohydrates, approximately 1 gm protein per kilogram of body weight, and sufficient fat to meet full caloric requirements.

Soft: A diet modified in consistency, which includes high-protein liquid foods and those solid foods which are low in fiber content and connective tissue.

Protein, low: For individuals with chronic renal failure of moderate severity or with subacute hepatic encephalophalopathy. Foods exclude milk, meat, protein foods, and include fruit or juice, low protein vegetables such as green beans, beetroot, cabbage, carrots, cauliflower, celery, cucumber, eggplant, lettuce, onions, pumpkin, radishes, summer squash, tomatoes and turnips; bread, cereals, cream, fat, sugar, jelly, syrup, hard candy, water ice, tea, coffee, and seasoning except salt, as desired.

Protein, high, restricted sodium: For individuals with nephrotic syndrome or hypoalbuminemia. Sodium intake is restricted by using no table salt and avoiding all highly salted foods, e.g., ham, bacon, sausages, corned beef, smoked fish, cheese, most ketchups and commercial sauces, canned and convenience foods.

Diabetic diets: Diabetic diets aim to restrict carbohydrate intake while meeting normal needs for protein and providing just sufficient energy to maintain normal weight in adults and to allow for growth in children.

Fat, very low; high carbohydrate: For individuals with nausea due to hepatitis or obstructive jaundice and for Type 1 hyperlipidemia. No butter, margarine, or cream should be taken. No cooking fat or oil should be used and the following foods should be avoided: whole milk, egg yolk, cheese, ice cream, cakes, potato crisps, pastries and cookies; sweets containing fat, e.g., fudge and milk chocolate; bacon, organ meats, fatty fish, e.g., herring, mackerel, sardines, and salmon, and all canned meat.

Fat, low; high energy: For individuals with malabsorption and steatorrhoea. It is recommended that the following foods be avoided: All fried foods, pork, organ meats, whole milk, cheese, cream and cream substitutes, ice cream, milk chocolate, cream soups, gravies, commercial cakes, pies, and cookies.

Low sodium, moderate energy: For individuals with edema from congestive heart failure, nephrotic syndrome, chronic glomerulonephritis and cirrhosis of the liver with ascites; may also be used for hypertension. No salt can be used in cooking or at the table. Avoid all cured meat and fish, e.g., bacon, ham, tongue, pickled brisket and silverside, smoked haddock, sardines, smoked salmon; all canned meats, fish and vegetables and soups; cheeses, bottle sauces, pickles, sausages, and all foods made with bicarbonate of soda or baking powder, e.g., cakes and biscuits. See *salt.*

diffusion. The word diffusion comes from the Latin word diffundere meaning "to spread" or "pour forth." It is the process by which particles in solution spread throughout the solution and across or throughout the solution and across separating membranes, from the place of highest soluble concentration to all spaces of lesser soluble concentration. It may be simple passive diffusion or it may be carrier-mediated which increases the rate of the diffusion process. See *active transport.*

digestibility, coefficient of apparent. The percentage of an ingested nutrient which cannot be recovered in the feces; hence the percentage of an ingested nutrient which is assumed to have been absorbed. The coefficient of digestibility of protein, fat, and carbohydrate in a mixed American diet have been estimated to be 92 percent, 95 percent, and 97 percent respectively.

digestion. Includes all the changes, physical and chemical, which food undergoes in the body, making it absorbable. In some instances no change is necessary. For example, water, minerals, and certain carbohydrates are absorbed without modification. In other instances cooking process initiates chemical changes in food before it enters the body. The digestive processes are controlled by both neural (nerve) and hormonal mechanisms. Strong unpleasant sensations may affect the nervous system and thus inhibit the secretion of the digestive fluids which in turn interferes with digestion. Pleasurable sensations on the other hand, aid digestion, hence there is value in attractively served food, pleasant surroundings, and cheerful conversation.

Site of Secretion	Important Constituents	Action
Mouth: saliva	Mucin	Lubrication
Salivary glands	Amylase (ptyalin)	Cooked starch—dextrins, maltose
Submaxillary		Enzyme activity in the mouth is not important
Sublingual		
Parotid		
Stomach: gastric juice	Hydrochloric	Pepsinogen—pepsin
Parietal cells	acid (HCl)	Bactericidal
		Reduces ferric iron to ferrous iron
Chief cells	Pepsinogen	Inactive form of pepsin
	Pepsin	Proteins—protose, peptones, polypeptides
	Mucin	Lubrication: protects gastric and duodenal
Liver: bile	Bile Salts	Neutralizes acid chyme
	Bile acids	Emulsifies fats for action of lipase
	Bile pigments	Facilitates absorption of fats and fat-soluble vitamins
Pancreas: pancreatic juice	Thin, watery, alkaline	Neutralizes acid chyme
	Enzyme	
	Amylase	Starch, dextrins, maltose
	Chymotrypsinogen	Inactive form of enzyme
	Chymotrypsin	Proteins—proteoses, peptones, polypeptides.
	Trypsinogen	Inactive enzyme
	Trypsin	Proteins—proteoses, peptones, polypeptides.
	Peptidase	Polypeptides—small peptides, amino acids.
	Lipase	Fats—monoglycerides, fatty acids, glycerol
Small intestine	Enterokinase	Trypsinogen—trypsin
intestinal juice	Peptidases	Polypeptides—amino acids
(succus entericus)	Nucleinases	Nucleic acid—nucleotides
	Nucleotidases	Nucleotides—nucleosides + phosphoric acid
	Lecithinases	Licithin—diglycerides + choline phosphate
	Cholerystokinin	
Within mucosal cells	Sucrase (invertase)	Sucrose—glucose + fructose
	Maltase	Maltose—glucose + glucose
	Lactose	Lactose—glucose + galactose

digestive juices and enzymes.

Juices and Glands	Place of Action	Enzymes	Changes in Foods
Saliva from 3 pairs of salivary glands	Oral cavity	Ptyalin	Begins starch digestion
Gastric juice from the gastric stomach wall	Stomach	Pepsin	Begins protein digestion
		Lipase	Digestion of fats
		Rennin	Curdling of milk protein
Pancreatic juice from pancrease	Small intestine	amylopsin	Acts on starches
		Trypsin	Acts on proteins
		Lipase	Acts on fats
Intestinal juice	Small intestine	Lactase	Breaks down complex sugars into simpler forms
		Maltase	
		Sucrase	
Bile from the liver	Small intestine	None	Breaks down fats physically so that lipase can digest them

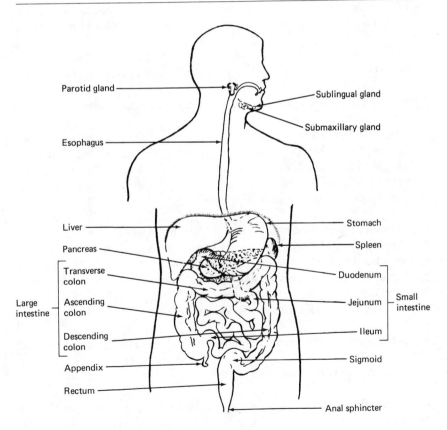

digestive system. The digestive system is made up of the alimentary canal or tract (food passage) and the accessory organs of digestion. Its main functions are to ingest and carry food so that digestion and absorption can occur and to eliminate unused waste material. The products of the accessory organs help to prepare food for its absorption and use (metabolism) by the tissues of the body. Digestion consists of two processes, one mechanical and the other chemical. The mechanical part of digestion may be broadly divided into chewing and swallowing, *peristalsis,* and *defecation.* The chemical part of digestion consists of breaking foodstuffs into simple components which can be absorbed and used by the body. In this process, foodstuffs are broken down by *enzymes,* or digestive juices, formed by digestive glands. *Carbohydrates* are broken into simple sugars. *Fats* are changed into fatty acids. Proteins are converted to *amino acids.* The accessory organs that aid in the process of digestion are, the *salivary glands, pancreas, liver, gall bladder,* and intestinal glands. A simple diagram of the digestive tract appears on p. 135.

digitalis. A drug that strengthens contractions of the heart muscles, slows rate of contraction of the heart, and promotes the elimination of fluid from body tissue.

diglyceride. A fat containing two *fatty acid* molecules as esters with *glycerol.*

dilatation. The condition of being stretched beyond normal dimension.

dill (*Anethum graveolens*). A hardy aromatic annual herb plant which reaches a height of about 3 feet. The branches have feathery leaves, and the flowers are yellow and very small. Dillseed is the dried fruit of the herb; dillweed, its dried leaves. Dill is used in preparing and serving soups, cheese, fish, meats, poultry, vegetables, potatoes, breads, and apple pie.

dioctyl sodium sulfosuccinate (DSS). A chemical involved in getting certain powdered foods to dissolve in water by coating the powder with a very small amount of a detergent like chemical or emulsifier such as DSS. It is used in powdered soft drink mixes in which it helps fumaric acid dissolve in water. Manufacturers also use it in some canned milk beverages containing cocoa fat, and in foods that contain hard-to-dissolve thickening agents.

diploid (duplex). With two sets of chromosomes. In human beings a fertilized egg, normally with 46 chromosomes, or 23 pairs, is in the diploid state as the resulting body cells are also diploids. The opposite of the *haploid state.*

direct calorimetry. The actual energy expended by the body throughout a given period may be determined by placing a human subject in a special calorimeter. The heat given off by the subject is absorbed by the water in the coils surrounding the well insulated chamber, where by an accurate mechanism, the total heat may be measured directly. This procedure is known as direct calorimetry, and is used only for scientific research.

disaccharidase. An enzyme which hydrolyzes disaccharides. *Sucrase* is a disaccharidase.

disaccharide. A carbohydrate that yields two sugars upon hydrolysis. *Sucrose**, *maltose**, *lactose**, are examples of disaccharides. The formula, $C_{12}H_{22}O_{11}$ shows that disaccharides consist of two *monosaccharides* or simple sugar groups. During the process of digestion they are split into their component monosaccharides. For example, sucrose* splits into glucose* and *fructose*;* lactose* splits into glucose* and *galactose*;* and maltose* splits into two molecules of glucose*.

disodium guanylate (GMP), and disodium inosinate (IMP). Belongs to the same family of food additives as *monosodium glutamate**, the flavor enhancer. Flavor enhancers have little or no taste of their own but accentuate the natural flavor of foods. They are used by manufacturers in place of more expensive natural ingredients. Disodium guanylate* and disodium inosinate* are found in powdered soup mixes, ham and chicken salad spread, sauces and canned vegetables. Manufacturers often use them together with monosodium glutamate, because of a synergistic action that exists between the three chemicals. They cannot be used in many moist foods, because enzymes in the food slowly convert the flavor enhancers to inert substances. See *guanosine triphosphate** (GTP) and *inosine triphosphate** (IMP).

disperse. To scatter or distribute over an area or to separate a substance into smaller parts. For example, in making mayonnaise, the oil is separated into small particles by beating and is distributed throughout the egg-acid mixture.

distill, distilled. The process of vaporizing a liquid by heat or reduced pressure and collections of the vapors by cooling. The resulting liquid is called the distillate.

distilled liquors. Distilled liquors or spirits are those produced by distillation of an alcoholically fermented product. Rum is the distillate from alcoholically fermented sugar-cane juice, syrup, or molasses. Whiskeys are distilled from saccharified and fermented grain mashes, e.g., rye whiskey, from wheat mash, etc. Rums and whiskeys are made from mashes fermented by special distillers' yeast, strains of *Saccharomyces cerevisiae* var. *ellipsoideus* which give high yields of alcohol. The grain mashes usually are acidified to favor the yeasts.

The aging of the distilled liquors in charred oaken barrels or tuns is a chemical rather than a biological process. See *yeasts*.

disulfide bond. Chemical bond formed between two sulfur atoms. In protein chemistry, disulfide bonds formed between cysteine residues and hold together separate polypeptide chains or separate parts of the chain. An example of a disulfide bond is *cystine**.

diuresis. Increased secretion of *urine*.

diuretic. A chemical given to increase *urine* output.

diverticulitis. From Latin divertere, "to turn aside." A diverticulum is an out-pouching or sac that protrudes from the intestinal lining into the intestinal wall. There can be scores of such outpouchings or diverticula, especially in the colon. Diverticulosis is always benign at the outset and usually remains so. When inflammation develops and when the inflammation is severe, the result is acute diverticulitis.

diverticula. Refers to small blind pouches resulting from a protrusion of the mucous membranes of a hollow organ through weakened areas of the organ's muscular wall. Diverticula occur most often in the intestinal tract, especially in the esophagus and colon. When they are present the individual is said to have a diverticulosis. If the diverticula become inflamed or infected, the condition is referred to as diverticulitis.

doughnut. A doughnut is a small cake, deep fried or baked and leavened with yeast or baking powder. Doughnuts are ring shaped with a hole in the center. Crullers and fried cakes are closely related to them. Both are made of the same kind of dough and deep fried, but technically crullers are shaped in a twist, and fried cakes are made round or square, without a hole. One baking powder or cake doughnut = 200 calories. 1 yeast or raised doughnut = 168 calories.

dried fruits. Fruits, of which the solids have been greatly concentrated by evaporating a large portion of the original water content, are called dried fruits. The purpose of drying is preservation. Dried fruits have a great variety of uses. They may be eaten as is, cooked and used as a sauce, used in pies, puddings, and stuffings, or served as meat accompaniments. In the drying, over 50 percent of the water is removed, but practically all the food nutrients remain. Dried fruit contain a variety of vitamins and minerals. The caloric value per pound of dried fruit is four to five times that of the fruit when fresh. However, this is true only if the dried fruit is eaten as purchased. When cooked the fruit regains much of the water lost and approximates the fresh fruit in composition.

Apples, 1 cup = 315 calories
Apricots, 1 cup = 423 calories
Currants, 1 cup = 536 calories
Dates, 1 cup = 505 calories
Figs, 1 cup × 453 calories
Nectarines, 1 cup = 424 calories
Peaches, 1 cup = 424 calories
Pears, 1 cup = 405 calories
Prunes (medium), 1 cup = 375 calories
Raisins, 1 cup = 429 calories

drug-nutrient interaction. Several therapeutic drugs have direct effects on nutritional status. In many instances the drugs counteract vitamin activities and lead to symptoms of vitamin deficiencies. The table below gives some of the known drug-nutrient effects and the clinical symptoms. Of interest in this category is the effect of substances such as *tyramine* * and the interaction with some antidepressants. See *tyramine toxicity.*

Major Drug Effects on Vitamins and Minerals

Therapeutic Class	Major Drugs	Nutritional Effect	Clinical Effect
Anticonvulsants and sedatives	Diphenylhydantoin Phenobarbital Glutethimide	Accelerated vitamin D metabolism	Rickets Neonatal hemorrhaging
		Accelerated vitamin K metabolism	Megaloblastic anemia Gingival hyperplasia (?)
		Folic acid deficiency	Neurologic deterioration (?)
			Congenital malformations (?)
Corticosteroids	Cortisone Prednisone	Vitamin B_6 deficiency	None established
		Accelerated vitamin D metabolism	Accelerated bone loss None established
		Increased vitamin C excretion	Abnormal glucose tolerance (?)
		Increased vitamin B_6 requirement	Mental depression (?)
		Increased zinc excretion	Slow wound healing
		Increased potassium excretion	Muscle weakness
Alcohol		Vitamin B_1 deficiency	Wernicke's encephalopathy Korsakoff's psychosis
		Impaired vitamin B_6 activation	Peripheral neuropathy (?) Sideroblastic anemia (?) "Rum fits" (?)
		Folic acid deficiency	Anemia (?)
		Increased magnesium excretion	ECG changes Delirium tremens

Major Drug Effects on Vitamins and Minerals (Continued)

Therapeutic Class	Major Drugs	Nutritional Effect	Clinical Effect
Nonabsorbed antibiotics	Neomycin Kanamycin	Reduced lactase levels	Lactose intolerance
Antitubercular drugs	Isoniazid	Vitamin B_6 deficiency Niacin deficiency	Polyneuritis Pellagra symptoms
Diuretics	Chlorthiazide	Increased potassium excretion Increased magnesium excretion	Muscle weakness Magnesium depletion
	Spironolactone	Reduced potassium excretion	Hyperkalemia
Hypotensives	Hydralazine	Vitamin B_6 depletion	Polyneuritis
Antiinflammatory drugs	Aspirin Indomethacin	GI bleeding	Iron deficiency anemia
	Phenylbutazone	Folic acid deficiency	Megaloblastic anemia
Oral contraceptives and estrogens	Mestranol Ethinyl estradiol	Vitamin B_6 depletion	Mental depression Abnormal glucose tolerance
	Conjugated estrogens	Folic acid deficiency	Megaloblastic anemia Megaloblastic cervical cytology Increased megaloblastic anemia in subsequent pregnancy
		Reduced calcium excretion	Reduced bone loss

dry weight. The weight of the residue of a substance that remains after virtually all the moisture has been removed from it. Also called dry matter.

dulcitol. Mol. Wt. 182. Obtained by hydrogenation or reduction of *galactose* in the same manner as *sorbitol* from *glucose*. A sugar which has a variety of industrial uses, sometimes employed in the manufacture of foods as improvers. See *sorbitol*.

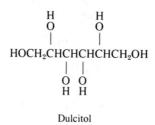

Dulcitol

duodenal drainage test. An intestinal specimen is obtained via a swallowed tube and examined for diagnosis of gallbladder and pancreas diseases.

duodenal ulcer. A common disease of the duodenum. The ulcer is a defect in the duodenum wall, commonly about the size of a dime, believed to be caused by the digestive action of the acidic gastric juice. Epigastric pain or distress is the most characteristic symptom. Pain usually occurs an hour or two after meals or when the stomach is empty. Pain is generally chronic and recurs frequently. When the ulcer is chronic there is also a deformity of the duodenum so that its bulb looks like a clover leaf instead of a chocolate drop on an x-ray film.

duodenum. First portion of the small intestine, extending from the plyorus to the jejunum. See *digestive system*.

durum wheat. (*Triticum durum*) A variety of wheat, often called "hard" or "macaroni" wheat, with hard translucent kernels. It is used chiefly for making macaroni and other pastas. Pasta products made from it do not disintegrate in cooking, but become tender while remaining firm.

dyspepsia. Indigestion or upset stomach.

dysmenorrhea. Refers to the association of pain with the menstrual flow.

dysphagia. Difficulty in swallowing.

dyspnea. Difficult or labored breathing.

dyssebacea. A term given to appearance of enlarged follicles around the sides of the nose, sometimes extending over the cheeks and forehead. The follicles are plugged with dry sebaceous material which often has a yellow color. Commonly found in Africans with *pellagra* and may be related to *riboflavin* * deficiency.

dysuria. Painful or difficult urination.

E

eczema. See *dermatitis*.

edema. The presence of an abnormally large volume of fluid in the intertissue (interstitial) spaces. Swelling of a part of or the entire body due to the presence of an excess of water. Edema is most noticeable at the end of the day around the ankles, which increase in size. Edema is a common condition of many nutritional diseases or conditions such as wet *beri-beri* and *marasmus*.

edible portion (E.P.). As used in food tables, term refers to that part of a food which is most commonly eaten. Some parts, such as parings of potatoes which are edible but not usually eaten are excluded.

EEG. See *electroencephalogram*.

EFA. See *essential fatty acid*.

eggs. Eggs are rich in essential nutrients. An average chicken egg contains 6 gm of protein and 6 gm of fat and yields 80 kcal. The proteins most of which are

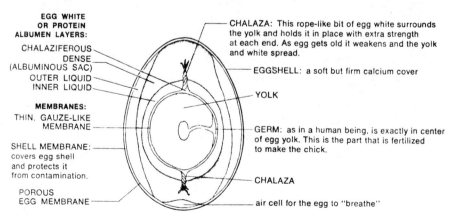

EGG WHITE OR PROTEIN ALBUMEN LAYERS:

CHALAZIFEROUS
DENSE (ALBUMINOUS SAC)
OUTER LIQUID
INNER LIQUID

MEMBRANES:
THIN, GAUZE-LIKE MEMBRANE

SHELL MEMBRANE: covers egg shell and protects it from contamination.

POROUS EGG MEMBRANE

CHALAZA: This rope-like bit of egg white surrounds the yolk and holds it in place with extra strength at each end. As egg gets old it weakens and the yolk and white spread.

EGGSHELL: a soft but firm calcium cover

YOLK

GERM: as in a human being, is exactly in center of egg yolk. This is the part that is fertilized to make the chick.

CHALAZA

air cell for the egg to "breathe"

The fatty acids and cholesterol content is as follows:

	Total Saturated		Unsaturated Fatty Acid (μg)		Cholesterol μg
	Total Fat	Fat μg	Oleic	Linoleic	
Eggs, whole	11.5	6	5	1	468
yolks only	30.6	10	13	2	1500

The nutrient value of an egg is as follows:

Food and Description	Wt. gm	Approximate Measure	Food Energy cal	Protein gm	Fat gm	Carbohydrate Total gm	Carbohydrate Fiber gm	Water gm
Eggs, fresh, stored or frozen:								
Raw or cooked:								
Whole	100	2 medium	163	13	12	1	0	74
	50	1 medium	81	7	6	tr.	0	38
White	100	3 medium	51	11	0	1	0	89
	31	1 medium	16	3	0	tr.	0	27
Yolk	100	6 medium	348	16	31	1	0	51
	17	1 medium	58	3	5	tr.	0	9

Food and Description	Wt. Gm.	Approximate Measure	Minerals Calcium μg	Minerals Phosphorus μg	Minerals Iron μg	Vitamins Vitamin A I.U.	Vitamins Thiamine μg	Vitamins Riboflavin μg	Vitamins Niacin μg	Ascorbic Acid μg
Whole	100	2 medium	54	205	2.3	1,180	0.10	0.29	0.1	0
	50	1 medium	27	102	1.2	590	0.05	0.15	tr.	0
White	100	3 medium	9	15	0.1	0	0	0.27	0.1	0
	31	1 medium	3	5	tr.	0	0	0.08	tr.	0
Yolk	100	6 medium	141	569	5.5	3,400	0.27	0.44	0.1	0
	17	1 medium	24	96	0.9	580	0.05	0.07	tr.	0

† One whole egg contains about 2 μg of *cobalamin* * (vitamin B_{12})

albumins in the white of the egg, have the highest *biological value* (BV) for human adults of all food proteins and serves as a standard for comparison with other proteins. One large egg = 80 calories. See *biological value*. Most of the yellow color of yolks is xanthophyll (lutein) which is a carotenoid but not a *retinol* * (vitamin A) *precursor*. There is little or no *ascorbic acid* * (vitamin C). An egg contains about 300 mg of *cholesterol* * and when eaten in large numbers may raise the blood cholesterol level. The anatomy of an egg is shown below.

eggplant (*Solanum melongena*). The eggplant is an erect branching plant closely related to the potato. It is cultivated for its fruit which is eaten as a vegetable. The fruit, which in reality is a berry, varies in length from 2 to 12 inches. Its shiny surface may be dark purple, white, red, yellowish, or even striped, depending upon the variety. Eggplant is grown in different sizes and shapes; round, oblong, pearshape and long. Little nutritive value can be found in eggplant, but it adds variety to the menu. Raw, 100 gm = 25 calories.

EKG. See *electrocardiogram*.

elastic tissue. A fibrous connective tissue composed of elastic fibers and found in the walls of blood vessels, in the lung, and in certain ligaments. The protein content of elastic tissue is mostly *elastin* and *collagen*.

elastin. Insoluble yellow elastic protein in connective tissue.

elderberry. A fruit of the elder (*Sambucus*), a wild shrub of the Sambucus family, with white flowers and purple-black or red berries. There are several varieties, with the flowers growing in saucerlike flat clusters and the berries growing in heavy clusters. Elderberries lack acid and eaten raw have a rank flavor and odor. When properly prepared with the addition of lemon juice, crab apples or sour grapes, they are excellent. They are used for making jellies and jams, and most famous for homemade wines. Elderberries can also be dried or stewed and used for making muffins and pies. Raw, 100 gm = 72 calories.

electrocardiogram (EKG). An electrical test used both as screening test for heart disease, and as a diagnostic test in heart disease. The K in EKG derives from the German spelling.

electroencephalogram (EEG). An electrical test based on "brain waves"; used in neurological examinations.

electrolytes. Chemical compounds that dissociate in water, breaking up into separated hydrated particles carrying a charge called *ions*, are known as electrolytes and the process is referred to as ionization. Salts, acids, and bases are electrolytes. Compounds such as *glucose* * and *urea* *, are called nonelectrolytes because they are molecules that do not ionize, i.e., they carry no charge. Each ion, the dissociated particle of an electrolyte carries an electric charge, either negative or positive. Positive ions (cations) in the body fluids include *sodium* (Na^+), *potassium* (K^+), *calcium* (Ca^{++}), and *magnesium* (Mg^{++}). The negative ions (anions) include *chloride* (Cl^-), *bicarbonate* HCO_3^-), *phosphate* (PO_4^{---}), and sulfate (SO_4^{--}), ions or organic acids such as *lactate* *, *pyruvate* *, and *aceto-acetate* *. Proteins are polyelectrolytes (carry many charges) and may be positively or negatively charged. Sodium ion (Na^+) is the major cation in plasma and *interstitial fluid* and chloride ion (Cl^-) is the major ion. The major cation in intracellular fluid is potassium ion (K^+) and the major anion is phosphate (PO_4^{---}). Other ions are present in varying amounts in the different body fluids.

electron transport (terminal respiratory chain). A complex sequence of enzymes that transfers electrons to oxygen to reduce it to and form water immediately. The oxygen comes from the respiration (the air breathed in) and the electrons come from the food and from metabolites being oxidized to carbon dioxide (CO_2), water (H_2O) and energy. See *terminal respiratory chain*.

electrophoresis. A method for separating molecules or compounds or metals based upon their electric charge (positive or negative) under a given set of conditions. The rate of migration of a molecule in an electric field is determined by its size and the number and kind (positive or negative) charged groups per molecule.

elemental analysis. Human body elementary composition (adult).

Oxygen	65%	Sulfur	0.25%
Carbon	18%	Sodium	0.15%
Hydrogen	10%	Chlorine	0.15%
Nitrogen	3.0%	Magnesium	0.05%
Calcium	1.5–2.2%	Iron	0.004%
Phosphorus	0.8–1.2%	Manganese	0.0003%
Potassium	0.35%	Copper	0.00015%
		Iodine	0.00004%

emaciation. A wasted condition of the body.

Embden-Meyerhoff pathway. See *glycolysis*.

emboli. Blood clots which form inside a blood vessel, contract and tend to become adherent to the vessel wall. When the free margin comes in contact with fluid blood, fresh blood clots may form. At this stage the clot is very liable to break away. Free-floating blood clots are called emboli and obstructions of a blood vessel by emboli are called embolic obstructions. Such embolic obstructions in the heart are called *myocardial infarcts* and in the brain are called strokes.

embolism. The obstruction of a blood vessel by a clot, plug of fat or other substance brought there by the blood. An obstruction due to a bubble of air or gas is an air embolism.

emesis. See *vomiting*.

emollients and protectives. Drug preparations used on the skin and mucous membrane for a soothing effect. Emollients are fatty preparations that soften the skin. An example is cold cream. Protectives are preparations that form a film on the skin. An example is compound tincture of benzoin.

emphysema. From Greek words meaning "overinflated." The overinflated structures are microscopic air sacs of the lungs. Tiny bronchioles through which air flows to and from the air sacs have muscle fibers in their walls. These structures may become hypertrophied and lose elasticity. The air flows into the air sacs easily but cannot flow out easily because of the narrowed diameter of bronchioles. As pressure builds up in the air cells their thin walls are stretched to the point of rupture, the ultimate result is shortness of breath, overwork of the heart, and sometimes death.

empyema. When the fluid within the pleural cavity becomes infected the exudate becomes thick and purulent, and the individual is said to have empyema. The organisms often causing the infection are staphylococcus, streptococcus, or pneumococcus.

emulsification. A process of breaking up large particles of liquid into smaller ones, which remain suspended in another liquid. Emulsification may be done mechanically, as in the homogenization of milk. It may be hastened by chemicals, as by the use of acid and *lecithin* (from egg yolk) in emulsification of oil for mayonnaise. Emulsification occurs naturally in body processes, as when *bile salts* emulsify fats during digestion.

emulsifiers. A group of additives used in the processing of food which permits the dispersion of tiny particles or globules of one liquid in another liquid. For example, oil and vinegar used in a salad dressing will begin to separate as soon as mixing stops. With the addition of an emulsifier, they stay combined long after mixing stops. Similarly an emulsifier enables oil and water to mix and stay mixed. Emulsifiers, sometimes called "surfactants" (for surface active agents), are used to improve keeping qualities and homogeneity of certain candies and confections. Emulsifiers usually contain water soluble and fat soluble portions in the same molecule. *Lecithin*, for example, contains fatty acid as the fat-soluble portion, and phosphate and choline as the water-soluble portion, and is a commonly used emulsifier.

emulsify. To make into an emulsion. When small drops of one liquid are finely dispersed (distributed) in another liquid, an emulsion is formed. These drops are held in suspension by emulsifiers, which surround each drop and make a coating around it. Soap's cleansing action results from emulsifying oily dirt.

emulsion. A system of two immiscible liquids such as oil and water, in which one is finely divided and held in suspension by another. The fine division may be by mechanical means as in *homogenization* or by the action of an *emulsifier*.

endergonic. A reaction that proceeds only with an input of energy. The opposite of exergonic. Most anabolic (biosynthetic) reactions are endergonic.

endive (*Cichorium endiva*). A salad green which is a member of the family of plants to which *chicory* also belongs. The endive is a plant with narrow, finely divided, curly leaves and is often called "curly endive." It grows in a loose-leaved head. Two other salad greens closely related to endive are escarole, which has broad waved leaves and a blanched heart, and witloof, or Belgian endive, which is 4 to 6 inches in length and 1 to 2 inches thick. The leaves of Belgian endive are white with light-green tips press close together to form a cylinder which tapers off to a point. Endive has a slightly bitter flavor and is used practically only in salads. A good source of vitamin A and a fair source of iron. Curly endive, raw, 100 gm = 20 calories. Belgian endive, raw, 100 gm = 17 calories.

endocrine. Applied to organs whose function it is to secrete internally a *hormone* which plays an important role in metabolism.

endocrine glands. All glands are organs made up of a variety of tissues that aid in secretion of substances needed by the body. These endocrine glands, or ductless glands, have no "pipelines" for their secretions. Endocrine glands discharge their secretions directly into the blood vessels that pass through them. The endocrine gland secretions, called *hormones,* are carried throughout the body by the circulatory system. Depending on the nature of the hormone produced and the characteristics of the cells it encounters, an endocrine gland may affect the functioning of cells, organs, and tissues in widespread locations throughout the body. Therefore, a gland is endocrine if it produces a hormone that (1) is specific to that gland, (2) is distributed by the bloodstream throughout the body, and (3) has a specific influence on some other part of the body, a target tissue or organ. See *endocrine system.*

endocrine system. The endocrine system is made up of the endocrine glands (ductless glands). These glands are located in different parts of the body. Secretions produced by endocrine glands are *hormones,* which are secreted directly into the circulatory blood, reach every part of the body and influence the activities of specific organs and tissues, as well as the activities of the body as a whole. Small in quantity but powerful in action, hormones are part of the body's chemical coordinating and regulatory system. There are six recognized endocrine glands; the *thyroid, parathyroid, adrenals, pituitary* (hypophysis),

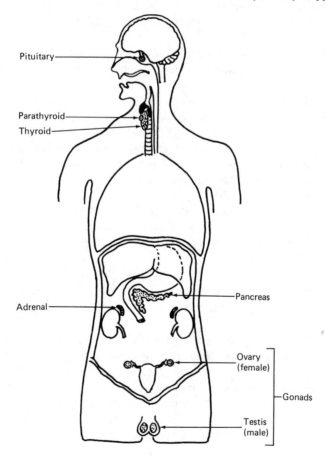

the *testes* or *ovaries* (the male and female gonads respectively), and the *pancreas*. Shown are the endocrine organs.

endogenous. Originating in the cells or tissues of the body.

endogenous carbohydrates. Carbohydrates synthesized from materials within the tissues. Even when the principal supply of carbohydrate for body use comes from dietary or *exogenous* sources, glucose is synthesized within the body. In the breakdown of *fat, protein* and *carbohydrate,* they may be converted to the simple sugar, glucose. Approximately 10 percent of dietary fat and approximately 50 percent of dietary protein may be transformed into carbohydrate in this way.

endoplasmic recticulum. Found within many areas of *cytoplasm* as a network of *vesicles*. These are pairs of parallel membranes sometimes studded with *ribosomes* which contain *ribonucleic acid* (RNA). In certain cells ribosomes are present without the endoplasmic reticulum. They are the site of protein synthesis and are crucial elements in the cell.

endosperm. The nutritive substance within the embryo sac of plants. The starchy portion within the kernel of wheat, corn, or other cereal, from which refined flavor is produced after the germ and fibrous outer layers are removed.

endosteum. The narrow cavities and *haversian canals* in bony tissue are lined with a membrane called endosteum. During bone growth it is formed by a delicate layer of connective tissue. Beneath it lies a layer of osteoblasts. After growth ceases, the cells become flattened and the two layers are indistinguishable. A stimulus for bone formation, such as an injury, activates these cells.

endothelium. A smooth, thin, glistening tissue made up of flat pavementlike cells which, in continuity, line the chambers of the heart, arteries, arterioles, capillaries, and veins of the entire body.

energy. The capacity of a system for doing work; available power. Energy is manifested in various forms, motion, position, light, electrical, heat, chemical, and sound. Energy is interchangeable among the various forms and is constantly being transformed and transferred among them. Energy metabolism may be defined as the chemical reactions in the oxidation of the foodstuffs (*protein, fat,* and *carbohydrate*) by which energy is interchanged, produced, used, and heat given off. The energy or caloric value of foods depends primarily upon the chemical composition, i.e., upon the relative amounts of the three primary energy nutrients, *carbohydrates, fats* and *proteins* that they contain. The energy value of food is determined either by complete combustion in a *calorimeter* experimentally or by calculations from its content of the primary energy nutrients. The average heat of combustion of pure energy nutrients experimentally determined in kcal per gram are as follows: carbohydrate, 4.1; fat, 9.45; protein, 5.65; and alcohol, 7.1. In body, the energy retained by combustion is slightly less, due to incomplete absorption or incomplete combustion or both. Foods with high energy value on the basis of a unit of weight are either rich in fat or low in water content. Thus, all the fatty foods, such as butter, nuts, cream cheese, mayonnaise, bacon, are relatively high in calorie value, as are foods low in moisture content, such as dried fruits, cookies, candy bars, etc. Foods of low-energy value include most fresh fruits and vegetables, especially green leafy vegetables, since these foods have a high content of both water and fiber. Lean meats, cereal foods, and starchy vegetables are intermediate in energy value

energy balance. In metabolism, the energy balance follows the first law of thermodynamics which under ideal conditions states that the work energy done is equal to the heat energy produced. It is a statement of the law of the conservation of energy. In an elegant study by Atwater and Benedict, it was shown that a balance exists between the energy taken in a food and the energy used by man in its various forms. In other words, the first law of thermodynamics applies to man. When the energy balance is perfect, there is a balance of weight, that is, the weight remains constant. When the energy in foodstuffs (fat, carbohydrates, and protein) exceeds the expenditure of energy, then the excess energy is stored in the body in the form of fat, and there is a gain in weight. When the energy in foodstuffs is less than the expenditure of energy, then there is a weight loss. During a diet, for example, the energy intake is less than the energy used and the difference is made up by burning the fat in the body and there is a weight loss equivalent to the fat metabolized. While in practice weight loss follows these simple conditions, the observed weight loss, in particular, or weight gain in an individual is often complicated by water retention. Water retention is influenced by the type of diet, and the tendency to retain water varies among individuals. (See *water balance.*) In computing an energy balance, the energy intake is easily determined by measure of the total calories in the food ingested. The energy used up or expended is more difficult to determine exactly. A *basal metabolic rate* (BMR) must be determined plus the energy consumed by the activities of the individual which produces heat. The Recommended Dietary Allowance for energy takes into account sex, body size, age and activity. Unlike the Recommended Daily Allowance, there is no margin for error in the energy allowance since increase intake results in increased weight.

The chart below represents approximations of the heat production (energy expenditures) per day based on National Research Council findings.

Energy balance = Energy intake minus energy output (heat production).

       Energy intake = 1. Food energy

                      2. Metabolic heat

                      3. Environmental heat

    Energy output =   1. Energy in excreta*

                      2. Heat lost to the environment.

*This represents undigested food in the feces and foodstuffs only partially oxidized. Fat and carbohydrates are completely oxidized to carbon dioxide, water and energy. Protein is not completely oxidized and *urea* * in urine represents the unoxidized carbon (potential energy) of protein that is excreted.

The table below shows the heat production (energy expenditures) associated with various types of physical activity and can be used to calculate the amount of weight (fat) loss. An energy expenditure of about 3500 calories is equivalent to 1 pound (454 gm) of weight (fat).

Recommended Daily Dietary Allowances for Energy*

	Age Years	Weight kg	lb	Energy kcal		Age Years	Weight kg	lb	Energy kcal
Infants	0.0–0.5	6	14	kg × 117	Males (cont.)	23–50	70	154	2700
	0.5–1.0	9	20	kg × 108		51+	70	154	2400
Children	1–3	13	28	1300	Females	11–14	44	97	2400
	4–6	20	44	1800		15–18	54	119	2100
	7–10	30	66	2400		19–22	58	128	2100
Males	11–14	44	97	2800		23–50	58	128	2000
	15–18	61	134	3000		51+	58	128	1800
	19–22	67	147	3000	Pregnancy				+300
					Lactation				+500

*Food and Nutrition Board: *Recommended Dietary Allowances*, National Academy of Sciences—National Research Council, Washington, D.C., 1974.

enriched. A food may be labeled "enriched" if it contains added nutrients in kinds and amounts meeting standards established by the Food and Drug Administration. Enriched bread may be made from enriched flour or by the addition of the required substance to the baker's formula or by the use of special high-vitamin yeast and iron. Enriched flour is white flour enhanced in *thiamine* *, *riboflavin* *, *niacin* *, and iron value by changing the milling process to return these constituents or by the addition of chemical to white flour. (See *wheat*). The minimum levels in the standards of identity promulgated under the

Energy Expenditures by a 150-Pound Person in Various Activities

Activity	Gross Energy Cost— kcal. per hr
A. Rest and Light Activity	50–200 per hr.
Lying down or sleeping	80
Sitting	100
Driving an automobile	120
Standing	140
Domestic work	180
B. Moderate Activity	200–350 per hr.
Bicycling (5½ mph)	210
Walking (2½ mph)	210
Gardening	220
Canoeing (2½ mph)	230
Golf	250
Lawn mowing (power mower)	250
Bowling	270
Lawn mowing (hand mower)	270
Fencing	300
Rowboating (2½ mph)	300
Swimming (¼ mph)	300
Walking (3¾ mph)	300
Badminton	350
Horseback riding (trotting)	350
Square dancing	350
Volleyball	350
Rollerskating	350
C. Vigorous Activity	over 350 per hr.
Table tennis	360
Ditch digging (hand shovel)	400
Ice skating (10 mph)	400
Wood chopping or sawing	400
Tennis	420
Water skiing	480
Hill climbing	490
Skiing (10 mph)	600
Squash and handball	600
Cycling (13 mph)	660
Scull rowing (race)	840
Running (10 mph)	900

*The standards represent a compromise between those proposed by the British Medical Association (1950), Christensen (1953), and Wells, Balke, and Van Fossan (1956). Where available, actual measured values have been used; for other values a "best guess" was made. Prepared by Robert E. Johnson, M.D., Ph.D., and colleagues, Department of Physiology and Biophysics, University of Illinois, August, 1967. (From Exercise and Weight Control, Committee on Exercise and Physical Fitness of the American Medical Association, and the President's Council on Physical Fitness in cooperation with the Lifetime Sports Foundation.)

Food, Drug and Cosmetic Act are given in the table below. Certain levels of *vitamin D* * and calcium are permitted as optional ingredients. See *fortified* also.

Enrichment Standards Required for 1 Pound of Cereal-Bread Products

Name of Food	Minimum to Maximum Requirements For			
	Thiamine mg	Riboflavin mg	Niacin mg	Iron mg
Bread & rolls	1.1–1.8	0.7–1.6	10.0–15.0	8.0–12.5
Flour	2.0–2.5	1.2–1.5	16.0–20.0	13.0–16.5
Cornmeal grits	2.0–3.0	1.2–1.8	16.0–24.0	13.0–26.0
Macaroni-noodles	4.0–5.0	1.7–2.2	27.0–34.0	13.0–16.5

*Source: U.S. National Archives, Code of Federal Register, Title 21, Food and Drug, 1955, with supplement to 1957.

enteritis. Inflammation of the intestine.

entero. Combining term denoting intestine.

enterocrinin. Hormone of small intestine that stimulates secretion of *intestinal juice*.

enterogastrone. *Hormone* secreted by duodenal (*duodenum*) mucosa upon stimulation by the presence of fat in the small intestine. It also inhibits secretion of gastric juice and reduces intestinal motility (peristalis).

enterohepatic circulation. The circulation of *bile* from the liver to the *gallbladder*, then into the intestine, from which it is absorbed, and carried by the blood back to the liver to be returned to circulation. This continual circulation efficiently conserves the bile which is required. For the 20 to 30 gm of bile used daily by the body, only about 0.8 gm is eliminated in the feces and must be replenished by the liver.

enterokinase. A proteolytic enzyme which activates the *trypsin* by a partial hydrolysis of *trypsinogen* of the pancreatic fluid. Trypsin is one of several proteolytic enzymes (proteases) involved in the digestion of food protein.

enteropathy. Any disease of the intestine.

enterotoxin. A toxin specific for the cells of the intestinal mucosa and arising in the intestine.

enzymatic. Related to that class of protein substances called enzymes which serve as biological catalysts. See *enzyme*.

enzymes. Enzymes are biological catalysts. They speed up the rate of chemical reactions in the body. Enzymes are *proteins* and have all of the properties of proteins in general. The *amino acid* composition of the enzymes determine their physical, chemical and catalytic properties. Enzymes range in size from molecular weights of a few thousand to a few million. The structural complexity of enzymes also varies from simple *polypeptide* chains composed only of amino acids to complex proteins which may contain metals, carbohydrates, lipids, or other smaller organic molecules as integral parts of the structure. Many enzymes require a *cofactor* or *coenzyme* in order to be active. Most of the coenzymes are vitamins. An enzyme that requires a coenzyme is described as an *apoenzyme* when the coenzyme is absent and a *holoenzyme* when the coenzyme is attached to the apoenzyme. Each cell in the body contains a few thousand different enzymes. Without enzymes, the complex chemical changes which constitute the metabolism of the body would be impossible. They are responsible for a variety of chemical processes such as *oxidation, reduction, hydrolysis,* and the building up or synthesis of simpler molecules into more complex structures. Some of these processes involve numerous enzymes, each one performing one step in turn, until the end product is reached. Most enzymes act within their parent cells but some leave the cell to act in the surrounding fluids such as the enzymes of the *digestive system.* Enzymes are highly specific and react upon a limited number of chemical substances called *substrates,* to produce specific end products. Enzymes are usually named by adding ''ase'' to the name of the substrate or sometimes adding ''ase'' to the particular chemical reaction which they produce. Some important groups of enzymes are: (1) Esterases; (a) Lipases digest fats; (b) Cholinesterase hydrolyses acetyl-choline; (c) Phosphatases remove phosphate (PO_4); (2) Carbohydrates; (a) Amylase hydrolses *starch *;* (b) *Maltase* hydrolyses *maltose *;* (c) Lactase hydrolyses *lactose *;* (3) Proteases: (a) Proteinase, *pepsin* and *trypsin* which

Enzyme	Source	Reaction Catalyzed
Chymotrypsin	Pancreas	Proteins to polypeptides
Enterokinase	Duodenal mucosa	Trypsinogen to trypsin
Gastric lipase	Gastric glands	Fats to glycerides
Lactase	Intestinal glands	Lactose to glucose and galactose
Maltase	Intestinal glands	Maltose to glucose
Pancreatic amylase	Pancreas	Starch to disaccharides
Pancreatic lipase	Pancreas	Fats to fatty acids
Pepsin	Gastric glands	Proteins to polypeptides
Peptidase	Intestinal glands	Peptides to amino acids
Ptyalin	Salivary glands	Begins carbohydrate digestion
Rennin	Gastric glands	Clots milk
Sucrase	Intestinal glands	Sucrose to glucose and fructose
Trypsin	Pancreas	Proteins to polypeptides

break down proteins (b) Peptidases attack partially digested proteins (peptides). The major digestive enzymes are given below:

Many of the digestive enzymes occur in inactive forms and are given the general name *zymogen*. For example, *trypsinogen* is an inactive form (a zymogen) of *trypsin*. In the presence of *enterokinase,* a proteolytic enzyme, a *polypeptide* is removed from trypsinogen thereby converting it to the active enzyme trypsin. The trypsin will in turn degrade the protein in food to *polypeptides* during the digestive process. Several enzymes and *hormones* have active and inactive forms.

epidermis. A stratified squamous epithelium, consisting of a variable number of layers of cells. It varies in thickness in different parts, being thickest on the palms of the hands and on the soles of the feet. It forms a protective covering over every part of the true skin and is closely molded on the papillary layer of the corium. The four regions of the epidermis going from the outside inward, are the stratum corneum, the stratum lucidum, the stratum granulosum, and the stratum germinativum (mucosum).

epiglottis. The cartilage in the throat which guards the entrance to the trachea and prevents fluid or food from entering it when a person swallows.

epinephrine (adrenaline). Mol. Wt. 183. The "emergency of flight or fight hormone" is an enzyme activator AMP-cyclase which in turn initiates a series of enzyme activations. In times of stress, small amounts of epinephrine are discharged from the adrenal glands into the bloodstream. Epinephrine ultimately causes the release of a flood of glucose molecules from the liver into the bloodstream for quick energy for the muscles. One epinephrine molecule is thought to cause the release of about 30,000 molecules of glucose. Epinephrine is one of a pair of optical isomers. Only the isomer that rotates polarized light to the left, L-epinephrine, is effective in starting a heart that has stopped beating or in giving a person more energy during times of great emotional stress. Epinephrine is synthesized from the essential amino acid *tyrosine* * and also requires *ascorbic acid* * (vitamin C) for that synthesis.

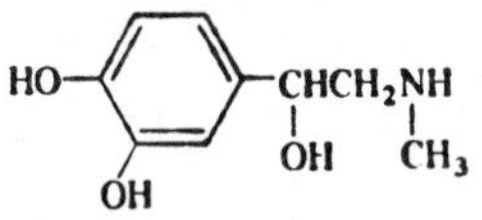

$$HO-\bigcirc-CHCH_2NH$$
$$\begin{matrix} | & | \\ OH & CH_3 \end{matrix}$$
$$OH$$

Epinephrine (adrenaline)

epithelial. Refers to those cells that form the outer layer of the skin, or epithelium.

epithelium. The outermost layers of the skin and the mucous membranes, consisting of cells of various forms and arrangement. The epithelium lines all the portions of the body that have contact with the external air (such as the eyes, ears, nose, throat, lungs), and those that are specialized for secretions as the *liver, kidneys, urinary* and *reproductive tracts.* Plain columnar epithelium are cells that have a cylindrical shape and are set upright on the surface which they cover. Columnar epithelium is found in its most characteristic form lining the stomach, small and large intestines, digestive glands, and gallbladder. The chief functions of the columnar epithelium are the secretion of digestive fluids and adsorption of digested food and fluids. See *tissue.*

ergocalciferol (vitamin D$_2$, calciferol). Mol. Wt. 397. Vitamin D$_2$ derived from *ergosterol* * by the action of light. Ergosterol comes from yeasts. The first crystalline *vitamin D* was obtained in 1931 and was synthesized shortly thereafter. Soon it became evident that there were at least 10 natural substances which exert vitamin D-like activity in varying degrees, but only two of these are of practical importance from the standpoint of their occurrence in foods, ergocalciferol (vitamin D$_2$) and cholecalciferol (vitamin D$_3$). See *vitamin D.*

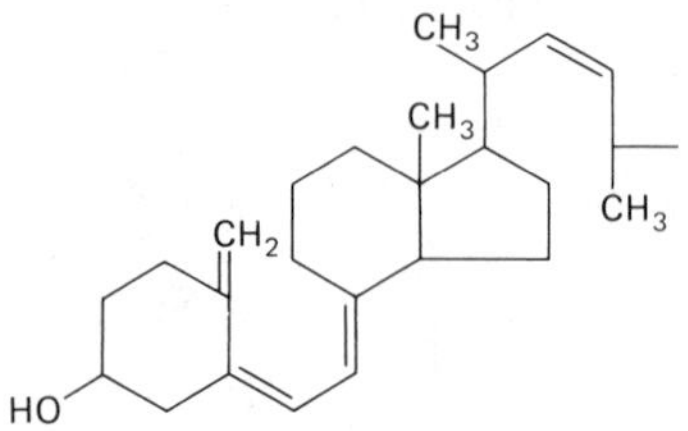

Ergocalciferol

ergosterol. Mol. Wt. 397. A substance belonging to the class of sterols that is found chiefly in yeasts and molds. It is white and crystalline and similar in appearance to the material that candles are made of. On exposure to ultra-violet light it is converted to vitamin D$_2$ (ergocalciferol). See *vitamin D.*

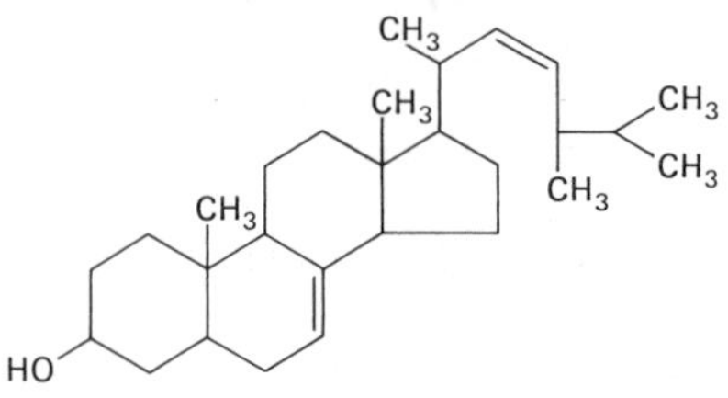

Ergosterol

ergot. A fungus found on cereal grain; used in medicine as a hemostatic.

erythrocyte. See *red blood cells.*

erucic acid. A fatty acid. Long been known as obtainable from the seed oils of cruciferous plants, such as the commercial fatty oils of rapeseed and of mustard seed. It also has been found in marine animal oils. Oleic and erucic acids are the best known members of the series $C_n H_{2n} O_2$.

erythema. Reddness of the skin produced by congestion or dilation of the capillaries.

Erythrocyte Sedimentation Rate (ESR). A test which measures the length of time it takes the red cells in a sample of whole blood to separate from the plasma and settle to the bottom of a glass test tube.

erythropoiesis. The formation of red blood cells.

Escherichia coli **(bacteria).** *Escherichia coli* belong to a group of true rod-shaped bacilli which normally live in the human intestinal tract. This bacillus is found in the intestinal tract and in the skin of the perineal area. When introduced into wounds, it produces infection characterized by light-brown plus with a fecal odor. *Escherichia coli* and other intestinal flora serve man by providing *vitamin K* and some of the B-vitamins.

esophagus. The esophagus is a musclar tube about 10 inches long, lined with a mucous membrane. It leads from the pharynx through the chest to the upper end of the stomach. Its function is to complete the act of swallowing. The involuntary movement of material down the esophagus is carried out by the process known as *peristalsis,* which is the wavelike action produced by contractions and relaxations of the muscular wall. Peristalsis is the method by which food is moved throughout the alimentary canal.

escarole (*Cichorium*). A salad green which is a type of *endive* with broad waved leaves. Often the heart is blanched. Its flavor is somewhat bitter. Escarole and endive can be used interchangeably in salads and in cooking. As a green leafy vegetable it provides a fair amount of iron, is rich in *retinol* * (vitamin A), and has small amounts of other vitamins and minerals. Raw, 100 gm = 20 calories.

essential amino acids. There are some 22 *amino acids,* each of them a separate chemical entity having certain characteristics in common with all others. Eight of these 22 are known as "essential" for adult human beings, because they must be supplied ready made in foods. The body cannot synthesize them from foods at the rate needed, nor can it derive enough of them from the breakdown of tissue proteins. The eight essential amino acids are, *lysine*, tryptophan*, phenylalanine*, methionine*, threonine*, leucine*,* and *valine**. An additional one, *histidine** is essential for infants. Practically all of the 22 amino acids are present in most proteins in greater or lesser amounts, but the amounts and proportions of the 8 essential amino acids determine whether proteins are of high or low quality.

essential fatty acids (EFA). An essential fatty acid is one which is necessary for normal nutrition and which cannot be synthesized by the body from other substances. *Linoleic acid** the polyunsaturated fatty acid most abundant in nature is the main essential fatty acid to be considered. *Linolenic acid** is also considered an essential fatty acid. The exact function of linoleic acid and its derivatives in the body is not well understood but such acids are known to be essential structural elements for synthesis of tissue lipids and *prostaglandins*.

esterase. An enzyme that catalyzes the hydrolysis of esters to form an organic acid and an alcohol. Acetylcholine esterase, for example, hydrolyzes *acetylcholine** to form *acetic acid** and *choline** an amino alchoool.

esters. Organic acids react with alcohols to form a class of compounds called esters. Esters are neutral. When ethyl alcohol is mixed with acetic acid in the presence of sulfuric acid, sweet-smelling ethyl acetate is formed. This reaction is a dehydration in which sulfuric acid acts as a *catalyst*. Ethyl acetate is a common solvent and is used in fingernail remover. Some of the odors of common fruits are due to the presence of mixtures of naturally formed volatile esters. In contrast, higher molecular weight esters often have a distinctly unpleasant odor. Fats and waxes are examples of esters with high molecular weights.

ACID	ALCOHOL		ESTER	
$CH_3CO(OH + H)O\ CH_2CH_3$		$\longrightarrow$	$CH_3COOCH_2CH_3 + H_2O$	
Acetic acid	Ethyl alcohol	Acid catalyst	Ethyl acetate	Water

estradiol-17β. Mol. Wt. 272. One of the class of steroid hormones called *estrogens* or female sex hormones. The steroid hormones are *cholesterol** derivatives. See *estrogens* and *estrone**.

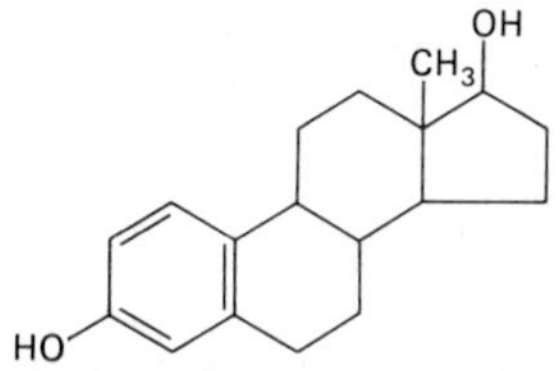

Estradiol-17β

estrogens. A class of steroid hormones that control the appearance of secondary female characteristics. They are the biological opposites of *androgens,* the male sex hormones. Estrogens are produced by the follicles of the ovaries. The compounds *estradiol** and *estrone** are examples of estrogens. The estrogens promote protein synthesis; cause a marked increase in phospholipid metabolism; and cause elevation of serum calcium and phosphorus with prolonged administrations.

estrone. Mol. Wt. 270. One of a class of steroid hormones called *estrogens* or female sex hormones. The steroid hormones are *cholesterol** derivatives. See *estrogens* and *estradiol**.

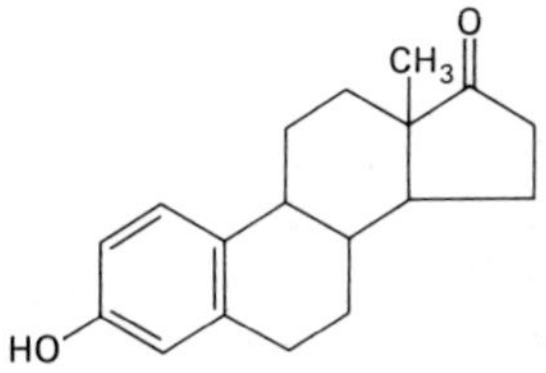

Estrone

etiology. The cause of a disease.

ethanol (ethyl alcohol, grain alcohol). Mol. Wt. 46. CH_3CH_2OH An alcohol which is distilled from the products of anaerobic fermentation of carbohydrate by microorganisms, yeast in particular, yields about 7 calories per gram, of which more than 75 percent is available to the body. Sugar or some form of carbohydrate is also frequently added to alcoholic beverages. A pint of beer, 4 percent alcohol, yields about 200 calories; a glass of wine 10 percent alcohol has about 75 calories, and an ounce of distilled liquor such as whisky, brandy, gin, or rum, yields from 75 to 80 calories. Ethanol is considered as "fattening" because it is burned in preference to fat. No individual substance is fattening, however, weight gain or loss depends upon total caloric uptakes and expenditures. (See *energy balance*.) Ethanol is addictive and is the major drug problem in many countries.

evaporated milk. See *milk products*.

exacerbation. Increase in severity of a symptom or disease.

excretion. The process by which the body rids itself of waste products. The pathways for the removal of waste products are the lungs, skin, kidneys, and intestine. True waste products fall into four general categories; materials that cannot be digested and absorbed; materials that, although absorbed, cannot be utilized; materials that are consumed or produced in the body in larger amounts than the body can use or is able to store; the end products of the metabolism of foodstuffs, chiefly urea and excess carbon dioxides. *Urea* and other soluble nitrogenous substances leave the body almost entirely in the urine through the *kidneys*. Excess carbon dioxide is excreted by the lungs.

exogenous. Originating or produced from an outside source.

exergonic. A reaction that proceeds with a release of energy. The opposite of *endergonic*. Many *catabolic* reactions (degradations) are exergonic.

extracellular. Situated or occurring outside the cells.

extracellular fluid (ECF). The body water is not a continuous mass but is divided roughly into two main compartments, the intracellular fluid (ICF) and extracellular fluid (ECF). About 60 percent of the total body water is found within the cells (the intracellular fluid); the other 40 percent is in various compartments outside the cells (the extracellular fluid). Less than one-fifth of the extracellular fluid is found in the *circulatory system* which is composed mainly of the *lymph* and *blood*.

extrinsic factor. *Cobalamin* * (vitamin B_{12}). Extrinsic factor was a term used prior to identification of the nature of the dietary factor that was required to prevent *pernicious anemia,* in association with an *intrinsic factor*. Literally it means a constituent from the outside. See *cobalamin* * and *pernicious anemia*.

exudate. Material that has escaped from blood vessels and has been deposited in or on tissue, usually as a result of inflammation.

exudation. More often associated with infection and the presence of large numbers of *leukocytes* and dead bacterial cells. The exudate is then known as pus and is composed of plasma and debris from the site of the inflammation. It is helpful in the removal of dead bacteria, tissue cells, and blood cells. It also brings antibodies into the area as well as necessary enzymes, all of which are helpful in removing the debris.

eye. The eye is specialized for the reception of light. Each eye is located in a bony socket or cavity called the orbit, which is formed by several bones in the skull. The orbit provides protection, support, and attachment for the eye and its muscles, nerves, and blood vessels. The interior of the eye is divided into the anterior cavity (anterior to the lens), where a clear watery solution, the aqueous fluid, is formed and circulated. A transparent, semifluid material, the vitreous fluid is contained in the posterior cavity. The globular form and firmness of the eyeball is maintained by its fluid contents, which also functions in the transmission light. The retina contains the rods (night vision) and cones (color vision). It is the rods that contain rhodopsin (visual purple) and which are early affected by a *retinol* * (vitamin A) deficiency known as night blindness (nyctalopia). Retinol (vitamin A) deficiency will also cause a condition known as *conjunctivitis* or inflammation of the conjunctiva.

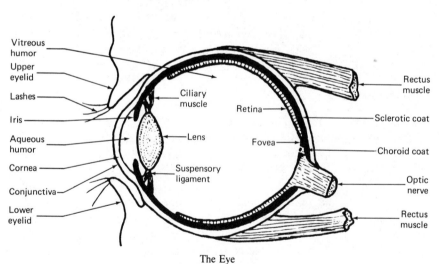

The Eye

F

factor. In nutrition, any chemical substance found in foods. A factor might be a vitamin, a mineral, or any other nutrient or nonnutrient. Usually it has some effect on animal growth or reproduction.

facultative. The ability of some microorganisms to live under *aerobic* or *anaerobic* conditions. *Yeast* is an example of a facultative organism.

FAD. See *flavin adenine dinucleotide.*

farina. A cereal made from hard (but not durum) *wheat,* from which the bran and most of the germ have been removed. It is creamy-colored, rich in protein, and very easily digested. Farina is used as a breakfast cereal, cooked in either water or molk. Dry, 100 gm = 371 calories; cooked 100 gm = 42 calories.

farnoquinone. See *vitamin K.*

fat (neutral fat). All true fats are alike in chemical nature and physical properties, have a greasy feel, are insoluble in water, but are soluble in such solvents as ether and gasoline. Every molecule of a true fat yields on hydrolysis one molecule of *glycerol** (a polyalcohol) and three molecules of *fatty acid.* Fats are glyceryl esters of *fatty acids,* and since *glycerol* contains three alcohol groups (—OH) and the fatty acids contain one carboxylic acid (—COOH) group, that is therefore a *triglyceride.* Hydrolysis yields three molecules of fatty acid and one molecule of glycerol. When the splitting of the fat is brought about by means of an alkali, the corresponding products are glycerol and the alkali salt of the fatty acid; and since alkali salts of the fatty acids are commonly known as soap, this reaction is usually called the *saponification* of the fat. Fats are a structurally distinct group of chemical compounds and the term applies equally to the solid and the liquid members of this group. As a matter of convenience, however, the liquid fats are called *oils.* Many food fats are of animal origin, butter, lard, fatty meats, fish, egg yolk, cream, and full milk cheese. *Palmitic** and *stearic acids** which enter largely into the composition of solid fats are saturated fatty acids. The more highly unsaturated fatty acids

162

(*linoleic**, *linolenic**, and *arachidonic** acids) have two, three and four double bonds per molecule, therefore they are said to be polyunsaturated. These have great nutritional importance. Listed below are some of the important fats and oils and the fatty acid composition.

Fat or Oil	Contains the Glyceryl Ester of	Source of Fat or Oil
Almond oil	Oleic, palmitic, linoleic acids, etc.	Bitter or sweet almonds
Butterfat	Butyric, caproic, capric, palmitic, stearic, oleic acids, etc.	Cow's milk
Cacao butter	Palmitic, oleic, stearic, myristic acids, etc.	Seeds of cacao nibs
Castor oil	Ricinoleic, stearic, oleic acids, etc.	Seeds of castor beans
Coconut oil	Caproic, caprylic, capric, lauric acids, etc.	Seeds of *Cocos nucifera,* kernel of nuts
Cod-liver oil	Oleic, myristic, palmitic, stearic acids, and cholesterol, etc.	Livers of codfish
Cottonseed oil	Oleic, stearic, palmitic, linoleic acids, etc.	Seeds of the cotton plant
Hemp oil	Isolinolenic, oleic acids, etc.	Seeds of hemp
Human fat	Stearic, palmitic, oleic, butyric, caproic acids, etc.	Human beings
Lard	Stearic, palmitic, oleic, linoleic acids, etc.	Body fat of swine
Linseed oil	Linoleic, linolenic, oleic, palmitic, myristic acids, etc.	Seeds of flax
Maize oil	Arachidic, stearic, palmitic, oleic acids, etc.	Seed germs of corn oil
Menhaden oil	Palmitic, myristic, oleic, stearic, and other unsaturrated acids, etc.	Bodies of menhaden fish
Mustard oil	Erucic, arachidic, stearic, oleic acids, etc.	Seeds of mustard
Neat's-foot oil	Palmitic, stearic, oleic acids, etc.	Hoofs of cattle
Olive oil	Linoleic, oleic, arachidic acids, etc.	Fruit of olive tree
Palm oil	Palmitic, lauric, oleic acids, etc.	Palm seed
Peanut oil	Arachidic, linoleic, hypogaeic, palmitic acids, etc.	Peanuts
Poppy oil	Linoleic, isolinolenic, palmitic, stearic acids, etc.	Poppy seeds
Rape oil	Erucic, arachidic, stearic acids, etc.	Rape seeds
Soybean oil	Oleic, linoleic, linolenic acids, etc.	Soybeans
Sperm oil	Oleic, palmitic acids, waxes, etc.	Head and blubber of sperm whale
Tallow	Stearic, palmitic, oleic acids, etc.	Fat of ox or sheep
Whale oil	Linoleic, isolinolenic acids, etc.	Blubber of whales

fat digestion. Digestion of fats takes place chiefly in the small intestine, where the emulsifying action of *bile* from the liver assists in bringing the fat into contact with fat-splitting digestive enzymes from the *pancreas,* and from the intestinal walls. The final products of these actions are two simpler processes, *fatty acids* * and *glycerol* *. These are absorbed through the walls of the small intestines and resynthesized within the intestinal cells to reform fat. During the passage, some of the fat enters the circulation as microscopic droplets of fat called *chylomicrons.* Some small portions of dietary fat passes into the circulation without hydrolysis. The droplets of fat are not in true solution in the blood but are in suspension, much like fat of homogenized milk. The end products of fat digestion pass into the lymph vessels and are carried by the blood directly to the body tissues.

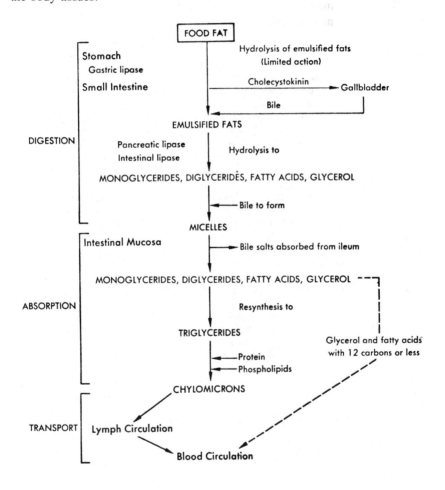

In the tissues fat oxidation is used to supply energy for work and the internal activities of the body. Fats from all sources are digested easily, and almost entirely, if eaten in moderation. Fat that is not needed immediately is stored as body fat. When needed, it is moved into the bloodstream again and is available to the cells for energy. Body weight gains and losses due to diet are almost entirely gains and losses in fat and/or water. The satiety value of fats depends on the fats' slow digestion and the emptying time of the stomach; meals that contain considerable fat remain longer in the stomach and prevent the early recurrence of ''hunger pangs'' that occur when it is empty.

fat metabolism. Fats are constantly being broken down and resynthesized, but they are at equilibrium when the caloric intake is in balance with the heat production. It does not matter from where calories come, fat, carbohydrate, or protein, an excess of caloric intake above energy expenditures will result in the accumulation of fat and a weight gain. When the caloric intake is less than the energy expended, weight is lost. Fat oxidation is the principal source of energy under most circumstances and certainly the major energy source over long periods of time. About 70 percent of the caloric needs of the body derive from fat oxidation. In times of an emergency when a rapid burst of energy is required, the oxidation of *glucose* * meets this temporary need. The oxidation of fat occurs in all tissues, but the liver and the adipose tissue are the principal organs of fat metabolism. The diagram below shows the roles of liver and adipose tissue in fat metabolism.

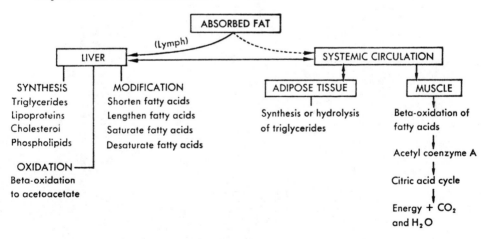

fat-soluble. Refers generally to substances that cannot be dissolved in water but can be in fats and oils, or in fat solvents such as ether or petroleum products.

Fat-Soluble Vitamins

	A	D	E	K
Active Chemical Forms	*Retinol* *Retinal* *Retinoic acid*	Cholecalciferol Ergocalciferol	*Tocopherols* α, β, γ, etc.	Phylloquinone, menaquinone, menadione, watersoluble synthetic forms
Important Food Sources	*Liver* *Egg yolk* *Butter, cream* *Margarine* Green and yellow vegetables *Apricots* *Cantaloupe*	Irradiated foods Small amounts in: *Butter* *Egg yolk* *Liver* *Salmon* *Sardines* *Tuna fish*	*Wheat germ* Leafy vegetables *Vegetable oils* *Egg yolk* *Legumes* *Peanuts* *Margarine*	*Cabbage* *Cauliflower* *Spinach* Other leafy vegetables *Pork liver* *Soybean oil* and other *vegetable oils*
Stability to Cooking, Drying, Light, etc.	Gradual destruction by exposure to air, heat and drying, more rapid at high temperatures	Stable to heating, aging and storage Destroyed by excess ultraviolet irradiation	Stable to methods of food processing Destroyed by *rancidity* and ultraviolet irradiation	Stable to heat, light and exposure to air Destroyed by strong *acids, alkalis* and oxidizing agents
Function	Maintains function of epithelial cells, skin, bone, mucous membranes, visual pigments	*Calcium* and phosphorus absorption and utilization in bone growth	*Antioxidant* in tissues, related to action of selenium	Necessary in formation of prothrombin, essential for clotting of blood
Deficiency: Signs and Symptoms	Night blindness Glare blindness Rough, dry skin Dry mucous membranes *Xerophthalmia*	*Rickets* Soft bones Bowed legs Poor teeth Skeletal deformities	Increased hemolysis of red blood cells *Macrocytic anemia* and dermatitis in infants	Slow clotting time of blood Some hemorrhagic disease of newborn Lack of prothrombin
Recommended Dietary	5000 I.U., when ⅓ from animal sources	Children and adolescents, 400 I.U.	Adult male, 30 I.U. Adult female, 25 I.U.	Unknown

fat-soluble vitamins. The fat soluble vitamins are *retinol* * (vitamin A), *vitamin D* *, *tocopherol* * (vitamin E) and *vitamin K* *. The table on p. 166 is a summary of the fat soluble vitamins, their derivatives, functions, sources, and *Recommended Daily Allowances* (RDA).

fatty acid. A fatty acid is a monocarboxylic acid with a hydrocarbon residue, which may be saturated or unsaturated (containing one or more double bonds). The most abundant of the unsaturated fatty acids is *palmitic acid* * which contains 16 carbons (C_{16}) and *stearic acid* * which is next (C_{18}). Naturally occurring fatty acids up to C_{28} have been shown in animal tissues. *Acetic acid* * (C_2) is also a fatty acid. The most abundant unsaturated fatty acids are *palmitoleic* (C_{16}), *oleic* * (C_{18}), *linoleic* * (C_{18}) and *linolenic* * (C_{18}). Linoleic and linolenic are *essential fatty acids*. The table on pp. 168–169 shows the fatty acid content of several common foods and the calories associated with the fatty acid.

fatty acid synthetase. A complex of seven *enzymes* involved in the synthesis of *fatty acids*, from two carbon units, acetyl-CoA. Two vitamins as coenzyme derivatives are involved in these complex series of reactions. *Pantothenic acid* * is a part of *Coenzyme A* * and as a part of the 4'-phosphopantetheine residue of the protein in the fatty acid synthetase complex called the acyl carrier protein (ACP). Niacin is a part of nicotinamide *adenine dinucleotide phosphate* (NADP) which in its reduced form, NADPH, is required as a cofactor in two steps of the synthesis. The unusual feature of this biosynthetic mechanism is that intermediate stages of the synthesis are not normally observed, and nothing is released from the enzyme until a chain length of 16 carbons is attained.

fatty oils. See *oils,* and *fats*.

favism. Condition caused by eating certain species of fava beans (*Vicia faba*) also known as broadbeans. The symptoms include fever, abdominal pain, headache, anemia, coma.

febrile. Pertaining to fever; feverish, having a fever.

feces. Term feces means "dregs," worthless residue. The quantity of feces formed varies with the quality and quantity of food ingested. Feces is primarily dried digestive juices, it contains about 75 percent water. Bacterial remains makes up about 25 percent of the solid material. The color of feces is due to bacterial action on *urobilinogen* * from bile which is oxidized to urobilin and sterobilin. On an average diet, about 200 gm of feces is excreted in a day. In disorders of the biliary system, feces may appear white, clay-colored, or gray.

Comparison of Fatty Acids and Calories in Common Foods*

Food	Measure	Saturated Fatty Acid		Linoleic (Polyunsaturated) Fatty Acid		Oleic (Monounsaturated) Fatty Acid	
		Grams	Calories	Grams	Calories	Grams	Calories
Fats							
Margarine, soft	1 T.	2	18	4	36	4	36
Butter	1 T.	6	54	trace		4	36
Margarine, firm	1 T.	2	18	3	27	6	54
Lard	1 T.	5	45	1	9	6	54
Corn oil	1 T.	1	9	7	63	4	36
Cottonseed oil	1 T.	4	36	7	63	3	27
Soybean oil	1 T.	2	18	7	63	3	27
Olive oil	1 T.	2	18	1	9	11	99
Meats							
Pork							
bacon	2 slices	3	27	1	9	4	36
roast, fresh	3 oz.	9	81	2	18	10	90
Roast beef	3 oz.	16	144	1	9	15	135
Hamburger, regular	3 oz.	8	72	trace		8	72
lean		5	45	trace		4	36
Steak, broiled	3 oz.	13	117	1	9	12	108
Lamb roast, leg	3 oz.	9	81	trace		6	54
Chicken, flesh only broiled)	3 oz.	1	9	1	9	1	9
Veal breast	3 oz.	7	63	trace		6	54
Salmon, pink, canned	3 oz.	1	9	trace		1	9

Nuts	Almonds, shelled	⅓ c.	2	18	5	45	17	153
	Peanuts, halved	⅓ c.	5	45	7	63	10	90
	Peanut butter	1 T.	2	18	2	18	4	36
	Walnuts, shelled	⅓ c.	1.3	12	12	108	9	81
Other	Milk, whole	1 c.	5	45	trace		3	27
	Milk, nonfat or skim	1 c.	0	0	0		0	0
	Egg, large	1	2	18	trace		3	27
	Avocado	1	7	63	5	45	17	153
	Bread	1 slice						
	white enriched		trace		trace		trace	
	whole wheat		trace		trace		trace	
	Corn muffin	1	2	18	trace		2	18

* Adapted from *Nutritive Value of Foods*, Bulletin No. 72 (Washington, D.C.: USDA, revised 1970).

Fatty stools, usually very light in color, usually indicate a disfunction in the absorption of fatty foods.

feedback control. Feedback control is the regulation of a series of biochemical reactions by the effect of an end product of the series on one of the reaction rates at the beginning of the series of reactions. The series of reactions in the body leading to *cholesterol* * synthesis is an example of a feedback control mechanism. Dietary cholesterol, the *bile salts* * (cholesterol derivatives) and cholesterol synthesized in the body, all serve to inhibit the synthesis of more cholesterol by inhibiting reactions at the beginning of the biosynthetic pathway. Feedback controls usually involve increases in reaction rates.

fennel (*Foeniculum vulgare*). An aromatic plant belonging to the carrot family, native to the Mediterranean. There are three types of fennel, all of which have bright green feathery foliage. Common fennel, is a tall perennial with finely divided feathery leaves and yellow flowers. It has a flavor reminiscent of anise. All parts of the plant can be utilized. The shoots are eaten raw or cooked; the leaves are used for salads and seasoning; and the seeds, which are oval, greenish- or yellowish-brown, are used as a culinary spice for cooking, candy and liqueurs. Fennel oil is used in medicine, perfume and soaps.

fenugreek (*Trigonella foenumgraecum*). An annual plant of the pea family cultivated chiefly for its aromatic seeds. The seeds are formed in a slender, beanlike pod with a beaked point. They are threshed from the pods and dried by artificial heat. They are small, irregularly shaped, and yellow-brown in color. Their flavor is pleasantly bitter, somewhat like burnt sugar. The seeds are used for curry powders, chutney, and spice blends.

fermentation. Fermentation is the result of the enzymatic reactions of microorganisms with carbohydrates, particularly *glucose*. For example, the end product of glucose fermentation by yeast is alcohol and serves as the basis for the wine production where the source of the glucose is the grape. Another example of fermentation is the souring of milk where *lactic acid* * is formed by the action of *Lactobacillus casei* on *lactose* * (milk sugar). In the pathways of fermentation, except for the final step, are almost identical in man and yeast. In man, *lactic acid* * is formed in muscle and in yeast it is *ethanol* *. The vitamin *niacin* * is important in this fermentation path, in yeast and man, as the *coenzyme nicotinamide adenine dinucleotide* * (NAD).

ferritin. An iron-containing protein with a molecular weight 450,000. Ferritin is the form in which iron is stored in the liver, spleen, intestinal mucosa, and recticuloendothelium of cells. The normal male liver contains about 700 mg of iron. Once iron is inside the intestinal mucosal cell, it can be either transferred (and later released) to the tissues with the aid of a serum protein known as *transferrin,* or it can be stored in the mucosal cell or other body cells in the form of ferritin. Discovered in 1937, ferritin is the major form in which iron is stored in the body, representing about 10 to 20 percent of iron by weight in its molecule. The iron is in the oxidized or ferric state. No other biological substance has this great capacity to store a heavy metal.

ferrous gluconate. Mol. Wt. 482. The iron salt of *gluconic acid*,* a chemical which is present naturally in the body. Used by the pharmaceutical industry as an iron supplement in vitamin pills and by olive growers as an artificial coloring. Gluconic acid is a natural product of *glucose** metabolism.

$$\left[\begin{array}{c} COO^- \\ | \\ H\!-\!C\!-\!OH \\ | \\ HO\!-\!C\!-\!H \\ | \\ H\!-\!C\!-\!OH \\ | \\ H\!-\!C\!-\!OH \\ | \\ CH_2OH \end{array} \right]_2 Fe^{++}$$

Ferrous gluconate

fever. Any body temperature above the normal body temperature. Normal body temperature is generally 98.7°F (37°C), although some individuals may vary slightly above or below this value. Hyperthermic fever is a fever marked by exceedingly high temperature of 105°F or more. Intermittent fever is a fever that falls to normal or below during the day, but then rises again. Relapsing fever is fever that may disappear for a day or several days and then return in alternating episodes. Sustained fever is fever in which the average daily temperature remains above normal.

fiber. As used in reference to therapeutic diets, this term includes indigestible organic tissue, either plant or animal. Crude fiber is made up largely of *cellulose** which is not readily soluble, and *lignin.* The fiber content is usually determined as that portion of a food sample which resists solution when boiled in dilute acid and dilute alkali.

fiber, meat. Meat fibers are the long cells in muscles of the meat. The size and shape of the fibers determine the physical structure and grain of the meat. Meat fibers are cells and are not related to the insoluble fiber of plants.

fibrin. A whitish, insoluble protein network that forms the essential protein of a blood clot, fibrinogen. Fibrin derives from fibrinogen by the proteolysis of the enzyme thrombin. It is the formation of thrombin that depends upon *vitamin K**. See *vitamin K**, *thrombin,* and *blood clot.*

fibrinogen. The soluble protein precursor to *fibrin.* The transformation from fibrinogen to fibrin is brought about by the *protease thrombin,* which itself is initially in the *zymogen* form prothrombin. *Calcium* is required for the conversion of prothrombin to thrombin. *Vitamin K** is responsible for the formation of normal thrombin by participation of a carboxylation reaction. See *vitamin K**, *thrombin,* and *blood clot.*

fibroblasts. Numerous and large, flat branching mesenchymal cells with many processes. They play a part in the formation of the *collagen* fibers. After tissue injury, these cells enlarge and become active in forming collagen fibers which fill the injured area.

fibrosis. The formation of fibrous connective tissue in repair processes.

fibrous proteins. Long coiled or folded chains of amino acids bound together by peptide linkages. They are found in the protective and supportive tissues of animals such as skin, hair, feathers, tendons, and the fins and scales of fish. The fibrous proteins in such tissues are very insoluble in water and for the most part indigestible. They are a valuable by-product of the food industry since gelatin and other nitrogenous substances can be extracted from them. Some fibrous proteins are *keratin,* the chief protein of hair; *collagen* of connective tissue; *fibrin* of a blood clot, and *myosin* of the muscles.

fig (*Ficus carcia*). Figs are the fruit of a tree. The fruit consists of a soft pulp covered by a thin skin. There are between 600 and 800 varieties of figs, varying in shape from round to oblong, and in color from almost white to purple-black. Fresh figs contain moderate amounts of potassium, riboflavin, phosphorus, calcium, and thiamin. Dried figs are a source of quick food energy, high in iron, with good amounts of calcium and phosphorus. They supply bulk for a natural laxative.

Fresh, 100 gm, raw = 80 calories
Dried, 100 gm = 274 calories
Preserved, 100 gm, canned in water = 48 calories
Preserved, 100 gm, canned in light syrup pack = 65 calories
Preserved, 100 gm, canned in heavy syrup pack = 84 calories

filbert. (*Corylus*). A nut which is the fruit of shrubs of small trees. It is also known as hazelnut or cobnut. Generally speaking the name "filbert" is applied to the oblong nuts of two varieties of hazel nuts native to Europe. *C. ovelana pontica* and *C. maxima;* "cobnut" to another native variety, *C. avelana grandis* which produces a large roundish nut; and "hazelnut" to the American varieties *C. americana* and *C. cornuta,* which bear small roundish nuts. The nuts are borne in clusters and each nut is enclosed in a husk which opens at the nut ripens. Filberts are eaten dried more than almonds or walnuts. Filberts provide protein, fat, *iron,* and *thiamine**. 100 gm = 634 calories.

firming agents. Add firmness to processed fruits and vegetables which otherwise might become soft. They also aid in the coagulation of certain cheeses. These substances may be added to foods such as pickles, maraschino cherries, canned peas, tomatoes, potatoes, and apples.

fish. Fish are coldblooded aquatic animals and, broadly speaking include shellfish as well as the tapered, scaly animal with backbone, gills, and fins. From a nutritional viewpoint we are concerned with the edible types of fish, which are usually divided into three groups: saltwater fish such as sea bass, pompano, cod, haddock, halibut, herring, mackerel, salmon, shad, sole, sturgeon, swordfish, tuna; freshwater fish such as bass, catfish, trout, perch; and shellfish such as abalone, clams, crabs, crayfish, lobsters, mussels, oysters, scallops and shrimps. Depending on the type, fish is a very good to excellent source of easily digested protein. Fish contains varying amounts of fluorine, iron, calcium, and B vitamins. Saltwater fish provides iodine. Fish-liver oils are rich in vitamins A and D. Roe and livers are rich in riboflavin and thiamine. The food value of canned fish is similar to that of fresh fish, except when oil is added. Curing destroys much of the vitamin content of the fish and sometimes increases the caloric value. The table on pp. 174–175 gives the nutrient content of fish and shellfish.

fistula. A tuberlike ulcer leading from an abscess cavity or organ to the surface, or from one abscess cavity to another.

fixation. (1) Generally, fixation refers to the incorporation of carbon dioxide (CO_2) or nitrogen (N_2) into a biologically usable form. The incorporations are of CO_2 into *carbohydrates* by photosynthetic plants and the incorporation of N_2 into more complex molecules by nitrogen-fixing bacteria. (2) The process of treating tissue in preparation for microscopic examination.

flavine adenine dinucleotide (FAD). Mol. Wt. 786. A coenzyme that contains the vitamin *riboflavin.* The coenzyme FAD functions in cell respiration as a part of the *terminal respiratory chain* and in the oxidative decarboxylations of *pyruvic* acid* and alpha (α)-*ketoglutaric acid**. The enzymes and proteins which associate with FAD come under the general classification of flavopro-

Fish and Shellfish

Food and Description	Wt. gm	Approximate Measure	Food Energy cal	Protein gm	Fat gm	Carbohydrate Total gm	Carbohydrate Fiber gm	Water gm	Calcium µg	Phosphorus µg	Iron µg	Vitamin A I.U.	Thiamine µg	Riboflavin µg	Niacin µg	Ascorbic Acid µg
Crabs, Atlantic and Pacific, hard shell, steamed	100	3½ ozs.	93	17	2	1		79	43	175	0.8	2,170	0.16	0.08	2.8	2
Canned, meat only	100	3½ ozs.	101	17	3	1		77	45	182	0.8		0.08	0.08	1.9	
Eels, raw, American	100	3½ ozs.	233	16	18	0	0	66	18	202	0.7	1,610	0.22	0.36	1.4	
Fish:																
Bluefish:																
Baked or broiled	100	3½ ozs.	159	26	5	0	0	68	29	287	0.7	50	0.11	0.10	1.9	
Fried	100	3½ ozs.	205	23	10	5	0	61	35	257	0.9		0.11	0.11	1.8	
Cod:																
Broiled	100	3½ ozs.	170	29	5	0	0	65	31	274	1.0	180	0.08	0.11	3.0	
Dried	100	3½ ozs.	375	82	3	0	0	12		891	3.6	0	0.08	0.45	10.9	0
Flounder, baked	100	3½ ozs.	202	30	8	0	0	58	23	344	1.4		0.07	0.08	2.5	
Haddock, fried	100	3½ ozs.	165	20	6	6	0	67	40	247	1.2		0.04	0.07	3.2	2
Halibut, broiled	100	3½ ozs.	171	25	7	0	0	67	16	248	0.8	680	0.05	0.07	8.3	
Herring:																
Atlantic, raw	100	3½ ozs.	176	17	11	0	0	69		256	1.1	110	0.02	0.15	3.6	
Pacific, raw	100	3½ ozs.	98	18	3	0	0	79		225	1.3	100	0.02	0.16	3.5	
Canned in tomato sauce	100	3½ ozs.	176	16	11	4	0	67		243				0.11	3.5	
Smoked, kippered	100	3½ ozs.	211	22	13	0	0	61	66	254	1.4	30		0.28	3.3	
Mackerel:																
Atlantic, broiled	100	3½ ozs.	236	22	16	0	0	62	6	280	1.2	530	0.15	0.27	7.6	
Pacific, canned, solids and liquid	100	3½ ozs.	180	21	10	0	0	66	260	288	2.2	30	0.03	0.33	8.8	

Food	g	Measure	Cal.	Protein (g)	Fat (g)	Carboh. (g)	Water (%)	Calcium (mg)	Phosph. (mg)	Iron (mg)	Vit. A (I.U.)	Thiamine (mg)	Ribofl. (mg)	Niacin (mg)	Ascorbic (mg)
Salmon:															
Cooked, broiled or baked	100	3½ ozs.	182	27	7	0	63		414	1.2	160	0.16	0.06	9.8	0
Canned: solid & liquid															
Chinook or King	100	3½ ozs.	210	20	14	0	65	154	289	0.9	230	0.03	0.14	7.3	0
Pink or humpback	100	3½ ozs.	141	21	6	0	70	196	286	0.8	70	0.03	0.18	8.0	0
Sockeye or red	100	3½ ozs.	171	20	9	0	67	259	344	1.2	230	0.04	0.16	7.3	0
Smoked	100	3½ ozs.	176	22	9	0	59	14	245						
Sardines:															
Atlantic type, canned in oil. drained solids	100	3½ ozs.	203	24	11	Tr.	62	437	499	2.9	220	0.03	0.20	5.4	Tr.
Pacific type,															
In brine or mustard	100	3½ ozs.	196	19	12	2	64	303	354	5.2	30	0.01	0.30	7.4	
In tomato sauce	100	3½ ozs.	197	19	12	2	64	449	478	4.1	30	0.01	0.27	5.3	
Shad, baked	100	3½ ozs.	201	23	11	0	64	24	313	0.6	30	0.13	0.26	8.6	0
Swordfish, broiled	100	3½ ozs.	174	28	7	0	65	27	275	1.3	2,050	0.04	0.05	10.9	0
Tuna fish, canned in oil															
drained solids	100	3½ ozs.	197	29	8	0	61	8	234	1.9	80	0.05	0.12	11.9	0
Canned in water															
solids and liquid	100	3½ ozs.	127	28	1	0	70	16	190	1.6			0.10	13.3	
White fish, cooked															
baked, stuffed	100	3½ ozs.	215	15	14	6	63		246	0.5	2,000	0.11	0.11	2.3	Tr.
Lobster:															
Raw	100	3½ ozs. meat	91	17	2	1	79	29	183	0.6		0.40	0.05	1.5	0
Canned or cooked	100	3½ ozs.	95	19	2	0	77	65	192	0.8		0.10	0.07		0
Oysters, meat only, raw															
Av. Eastern	100	5-8 medium	66	8	2	3	85	94	143	5.5	310	0.14	0.18	2.5	
Oyster stew:															
1 part oysters to 3 parts milk by volume	100	½ c. scant	86	5	5	5	84	117	109	1.4	280	0.06	0.18	0.7	
Scallops, cooked, steamed	100	3½ ozs.	112	23	1	1	73	115	338	3.0					
Shrimp, French fried	100	3½ ozs.	225	20	11	10	57	72	191	2.0		0.04	0.08	2.7	0
Canned, dry pack or drained	100	3½ ozs.	116	24	1	1	70	115	263	3.1	60	0.01	0.03	1.8	0

teins, which in general catalyze oxidation-reduction reactions. See *flavine mon-onucleotide* * (FMN) and *riboflavin* *.

Flavine adenine dinucleotide (FAD)

flavine mononucleotide (FMN). Mol. Wt. 456. A coenzyme that contains the vitamin *riboflavin* *. The coenzyme FMN is involved in the oxidative *deamination* of amino acids in kidney *mitochondria*. In general, the coenzymes FMN and FAD bind so tightly to their *apoenzymes* that they cannot be removed without causing the protein to denature. Since they bind so tightly, they are often referred to as *prosthetic groups*. See *flavine adenine dinucleotide* * (FAD) and *riboflavin* *.

Flavine mononucleotide (FMN)

flavobacterium. Yellow- to orange-pigmented species of this genus may cause discolorations on the surface of meats and may be involved in the spoilage of shellfish, poultry, eggs, and butter and milk. Some of these organisms are able to grow at low temperatures and have been found forming on thawing vegetables.

flavoproteins. (1) Proteins containing *riboflavin* derivatives. They are important as enzymes in the *Krebs cycle*. (2) A conjugated protein that contains a flavin and is involved in tissue respiration.

flavor enhancers. Flavor enhancers have little or no taste of their own but amplify the flavors of other substances. They exert synergistic and potentiation effects. Potentiators were first used in meats and fish. They are also used now to intensify the flavor and cover unwanted flavors in vegetables, bread, cakes, fruits, nuts, and beverages. Common flavor enhancers are *monosodium glutamate** (MSG), *disodium guanylate** and *disodium inosinate**, and *maltol.*

flora (intestinal). The bacteria and other organisms that grow naturally in the intestine. Some of these bacteria are sources of vitamins, e.g., *vitamin K**.

flounder. The name is used for a large family of saltwater flatfish, including gray sole, summer flounder, winter flounder, lemon sole, and dabs. The most common flounders are dark gray on top and white on the bottom. The eyes are on top. Flounders are important food fish, the flesh is lean and sweetly flavored. Their weight generally ranges from one-half to 5 pounds. Fish is a very good source of protein and contains iron, calcium, *retinol**, (vitamins A) and the B vitamins. Cooked, 100 gm = 202 calories.

flour. Wheat ground to a powder. The outer layers of the wheat are generally removed as bran, and the central portion of the grain is made into flour by a process called milling. To remove more of the whole grain or bran, the flour is subjected to a series of sifting processes through finer and finer sieves. (See *wheat*) The unique properties of wheat flour that make a dough that will stick together and rise, derive from the presence of the proteins *gliadin* and *glutelin*. Except for rye, none of the other cereal grains contain these proteins. See *wheat.*

fluoridation. The use of *fluorine,* as in water to reduce the incidence of tooth decay. Fluoridated water is a dietary control of dental decay, with the recommended concentration of one part ppm of water. It is harmless, tasteless, odorless, and colorless. Studies indicate that fluoridated water drinkers have fewer acid-making germs in their mouth than drinkers of nonfluoridated water. When fluoride gets into the bloodstream it quickly incorporates into the bones and teeth. Medical studies indicate fluoride strengthens the bones and teeth that incorporate it. Dental studies show that the bloodstream also brings the fluoride to the gums. Any teeth growing there take up the fluoride. It is a chemical action. Teeth are made up largely of living apatite crystals which contain hydroxyl ions. Fluoride in contact with apatite replaces the hydroxyl ions. The apatite becomes fluorapatite. As the tooth develops in the gums, first the crown and then the root acquires fluorapatite. The fluoride is everywhere, in the pulp, dentine and enamel, from biting surface to root tip, strengthening the entire tooth and causing it to be more resistant to bacteria. When fluoridated water comes in contact with the surface of the teeth that are already formed and in place, it still forms fluroapatite, but only on the surface.

fluorine (F). Element No. 9. Atom. Wt. 19. There is no known metabolic role in the body for fluorine, although it is known to activate certain enzymes and to inhibit others. Fluorine should not be confused with the ionic form *fluoride*. The fluorine content of body tissues and foods varies widely. This trace element is present in minute amounts in nearly every human tissue but is found primarily in the skeleton and teeth. The organs contain more fluorine than do other soft tissues. Among the richer food sources of fluorine of animal origin are gelatin, the organs, seafoods, and infant foods which contain bonemeal. It has been estimated that an adult may secure from his food 0.5 to 1.0 mg fluorine daily.

Fluphenazine (Prolixin, Permitil). A powerful antiemetic (inhibits vomiting). A phenothiazine derivative used for sustained action over time.

foaming agents and inhibitors. Used for pressure-packed whipped toppings so that they squirt whipped from their containers. Adding a foam inhibitor, such as alginic acid (a seaweed derivative) prevents foaming.

folacin (folic acid). Mol. Wt. 441. The generic term for folic acid, pteroylglutamic and other compounds having the activity of folic acid is folacin. The name officially selected to replace the term folic acid. Folacin is a vitamin of the B-complex group necessary for the maturation of red blood cells and synthesis of nucleoproteins; also known as pteroylglutamic acid. Members of this group include folacin (or pteroylglutamic acid), pteroyltriglutamic acid, pteroylheptaglutamic acid, and folinic acid or citrovorum factor, a derivative of folic acid that occurs in natural materials in both free and combined form. Folacin participates in the formation of complex chemical compounds known as purines and pyrimidines that are components of *deoxynucleic acid* (DNA) and *ribonucleic acid* (RNA). The DNA is genetic material and RNA is required for protein synthesis. The necessity of folacin for hematopoiesis (the manufacture of blood cells) in man presumably resides in its function in the formation of purines and pyrimidines. Folacin stimulates the formation of blood cells in the treatment of certain *anemias*, which are characterized by oversized red cells and the accumulation in the bone marrow of immature red blood cells, called myoblasts. The bone marrow is the organ that manufactures blood cells. It cannot complete the process in the absence of folacin. *Cobalamin* * (vitamin B_{12}) also is needed for the formation of blood cells and is also effective in the treatment of many anemias. The best sources include liver, dry beans, lentils, cowpeas, asparagus, broccoli, spinach, and collards. Other good sources include kidney, peanuts, filberts, walnuts, immature or young lima beans, cabbage, sweet corn, chard, turnip greens, lettuce, beet greens and wholewheat products. Folacin contains the pteridine group and one molecule each of glutamic acid and para-aminobenzoic acid. It is a yellow crystalline substance, slightly soluble in water, relatively unstable to heat, and labile to acid and to sunlight when in solution. Folacin occurs in foods of animal and plant origin, some of it in the free form but usually as a conjugate in which it is combined with two or six additional molecules of glutamic acid. A derivative of folic acid, folinic acid, often called the citruvorum factor, leucovorum, or N^5-formyltetrahydrofolic acid, also occurs in foods usually conjugated with additional glutamic acid molecules.

Folacin (folic acid)

Folic acid dietary sources—(Micrograms per 100-gm edible portion)

Apricots	3.6	Bread, cracked wheat	27
Avocados	4–57	Bread, rye	20
Bananas	9.6	Bread, Vienna	11
Beans, lima	10–56	Bread, white	15
Beans, lima, dry	100	Buttermilk	11
Beans, snap	13–56	Brazil nuts	4.5
Beans, navy, dry	130	Cherries	3–8
Beans, wax	15–39	Cheese, cheddar	15
Beets	13	Cheese, cottage	21–46
Blackberries	6–18	Cheese, processed	11
Blueberries	7.6	Chuck	15
Broccoli	34	Chicken liver	380
Brussel sprouts	27	Coconuts	28

Folic acid dietary sources (*continued*)

Cabbage	6–42	Lentils, dry	99
Carrots	8	Lettuce	4–54
Cauliflower	29	Mushrooms	14–29
Celery	7.2	Oranges	5.1
Corn, sweet	9–70	Orange juice	4.8
Cucumbers	6.7	Oats, white	23–66
Dates, dry	25	Okra	24
Eggs, whole	5.1	Onions, green	13
Egg yolk	13	Onions, mature	6–14
Egg white	0.6	Prunes, dry	5.4
Figs	6.7	Pork sausage	12
Flour, cake	6.6	Parsnips	8–37
Flour, white, enriched	8.1	Peas	5–35
Flour, whole wheat	38	Peas, dry split	22
Filberts	67	Peppers, green	4–11
Grapes, green	4.5	Potatoes, peeled	4–12
Grapes, red	4.9	Potatoes, whole	2–130
Grains, barley	50	Pumpkin	5–10
Grains, yellow corn	24	Radishes	3–10
Grains, rice, brown	22	Red raspberries	5.1
Grains, rye	34	Round steak	7–17
Grains, wheat	27–51	Strawberries	4.3
Hamburger	5	Sweetbreads	22.8
Ham, smoked	7.8	Squash, acorn	16.7
Kidney	58	Squash, crookneck	7–16
Lemons	7.4	Sweet potatoes	5–19
Limes	4.6	Tangerines	7.4
Liver, calf	290	Tomatoes	2–16
Liver, lamb	280	Turnips	4.3
Liver, pork	220	Zucchini	11

folic acid deficiency. As iron is essential for the formation of hemoglobin, two vitamins, folacin (folic acid) and *cobalamin* * (vitamin B_{12}) are necessary for the formation of red blood cells. They are both involved in the building of the nucleoproteins needed for red blood cell structure and maturation. In a deficiency of either of these vitamins, the number of red cells is markedly reduced. The red cells present in the blood are large and filled with hemoglobin since there is no deficiency of iron. These anemias are therefore called hyperchromic macrocytic (large cell) anemias. Free folic acid does not occur naturally but can be made synthetically and used as a medication. See *pernicious anemia* and *cobalamin*.

follicle. Small excretory sac, cavity or gland, e.g., hair follicle, ovarian follicle.

follicle-stimulating hormone (FSH). A hormone of the adenohypoptysis (anterior pituitary gland) that stimulates the gonads to produce reproductive cells (*sperm* or *ova*).

follicular hyperkeratosis. A *retinol** (vitamin A) deficiency condition in which the skin becomes dry and scaly and small pustules or hardened, pigmented, papular eruptions form around the hair follicles.

follicular keratosis. Normal human skin contains pores which are the openings of microscopic follicles, a small cavity or depression. The secretions of the sebaceous and sweat-producing glands enter the follicles and reach the surface through these pores. Hairs emerge from their roots through the same follicles. In follicular keratosis the follicles become blocked with plugs of keratin, a major protein of the skin, derived from their surface epithelial cells which have undergone a change to a squamous or flat type. The change is called a squamous metaplasia. This pathological change is characteristic of vitamin A deficiency.

food. Edible material containing the nutrients from which the body derives nourishment for growth or maintenance of a nutritionally healthy condition. Food contains fats, carbohydrates, proteins, vitamins, and minerals necessary for good health. There are more than 40 known nutrients required in foods.

food additives. Hundreds of different substances come under the heading of intentional food additives. These are added purposely to better the product in some way or to enhance its use. Nonnutritive substances added to foods to improve in appearance, texture, flavor, and keeping qualities include stabilizers, preservatives, coloring, sweeteners, and flavoring. They perform essential functions in the production process and marketing of acceptable products. Incidental additives are those that become part of foods unintentionally. This may occur at different stages in the growing, harvesting, or marketing of foods. Residues from pesticide sprays used in the growing of vegetables are an example of undesirable incidental additives. In a broad sense, radioactive materials in the atmosphere become incidental additives to food. They are always present in the air and soil to some degree, and food and water become carriers. The following table lists some typical uses of intentional additives.

Technical Effects of Food Additives

Technical Effect*	Typical Additives in Current Use to Achieve These Effects‡§
Anticaking agents, free-flow agents, keep seasoning salts and other mixes from turning into a solid chunk during damp weather	Calcium stearate, cornstarch, sodium aluminosilicate, tricalcium phosphate, calcium silicate, magnesium carbonate, silica aerogel
Antigushing agents prevent the beer or other carbonated beverage from "gushing" from the container when it is first opened	None now known to be in use
Antioxidants include substances that keep edible fats and oils from turning rancid and others that prevent cut fruits and vegetables from turning brown	BHA, BHT, ascorbic acid (Vitamin C), ethoxyquin
Boiler water additives are chemicals added to boiler feed water to prevent scale from forming as a result of the hardness of the water; when steam from the boiler is used in food processing, small amounts may be carried over into the final food	Acrylamide-sodium acrylate resin, polyethylene glycol, sodium tripolyphosphate, morpholine
Clouding and crystallizing agents and inhibitors	Methyl glucoside-coconut oil ester, oxystearin
Colors, coloring adjuncts (including color stabilizers, color fixatives, color-retention agents, etc.) consist of synthetic colors, synthesized colors that also occur naturally, and other colors from natural sources	FD&C Blue No. 1, FD&C Red No. 3, and other certified synthetic colors; β-carotene; iron oxide and other exempt synthetic colors; beet powder; grape skin extract; caramel, turmeric, and other natural colors
Compounds in the manufacture of other food additives are substances that perform no function in the final food but are necessary in the manufacture of some other additive, and traces of which may survive into the final food; it is an unintentional "additive in an additive	Any common inorganic compounds, such as sodium hydroxide, sulfuric acid, food color intermediates, synthetic fatty alcohols
Curing, pickling agents preserve (cure) meats, give them desirable color and flavor, discourage the growth of microorganisms, and prevent toxin formation	Sodium nitrate, sodium nitrate, salt, sodium metaphosphate, sodium tripolyphosphate; sodium erythorbate, ascorbic acid
Dough conditioners, strengtheners are both simple chemicals and also enzymes which modify the protein and cellulose in such a way as to reduce the "toughness" or "springiness" of dough and make it both easier to handle and more appealing to consume	Potassium bromate, acetone peroxide, calcium sulfate, glyceryl monostearate, ammonium sulfate, monocalcium phosphate, locust (carob) bean gum
Drying agents are intended to absorb moisture from other food components	Specially dried cornstarch, anhydrous dextrose

Technical Effects of Food Additives

Technical Effect*	Typical Additives in Current Use to Achieve these Effects ‡ §
Emulsifiers are an important group of substances used to obtain stable mixture of liquids that otherwise would not mix or would separate quickly	Mono- and diglycerides; lecithin; propylene glycol monostearate; sorbitan monostearate; polysorbates 60, 65, and 80
Enzymes are complex proteins which promote almost all the chemical reactions that occur in all living things; some of these can be adapted to specific processing needs	Rennet for producing cheese curd, papain for tenderizing meat, pectinase for clarifying beverages
Fermentation aid, malting aid are yeast nutrients and other substances that promote rapid and proper fermentation	Gibberellic acid, potassium gibberellate, potassium bromate
Firming agents produce desirable crispness or texture	Calcium salts, aluminum sulfate, calcium lactobionate
Flavor enhancers do not themselves contribute significant flavors but increase the effect of certain kinds of other flavors	Soy sauce, MSG, disodium inosinate, disodium guanylate
Flavoring agents, adjuvants are the ingredients, both naturally occurring and added, which give the characteristic flavor to almost all the foods in our diet; flavor adjuvants are substances not themselves flavors, which improve the usefulness of flavors, such as solvents and fixatives	Many of the traditional spices and herbs plus nearly 1500 individual chemical entities, most of which have been identified as the constituents responsible for the flavor of natural food products
Flour-treating agents (including bleaching and maturing agents) usually both bleach and "mature" the flour; i.e., they provide the same effect as increased age. They oxidize some of the proteins and lead to better handling characteritics and larger loaf volume	Acetone peroxide, benzoyl peroxide, azodicarbonamide, potassium bromide
Formation aids cover a hodgepodge of substances which simply allow foods to be put together in a useful way with retention of quality during transportation and storage	Carrier solvents for dissolving and standardizing flavors, starch as a binder, modified starch, gum acacia, magnesium stearate, sodium caseinate, mannitol, propylene glycol, corn syrup, dextrose
Freezing agents are extremely volatile liquids—gases at ordinary temperatures and pressures—which evaporate rapidly and chill the food exposed to the cold vapor	Liquid nitrogen, dichlorodifluoromethane
Fumigants kill undesirable organisms	Methyl bromide, ethylene oxide, phostoxin
Humectants, moisture-retention agents, and antidusting agents retain the texture of food by preventing it from drying out	Sorbitol, propylene glycol, sodium tripolyphosphate
Ion-exchange resins are long, insoluble molecules (polymers) which have an affinity	A long list of resins, including acrylate-acrylamide resins, sulfonated copolymer of

Technical Effects of Food Additives

Technical Effect*	Typical Additives in Current Use to Achieve These Effects ‡ §
for certain positively or negatively charged ions, and which can be used to remove these ions from water or a solution or juice	styrene and divinyl benzene, sulfonated anthracite coa, sulfite-modified cross-linked phenol-formaldehyde, etc.
Leavening agents produce light, fluffy baked goods	Yeast, monocalcium phosphate, sodium aluminum, phosphate, sodium acid phosphate, sodium carbonate, calcium carbonate and other baking powder ingredients
Lubricants, release agents allow the extrusion of foods and rapid, economical production of bread by permitting it to come cleanly out of the baking pan	Oleic acid, hydrogenated sperm oil, mineral oil
Masticatory substances for chewing gum give the bulk, plasticity, and resistance required for proper mouth feel	Chicle, rubber, paraffin, glycerol esters of rosin
Nonnutritive sweeteners having less than 2 percent of the caloric value of sucrose per equivalent unit of sweetening capacity, replace sugar or corn syrup in dietetic foods	Saccharin, cyclamate (in many countries)
Nutrient supplements restore values lost in processing or storage or insure higher nutritional value than nature may have provided	All the known essential nutrients such as vitamin A and other vitamins, iron and other trace minerals, amino acids and essential fatty acids
Nutritive sweeteners are any digestible sweeteners yielding more than 2 calories per gram	Dextrose, fructose, sucrose, corn syrup, molasses, honey
Oxidixing and reducing agents perform these chemical operations on food components to get rid of an undesirable component or contaminant	Peroxidase (enzyme) to destroy glucose in dried egg, so that it will store well; hydrogen peroxide added as a bleaching or antimicrobial agent
pH control agents (including buffers, acids, alkalies, neutralizing agents) reduce or increase the acidity or sourness of a food	Vinegar (acetic acid), sodium bicarbonate, hydrogen chloride, citric acid sulfuric acid, sodium citrate, sodium hydroxide, adipic acid
Preservatives, antimicrobial agents prevent bacteriological spoilage	Sodium benzoate, calcium propionate, potassium sorbate
Processing aids are added, not for the continuing effect they exert on the food, but to help make it better in the first place, for example, by aiding filtration or removing unwanted color	Charcoal, diatomaceous earth, hydrochloric acid, papain, polyvinylpolypyrrolidone, dioctyl sodium sulfosuccinate
Propellants, aerating agents, gases push the whipped cream topping from the can and make it fluffy, or exclude oxygen and prolong the shelf life and nutritional value of a packaged food	Chlorinated, fluorinated hydrocarbons; carbon dioxide; nitrous oxide; nitrogen; combustion gases

Technical Effects of Food Additives

Technical Effect*	Typical Additives in Current Use to Achieve These Effects‡§
Sequestrants combine chemically with traces of metals present naturally in all foods, which if uncombined, would promote instability and off-flavors	Citric acid, *EDTA*, phosphoric acid, sodium metaphosphate
Solvents, vehicles dissolve or suspend flavors, colors, and many other ingredients in an easy-to-use form	Alcohol, propylene glycol, glycerine, triethyl citrate, triacetin, acetone
Stabilizers, thickeners give desirable viscosity and mouth feel, prevent emulsions from separating, and prevent a pudding from being "sloppy"	Starch, modified food starches; natural and synthetic gums, such as guar, acacia, carrageenan, carob bean
Surface-active agents are related to the emulsifiers and permit rapid wetting of dry ingredients and better whipping of toppings; they promote foam where it is wanted or prevent it where it is not	Dioctyl sodium sulfosuccinate, sodium lauryl sulfate, lactylic esters of fatty acids, dimethyl polysiloxane
Surface-finishing agents are used on fruits, candies, and baked goods both for protection and appearance	Beeswax, carnauba wax, gum acacia, shellac wax, rice bran was, oxidized polyethylene, rosin, polyvinylpyrrolidone
Synergists is a catch-all category of substances which produce no particular effect in themselves but help those of other additives	Citric acid, tricalcium phosphate, and other phosphates
Texturizers contribute or preserve desirable appearance or mouth feel; e.g., a smooth, slick sauce or pudding produced with normal starch is often less attractive than one with a somewhat pulpy appearance and feel produced by modified starches.	Sodium bicarbonate, glycerine, corn syrup, modified food starch
Washing-peeling aids, vegetable cleaning agents are substances that soften or dissolve the peel of a fruit or vegetable or that soften or loosen dirt; they save hand labor by making mechanical peeling and washing more effective, and they waste less food than hand processing	Sodium hydroxide (lye), sodium metasilicate, aliphatic acids, sodium hypochlorite, sodium *n*-alkylbenzene sulfonate, odorless light petroleum hydrocarbons

*R. L. Hall, "Food Additives," Nutrition Today, Vol. 8, No. 4, Jul/Aug 1973).
‡NRC "A Comprehensive Survey of Industry on the Use of Foods General Recognized as Safe (GRAS), Table 6, PB-221 929 (Apr. 1973.
§Code of Federal Regulations, 21 Food and Drugs, Part 10 to 199, Rev. Apr. 1, 1976 (Wash. D.C. Gov. Print. Office).

food energy. Expressed in terms of calories per unit weight. Food energy represents the energy available from its oxidation after deductions have been made for losses in digestion and incomplete oxidation. Energy values stated in food composition tables have been computed on the basis of the specific fuel factor experimentally determined in a *bomb calorimeter* for the individual foods. The commonly used physiological fuel factors, when applied to the total daily intake of protein, fat, and carbohydrate from a typical American diet, provide a good estimate of the energy value of the diet. See *metabolism, basal metabolism, oxidative phosphorylation,* and *terminal respiratory chain.*

food poisoning. Any disease or toxin production by microorganisms that is transmitted through food is food poisoning. Food poisoning is produced by microorganisms that are: (1) Naturally occurring animal infections that can be transmitted to man. This group of microorganisms includes *bacteria, fungi, viruses,* worms and *protozoa.* (2) Microorganisms that may cause infections or present toxic effects in man but are not normally present in food. The table below gives some diseases produced by common microorganisms associated with food poisoning.

Disease	Mode of Spread
Food poisoning	
Salmonella	From rats, mice, cattle, and occasionally other animals
Staphylococcal	From a human carrier
Clostridial	From dust, feces, flies, etc.
Botulism	From dust, soil, etc., improperly canned foods.
From milk	
Brucellosis (undulant fever)	From infected cows or goats.
Bovine tuberculosis	From infected cows or goats
From infected meats	
Trichinosis	From pork
Tape worms	From beef
Cysticercosis	From pork
Clonorchiasis	From fish in the Far East
Opisthorchiasis	From fish in S.E. Europe and Asia
Laragonimiasis	From crayfish and crabs
Diphyllobothriasis	From fish
Balantidiasis	From pigs
From vegetables	
Fascioliasis	From pigs and ruminants

food spoilage. Food spoilage has several causes. (1) Growth and activity of microorganisms. Often a succession of organisms are involved. (2) Insects. (3) Action of the enzyme of the plant or animal food. (4) Purely chemical reactions, that is, those not catalyzed by enzymes of the tissue or of microorganisms. (5) Physical changes, such as those caused by freezing, burning, drying, pressure, and humidity which may in turn promote the growth of microorganisms, chemical reactions, or the action of enzymes.

food toxins. There occurs in foods a number of compounds that are toxic or carcinogenic or have pharmacological effects. The food toxins are grouped as: (1) natural carcinogens, (2) as having toxic or pharmacological effects, and (3) as nutritional inhibitors. (1) Natural carcinogens in commonly eaten foods:

Source	Carcinogens
Agricultural products	Aflatoxin
Barbecued meats	Benzopyrene
Beverages, tea and wine	Tannins
Cabbage	Thiourea
Coffee	Caffeine and/or phenolic compounds (latter as catalysts)
Corn	Zearalenone (estrogenic)
Flour	Patulin
Herbs	Various alkaloids
Meats, eggs, dairy products, wheat germ, and leafy vegetables	Estrogens
Orange and apple juice	Patulin
Proteins	Tryptophane
Fermented products including bread, beer, and wine	Ethyl carbamate
Vegetables plus Protein sources: meat, fish, milk, eggs, etc.	Nitrates and nitrites plus Secondary amines } ⟶ nitrosamines

(2) Some possible toxic or pharmacological effects of foods:

Occurrence	Active Agent	Effects
Bananas and some other fruits	5-hydroxytryptamine; adrenaline; nonadrenaline	Effects on central and peripheral nervous system
Some cheeses	Tyramine	Raises blood pressure; enhanced by monoamine oxidase inhibitors
Almonds, cassava, and other plants	Cyanide	Interfers with tissue respiration
Quail	Due to consumption of hemlock	Hemlock poisoning
Mussels	Due to consumption of dino-flagellate, *Gonyaulax*	Tingling, numbness, muscle weakness, respiratory paralysis
Cycad nuts	Methylazoxymethanol (cycasin)	Liver damage; cancer

Occurrence	Active Agent	Effects
Some fish, meat, or cheese	Nitrosamines	Liver damage; cancer
Mustard oil	Sanguinarine	Edema (epidemic dropsy)
Legumes	Haemagglutinins	Red cell and intestinal cell damage
Some beans	Vicine	Hemolytic anaemia (favism)
	β-aminopropionitrile	Interferes with collagen formation
	β-N-oxalyl-amino-alanine	Toxic effects on nervous system Lathyrism
Ackee fruit	α-amino-β-methylene cyclopropane propionic acid	Hypoglycemia, vomiting sickness
Brassica seeds and some other Cruciferae	Glucosinolates, thiocyanate	Enlargement of thyroid gland (goiter)
Rhubarb	Oxalate	Oxaluria
Green potatoes	Solanine; possibly other sapotoxins	Gastrointestinal upset
Many fish	Various, often confined to certain organs, or seasonal	Mainly toxic effects on nervous system
Many fungi	Various mycotoxins	Mainly toxic effects on nervous system and liver

(3) Some nutritional inhibitors naturally present in common foods:

Source	Inhibitor	Action	Counteraction
Beans, lima, and soy-beans	Antitrypsin	Prevents protein digestion	Heat inactivation
	Hemagglutinins	Retards growth	Heat inactivation
	Lipoxidase	Destroys vitamin A	Heat inactivation
Cabbage, kale, rutabagas	Goitrogens	Prevents synthesis of thyroxine	Additional iodine
Cereals	Unknown (niacinogen)	Binds niacin	Additional niacin or tryptophane
Corn, millet	Unknown (leucine?)	Decreases effectiveness of niacin	Additional niacin or tryptophane
Cottonseed oil	Sterculic acid	Interferes with reproduction	Heat or hydrogenation
Egg white	Ovamucoid	Prevents protein digestion	Heat inactivation
	Avidin	Binds biotin	Heat inactivation
	Conalbumin	Binds iron	Heat inactivation
Fish, clams	Thiaminase	Destroys thiamine	Heat inactivation
Milk, yogurt	Lactose	Diarrhea and loss of nutrients	Enzymic hydrolysis of lactose
Oatmeal	Phytin	Binds calcium	Additional calcium
		Binds iron	Additional iron

Source	Inhibitor	Action	Counteraction
Onions	Unknown	Produces anemia	Avoid excessive intake
Peas	Nitrile compound	Interferes with sulfur metabolism (collagen formation)	Avoid excessive intake
Plant products	Molybdenum	Increases requirement for copper	Additional copper
Potatoes (immature or sprouting)	Solanine	Vomiting and diarrhea resulting in loss of nutrients	Avoid such potato products
Rhubarb, spinach	Oxalic acid	Binds calcium	Additional calcium
Vegetables and fruits	Ascorbic acid oxidase	Destroys vitamin C	Heat inactivation or additional vitamin C

formic acid. Mol. Wt. 46. HCOOH. The simplest organic acid in which the carboxyl group is attached directly to a hydrogen atom. This acid is found in ants and other insects and is part of the irritant that produces itching and swelling after a bite. Formic acid derivatives occur in the body naturally and are important in protein synthesis. Transfer of the formic acid or formyl group requires the participation of the vitamin *folacin* * as in the formation of *formiminoglutamic acid.*

formiminoglutamic acid (FIGLU). Intermediary product of *histidine* * breakdown (catabolism). *Folacin* * is necessary for its breakdown, the urinary excretion of FIGLU may be measured to determine the folacin status of an individual.

fortified or fortification. The addition of a nutrient or nutrients to a food in amounts sufficient to make the total content larger than that contained in any natural (unprocessed) food of its class; for example, vitamin D milk, fortified margarine, fortified fruit juices. In general, no standards of identity have to be met when a food is labeled "fortified." See *enriched.*

fortify. To add nutrients to a food so that it contains more of the nutrients than was present before processing. Milk often is fortified with vitamin D.

fractionation. A term used by chemists when a complex of natural materials are separated in the laboratory by physical or chemical means. It is done usually to isolate or purify some specific compound present in feeds or foods.

frankfurters (weiners or hot dogs). A type of sausage made from beef, pork, and sometimes veal or combinations of these meats. The meats are combined with seasonings and curing nitrates and in some cases fillers; then stuffed into casings, smoked, cooked in steam, and quickly chilled. Good source of protein, some vitamins of B-group, *thiamine**, *riboflavin** and *niacin**. Fair source of calcium and iron. All meat, 100 gm = 296 calories.

friable. Easily broken or crumbled.

fructose (levulose). Mol. Wt. 180. Fructose occurs in plant juices, in fruits, and especially in honey, of which it constitutes about one-half the solid matter. It results in equal quantity with *glucose** from the hydrolysis of cane sugar and in smaller proportions from some other less common sugars. Fructose serves like glucose for the production of glycogen. Glucose and fructose are convertible chemically under the influence of very dilute alkalies and biochemically by enzymes (an isomerase) that interconvert the phosphate derivatives, glucose-6-phosphate to fructose-6-phosphate.

CH$_2$OH O CH$_2$OH OH OH OH

Fructose (levulose)

fruits. The edible portion of the reproductive body of the seed of a plant, which usually involves the pulp associated with the seed. In fruits, the carbohydrate is mostly in the form of the monosaccharides *glucose** and *fructose**. The disaccharide, *sucrose** may be found in a few fresh fruits. The sugar content of fruits may vary from 6 to 20 percent, those of canteloupe and watermelon being the lowest, and that of banana one of the highest. The *caloric value* of fruits, fresh, canned, or frozen, is determined largely by their sugar content. The table starting on page 192 gives the nutritive content of some common fruits and fruit products.

fungi. Fungi are simple plant organisms which are larger than bacteria. They most often attack the skin, including the hair and nails, causing such chronic infections as ringworm and athlete's foot. Infections caused by fungi are called mycotic infections and can be serious when internal organs are involved. Mushrooms and yeasts are examples of fungi. Some fungi benefit man as in the production of antibiotics, cheese and wine, while other fungi cause diseases.

fumaric acid (fumarate). Mol. Wt. 116. A solid at room temperature, inexpensive, highly acidic, and does not absorb moisture readily. A source of tartness and acidity in such products as gelatin desserts, puddings, pie fillings, candy, instant soft drinks, and leavening agents. Fumaric acid is an important metabolite in the *Kreb's (tricarboxylic acid) cycle* * and is present in every cell of the body.

$$\underset{\text{HOOC}}{\overset{\text{H}}{\diagdown}} C = C \underset{\text{H}}{\overset{\text{COOH}}{\diagup}}$$

Fumaric acid (fumarate)

furcellaran. A vegetable gum whose composition and properties are similar to that of *carrageenin*. Like carrageenin this food additive is obtained from seaweed and is used by food manufacturers as a gelling agent in milk puddings and as a thickening agent in many foods.

Food, Approximate Measure, and Weight (in grams)		Grams	Water Per-cent	Food Energy Calo-ries	Protein Grams	Fat Grams

Fruits and Fruit Products

Food, Approximate Measure, and Weight (in grams)		Grams	Per-cent	Calo-ries	Grams	Grams
Apples, raw (about 3 per lb)[5]	1 apple	150	85	70	Trace	Trace
Apple juice, bottled or canned	1 cup	248	88	120	Trace	Trace
Applesauce, canned:						
Sweetened	1 cup	255	76	230	1	Trace
Unsweetened or artificially sweetened	1 cup	244	88	100	1	Trace
Apricots:						
Raw (about 12 per lb.)[5]	3 apricots	114	85	55	1	Trace
Canned in heavy sirup	1 cup	259	77	220	2	Trace
Dried, uncooked (40 halves per cup).	1 cup	150	25	390	8	1
Cooked, unsweetened, fruit and liquid	1 cup	285	76	240	5	1
Apricot nectar, canned	1 cup	251	85	140	1	Trace
Avocados, whole fruit, raw:[5]						
California (mid- and late-winter; diam. 3⅛ in.).	1 avocado	284	74	370	5	37
Florida (late summer, fall; diam. 3⅝ in.).	1 avocado	454	78	390	4	33
Bananas, raw, medium size.[5]	1 banana	175	76	100	1	Trace
Banana flakes	1 cup	100	3	340	4	1
Blackberries, raw	1 cup	144	84	85	2	1
Blueberries, raw	1 cup	140	83	85	1	1
Cantaloupes, raw; medium, 5-inch diameter about 1⅔ pounds.[5]	½ melon	385	91	60	1	Trace
Cherries, canned, red, sour, pitted, water pack.	1 cup	244	88	105	2	Trace
Cranberry juice cocktail, canned.	1 cup	250	83	165	Trace	Trace
Cranberry sauce, sweetened, canned, strained.	1 cup	277	62	405	Trace	1
Dates, pitted, cut	1 cup	178	22	490	4	1
Figs, dried, large, 2 by 1 in.	1 fig	21	23	60	1	Trace
Fruit cocktail, canned, in heavy sirup.	1 cup	256	80	195	1	Trace
Grapefruit:						
Raw, medium, 3¾-in. diam.[5]						
White	½ grape-fruit.	241	89	45	1	Trace

Fatty Acids										
	Unsaturated									
Satu-rated (total)	Oleic	Lin-oleic	Carbo-hy-drate	Cal-cium	Iron	Vita-min A Value	Thia-mine	Ribo-flavin	Niacin	Ascor-bic Acid
Grams	*Grams*	*Grams*	*Grams*	*Milli-grams*	*Milli-grams*	*Inter-national units*	*Milli-grams*	*Milli-grams*	*Milli-grams*	*Milli-grams*
—	—	—	18	8	0.4	50	0.04	0.02	0.1	3
—	—	—	30	15	1.5	—	0.02	0.05	0.2	2
—	—	—	61	10	1.3	100	0.05	0.03	0.1	[8]3
—	—	—	26	10	1.2	100	0.05	0.02	0.1	[8]2
—	—	—	14	18	.5	2,890	.03	.04	.7	10
—	—	—	57	28	.8	4,510	.05	.06	.9	10
—	—	—	100	100	8.2	16,350	.02	.23	4.9	19
—	—	—	62	63	5.1	8,550	.01	.13	2.8	8
—	—	—	37	23	.5	2,380	.03	.03	.5	[8]8
7	17	5	13	22	1.3	630	.24	.43	3.5	30
7	15	4	27	30	1.8	880	.33	.61	4.9	43
—	—	—	26	10	.8	230	.06	.07	.8	12
—	—	—	89	32	2.8	760	.18	.24	2.8	7
—	—	—	19	46	1.3	290	.05	.06	.5	30
—	—	—	21	21	1.4	140	.04	.08	.6	20
—	—	—	14	27	.8	[9]6,540	.08	.06	1.2	63
—	—	—	26	37	.7	1,660	.07	.05	.5	12
—	—	—	42	13	.8	Trace	.03	.03	.1	[10]40
—	—	—	104	17	.6	60	.03	.03	.1	6
—	—	—	130	105	5.3	90	.16	.17	3.9	0
—	—	—	15	26	.6	20	.02	.02	.1	0
—	—	—	50	23	1.0	360	.05	.03	1.3	5
—	—	—	12	19	0.5	10	0.05	0.02	0.2	44

Food, Approximate Measure, and Weight (in grams)		Grams	Water Per-cent	Food Energy Calo-ries	Protein Grams	Fat Grams
FRUITS and FRUIT PRODUCTS—Con.						
Pink or red	½ grape-fruit.	241	89	50	1	Trace
Canned, sirup pack	1 cup	254	81	180	2	Trace
Grapefruit juice:						
Fresh	1 cup	246	90	95	1	Trace
Canned, white:						
Unsweetened	1 cup	247	89	100	1	Trace
Sweetened	1 cup	250	86	130	1	Trace
Frozen, concentrate, unsweetened:						
Undiluted, can, 6 fluid ounces.	1 can	207	62	300	4	1
Diluted with 3 parts water, by volume.	1 cup	247	89	100	1	Trace
Dehydrated crystals	4 oz.	113	1	410	6	1
Prepared with water (1 pound yields about 1 gallon).	1 cup	247	90	100	1	Trace
Grapes, raw: [5]						
American type (slip skin).	1 cup	153	82	65	1	1
European type (adherent skin).	1 cup	160	81	95	1	Trace
Grapejuice:						
Canned or bottled	1 cup	253	83	165	1	Trace
Frozen concentrate, sweetened:						
Undiluted, can, 6 fluid ounces.	1 can	216	53	395	1	Trace
Diluted with 3 parts water, by volume.	1 cup	250	86	135	1	Trace
Grapejuice drink, canned	1 cup	250	86	135	Trace	Trace
Lemons, raw, 2⅛-in. diam., size 165.[5] Used for juice.	1 lemon	110	90	20	1	Trace
Lemon juice, raw	1 cup	244	91	60	1	Trace
Lemonade concentrate:						
Frozen, 6 fl. oz. per can	1 can	219	48	430	Trace	Trace
Diluted with 4⅓ parts water, by volume.	1 cup	248	88	110	Trace	Trace
Lime juice:						
Fresh	1 cup	246•	90	65	1	Trace
Canned, unsweetened	1 cup	246	90	65	1	Trace

Fatty Acids										
Saturated (total)	Unsaturated		Carbohydrate	Calcium	Iron	Vitamin A Value	Thiamine	Riboflavin	Niacin	Ascorbic Acid
	Oleic	Linoleic								
Grams	Grams	Grams	Grams	Milligrams	Milligrams	International units	Milligrams	Milligrams	Milligrams	Milligrams
—	—	—	13	20	0.5	540	0.05	0.02	0.2	44
—	—	—	45	33	.8	30	.08	.05	.5	76
—	—	—	23	22	.5	([11])	.09	.04	.4	92
—	—	—	24	20	1.0	20	.07	.04	.4	84
—	—	—	32	20	1.0	20	.07	.04	.4	78
—	—	—	72	70	.8	60	.29	.12	1.4	286
—	—	—	24	25	.2	20	.10	.04	.5	96
—	—	—	102	100	1.2	80	.40	.20	2.0	396
—	—	—	24	22	.2	20	.10	.05	.5	91
—	—	—	15	15	.4	100	.05	.03	.2	3
—	—	—	25	17	.6	140	.07	.04	.4	6
—	—	—	42	28	.8	—	.10	.05	.5	Trace
—	—	—	100	22	.9	40	.13	.22	1.5	([12])
—	—	—	33	8	.3	10	.05	.08	.5	
—	—	—	35	8	.3	—	.03	.03	.3	
—	—	—	6	19	.4	10	.03	.01	.1	39
—	—	—	20	17	.5	50	.07	.02	.2	112
—	—	—	112	9	.4	40	.04	.07	.7	66
—	—	—	28	2	Trace	Trace	Trace	.02	.2	17
—	—	—	22	22	.5	20	.05	.02	.2	79
—	—	—	22	22	.5	20	.05	.02	.2	52

Food, Approximate Measure, and Weight (in grams)		Water	Food Energy	Protein	Fat
FRUITS and FRUIT PRODUCTS—Con.	*Grams*	*Per- cent*	*Calo- ries*	*Grams*	*Grams*
Limeade concentrate, frozen:					
Undiluted, can, 6 fluid ounces.	1 can	218	50	410	Trace	Trace
Diluted with 4⅓ parts water, by volume.	1 cup	247	90	100	Trace	Trace
Oranges, raw, 2⅝-in. diam., all commercial, varieties.[5]	1 orange	180	86	65	1	Trace
Orange juice, fresh, all varieties.	1 cup	248	88	110	2	1
Canned, unsweetened	1 cup	249	87	120	2	Trace
Frozen concentrate:					
Undiluted, can, 6 fluid ounces.	1 can	213	55	360	5	Trace
Diluted with 3 parts water, by volume.	1 cup	249	87	120	2	Trace
Dehydrated crystals	4 oz.	113	1	430	6	2
Prepared with water (1 pound yields about 1 gallon).	1 cup	248	88	115	2	1
Orange-apricot juice drink	1 cup	249	87	125	1	Trace
Frozen concentrate:					
Undiluted, can, 6 fluid ounces.	1 can	210	59	330	4	1
Diluted with 3 parts water, by volume.	1 cup	248	88	110	1	Trace
Papayas, raw, ½-inch cubes.	1 cup	182	89	70	1	Trace
Peaches:					
Raw:					
Whole, medium, 2-inch diameter, about 4 per pound.[5]	1 peach	114	89	35	1	Trace
Sliced	1 cup	168	89	65	1	Trace
Canned, yellow-fleshed, solids and liquid:					
Sirup pack, heavy:					
Halves or slices	1 cup	257	79	200	1	Trace
Water pack	1 cup	245	91	75	1	Trace
Dried, uncooked	1 cup	160	25	420	5	1
Cooked, unsweetened, 10–12 halves and juice.	1 cup	270	77	220	3	1
Frozen:					
Carton, 12 ounces, not thawed.	1 carton	340	76	300	1	Trace

Fatty Acids										
	Unsaturated		Carbo-			Vita-				Ascor-
Satu-		Lin-	hy-	Cal-		min A	Thia-	Ribo-		bic
rated (total)	Oleic	oleic	drate	cium	Iron	Value	mine	flavin	Niacin	Acid
				Milli-	Milli-	Inter-national	Milli-	Milli-	Milli-	Milli-
Grams	Grams	Grams	Grams	grams	grams	units	grams	grams	grams	grams
—	—	—	108	11	.2	Trace	.02	.02	.2	26
—	—	—	27	2	Trace	Trace	Trace	Trace	Trace	5
—	—	—	16	54	.5	260	.13	.05	.5	66
—	—	—	26	27	.5	500	.22	.07	1.0	124
—	—	—	28	25	1.0	500	.17	.05	.7	100
—	—	—	87	75	.9	1,620	.68	.11	2.8	360
—	—	—	29	25	.2	550	.22	.02	1.0	120
—	—	—	100	95	1.9	1,900	.76	.24	3.3	408
—	—	—	27	25	.5	500	.20	.07	1.0	109
—	—	—	32	12	.2	1,440	.05	.02	.5	[10]40
—	—	—	78	61	0.8	800	0.48	0.06	2.3	302
—	—	—	26	20	.2	270	.16	.02	.8	102
—	—	—	18	36	.5	3,190	.07	.08	.5	102
—	—	—	10	9	.5	[13]1,320	.02	.05	1.0	7
—	—	—	16	15	.8	[13]2,230	.03	.08	1.6	12
—	—	—	52	10	.8	1,100	.02	.06	1.4	7
—	—	—	20	10	.7	1,100	.02	.06	1.4	7
—	—	—	109	77	9.6	6,240	.02	.31	8.5	28
—	—	—	58	41	5.1	3,290	.01	.15	4.2	6
—	—	—	77	14	1.7	2,210	.03	.14	2.4	[14]135

Food, Approximate Measure, and Weight (in grams)		Water	Food Energy	Protein	Fat
FRUITS and FRUIT PRODUCTS—Con.		*Per-cent*	*Calo-ries*	*Grams*	*Grams*
	Grams				
Pears:					
Raw, 3 by 2½-inch diameter.[5]	1 pear	182	83	100	1	1
Canned, solids and liquid:					
Pineapple:					
Raw, diced	1 cup	140	85	75	1	Trace
Canned, heavy sirup pack, solids and liquid:					
Crushed	1 cup	260	80	195	1	Trace
Sliced, slices and juice.	2 small or 1 large.	122	80	90	Trace	Trace
Pineapple juice, canned	1 cup	249	86	135	1	Trace
Plums, all except prunes:					
Raw, 2-inch diameter, about 2 ounces.[5]	1 plum	60	87	25	Trace	Trace
Canned, sirup pack (Italian prunes):					
Plums (with pits) and juice.[5]	1 cup	256	77	205	1	Trace
Prunes, dried, "softenized," medium:					
Uncooked[5]	4 prunes	32	28	70	1	Trace
Cooked, unsweetened, 17–18 prunes and ⅓ cup liquid.[5]	1 cup	270	66	295	2	1
Prune juice, canned or bottled.	1 cup	256	80	200	1	Trace
Raisins, seedless:					
Packaged, ½ oz. or 1½ tbsp. per pkg.	1 pkg.	14	18	40	Trace	Trace
Cup, pressed down	1 cup	165	18	480	4	Trace
Raspberries, red:					
Raw	1 cup	123	84	70	1	1
Frozen, 10-ounce carton, not thawed.	1 carton	284	74	275	2	1
Rhubarb, cooked, sugar added.	1 cup	272	63	385	1	Trace
Strawberries:					
Raw, capped	1 cup	149	90	55	1	1
Frozen, 10-ounce carton, not thawed.	1 carton	284	71	310	1	1
Tangerines, raw, medium, 2⅜-in. diam., size 176.[5]	1 tan-gerine	116	87	40	1	Trace
Tangerine juice, canned, sweetened.	1 cup	249	87	125	1	1
Watermelon, raw, wedge, 4 by 8 inches (¹/₁₆ of 10 by 16-inch melon, about 2 pounds with rind).[5]	1 wedge	925	93	115	2	1

Fatty Acids										
	Unsaturated									
Satu-rated (total)	Oleic	Lin-oleic	Carbo-hy-drate	Cal-cium	Iron	Vita-min A Value	Thia-mine	Ribo-flavin	Niacin	Ascor-bic Acid
Grams	Grams	Grams	Grams	Milli-grams	Milli-grams	Inter-national units	Milli-grams	Milli-grams	Milli-grams	Milli-grams
—	—	—	25	13	.5	30	.04	.07	.2	7
—	—	—	19	24	7	100	.12	.04	.3	24
—	—	—	50	29	.8	120	.20	.06	.5	17
—	—	—	24	13	.4	50	.09	.03	.2	8
—	—	—	34	37	.7	120	.12	.04	.5	[8] 22
—	—	—	7	7	.3	140	.02	.02	.3	3
—	—	—	53	22	2.2	2,970	.05	.05	.9	4
—	—	—	18	14	1.1	440	.02	.04	.4	1
—	—	—	78	60	4.5	1,860	.08	.18	1.7	2
—	—	—	49	36	10.5	—	.03	.03	1.0	[8] 5
—	—	—	11	9	.5	Trace	.02	.01	.1	Trace
—	—	—	128	102	5.8	30	.18	.13	.8	2
—	—	—	17	27	1.1	160	.04	.11	1.1	31
—	—	—	70	37	1.7	200	.06	.17	1.7	59
—	—	—	98	212	1.6	220	.06	.15	.7	17
—	—	—	13	31	1.5	90	.04	.10	1.0	88
—	—	—	79	40	2.0	90	.06	.17	1.5	150
—	—	—	10	34	.3	360	.05	.02	.1	27
—	—	—	30	45	.5	1,050	.15	.05	.2	55
—	—	—	27	30	2.1	2,510	.13	.13	.7	30

G

galactose. Mol. Wt. 180. A natural monosaccharide. One of the monosaccharides in milk sugar (*lactose**). The hydrolysis of milk sugar, either by acid or by digestive enzyme, yields galactose and *glucose**. Galactose is convertible to glucose in the body. Polymeric anhydrides of galactase, known as galactans are widely distributed in plants, and galactosides which are compounds containing galactose in chemical combination with radicles of other than carbohydrate in nature, are constituents of the brain and nerve tissues. Galactose has also been recognized as a minor constituent of several proteins. See *galactosemia*.

Galactose

galactose-1-phosphate. An intermediate product of galactose metabolism.

galactosemia. A rare genetic disease in which galactose is not properly metabolized because an enzyme, phosphogalactose uridyl transferase is missing. The result is an accumulation of galactose in the blood owing to a hereditary lack of an enzyme to convert galactose to glucose. The disease is accompanied by severe mental retardation which can be ameliorated if special diets are given after birth.

gall bladder. The gall bladder is a dark green sac, shaped like a black jack and lodged in a hollow on the underside of the liver. Its ducts join with the duct of the liver to conduct *bile* to the upper end of the small intestines. The main function of the gall bladder is the concentration and storage of the bile until it is needed for digestion, particularly of fats. See *bile* and *bile salts*.

gallstones. Accumulation of variable sized stones with high cholesterol concentrations or calcium combined with bile in the gall bladder ranging in size from a tiny speck to an inch or more in diameter. *Cholesterol* * may become so concentrated in the gallbladder that it tends to crystallize out, and these crystals form gallstones. The passage through the cystic and common bile ducts often causes severe pain called gallbladder colic. They are common especially at the age of 50 to 60 years. A low fat diet often is suggested as a treatment for gallstones, although no conclusive evidence indicates that such a diet will prevent such symptoms.

gamete. A reproductive cell; an *ovum* or a *spermatozoon.*

gamma globulins. A class of serum proteins some of which function as antibodies.

ganglia (ganglion). A collection of nerve cells which form a distinct mass in the nervous system.

garlic (*Allium sativum*). The garlic, a hardy bulbous plant, is a member of the lily family, which also includes leeks, chives, onions, and shallots. Like the *onion,* the edible bulb of the plant grows beneath the ground. This compound bulb is made up of small sections or bulblets called "cloves" which are encased in thin papery envelopes. One garlic bulb = 1 calorie.

gastric. Pertaining to the stomach.

gastric analysis. A specimen of stomach juice obtained by a stomach tube and examined chemically and microscopically as a screening test for ulcer and cancer.

gastric juice. Secreted by the gastric glands lining the mucous membrane of the stomach. It is a thin, colorless, or nearly colorless liquid containing the digestive enzyme pepsin, produced by the *chief cells,* and hydrochloric acid, produced by the *parietal cells.* The acid which is secreted by the parietal cells has a pH of about 0.9. In addition to salts, gastric juice also contains glycoproteins one of which is the *intrinsic factor* of the antianemia principle. About 700 ml of gastric juice is secreted with each meal. See *digestive system.*

gastric ulcer. An ulcer seated in the wall of the stomach, creating burning pain in the stomach area which is relieved by taking food, milk, or antiacids. Pain usually occurs when stomach is empty. Vomiting may occur.

gastrin. Hormone of the gastrointestinal tract which stimulates the secretion of *hydrochloric acid (HCl)* by the parietal cells of the gastric glands. Although the secretion of gastric juice and the motility of the stomach are sensitive to nervous and psychic influences, by far the strongest stimulus to the secretion of gastric juice comes from the presence of food in the stomach. The formation of a hormone called gastrin in the pyloric glands in the pyloric region of the stomach (under influence of the presence of food) stimulates the muscular activity of the stomach and the secretion of *gastric juice.*

gastritis. Signifies inflammation of the stomach. It occurs in all ages, but appears more common in older people. The term often is used loosely as a catch-all for any digestive complaint, particularly heartburn, belching, "sour stomach," and bloating. These symptoms more often reflect irritability rather than inflammation of the stomach. Chronic gastritis usually follows ingestion of highly spiced food or excessive amounts of alcohol over an extended period of time. See *heartburn.*

gastro ferrin. In the small intestine, the epithelial cell lining of the intestinal wall (the mucosal cell) is the key to the mechanism of iron absorption. This cell lining takes in iron by regulatory procedures not fully understood. It appears that a protein called gastroferrin present in normal *gastric juice,* is involved in the regulation of the absorption of iron by the intestinal mucosal cells.

gastrointestinal. Refers to the part of the digestive system made up of the stomach and the intestines. See *digestive system.*

gastrointestinal disturbances. Digestive and eliminative processes are subject to many kinds of disorders. There are disorders of appetite and excessive eating; at the other extreme anorexia nervosa, a loss of appetite so severe that it sometimes threatens life. *Gastritis* sometimes called "nervous stomach" is marked by gastric distress and pain, occasionally with vomiting. In gastritis there is irritation of the walls of the stomach but not sharply localized injury. *Peptic ulcer* is a focal lesion of the mucous lining of stomach or duodenum, an inflamed crater that may even cause the internal loss of blood. At the eliminative end of the tract the two possibilities are chronic constipation and chronic diarrhea. The latter is usually called *colitis* (inflammation of the colon); it may be associated with chronic spasm of the smooth muscle of the colon or it may invoke ulceration of the inner walls. None of these disorders is necessarily psychogenic. Infections, metabolic disorders, glandular malfunctioning, structural defects, long-continued faulty diet, and many other conditions can cause the gastrointestinal disturbance or distress.

gastrointestinal series (GI Series). A series of gastrointestinal x-ray tests after swallowing barium, which is used for the diagnosis of suspected *ulcer* and cancer of stomach and *duodenum*.

gastrointestinal tract (GI tract). Gastrointestinal tract which includes the *stomach* and *intestines* taken as a unit. See *digestive system.*

gastroscopy. A direct, visual examination of the stomach performed with the aid of a "gastroscope." Especially valuable in detecting *lesions,* such as *ulcers* and *tumors,* not seen in an x-ray examination and for permitting a better evaluation of lesions merely suspected on the basis of x-ray examination.

gavage. Feeding through a tube passed into the stomach through the esophagus.

gelatin. A protein substance which swells on contact with a liquid, dissolves in hot water and forms a jelly when it cools. The word gelatin and jelly both come from the Latin gelatus, meaning "frozen." In cookery gelatin is used as a thickening agent. Edible gelatin is made by a scientific process, from animal tissues, chiefly from veal and beef. Good gelatin is odorless and tasteless; when dissolved, it should make a clear solution. There are two main types of gelatin. The alkaline type found in unflavored gelatin and the acid type used in the flavored gelatin. Gelatin is pure protein, easily digested. It contains seven essential amino acids. However, it is not a complete protein as are meats, egg, cheese, and milk proteins. It is useful as a protein supplement. 1 envelope = 28 calories.

gene. The biological unit of hereditary information, self-reproducing and located in a definite position (locus) on a particular *chromosome*. The gene is the trinucleotide sequence of *deoxyribonucleic acid* (DNA) within the chromosome which determines the amino acid sequence of a polypeptide chain. See *genetic code.*

gene linkage. Refers to the fact that all the *genes* of a given chromosome are inherited together.

Generally Regarded As Safe (GRAS). GRAS refers to the Food and Drug Administration's list of food additives that have been used for relatively long periods, and thus are exempt from requirements for premarket clearance.

generic name drugs. The generic or official name of a drug is assigned by the producer of the drug in collaboration with the Food and Drug Administration and Council on Drugs of the American Medical Association. The generic name may be used by any interested party and is usually the name found in the USP and NF. The generic listing is usually used in the Federal Supply Catalog and in AMEDD pharmacies. A generic drug name is not capitalized; for example, *aluminum hydroxide*.

genetic. Congenital or inherited, or referring to the gene.

genetic code. The formal correspondence between the trinucleotide base sequence in *deoxyribonucleic acid* (DNA) and amino acid sequences in proteins which makes possible the synthesis of specific proteins according to hereditary information contained in the genes. Codes have been worked out for each of the amino acids. It is now possible to say exactly what combinations of *purine* and *pyrimidine* bases in the *nucleic acid* molecules instruct the *ribosomes* to attach a particular amino acid to a particular place in a growing protein or *polypeptide chain*.

genome. The sum of all the various genes present in an organism.

genotype. The genetic make-up of individuals. Persons with the same genes have the same genotype. When persons merely show the same physical traits, they are referred to as having the same phenotype. Sometimes persons with the same genotype may differ in phenotype, as with identical twins who have developed differently because of environmental or nutritional influences. Conversely, persons with the same phenotype, showing the same physical traits may or may not be carrying the same genes. For example, two dark-eyed persons, one of whom carries two "dark-eyed" genes, the other one carrying a dominant "dark-eye" gene plus a recessive "light eye" gene, may appear alike, that is they have the same phenotype but their genes are not identical. Therefore they are different genotypes.

germ. The part of a cereal seed that grows and produces new plants. See *cereal grains*. Also a common name for *bacteria*.

germ plasm. The material of the germ cells, in the testes of the male or the ovaries of the female, from which the sperms or eggs with their *chromosomes* are fashioned.

ghee. The anglicized version of the Hindustani for ghi, which means "clarified butter" and is a basic ingredient in the cooking of India. Indian butter is made from buffalo's or cow's milk. To clarify it, the butter is heated until the milk solids are separated from the clear fat. Then it is strained through a cloth and poured into a container for storage. The reason for clarifying butter in a hot climate is that it will keep without refrigeration for quite a long time, depending upon the temperature.

gibberellins. A group of growth-regulating substances (hormones) for plants that are produced by certain species of fungi of the genus *Gibberella*.

gin. A simple alcoholic liquor of pure ethyl alcohol (*ethanol,* grain alcohol), plus water and flavoring. The flavor is derived by allowing the alcoholic vapors to flow over the flavoring ingredients, usually juniper berries (although orange peel, caraway seeds, and other flavoring materials are used). The principal effects of gin are produced by the alcohol and have a toxic effect. The concentration of ethyl alcohol in beverages is expressed in proof, which is twice the percentage of the alcohol.

ginger (*Zingiber officnale*). Ginger is a spice obtained from a root. An erect perennial plant that grows to a height of 3 feet, and has large brilliant yellowish flowers with purple lips, which are borne in a spike. There are several hundred varieties of ginger. The pungent smell of ginger comes from an aromatic oil, the peppery taste from a substance called "gingerin." The root, or rhizone, of the plant is the part that is prepared for use. Ginger is used crystallized, preserved, or dried; whole, cracked, or ground to a powder.

ginger ale. A carbonated beverage flavored with ginger, sugar, capsicum, and other flavorings and colored with caramel. Ginger ale is also made with an artificial sweetener rather than with sugar. 100 gm = 31 calories; With artificial sweetener, 100 gm = less than 1 calorie.

ginger beer. A clear effervescent beverage made of ginger, sugar, and water, and fermented by yeast. It has a stronger ginger flavor than ginger ale.

gingiva. The mucous membrane and connective tissue that encircles the neck of the tooth, and overlies the crowns of those not as yet erupted. Commonly referred to as the gums. See *tooth*.

gingivitis. An inflammation of the gums (gingiva), beginning with a slight swelling along the gum margin of one or more teeth. The gum tissue in the area may have a slightly different color. As the condition grows worse, the "collar" of gum tissue loses its tight adaptation to the tooth surface, and the tissue bleeds on slight pressure. Usually there is no pain. Gingivitis is a common symptom of vitamin deficiencies, especially *ascorbic acid* (vitamin C) which leads to scurvy.

G.I. series. See *gastrointestinal series*.

G.I. tract. See *gastrointestinal tract*.

glands. Groups of cells which take certain materials from tissue fluid and make new substances of them. All cells in the body take from the surrounding fluid substances essential for their nutrition and give off products of their metabolism. A group of cells that have definite structure for the specific purpose of either secretion or excretion is called a gland. Glands may be classified as *exocrine,* or duct glands, which secrete into a cavity or on the body surface, and the *endocrine,* incretory, or ductless glands which secrete into the tissue fluid and blood.

glandular. Adjective of glands. A gland is an organ that makes and discharges a chemical substance that is used elsewhere in the body or eliminated.

gliadin. A plant protein fraction of wheat gluten. It belongs to a class of plant proteins called *prolamines*. It is gliadin and the protein *glutenin* in combination that gives wheat flour its characteristic stickiness when moistened and its bonding when baked. See *wheat, flour,* and *bread*.

globular proteins. A classification of proteins based upon their shape. Globular protein molecules tend to be nearly round in shape. The contrast of the globular proteins are the *fibrous proteins* which are long and thin in shape. Found in tissue fluids of animals and plants in which they readily disperse, either in true solution or colloidal suspension. Important globular proteins from the standpoint of nutrition are caseinogen in milk, albumin in egg white and albumins and globulins of blood, which are not only easily digestible, but which also contain in their structure a good proportion of the essential *amino acids*. See *globulin* and *proteins*.

globulin. A globular protein found throughout body tissues in various forms such as gamma (γ) globulins, serum globulins, alpha- (α) and beta- (β) globulins, etc. Simple proteins insoluble in pure water, but soluble in neutral salt. Examples are muscle globulin, serum globulin (blood), edestin (wheat, hemp seed, and other seeds), phaseolin (beans), legumin (beans and peas), vigin (cow peas), tuberin (potato), amandin (almonds), excelsin (Brazil nuts), arachin and conarachin (peanuts).

glomerulonephritis (kidney disease). The most frequently occurring kidney disease is probably *nephritis,* or Bright's disease, characterized by inflammation of kidney tissue. Since it is the glomeruli which are first affected, this type of kidney damage is called glomerulonephritis. It usually follows a hemolytic strepococcal infection in another part of the body, or may be precipitated by a generalized infection.

glomerulus (glomerular filtration). A network of *capillaries* that forms a tuft at the beginning of each tubule within the *kidney*. It is the glomerulus and the process of glomerular filtration that is responsible for the production of urine. The diagram below shows that the pressure developed in forcing blood through the small capillaries is greater than the opposing forces (colloidal osmotic pressure and hydrostatic pressure) by 50 mm of Hg. Blood is filtered and only small molecules can pass through the pores of the capillary walls. The pore size is estimated at 20 Å (angstroms) which is large enough to let small proteins (such as myoglobin through (Mol. Wt. 17,000) but not serum albumin (Mol. Wt. 66,500). The filtered blood then passes through the tubules where specific reabsorptions of the filtrate occurs. The glomerulus plus the tubule make up the filtration unit called the *nephron*. There are approximately one million nephrons in each kidney. See *urinary system, urine,* and *nephron.*

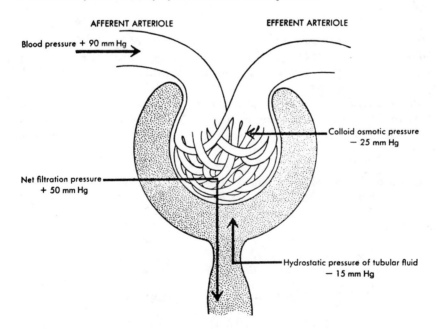

glossitis. Deficiencies of *niacin*, riboflavin*, cobalamin** (vitamin B_{12}), *folacin*,* and *iron* all give rise to glossitis, a feature of *pellagra,* sprue, and various types of nutritional anemias. In acute glossitis the tongue is swollen, the papillae are usually prominent, with the color of the tongue characteristically red.

Deep irregular fissuring is common and shallow ulcers may occur, especially in the sides or tips. The tongue is usually extremely painful creating a problem in eating. In chronic atrophic glossitis the tongue is small, with an atrophic mucous membrane and small or absent papillae so that its surface appears smooth, moist and abnormally clean. It is usually not painful.

glucagon. A hormone which is functionally the opposite of *insulin*. Its main role is to increase the amount of glucose in the blood. Glucagon initiates a series of reactions in which the glycogen store of the liver is mobilized to release glucose into the blood. Also, the enzyme systems that manufacture glucose from amino acids are stimulated to synthesize glucose. Glucagon in this respect is very similar to *epinepherine*. Both glucagon and epinepherine stimulate the formation of *cyclic- adenosine-nonophosphate (AMP)*, the so-called second messenger. Cyclic-AMP then stimulates a host of other enzymes. *Insulin* and glucagon work together in a seesaw mechanism to maintain the blood glucose at a required level. Glucagon increases blood glucose and insulin decreases blood glucose. Glucagon is a single chain of 29 amino acids strung end-to-end. See *insulin*.

glucocorticoid hormone. A class of hormones produced by the adrenal cortex which increases the rate of glucose formation raising the concentration of liver glycogen and blood glucose. See *cortisol* and *cortisone*.

gluconeogenesis. The anabolic formation or synthesis of glucose and glycogen from the intermediate compounds of metabolism is called gluconeogenesis. The formation of glucose from noncarbohydrate sources. The opposite of *glycogen-olysis*.

gluconic acid (gluconate, sodium or potassium). Mol. Wt. 196. Occasionally used as a component of leavening in cake mixes or as an acid in powdered gelatin and soft drink mixes. Occurs naturally in the human body as the phosphate derivative.

$$\text{HOCH}_2 - \underset{\underset{\text{OH}}{|}}{\overset{\overset{\text{H}}{|}}{\text{C}}} - \underset{\underset{\text{OH}}{|}}{\overset{\overset{\text{H}}{|}}{\text{C}}} - \underset{\underset{\text{H}}{|}}{\overset{\overset{\text{OH}}{|}}{\text{C}}} - \underset{\underset{\text{OH}}{|}}{\overset{\overset{\text{H}}{|}}{\text{C}}} - \text{COOH}$$

Gluconic acid

glucose or dextrose. Mol. Wt. 180. A hexose (six-carbon sugar). Glucose is often called dextrose in food preparations. It is one of the important *monosac-*

charides in intermediary metabolism. Glucose is the building block for *starches* and *amylopectons* in plants and for *glycogen* in animals. Glucose is a *precursor* to *ascorbic acid** (vitamin C) synthesis in plants and animals, with the exceptions of man, other primates, the guinea pig, and a species of fruit bat which cannot make ascorbic acid (vitamin C). Glucose is also a source of energy and under ordinary circumstances about 20 percent of the total energy needs derives from the oxidation of glucose. However, glucose is the major source of energy for the brain one of a few substances that can freely cross the blood-brain barrier to enter brain and nerve cells. The maintenance of blood sugar (glucose) levels is an important homeostatic process since severe low blood sugar, as in the case of *insulin* overdose, will cause shock. The shock is brought on because brain cells are derived of energy at very low blood sugar levels and the brain begins to function abnormally. The brain, which is 2 percent of adult body weight, utilizes 20 percent of the oxygen we breathe, and the utilization of oxygen by the brain is proportional to its oxidation of glucose. Glucose is also an emergency reserve in the form of liver glycogen. During emergencies liver glycogen breaks down (*glycogenolysis*) and glucose enters the blood to meet the immediate demand for more energy. A normal blood level of glucose is 80 to 100 milligrams per 100 milliters of blood. Since the body can readily synthesize glucose (*gluconeogenesis*) there is no dietary requirement for glucose.

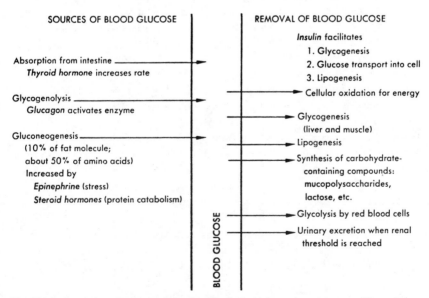

The blood glucose is maintained within physiologic limits by replacement as rapidly as it is removed to meet metabolic needs. Glycogenesis, lipogenesis, and excretion at the renal threshold are mechanisms that prevent hyperglycemia in the normal individual.

$$\text{(6)}\quad CH_2OH$$

Glucose (dextrose)

Glucose occurs in fruits and in chemical combinations with *fructose* * and *sucrose* * (table sugar). As a carbohydrate, glucose yields 4.0 calories per gram. The diagram on p. 209 shows how the blood glucose is maintained relatively constant by a balance of the sources and removal of glucose.

glucose oxidase. A highly specific enzyme produced by the submerged growth of *Aspergillus niger* and other molds. It is used to remove glucose from egg white or whole eggs to facilitate drying, prevent deterioration and improve the whipping properties (of the reconstituted dried whites). It has been employed also to extend the shelf life of canned soft drinks by retarding the pickup of iron and the fading of color. Oxidation of the glucose by glucose oxidase forms *gluconic acid* * and hydrogen peroxide, the latter then being decomposed by the catalase in the same preparation. A combination of glucose oxidase and *catalase* is used to remove small residues of oxygen in packaged foods. Glucose oxidase is the most specific enzyme known since it can catalyze the rapid oxidation of glucose only. The high specificity of glucose oxidase and its relatively high stability for an enzyme has made it ideal for detection of glucose in urine. The test depends upon the oxidation of a dye by the *hydrogen peroxide* (H_2O_2) produced by glucose oxidase action on glucose.

glucose test. A chemical test, either on blood or urine, used as a screening test and also for the diagnosis of diabetes mellitus and other metabolic diseases, and as a guide to treatment.

glucose tolerance test. A test to determine how effectively an individual can remove high levels of glucose from the blood. The person being tested drinks a concentrated glucose solution and the blood glucose levels are subsequently measured over a period of several hours. The test is unpleasant but often necessary in the diagnosis of *diabetes mellitus* (sugar diabetes) or *hypoglycemia*.

glucostatic theory. The theory that the level of blood sugar affects cells in the hypothalmus of the brain to arouse eating behavior when the blood sugar level is low.

glucosuria. The presence of glucose in the urine. It is often an indication of an abnormality.

glutamic acid (glutamate). Mol. Wt. 147. One of the amino acids found in proteins. Glutamic acid contains two carboxylic acid groups in the molecule. It is therefore classified as an acidic amino acid. It is one of the few substances that can readily pass through the *blood brain barrier*. Glutamate is a nonessential amino acid that can be synthesized by *transamination* to alpha (α) *ketoglutarate*. *Pyridoxine* * (vitamin B$_6$) participates in transamination as the coenzyme *pyridoxamine phosphate* *. A *Kreb's cycle* intermediate. *Monosodium glutamate* (MSG), the flavor enhancer, is a sodium salt of glutamic acid.

$$HOOC—CH_2—CH_2—\underset{\underset{NH_2}{|}}{CH}—COOH$$

glutamine. Mol. Wt. 146. One of the amino acids found in proteins. Formed from *glutamic acid* * by the addition of ammonia to the second carboxylic acid group to form an amide group. It is taken up by the brain in greater quantities than any other amino acid. See *blood brain barrier*.

$$\overset{\overset{O}{\|}}{H_2NC}—CH_2—CH_2—\underset{\underset{NH_2}{|}}{CH}—COOH$$

Glutamine

glutathione. A tripeptide coenzyme involved in metabolism; isolated from plant and animal tissue. A tripeptide of *glutamic acid* *, *cysteine* *, and *glycine* *, which is an important factor in the oxidation and reduction reactions of the cell by the virtue of the sulfhydryl (—SH) group.

glutelins. Simple plant proteins insoluble in all neutral solvents, but readily soluble in very dilute acids and alkalies. The best known and most important members of this group are the glutenin of wheat, hordenin from barley, and oryzenin from rice. See *wheat*.

gluten. A mixture of two proteins, *gliadin* and *glutenin*, found in many cereals and grains. A tough elastic substance that gives adhesiveness to dough. It is formed when the proteins in flour, especially those in wheat flour, absorb water. The result is to remove the starch in the flour. Gluten helps give shape to cooked products because it coagulates when heated. Gluten flour is higher in protein. "Hard" wheat is higher in gluten than "soft" wheat. See *wheat*.

glutenin. A protein of the classification *glutelin* found in *wheat*. It is the combination of glutenin and *gliadin* when mixed with water that gives the characteristic stickiness and doughy consistency. Heat bonds these proteins. Rye has only a small amount of glutenin but enough to make a bread loaf. Oats, barley, rice, and millets contain too little glutenin to permit them to be used to make breads. See *wheat*.

glycemia. Presence of sugar (in the form of *glucose*) in the blood.

glycerin. See *glycerol**.

glycerol (glycerin). Mol. Wt. 90.1. Glycerol is a polyalcohol containing three carbons and three hydroxy (—OH) groups. Glycerol is a colorless, odorless, syrupy sweet liquid, a major component of neutral fat molecules and obtained by the hydrolysis of fats. Chemically, glycerol has the properties of an alcohol. When esterified with fatty acids, glycerol forms *glycerides*. Glycerol is added to foods to maintain moisture and to prevent foods from drying out and becoming hard. Glycerol is used in marshmallows, candy fudge and baked goods in amounts ranging from 0.5 to 10 percent. Glycerol is also used as a solvent for oily chemicals, especially flavorings that are not very soluble in water.

$$H_2C—OH$$
$$|$$
$$HO—C—H$$
$$|$$
$$H_2C—OH$$

Glycerol (glycerin)

glycine. Mol. Wt. 75. A nonessential amino acid. It is the only amino acid that does not possess an asymmetric alpha (α) carbon. Glycine can be synthesized from *serine**, another nonessential *amino acid*, with the B-vitamin *folacin** acting as a *coenzyme*. Glycine gets its name from the Greek word meaning "sweet" and is in fact a sweet-tasting substance. During rapid growth the demand for glycine may be enormous. It is an important *precursor* in many syntheses in the human body, such as those of the *purine* bases, *porphyrins*, *creatine*, and the conjugated *bile acids*. It is utilized by the liver in the elimination of toxic phenols, and conjugated with the bile acid to form *bile salts*.

H
|
H—C—COOH
|
NH$_2$

Glycine

glycogen (animal starch). Mol Wt. up to 1,000,000. Name means "sugar former," given to this compound because whenever the body needs extra *glucose* * the liver glycogen can be converted back into glucose again and released into the bloodstream. The storage form of carbohydrates in animals. The only homopolysaccharide of importance in animal storage. Plants have *starch* * and *amylopectin*. Although the total quantity of glycogen in the animal body is low, its role is primarily that of storing carbohydrate, similar to the role of starch in plant cells. It occurs in all cells and predominantly in the liver where it is important to the mechanism that regulates the glucose level of the blood. Glycogen is a complex polymer of glucose. It functions as a storage form of glucose in all cells, but liver glycogen has a special role. Glycogen is a branched chain containing two types of linkages, the $\alpha 1 \rightarrow 4$ and the $\alpha 1 \rightarrow 6$. The branches occur about every 6–8 glucose units. Glucose is released from glycogen by the action of an enzyme called a phosphorylase which yields a phosphorylated derivative, glucose-1-phosphate. Glucose-1-phosphate can then be catabolized by a series of enzymes to yield carbon dioxide (CO_2), water, and energy. These events occur in all cells and the activation of the phosphorylase to breakdown glycogen can be initiated with hormones *epinephrine* or *glucagon*. Liver differs from other cells in that one of the phosphorylated derivatives of glucose, glucose-6-phosphate, can be converted to free glucose and thus leave the liver cell and enter the blood. The liver acts as a reservoir for glucose for the entire body. Tissues continually withdraw glucose from the blood for their own uses, and the glycogen in the liver must be converted to glucose to maintain blood glucose at the normal level. The amount of glycogen in the liver and muscle depends somewhat on the supply of carbohydrate in the diet. Glycogen molecules are similar in many respects to those of the branched form of plant starch (*amylopectin*) but glycogen has a shorter chain of glucose units and therefore a more complicated branched structure. Glycogen is therefore well adapted to being broken into smaller units or being rebuilt as needed from smaller units in the body tissues. Only limited amounts of glycogen can be stored in the liver and other tissues and this is used up rapidly during fasting or muscular work. Liver usually contains 1.5 to 5 percent glycogen by weight while shellfish (including oysters) have 0.5 to 5 percent. See *starch* *.

Glycogen (animal starch)

glycogenolysis. The specific term for conversion of glycogen into *glucose* * in the liver. Glycogenolysis is the complex series of enzymatic hydrolysis or breakdowns by which this conversion is accomplished. The hormones *epinephrine* * and *glucagon* stimulate glycogenolysis. Glycogenolysis is the opposite of *gluconeogenesis*.

glycolipids. (1) Compounds of fatty acids which are combined with carbohydrates and nitrogen. Because they are found chiefly in brain tissue, these substances are also called *cerebrosides*. (2) Compounds that have the solubility properties of a lipid and contain one or more molecules of a sugar. Often associated in biological systems. Many animal glycolipids are derivatives of a class of compounds known as *ceramides*.

glycolysis. The enzymatic conversion of sugar to *pyruvic acid* * and *lactic acid* * (lactate), and is also called Embden-Meyerhof-Parnas pathway. Glycolysis is an important part of metabolism (anaerobic metabolism). The enzymatic reactions involved in glycolysis, are much the same as those in fermentations to form alcohol in the products of beers and wines by yeast.

glycolytic. Pertaining to the breakdown of sugars.

glycoproteins. Biopolymers having proteins and sugar residues linked covalently to each other. They differ from *mucoproteins* in that they contain considerably less carbohydrate. The carbohydrate chains of glycoproteins are short, consisting of perhaps 8 to 10 monosaccharide units. The class of glycoproteins include a large number of biologically active substances such as enzymes, hor-

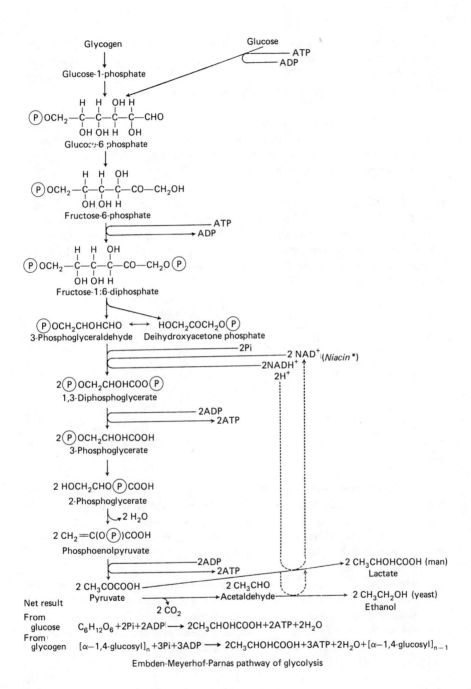

Embden-Meyerhof-Parnas pathway of glycolysis

mones, and immunoglobulins as well as structural components of blood vessels and skin. Of particular interest are the glycoproteins associated with the cell membrane surface. These cell surface glycoproteins are likely involved in active transport of ions and intercellular communication.

glycoside. A *monosaccharide* derivative chemically linked at the carbonyl group with an alcohol (OH) group. The linkage is called a *glycosidic linkage* *. Examples are *digitalis* derivatives, which form drugs essential to cardiac therapy, and steroids, the adrenal hormones.

glycosidic linkage. The link between the carbonyl group of a monosaccharide and an alcoholic group of another compound. Two monosaccharides can be joined in a glycosidic linkage. *Maltose* * is an example in which case the glycosidic linkage is sometimes referred to as a glucosidic linkage, which indicates glucose units are involved. The α 1 $\longrightarrow$ 4 shown is a glycosidic (glucosidic) linkage.

Glycosidic linkage

glycosuria. A general term for an abnormal amount of sugar in the urine. See *glucosuria*.

goiter. The enlargement of the *thyroid gland*. Simple goiter is a complex nutritional disease, brought about in part by an insufficient supply of *iodine*. The gland enlarges in an attempt to compensate by additional glandular tissue for the shortage of necessary material (iodine) for making its internal secretion (*thyroxine* *). See *thiocyanic acid* and *thiourea*.

goitrogens. A lack of iodine in the diet can lead to goiter. It is also known that eating cabbage, cauliflower, turnips, mustard, and collard greens, and Brussel sprouts may induce goiter formation in susceptible individuals. These plants and other of the Cruciferae family, including kale, broccoli, rutabaga, kohlrabi, radish, and horseradish, contain thioglucosides which under certain conditions can block the absorption of iodine. See thiocyanic acid and thiourea.

Golgi complex or apparatus. An internal structure of cells. Most noticeable in secreting cells, appears as a parallel arrangement of membranes and small vacuoles, somewhat like flattened bags, lying near the centrioles. It functions in regard to concentrating the cell secretion and in the formation of cell membranes. See *cell*.

gonad. A reproductive gland. The testicle in the male and the ovary in the female. See *Sex Glands*

gonadotrophic hormone (GTH). Hormones that stimulate the gonads to produce hormones and reproductive cells, and regulate the female estrus cycle, such as the follicle stimulating hormone (FSH), luteinizing hormone (LH), and *prolactin* of the *pituitary gland.*

gonadotropins. Hormones from embryonic sex glands.

gooseberry (*Ribes*). A round juicy berry, a first cousin of the fresh *currant*. It grows on a bush. The flavor is tart, yet sweet when the berries are fully ripened. Gooseberries can grow as large as 1 inch in diameter and 1½ inches in length. There are a number of varieties; red, green, white, or yellow, and smooth or hairy. Raw, 100 gm = 39 calories; canned, heavy syrup, 100 gm = 90 calories.

gout. A metabolic disease, the result of a defect in the metabolism of *purines,* which are products of the digestion of *nucleic acids*. The faulty mechanism results in an elevation above normal of *uric acid* * in the blood (hyperuricemia). Eventually there are deposits of the sodium salt of uric acid crystals in the joints, kidneys, cartilage of the ear and sometimes in the heart or other internal organs. Subcutaneous deposits of *urate* * crystals are called tophi, and they appear in about one-third of those who have gout. Meats have a high *nucleic acid* content and thus a high purine content. A part of the treatment is a special diet. The 95 percent of individuals with gout are males.

grade. The grade of a food is an indication of the general size, palatability, appearance and maturity of the food. The grade is not related to the nutrient value. In the United States, grading is voluntary. It is not required by law and processors and packers pay a fee for the grading service. The grading of food should not be confused with the inspection of food for its fitness to be consumed. The inspection of food passing over state lines is mandatory. Both grading and inspection are done by government employees.

grain alcohol. See *ethanol.*

grapefruit (*Citrus paradisi*). A member of the citrus family, large and round with a rind colored from pale yellow to bronze; a juicy pulp which may be yellowish-white or pink, and a slightly bitter flavor. Grapefruit can weigh from 2 to 12 pounds and have a diameter of 4 to 6 inches. Grapefruit is a good source of vitamin C and is also low in calories. Fresh grapefruit or juice should be used as soon as possible as long storage or exposure to air decreases vitamin C content.

Grapefruit, fresh, 100 gm = 41 calories
Canned, segments and liquid, water pack, 100 gm = 30 calories
Canned and frozen, segments and liquid, sugar pack, 100 gm = 70 calories
Fresh juice, 100 gm = 39 calories
Canned juice, and frozen juice diluted with 3 parts water, unsweetened, 100 gm = 41 calories
Canned juice, sweetened, 100 gm = 53 calories
Frozen juice, sweetened, diluted with 3 parts water, 100 gm = 47 calories
Canned grapefruit and orange juice, unsweetened, 100 gm = 43 calories
Canned grapefruit and orange juice, sweetened, 100 gm = 50 calories

GRAS. See *Generally Regarded as Safe.*

greengage (*Prunus*). A fine-quality dessert plum, round in shape and greenish yellow in color. The flesh is juicy and sweet, yet it has a tang. The stone is small and round and the flesh clings to it. Greengages should be tree ripened as they do not ripen well after picking. Caloric values: Fresh, 100 gm = 75 calories; canned, water pack, 100 gm = 33 calories; canned, heavy syrup, 100 gm = 70 calories. See *Plum.*

grits, groats. Both words refer to hulled and coarsely ground cereal grains and both have the meaning of "fragment" or "part." Grits are smaller than groats, more finely ground, usually from corn, but also from buckwheat, rye, oats, or rice. Grits ground from corn are known as hominy grits. Groats are most often ground from buckwheat, oats, barley, and wheat, as well as corn. Cracked wheat is another name for wheat groats or grits. Buckwheat grouts are the most commonly used. They are also called kasha, a Russian word, and are a staple of Russia's diet.

grouper (*Epinephelus* and *Mycteroperea*). Salt water fish which live in warm waters, at the bottom of the sea, and in rocky nooks and crevices. They resemble sea bass, and are an important food fish. Groupers can grow to a great size, about 40 to 50 pounds. They can be cooked like sea bass or red snapper. Raw, 100 gm = 87 calories.

growth hormone (GH, Somatotropin). (1) The only hormone of the anterior *pituitary gland* that does not exert its effect on other endocrine glands. Growth hormone or somatotropin is a protein. Unlike other hormones that influence growth, GH merely affects the rate of the process. It does not control the actual process of maturation or the development of tissues. GH also influences the level of glucose and fat in the blood. (2) GH stimulates growth, increases protein synthesis, decreases carbohydrate utilization and increases fat catabolism. GH facilitates the transport of many amino acids through the cell membrane. Once in the cell, they are available for protein synthesis. As a result of the suppression of carbohydrate utilization under the influence of GH blood glucose increases. This stimulates the secretion of insulin. The level of GH in plasma is normally about 2μ g/liter during the day, rising to peaks of 10 to 15μ g/liter during sleep. Secretion is controlled by two factors from the *hypothalamus;* (1) the growth hormone releasing factor (GRF) and, (2) the growth hormone release inhibiting factor (GRIF). During protein deficiency, GH secretion increases as it does when blood sugar level falls. Exercise increases secretion.

guanosine triphosphate (GTP). Mol. Wt. 523. A high-energy phosphate compound equivalent in energy to *adenosine triphosphate* * (ATP). The guanosine nucleotides, GTP, GDP, and GMP are important in several specific reactions. The chemical energy of GTP is required for protein synthesis and GDP is required in the oxidation of alpha (α) *ketoglutaric acid* * in the *Kreb's* (tricarboxylic acid) *cycle.* * The GMP moiety is in all nucleic acids.

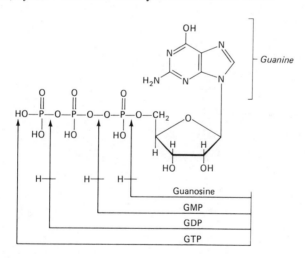

Guanosine triphosphate (GTP)

guar gum. A vegetable gum stabilizer which will dissolve in cold water. A guar gum solution will turn into a rubbery gel if borate is added as a cross-linking agent. Serves as a thickening agent in beverages, ice cream, frozen puddings, and salad dressing. Used to increase the resiliency of doughs and batters and in the production of artificial whipped cream.

gum arabic. A soluble gum obtained from several species of acacia trees. Used by food processors to prevent sugar crystals from forming in candy, helps citrus oils dissolve in drinks, encapsulates flavor oils in powdered drink mixes, stabilizes foam in beer and improves the texture of commercial ice cream. Gum arabic is very soluble in water; solutions become very viscous only when they contain 10–20 percent gum.

gum ghatti. A vegetable gum used by food manufacturers to keep oil and water ingredients from separating out into two layers in such products as salad dressing and butter-in-syrup.

H

haddock (*Melandogrammus Aeglefinus*). A saltwater fish, an important food fish. It is closely related to the cod, but the two fish can easily be told apart. The haddock is much smaller than the cod. The flesh is firm and white, with a pleasant flavor which is on the bland side. Smoked haddock is called finnan haddie. Haddock is a very good source of protein and contains phosphorus, potassium, niacin, and thiamine. Raw, 100 gm = 79 calories; Fried, 100 gm = 165 calories; Smoked 100 gm = 103 calories. See *fish*.

haeme. See *heme*. The prefix hem- is used in lieu of haem-.

hake (*Merluccius* and *Urophycis*). Saltwater food fish, relatives of the *cod*. Hakes are slender, dark-gray fish with fins on their backs. Their average market weight is between 1 and 4 pounds. The meat is soft and white with a delicate flavor. Raw, 100 gm = 74 calories.

halibut (*Hippoglassus*). Cold-water fish which lives in all the seas of the world and is one of the most important food fishes. There several varieties. The fish is flat and resembles a gigantic flounder. The flesh is white and excellent in flavor and texture. Chicken halibuts, weighing up to 10 pounds are considered the finest. A very good source of protein, low in fat. Halibut liver oil is a rich source of *retinol* (vitamin A). Raw, 100 gm = 100 calories; broiled, 100 gm = 171 calories. See *fish*.

ham. The rear leg of a hog, from the aitchbone (hipbone) through the meaty part of the shank bone is called a ham. Fresh ham is a very good to excellent source of high quality protein and thiamine, a fair to good source of iron and niacin, and a fair source of riboflavin. Fat, roasted, 100 gm = 394 calories. Medium-fat, roasted, 100 gm = 374 calories. Lean, roasted, 100 gm = 346 calories. See *meat*.

Hamburger. This term describes ground beef prepared from the less tender cuts. Good source of protein and a variable source of fat, depending on the type of meat ground. Market ground, raw, 100 gm = 268 calories. Ground lean, raw, 100 gm = 179 calories. See *meat.*

hanseniaspoia. Lemon-shaped (apiculate) yeasts which grow in fruit juices. Nadsonia yeasts are large and lemon-shaped.

haploid. Having a single set of chromosomes. In human beings each sperm or egg is a haploid cell, containing only one set, or 23 single chromosomes, in contrast to a developed cell with two sets.

haverisian canals. Vascular canals in bone or bony tissue.

hazelnut. A grape-size, smooth-shelled nut growing on shrubs and trees. (*Corylus.*) The nuts grow in clusters and each is wrapped in a fuzzy outer husk that opens as the nut ripens. The hazelnut is also known as a cobnut or filbert. Hazelnuts provide protein, fat, iron, and *thiamine.** 100 gm = 634 calories.

head cheese. A well-seasoned cold cut made of the edible parts of a calf's or a pig's head such as the cheeks, snouts, and underlips to which sometimes brains, hearts, tongues, and feet are added. The meat is boiled, stripped from the bones, skinned, cut into pieces, and seasoned with onions, herbs and spices. Then it is put into a mold and pressed into a firm, jellied mass.

heart. A cone-shaped muscle about the size of the fist. It lies in the chest, between the lungs, in a cavity called the mediastinum. The heart is really two pumps in a single organ. It is made up of four chambers, two atria or auricles and two ventricles. The right atrium and right ventricle are completely separated from the left artrium and left ventricle. Blood with low oxygen content flows from the body into the right atrium by the way of large veins, the inferior and superior vena cava. The blood with low oxygen content goes from the right atrium to the right ventricle through the atrioventricular opening. The pulmonary *artery* carries the blood from the right ventricle to the lungs where it is oxygenated. The oxygenated blood is returned to the heart by way of the pulmonary veins and enters the left atrium and from there into the left ventricle. The oxygenated blood moves from the left ventricle through the aorta and from there to all parts of the body, giving up its oxygen to the cells in its course and returning again to the heart. The total blood volume of the average man is about 6 liters. An average man has a cardiac output of about 5.5 liters/min. The table below shows the blood flow through various organs in the body. The heart is a *muscle* and like other muscles it uses *creatine phosphate** as an energy reserve to form *adenosine triphosphate** (ATP). The enzyme that catalyzes the reaction forming ATP is creatine *phosphokinase* (CPK). During a *myocardial* *infarction,* heart cell tissues die and CPK is released into the blood. The detection of high levels of CPK activity in the blood is evidence for a heart attack.

Partition of left ventricular output and pulmonary oxygen intake in man at rest under basal conditions is shown below.*

Region	Mass (kg.)	Blood Flow (ml./min.)	(ml./100 Gm./min.)	A-V O: Difference (ml./L.)	Oxygen Use (ml./min.)	(ml./100 Gm./min.)
1. Hepatic-portal	2.6	1,500	57.7	34	51	1.96
2. Kidneys	0.3	1,260	420.0	14	18	6.00
3. Brain	1.4	750	53.6	62	46	3.30
4. Skin	3.6	462	12.8	25	12	0.33
5. Skeletal muscle	31.0	840	2.7	60	50	0.16
6. Heart muscle	0.3	252	84.0	114	29	9.66
7. Residual tissue	23.8	336	1.4	129	44	0.18
Entire body	63.0	5,400	8.6	46	250	0.40

*Weighs 63 kg., has a surface area of 1.8 sq.M., a mean arterial pressure of 90 mm. Hg, a cardiac output of 5,400 ml., and an oxygen consumption of 250 ml./min.

The diagram on p. 224 shows the chambers of the heart and the valves.

heart. The hearts of beef, veal, lamb, and pork are used in cookery. Hearts are used in any recipe calling for sliced, diced, or ground meat. Heart is high in protein, iron, *riboflavin*, and *niacin*, and has fair amounts of *thiamine*.

Beef, raw, 100 gm = 108 calories
Veal, raw, 100 gm = 124 calories
Pork, raw, 100 gm = 113 calories
Lamb, raw, 100 gm = 162 calories

heartburn. A burning sensation under the breastbone or in the pit of the stomach is a common complaint, usually relieved by any one of the many antacid preparations. The most common cause is an irritable digestive tract or so-called "acid indigestion." When the junction between the esophagus and stomach is relaxed, the acid stomach juice flows back into the esophagus and causes irritation of its surface (esophagitis). A common cause of chronic heartburn is a rupture or weakness of the diaphragm which separates the chest from the abdomen; this weakness is called a diaphragmatic or hiatus hernia, allowing part of the upper portion of the stomach to move up into the chest. Simple measures to relieve the heartburn of diaphragmatic hernia are the use of antacids, avoiding or correcting obesity, eating smaller meals, avoiding highly sweetened foods, and sleeping with the head of the bed raised. See *gastritis.*

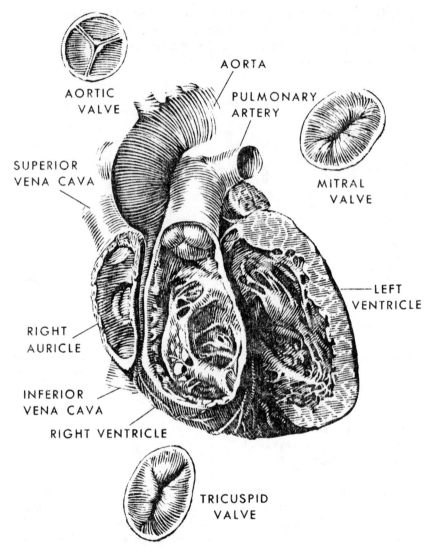

Section of heart showing chambers and valves

heat labile. Changeable by heat; unstable to heat.

heat of combustion. The heat of combustion of a substance is the amount of energy in the substance measured in terms of the amount of heat released by its oxidation. By burning each of the foodstuffs in a *bomb calorimeter,* it has been found that carbohydrate has an average fuel value of 4.1; fat, 9.45; and protein

5.65 calories per gram. The differences in energy content exists in the chemical composition of the three materials. In carbohydrates there is enough oxygen in the molecule to combine with all the hydrogen, and only the carbon present in small proportion remains to be burned; a correspondingly small amount of heat will be produced. With fats which have little oxygen in the molecule, the carbon and nearly all the hydrogen are oxidized and much heat is involved. Nitrogen when burned has no fuel value. The heat of combustion of an average meal, i.e., a mixture of foodstuffs, is usually estimated at 4.8 calories per liter of oxygen. See *energy balance* and *Appendix 9.*

heat production. See *basal metabolism.*

helix. A coil or spiral; the shape assumed by some large molecules, including *proteins* and *nucleic acids*. The alpha (α)helix is a particular conformation of protein. *Deoxyribonucleic acids* form double helixes.

hematinic. An agent that increases the hemoglobin level and the number of red blood cells.

hematocrit. A measure of the volume of blood cells in relation to the volume of plasma. When there has been a loss of body fluids but no cell loss, as in dehydration, the cell volume is high in proportion to the amount of liquid (plasma) in the bloodstream, i.e., the hematocrit is above normal. When either hemorrhage or anemia has depleted the supply of cells, the blood is "thinned," and the hematocrit or cell volume is low. The normal range for the hematocrit is 38 to 54 ml per 100 ml for men and 36 to 47 ml per 100 ml for women. Hematocrit determinations are used as a screening procedure, and for the diagnosis of anemia and also as a guide to treatment.

hematoma. A localized mass of blood that has escaped from injured blood vessels and has entered an organ or spaces between the cells of a tissue. The blood is often clotted or partly clotted and discolored. The decoloration is due to the breakdown products of the *heme* in hemoglobin. See *heme.*

hematopoiesis. The formation of blood.

hematopoietic. Affecting the formation of blood cells.

heme (haeme, protoheme). Mol. Wt. 616. A complex ring structure called protoporphyrin-α containing the metal iron in the ferrous (Fe^{+2}) state. Heme is a component of *hemoglobin* and is responsible for absorption of oxygen from the blood. The heme structure is also a component of cytochrome C and modifications of heme are present in other members of the *terminal respiratory chain*, a complex of enzymes in the *mitochondria* responsible for cell utilization of oxygen. Among the breakdown products of heme are *biliverdin*, a green *bile* pigment; *bilirubin*, a red bile pigment; and *urobilin*, an orange pigment. *Jaundice* is characterized by a hyperbilirubinemaia.

Heme

heme iron. Iron which is bound to porphyrin in hemoglobin and myoglobin. Unlike iron salts, the absorption by the intestinal mucosa of heme iron is not affected by phosphate or *phytic acid**, nor by *ascorbic acid** (vitamin C)). The heme complex is absorbed intact into the intestinal epithelial cell and only then is the iron split off. Its absorption is more efficient than that of ionic iron, i.e., iron occurring as a salt.

hemicelluloses. A heterogeneous group of polysaccharides closely associated with cellulose in plant tissues but can be separated by oxtraction with aqueous alkali. The largest chemical group are the pentosans (pentose polymers), xylans and arabinoxylans; a second group consists of *hexose* polymers such as the galactans, and a third group are the acidic hemicellulose which contain galacturonic or glucuronic acid. The hemicelluloses are not digested in the small intestine but are broken down by microorganisms in the colon more readily than cellulose.

hemochromatosis. A disturbance of iron metabolism in which excessive iron storage causes a bronze discoloration of skin and viscera, liver and pancreas damage and diabetes (bronzed diabetes). The condition is believed to be genetically transmitted by a defect occurring chiefly in males.

hemoglobin. The major protein in *red blood cells* (erythrocytes). It is a *globulin* and contains *heme**. The iron content of the red blood cells has its highest concentration in the heme or hemoglobin. Hemoglobin consists of four poly-peptide chains, two alpha (α) chains, plus two beta (β) chains, each chain has one heme. The red, iron-containing protein pigment of the erythrocytes that transfers oxygen and carbon dioxide and aids in regulation of pH. Comprised of a complex portein molecule named globin and a nonprotein portion named *heme* (hematin), which contains iron. One red cell contains several million molecules of hemoglobin. Since one molecule of hemoglobin contains four molecules of iron, it can carry four molecules of oxygen. Hemoglobin com-bines with oxygen to form oxyhemoglobin. Under normal circumstances the adult body produces about 6.25 gm of hemoglobin per day. Normal hemoglo-bin values are 14–18 gm% (14–18 grams per 100 ml of blood) for men; 12–16 gm% for women; 12–14 gm% for children; and 14.5–24.5 gm% for newborns. The entire function of hemoglobin depends upon its capacity to combine with oxygen in the lungs and then release it readily in the capillaries of the tissues. In the tissues it picks up carbon dioxide. Genetic variants of he-moglobin can give rise to several diseases (hemoglobinopathies), including sickle cell anemia and thalessemia. These hemoglobinopathies are the result of a mutation or error in the genetic code, that causes the substitution of a single amino acid out of the 574 with profound changes in the ability of hemoglobin to function normally. There are over 500 known abnormal variants of normal hemoglobin.

hemolysis. The disintegration of red blood cells which results in the appearance of hemoglobin in the surrounding fluid.

hemolytic. Causing the destruction of the red blood cells.

hemolytic anemia. In this type of anemia, red blood cells are destroyed at rates faster than normal. Hemolytic anemia may be congenital or acquired, acute or chronic. In addition to symptoms common to other anemias such as fa-tigue and shortness of breath, hemolytic anemia usually produces some degree of jaundice because the destroyed red cells release their hemoglobin which is converted into bile pigments at rate faster than they can be removed. The increased bile pigments give the skin a yellow color, a condition known as jaundice. Some hemolytic anemias are chronic and may last for years. If ne-glected they may lead to development of *gallstones,* and in some cases leg ul-cers.

hemopoietic. Concerned with the formation of blood.

hemorrhage. Hemorrhage is bleeding, particularly excessive bleeding, from blood vessels due to a break in their walls. It may be caused by a wound or disease. Hemorrhage can occur externally or internally. Bleeding in some internal areas is evidenced, however, when blood accumulates in tissues (forming a hematoma), or is vomited, coughed up, or excreted in urine or feces.

hemorrhoids (piles). Stretched or dilated veins, varicose veins under the mucous membrane lining of the anal and rectal area. When they occur in the wall of the rectum above the sphincter muscle, they are classified as internal; those below, in the anal canal are called external.

hemosiderin. An insoluble iron oxide-protein compound, in which iron is stored in the liver if the amount of iron in the blood exceeds the storage capacity of *ferritin*. See *hemosideroisis*. Such accumulation of excess iron occurs in diseases that are accompanied by rapid destruction of red blood cells (malaria, hemolytic anemia).

hemosiderois. A condition in which large amounts of the iron storage compound *hemosiderin* are deposited, especially in the liver and spleen. Hemosiderosis may occur as the result of excessive breakdown of red blood cells in diseases such as malaria and hemolytic anemia, or after multiple blood transfusions.

heparin. The naturally occurring anticoagulant in blood and other tissues containing glucosamine, glucuronic acid, and varying proportions of sulfate and acetyl groups. Its structure is not entirely clear. It is produced by the *mast cells* of the connective tissue and is stored as granules within the cells. The heparin content of tissues correlates with the number of mast cells present. Heparin is secreted into the intercellular substance and functions there to prevent the *fibrinogen* that escapes from capillaries from forming *fibrin* clots. It also functions in the formation or activation of lipoprotein *lipase,* which clears *chylomicrons* from the blood plasma.

hepatic. Pertaining to the liver.

hepatic coma. A syndrome of progressive confusion, apathy, personality changes, muscle contractions, spasticity, loss of consciousness, leading to eventual death. In hepatic coma, toxic nitrogenous materials from the bowel, primarily ammonia, enter the systematic circulation and reach the central nervous system without prior detoxification by a normally functioning liver.Blood ammonium-ion levels are characteristically increased in hepatic coma. A major feature of hepatic coma is ammonia intoxication of the central nervous system caused by failure of the liver to convert ammonia to nontoxic *urea*. Impaired ability of the liver to convert ammonia to urea, which is secreted by the kidney is the primary cause of hepatic coma.

hepatomegaly. Enlargement of the liver.

hermetic. Food containers that do not permit gas or micro-organisms to enter the container or to escape from it. A properly sealed tin can is a hermetic container.

herring (*Clupea harengus*). A small, salt water fish. The shad, alewife, and sardine are related to them. Also related to this family is a freshwater variety, lake herring, sometimes called "cisco." Herring is an important food fish. Herring have small heads; they are streamlined and covered with silvery, irridescent scales. Mature herrings measure 10 inches in length. Herring is a good source of protein and fat. Fresh herring is high in phosophorus. The caloric value of 100 gm of fresh saltwater herring can vary from 98 to 176 calories depending on the variety. The value of 100 gm of smoked herring varies from 196 to 300 calories, depending upon variety and method of smoking. Freshwater herring (cisco), raw, 100 gm = 211 calories.

heterocrine. Referring to glands or other tissues that secrete more than one type of substance, such as the pancreas which produces both *endocrine* and *exocrine* secretions.

heterogeneous. Made up of differing ingredients or not of uniform quality throughout.

heteropolysaccharide. A polysaccharide containing more than one type of monosaccharide.

heterotrophic. Incapable of manufacturing organic compounds from inorganic raw materials, therefore requiring organic nutrients from the environment.

heterotrophs. Organisms that require carbon in the form of carbon-hydrogen bonds in such organic substances as *carbohydrates, fats,* and *amino acids.*

heterozygote. A fertilized egg of individual in which paired genes differ, because of different contributions from the two parents. A person who is heterozygous for eye color, will be carrying two different "eye-color" genes, as for instance one "blue-eye" gene and one "brown-eye" gene. In a person who is homozygous the two "eye-color" genes would be the same.

heterozygous. Possessing dissimilar pairs of genes for any hereditary trait.

hexose. A class of simple sugars (monosaccharides) that contain six carbon atoms. The most common members are *glucose* * (dextrose), *fructose* * (levulose), and *galactose.* *

hiccups (singultus). Short, sharp, inspiratory coughs involving spasomodic lowering of the diaphragm. May be due to indigestion, overloaded stomach, irritation under the surface of the diaphragm, alcoholism, or other causes.

histamine. Mol. Wt. 111. A nitrogenous substance found in all animal and vegetable tissues. A stimulator of the autonomic nervous system and a potent stimulant of gastric secretion. The *essential amino acid histidine* * is a precursor to histamine. Histamine is believed to be liberated especially from injured and dying cells. Histamine causes dilation of capillaries and arterioles and a fall in blood pressure. Antihistamines counteract the effects of histamine.

$$\overset{\displaystyle \text{---CH}_2\text{CH}_2\text{NH}_2}{\underset{N\diagdown\diagup NH}{\square}}$$

Histamine

histidine (HIS). Mol. Wt. 155. An amino acid apparently essential for growth and possibly for repair of human tissue because the body is unable to make the basic ring structure of its molecule. Once provided with this structure it can add on the amino group without difficulty. By losing its carboxyl group, histidine is converted to *histamine* * an important physiological substance which is normally freely present in the intestine and in basophil granules in cells of the reticuloendothelial system. Histamine stimulates the secretion of hydrochloric acid by the stomach.

$$\overset{\displaystyle \text{---CH}_2\text{---CH---COOH}}{\underset{N\diagup\diagdown N \qquad NH_2}{\square}}$$

Histidine

histones. A class of basic proteins that are soluble in water, and insoluble in very dilute ammonia. Histones often yield precipitates with solutions of other proteins and a coagulum on heating which is easily soluble in very dilute acids. On hydrolysis histone yields several amino acids, among which the basic ones predominate. The only member of this group which may have any considerable importance in terms of food are the thymus histones and the globin of hemoglobin.

hives (uritcaria). Hives are raised red bumps (weals) in the skin with sharp, serpentlike borders surrounded by a red halo in the adjacent skin. The duration is no more than 8 to 12 hours. However, during the interval of one attack, they characteristically appear and disappear in different places on the skin. Hives cause an intense itch, stinging, or prickling as the major symptom. The typical attack of hives lasts for no more than several days and often less. Such an episode is known as acute urticaria. An attack of hives lasting for more than 6 weeks is called chronic urticaria. Acute urticaria is usually a type of allergic reaction to some environmental factor such as an insect bite, a food, a medication or as one part of the reaction to many different allergens.

homeostatis. A balanced, dynamic state or concentration of substances. Homeostasis differs from equilibrium in that no energy is required to maintain equilibrium while homeostasis requires energy because the conditions while constant are displaced from equilibrium. Examples of homeostasis are body temperature and blood pressure.

homeostatic. Steady states in the body, maintained by physiological processes.

hominy. Kernels of hulled dried corn from which the germ has been removed. It is also known as "samp." Ground hominy is called *grits*. Hominy is cooked in water or milk, and may then be fried, baked or served with a sauce. Hominy is a good source of carbohydrate. Nutritive food values: hominy and hominy grits, cooked, 100 gm = 51 calories.

homogenize. A word of Greek origin, composed of homos, meaning "the same" and "genos," kin or kind. In culinary language, "to homogenize" is to reduce an emulsion to particles of the same size and to distribute them evenly. The word is most frequently used for milk, but also for salad dressings and mayonnaise. Most whole milk that has been homogenized has been put through a process that breaks up the fat into such fine particles that it remains evenly distributed in the fluid. Fats that are in small droplets in a fluid (emulsified), as in milk and egg yolk are more readily digestible because the tiny droplets can be surrounded and attacked by digestive enzymes.

homologous chromosomes. Paired chromosomes with matching genes, one of the pair from the father, one from the mother.

homozygote. A fertilized egg or individual in which given paired genes are the same.

homozygous. Having identical pairs of genes for any given pair of hereditary traits.

honey. A sweet sticky liquid made by honeybees from the nectar of plants. The bees suck the nectar from the flowers and store it in their honey sacs where it undergoes certain changes. Later the bees deposit the liquid in honey combs where with other changes, it becomes honey. Honey is almost pure carbohydrate. It is a predigested sweetener, and as such is valuable in certain special diets. Extracted, 100 gm = 304 calories.

honeydew melon (*Cucum*). Melons which belong to the muskmelon family, whose varieties include cantaloupes, honeydews, casaba, and Persian melons. Honeydews have a smooth yellowish-white rind, and their flesh is sweet and green. Honeydew contains *ascorbic acid** (vitamin C). Fresh, 100 gm = 33 calories; frozen melon balls, syrup pack, 100 gm = 62 calories. See nutritional table for *fruits*.

hookworm. Small worms which attach themselves to the lining of the small intestine. The larvae of the worms generally get through the skin of the feet and lower legs and produce a "ground itch." As they pass to other parts of the body, they may produce bronchitis, big appetites, dirt-eating, constipation, headache, weakness, stupor, dropsy, and even death. Can be cured with tetrachloroethylene.

hops. See *malt* and *malt beverages*.

horehound (*Marrubium vulgare*). Horehound is a member of the mint family, a large family of plants including herbs such as thyme, marjoram, and basil. It shares an aromatic odor with its better-known relatives, but is very bitter in taste. Horehound also refers to the extract or candy made from the plant and used for coughs and colds.

hormones. Hormones are specific substances synthesized by specific cells or organs and secreted directly into the blood stream to produce an effect on cellular processes in other cells or organs. Most hormones are produced in *endocrine glands* in contradistinction to *exocrine glands* which secrete substances through ducts that lead to surfaces or other ducts that are continuous with the outside of the body, e.g., the *salivary glands* secrete into the digestive tract and the *prostate gland* secretes into the urethra. Hormones regulate a number of familiar body functions like growth, sexual development, and lactation (milk production). Less familiar activities regulated by hormones include control of the levels of calcium, sugar, and salt in the blood, the texture of the skin and hair, and the excretion of water by the kidneys. Over- or underproduction of a hormone makes itself apparent by changes in body functions. The glands that produce hormones are known as *endocrine glands,* and they include the *pituitary, thyroid, parathyroid, pancreas, adrenal, ovaries,* and *testes.* Hormones are also produced by nerve cells of the autonomic nervous system and of the hypothalamus, a portion of the brain that lies just above the pituitary gland. Each gland produces and secretes into the bloodstream a characteristic hormone or hormones. The following are hormones that regulate secretory and motor activity of the digestive tract.

Hormone	Where Produced	Stimulus to Secretion	Action
Gastrin	Pyloric and duodenal mucosa	Food in stomach especially proteins, caffeine, spices, alcohol	Stimulates flow of gastric juices
Enterogastrone	Duodenum	Acid chyme, fats	Inhibits secretion of gastric juice;reduces motility
Cholecystokinin	Duodenum	Fat in duodenum	Contraction of gallbladder and flow of bile to duodenum
Secretin	Duodenum	Acid chyme; polypeptides	Secretion of thin, alkaline, enzyme-poor pancreatic juice.
Pancreozymin	Duodenum	Acid chyme; polypeptides	Secretion of thick enzyme-rich pancreatic juice
Enterocrin	Upper small intestine	Chyme	Secretion by glands of intestinal mucosa

humectant. A chemical that is incorporated into a food (marshmallows, shredded coconut, candies, etc.) to maintain the desired level of moisture. For example, glycerol and polyalcohols are humectants. See *sorbitol.*

hubbard squash (*Cucumis*). A large winter squash. See *squash.*

huckleberry (*Gaylussacia*). The huckleberry is dark blue to black edible berry and there are a number of varieties which grow in an acid soil on low or high bushes. Each huckleberry contains 10 hard little seeds. 100 gm = 62 calories.

hunger. Hunger is a compelling need or desire for food accompanied sometimes with a painful sensation or state of weakness. Hunger differs from appetite in the degree of desire. Appetite is usually associated with the pleasurable sensations of food intake. With continued deprivation of food, an appetite becomes hunger. When the stomach has emptied and the food has been digested, the stomach undergoes rhythmic contractions which give rise to a sensation of hunger. These contractions are normally known as "hunger pangs." The longer the period of time following a meal, the more frequent the contractions. To a limited extent they are controlled by the level of glucose in the blood.

hyaluronic acid. A mucopolysaccharide that is a component of the ground substance of intercellular material. The human unbilical cord, and cattle synovial fluid, and vitreous fluids are the most common sources of hyaluronic acid, but it is widely distributed and is found in most connective tissues. Its name is derived from hyaloid (vitreous) and uronic acid. Hyaluronic acid is composed of equimolar proportions of D-glucuronic acid and acetyl glucosamine occupying alternating positions in the molecule.

hydrocarbon chains. Molecular units made up solely of carbon and hydrogen atoms. See *fatty acid, oleic acid*, stearic acid**.

hydrochloric acid (HCl). Mol. Wt. 36. The parietal cells of the gastric glands secrete the hydrochloric acid from chlorides such as sodium chloride (table salt), found in the blood. The chloride ion combines with the hydrogen ion and is then secreted upon the free surface of the stomach as hydrochloric acid. In normal *gastric juice* it is found in the proportion of about 0.5 percent, having a pH value of about 1. It serves to activate *persinogen* and convert it to *pepsin*, a digestive, *proteolytic* enzyme, and to provide an acid medium which is necessary for the pepsin to carry on its digestive functions; to swell and denature the food protein giving easier access to pepsin; to help in the hydrolysis of sugar and starch; and to destroy organisms that enter the stomach.

hydrocortisone (cortisol). See *cortisol**

hydrogen (H). Element No. 1. Atomic Wt. 1. Hydrogen has the smallest atomic weight. Present in *proteins, carbohydrates, fats* and water. Hydrogen makes up approximately 10 percent of the human body and more than 90 percent of the universe.

hydrogenation. Generally referred to as a type of chemical processing which adds hydrogen to unsaturated bonds of carbon or oxygen. In the fatty acid chains hydrogenation increases the degree of saturation of the fat. Oils, for example, are converted to fat by hydrogenation. Hydrogenation also prevents oxidative rancidity and thus greatly prolongs the storage life of the fat by converting unsaturated fatty acids to saturated fatty acids. One practice is to expose fats or oils in a continuous controlled process so that more fatty acids are saturated but not completely. This process tends to convert most of the essential fatty acid, linoleic acid, to oleic acid.

Hydrogenation

hydrogen bonds. Weak chemical attraction between hydrogen atoms and other atoms, chiefly oxygen and nitrogen. Hydrogen bonds are important in giving enzymes their characteristic shapes. Hydrogen bonds are one of a class of weak bonds or interactions also known as secondary valence forces.

hydrogenic sediments. Precipitate from solution in water.

hydrolysate. The product of hydrolysis, e.g., protein hydrolysate is a mixture of the constituent amino acids when the protein molecule is split by acids, alkalies, or enzymes.

hydrolysis. A chemical reaction in which the rupture of a chemical bond may be interpreted as the incorporation and splitting of water molecules which result in the formation of two new compounds.

Peptide   Hydrolysis   Hydrolytic
bond   products

The splitting of a substance by hydrolysis can be catalyzed by *enzymes* (proteolysis), *acids* (acid hydrolysis), or *alkalis* (alkaline hydrolysis). In all cases the products appear to have incorporated hydrogen ion (H^+) in one and hydroxyl (OH^-) in the other product. For example, the digestion (hydrolysis) of proteins by acid, alkali or enzymes yields *hydrolysates* composed of amino acids that are the result of a rupture of the *peptide bond* by water.

hydrolyzed vegetable protein (HVP). Used to bring out the natural flavor of food. Consists of vegetable (usually soybean) protein that has been chemically degraded to the amino acids of which it is composed. It can be found in instant soups, beef stew, frankfurters, gravy and sauce mixes, and canned chili.

hydrophilic. Soluble in water. See *micelle*.

hydroponics. Soiless culture of plants. The roots are immersed in a nutrient-rich aqueous medium.

hydroxocobalamine. *Cobalamin* * (vitamin B_{12}) with a hydroxyl group (—OH) in place of a cyano group (—CN). See *cobalamin* * (vitamin B_{12}).

hydroxylated lecithin. Manufactured by treating soybean lecithin with peroxide. Used by the food industry as an emulsifier/antioxidant in baked goods, ice cream and margarine.

hydroxyproline (HYP). Mol. Wt. 131. A nonessential amino acid occurring abundantly in collagen.

$$\begin{array}{c} \text{H} \\ \text{HO—C——CH}_2 \\ \mid \qquad \mid \\ \text{H}_2\text{C} \quad \text{CH—COOH} \\ \diagdown \diagup \\ \text{N} \\ \text{H} \end{array}$$

Hydroxyproline

hypercalcemia. An excess of calcium in the blood.

hypercalciuria. Abnormal calcium excretion in the urine.

hyperchlorhydria. Excessive secretion of hydrochloric acid in the stomach.

hypercholesteremia. Excess of cholesterol in the blood.

hyperchromic. Highly or excessively colored.

hyperglycemia. An excess of sugar in the blood.

hyperinsulinism. Excessive secretion of insulin by the pancreas which results in hypoglycemia.

hyperkalemia. Excessive amounts of potassium (k) in blood plasma. Hyperkalemia is a serious complication of kidney (renal) failure, severe dehydration, or shock. Hyperkalemia causes the heart to dilate, and the heart rate is slowed by weakened contractions. Potassium ion (K^+) plays a vital role with ionized sodium (Na^+) and calcium (Ca^{++}) in regulating neuromuscular stimulation, transmission of electrochemical impulses and contraction of muscle fibers.

hyperlipemia. Excess of fat or lipids in the blood.

hyperphagia. Ingestion of greater than optimal quantity of food; an increased and abnormal hunger.

hyperphosphatemia. A high serum phosphate ion (PO_4) concentration. Hyperphosphatemia may be caused by kidney (renal) insufficiency because the kidney cannot excrete phosphorus adequately or by *hypoparathyroidism* which causes an insufficient secretion of *parathyroid hormone,* which regulates the renal excretion of phosphorus. When serum phosphate ion concentration rises, serum calcium ion falls, causing tetany (a muscle malfunction).

hyperplasia. Abnormal multiplication of cells with increase in size of an organ, but without formation of a tumor.

hypertension (high blood pressure). Said to exist when the systolic pressure is consistently above 150 mm of mercury or when the diastolic pressure exceeds 99 mm of mercury. A high diastolic pressure reading that is constant, meaning that the blood vessels are under relentless pressure at all times, indicates that the person is a good candidate for heart disease or vascular disorder of some kind. Systolic hypertension may be due to increased cardic output of blood, as in hyperthyroidism, or to loss of elasticity in the larger arteries. Diastolic hypertension is a result of a narrowing of the small arterioles that control the flow of blood out of the larger arteries. Hypertension heart disease is an increase in the blood pressure placing an extra burden on the heart, as it works harder to force the blood through the blood vessels. This brings about an increase in the size of the heart and impaired function as a result of fatigue of the heart muscle. Hypertension may result from chronic kidney infection or diseases of the arteries such as arteriosclerosis. It may occur without any apparent cause, having no known relationship with any other disease.

hyperthyroidism. A systemic condition resulting from overactivity of the thyroid gland and overproduction of the hormone *thyroxine**. This disorder is also known as Grave's disease, toxic goiter and thyrotoxicosis. The result of an overactive thyroid gland is an increased *basal metabolic rate* (BMR), hyperactivity in some instances and general weakness and weight loss in the extreme. See *thyroxine**.

hypertonic dehydration. Loss of water from the cell as a result of excess solutes hence greater osmotic pressure in the surrounding extracellular fluid. The osmotic pressure of the extracellular fluid is higher than that of the intracellular fluid and water moves in the direction of the higher osmotic pressure. The imbalance in osmotic pressure causes water to shift from the cell into the extracellular fluid spaces. This situation can occur from either excess water loss or water restriction.

hypertropic. Pertaining to enlargement of an organ due to increase in size of its constituent cells.

hyperuricemia. Excess of *uric acid** in the blood; one of the characteristics of the disease, *gout*.

hypervitaminosis. A pathology or toxicity due to an excess of one or more vitamins. The fat-soluble vitamins, especially *retinol** (vitamin A) and *vitamin D,** have the distinct potential to poison at high dosages because they are stored by the body. The danger of toxicity does not hold for water-soluble vitamins, as the body eliminates any excess in the urine. See *vitamin toxicity*.

hypoalbuminemia. Abnormally low albumin content of the blood.

hypocalcemia. Abnormally low blood calcium.

hypochloremic alkalosis. A condition of alkalosis caused by a loss of lowered blood chlorides. Excessive loss of gastric secretion (*hydrochloric acid**), results in loss of chlorides, with bicarbonate replacing the depleted chloride ions. Hypochloremic alkalosis (a type of metabolic alkalosis) results. Such gastrointestinal disorders as excessive vomiting may lead to hypochloremic alakalosis. Therefore prompt replacement of chloride is essential to treatment.

hypochlorhydria. Diminished secretion of *hydrochloric acid* * in the stomach.

hypochromic. Decrease in color; usually applied to decrease in hemoglobin content of the erythrocytes.

hypoglycemic. An agent that acts to lower the amount of glucose in the blood.

hypoglycemia. Refers to an abnormally low level of glucose in the circulating blood. The person with this condition utilizes the available glucose in his blood to a seriously low level within a few hours after he has eaten a meal or after exercise. Persons with chronic hypoglycemia are considered to be predisposed to diabetes, but the condition is relatively rare. Evidence for hypoglycemia is obtained by a *glucose tolerance test.*

hypokalemia. Low blood potassium. Hypokalemia is a serious complication of severe diarrhea, for example, in which large amounts of potassium are lost in intestinal secretions. Hypokalemia may also result from rapid glycogenesis during the recovery of diabetic acidosis. Replacement therapy in both instances should involve added potassium.

hypophosphatemia. Low serum phosphorus, which may be caused by decreased absorption of phosphorus as in intestinal diseases (*sprue, celiac disease*); or to an upset serum calcium to phosphorus ratio as in bone disease (*rickits, ostemalacia*); or to excess secretion of parathyroid hormone with resulting excessive renal excretion of phosphorus.

hypoproteinemia. Decrease in the normal quantity of serum protein in the blood.

hypoprothrombinemia. Deficiency of *prothrombin* in the blood. Prothrombin is required for normal blood clot formation.

hypothalamus. A small collection of nerve cells and fibers arranged in a complicated system of nuclei in the center of the brain at the upper end of the brain stem. Closely related to the *pituitary gland*—many nerve fibers connect the two organs. It is essential for the regulation and control of visceral activity, body temperature, water and electrolyte balance, blood pressure, sexual and reproductive activity, and possibly body weight. It is also important in the expression of various emotions such as anger, fright, and embarrassment. The hypothalamus controls these varied activities by means of patterns of nerve impulses which are conveyed to their destination in sympathetic and parasympathetic nerve fibers.

hypothyroidism. Underactivity of the *thyroid gland* with a deficiency in the production of the hormone *thyroxine.* When the thyroid does not produce enough thyroxin to maintain a normal metabolic rate hypothyroidism occurs. The effects of hypothyroidism depend on whether the condition occurs during growth or after maturity. Adult hypothyroidism is called *myxedema.* The name comes from the collection of body fluid in connective tissue (edema) that gives the individual a puffy bloated appearance. Myxedema, caused by an onset of thyroid inefficiency in the adult reduces the basal metabolic rate (BMR) by 35 to 40 percent. This results in sluggishness, chills from inability to maintain body temperature, and reduced muscle tone. Motivation, vigor, and alertness diminish, and the individual sleeps much of the time. The central nervous system may deteriorate until the individual becomes an imbecile. Supplementary thyroxine can effect complete recovery.

I

ice crystals. When food is exposed to a low enough temperature the water in food solidifies and forms ice crystals. The formation of large ice crystals in foods such as fruits, vegetables, or meats may rupture the cell walls and affect the appearance and texture of the food. Pure water freezes at 32°F. (0°C).

idiopathic. Pertaining to a disease of unknown origin.

idiopathic steatorrhea. When individuals exhibit only the gastrointestinal symptoms of sprue, but not the complete symptomology of the sprue syndrome, including the *megaloblastic anemia*. The disorder has been called idiopathic *steatorrhea* after pancreatic disorders, intestinal lipodystrophy, lymphomata of the small intestine, amyloidosis, and chronic inflammatory disease of the small intestine have been ruled out. In many cases of idiopathic steatorrhea the course of the disorder is unpredictable. It is believed that a majority of cases in the adult are linked to the basic underlying *celiac disease* of childhood.

ileum. One of the sections of the small intestine that joins with the cecum (large intestine). Most of the absorption of food takes place in the ileum. The walls of the ileum are covered with extremely small, fingerlike structures called villi (*villus*) which provide a large surface for absorption. After food has been digested, it is absorbed into the capillaries of the villii. It is then carried to all parts of the body by the blood and lymph. See *digestive system.*

impermeable. Not capable of being penetrated. It is always necessary to name the substance to which a food wrapping material is impermeable. It may be impermeable to water vapor only or to water vapor and air (or other gases).

inactivate. To suspend or terminate certain biological activities such as by heat, irradiation, or other forms of energy.

indigestion. Usually refers to almost any symptoms involving or related to digestive system distress. The term in one sense is a misnomer since usually digestion, the process of breaking down food into small particles for absorption is normal. Acute indigestion may occur after eating irritating or spoiled food. Difficulties such as belching, gas, abdominal rumblings and gurgling, passing gas by rectum, heartburn and vague feelings of discomfort, heaviness and unrest in the abdomen, often are termed indigestion or *"gastritis."* The most common cause of an irritable bowel is emotional tension. The treatment for an irritable bowel includes the use of bland diet, adapted to individual requirements. The production of gas by certain foods such as onions, cabbage, and beans, and the passage through the rectum of gas which may have a foul odor is due to production of gas by bacteria as they act on food in the large intestine (bowels) together with the accumulation of swallowed air.

indirect calorimetry. The rate of metabolism or heat production is calculated from the oxygen intake or from the oxygen intake and carbon dioxide content of the expired air, as measured by a respiration apparatus. By determining either the oxygen consumed or the carbon dioxide exhaled in a given number of minutes, the caloric expenditure can be calculated. This principle may be applied to persons engaged in various types of activities or when lying at rest. If the subject is moving about he has to carry his respirator with him. A caloric equivalent of 4.8 calories per liter oxygen consumed is a value used to convert oxygen utilization into heat produced. See *energy balance.*

induction. Stimulation of enzyme formation by certain lower molecular weight substances (inducers). The actuation of new stages of development during the evolution of individual (ontogeny) of more complex organisms is also known as induction. Several hormones effect the development type of induction and the induction of enzyme formation.

inedible. A substance that is not fit for food, such as poisonous or unpleasant tasting nuts and plants. Tough skins, seeds, and decayed spots of fruits and vegetables, and bones of meat are considered inedible parts, because they are not suitable for human consumption.

inert gas. Gas which does not react with the materials in food. Nitrogen is an inert gas that may be used to replace air (oxygen) in packages of food in order to slow down the deterioration of the food.

infarction. The formation of an area of dead tissue resulting from the obstruction of blood vessels supplying the part. See *myocardial infarction.*

inflammation. Inflammation is the local reaction of the body to irritation or injury. It occurs in tissue that is injured but not destroyed. It is a defensive and protective effort by the body to isolate and eliminate the injuring agent and to repair the injury. A certain degree of inflammation takes place following any type of injury, including a wound made under aseptic conditions by a surgeon.

ingest. To eat or take in through the mouth. To take food into the body.

inhalents. Drugs which are inhaled and absorbed through the lungs. An example is aromatic spirits of ammonia.

inhibition. The reduction or stoppage of the action of enzymes or chemical processes by substances called inhibitors. A competitive inhibitor competes with the *substrate* for the active site of an *enzyme*.

inorganic compounds. Chemical compounds that do not contain carbon. The inorganic compounds exist in cells partly as dissolved salts and partly in combination with the organic compounds. In chemical analysis of cells, the mineral elements remain either wholly or largely in the ash when the cells are incinerated; hence, they are grouped as ash constituents. Only small amounts of these elements are needed, but they are essential parts of the cells.

inorganic nutrients. Mineral elements and water are sometimes called inorganic nutrients. See *minerals*.

inosine diphosphate (IDP). See *inosine triphosphate* * (ITP).

inosine monophosphate (IMP). See *inosine triphosphate* * (ITP).

inosine triphosphate (ITP). Mol. Wt. 506. A high-energy phosphate compound equivalent to *adenosine triphosphate* * (ATP) as a source of chemical energy. The pyruvate kinase reaction in *glycolysis* forms ITP from IDP. The disodium salt of IMP, disodium inosinate, and *disodium guanylate* are flavor enhancers.

inositol (myo-inositol). Mol. Wt. 180. A cyclic alcohol with six hydroxyl radicals allied to the hexoses. It occurs in many foods and especially in the bran of cereal grains. Inositol in combination with six phosphate molecules forms the compound *phytic acid* * which hinders intestinal absorption of calcium and iron. Like *biotin* *, inositol is found in the vitamin-B complex, but its role as a vitamin is not clear. It can be synthesized in the intestines of most animals. It

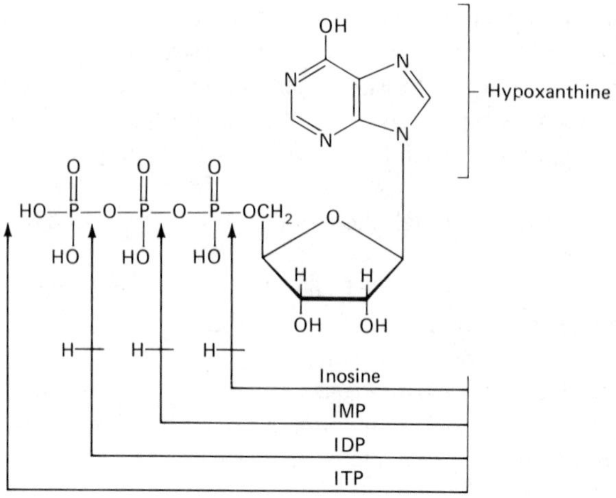

Inosine triphosphate (ITP)

may act in the utilization of carbon dioxide in certain chemical reactions within the cell. Good sources are liver, heart, yeast, and peanuts. Chemically, inositol is a colorless water-soluble crystalline material with some *carbohydrate* properties.

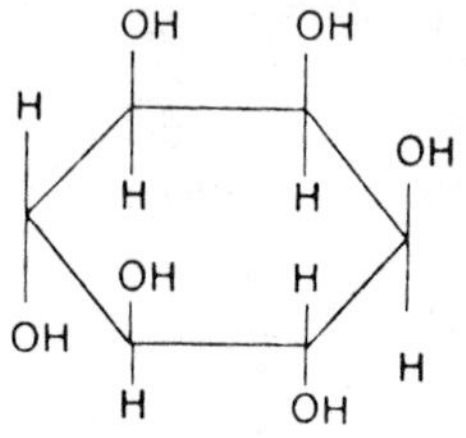

Inositol

insalivation. During the process of mastication, saliva is poured in large quantities into the mouth, and mixed with the food, helps lubricate, moisten, and reduce it to a softened mass known as a *bolus,* which can be readily swallowed.

insulin. A protein secreted into the blood by the beta (β) cells in the Islets of Langerhans of the *pancreas.* The normal stimulus to insulin secretion is the ingestion of carbohydrates and the consequent rise in blood sugar. Secretion is also stimulated by the amino acids and by the intestinal hormone pancreozymin. Insulin is the only hormone that lowers blood sugar. Insulin fosters glycogenesis by conversion of *glucose* * to *glycogen* * in the liver, where the glycogen is stored. Insulin also fosters lipogenesis, which is the formation of fat. Glucose is converted to fat for storage in adipose tissue (fat depository). This conversion takes place mainly in the adipose tissue itself, but some glucose is converted to fat in the liver. Insulin increases cell permeability to glucose in liver, muscle, and adipose tissues and allows glucose to pass from the extracellular fluids into the cells for oxidation to supply needed energy. It is insulin's function to direct the distribution of glucose within the body and to maintain a constant level of glucose in the blood. When insulin is secreted it stimulates the liver to increase the uptake of glucose and to increase its synthesis of glycogen from glucose. At the same time the liver and the muscle cells react by stepping up their intake of glucose and by increasing the conversion of glucose to glycogen. Insulin seems to be important in stimulating protein synthesis in conjunction with growth hormone. The manufacture of large fat molecules is also enchanced by insulin. Insulin does not affect the rate of uptake of glucose in the brain.

insulin shock. This type of shock is produced by an intravenous or a deep muscular injection of excessive amounts of insulin. The presence of the abnormal excess of insulin produces *hypoglycemia* (lowered blood sugar level), which results in vast changes in the entire physiological reactions of the organism. The central nervous system reacts most strongly to such a condition of hypoglycemia, because glucose is the primary metabolic fuel of the central nervous system. In hypoglycemia, there is a profound metabolic depression which chiefly affects the brain. The brain itself is affected differently by the hypoglycemic reaction following the injection of insulin. Those parts of the brain with the highest metabolism rates suffer first. Insulin shock is used as therapy in certain mental diseases also.

intake. Substances or amounts of substances which are taken in by the body, e.g., the intake of food. See *ingestion.*

interferon. A protein formed during the interaction of animal cells with viruses, which is capable of conferring resistance to infection with a wide range of viruses.

intermediate metabolism. A general term that refers to any series of biochemical reactions, *anabolic* or *catabolic* that occur with cells, tissues, or organs.

International Units (IU). The measure commonly used for vitamins. The amount of the vitamin comprising a unit is determined by its biological activity; that is, the amount of the vitamin required to cure or prevent a disease that is associated with a deficiency of that specific vitamin. Such units have been established for *retinol** (vitamin A) *ascorbic acid** (vitamin C) *vitamin D**, and *thiamine**, but are used principally for vitamins A and D.

Vitamin	One International Unit (I.U.)
Retinol (vitamin A)*	0.30 μg
Beta (β)-carotene	0.60 μg
Retinyl acetate	0.34 μg
Retinyl palmitate	0.55 μg
Thiamine-Hydrochloride (vitamin B$_1$)	3.0 μg
Ascorbic acid (vitamin C)	50 μg
Vitamin D$_2$ (ergocalciferol)	0.025 μg
Vitamin D$_3$ (cholecalciferol)	0.025 μg

*The Food and Nutrition Board has recommended the use of retinol equivalents (R.E.) for vitamin A. The R.E. takes into account the losses of *carotene** during absorption and the losses inconversion to retinol:
1 R.E. for retinol is 1 μg (3.33 I.U.)
1 R.E. for β-carotene is 6 μg (10 I.U.)

interstial space. Space between cells, exclusive of the lymphatics and blood vessels.

intestinal juice. The mucosa of the small intestine secrete a fluid termed succus entericus, or simply, intestinal juice. It is secreted by intestinal glands. Pure intestinal juice contains two enzymes; (1) *enterokinase,* which activates *trypsin,* and (2) a weak *amylase.* Intestinal juice, which is secreted at a rate of about 3000 ml/day, may function primarily to carry substances to be digested to the epithelial cells, where, while these substances are being absorbed, undergo final digestion by the enzymes in those cells.

intestine, large (colon). The large intestine is about 5 feet long. The cecum, located on the lower right of the abdomen is the first portion of the large intestine into which food is emptied from the *ileum,* the lower portion of the *small intestine.* The appendix extends from the lower portion of the cecum and is a blind sac. Although the appendix usually is found lying just below the cecum, by virtue of its free end, it can extend in several different directions depending upon its mobility. The colon extends along the right side of the abdomen from the cecum up to the region of the liver (ascending colon). There the colon bends (hepatic flexure) and is continuous across the upper portion of the abdomen (transverse colon) to the spleen. The colon bends again (splenix flexure) and goes down the left side of the abdomen (descending colon). The last portion makes an S curve (Sigmoid) toward the center and posterior of the abdomen and ends in the rectum. The main function of the large intestine is the recovery of water from the mass of undigested food and intestinal juices it receives from the small intestine. As the mass passes through the colon, water is absorbed and returned to the tissues. Waste materials, or feces, become more solid as they are pushed along by the peris*taltic movements*. Constipation is caused by delay in movement of intestinal contents and removal of too much water from them. Diarrhea results when movement of the intestinal contents is so rapid that not enough water is removed. See *digestive system*.

intestine, small. The small intestine is a tube about 22 feet long. The intestine is attached to the margin of a thin band of tissue called the *mesentery,* which is a portion of the *peritoneum,* the membrane lining in the abdominal cavity. The mesentery is a tissue membrane that supports the intestine and the vessels which carry blood to and from the intestine. The other edge of the mesentery is drawn together like a fan; the gathered margin is attached to the posterior wall of the abdomen. This arrangement permits the folding and coiling of the intestine so that this long organ can be packed into a small space. The small intestine is divided into three continuous parts; duodenum, jejunum, and ileum. It receives digestive juices from three accessory organs of digestion; the *pancreas, liver,* and *gall bladder.* See *digestive system.*

intracellular. Within the cell.

intracellular fluid compartment (IFC). The total water inside the body cells amount to about twice that outside the cells. The cell is the basic unit of structure of the entire body, and the cells are the sites of the vast basic metabolic activity of the body. The intracellular fluid compartment makes up about 40 percent of the total body weight. The water compartment outside of the cell is called the *extracellular fluid.*

intravenous. Into or from within a vein.

intrinsic factor. A *glycoprotein* (mucoprotein) normally synthesized in the stomach and required for the absorption of the extrinsic factor, *cobalamin* * (vitamin B_{12}) from food. Persons lacking the ability to synthesize intrinsic factor develop a condition called *pernicious anemia.*

inulin. A *polysaccharide* composed of *fructose* * units which has little dietary significance. Found only in a few common foods such as onions, garlic, and artichokes. The carbohydrate inulin is only partially digested, although further breakdown by bacteria may occur in the large intestine. Storage of inulin-containing foods also affects this carbohydrate. Fresh food may have much of its carbohydrate in this unavailable inulin form, however, upon storage much of the inulin may be converted to available sugar. Although inulin is of small dietary significance, it is of interest and importance in medicine and nursing because it provides a test of kidney function. Since inulin is filtered at the *glomerulus* during the formation of urine, but is neither secreted nor reabsorbed by the tubule, it can be used to measure glomerular filtration rate.

invert sugar. Invert sugar forms when sucrose is split into the two monosaccharides, *glucose** and *fructose** by an enzyme (invertase), or an acid. It is called "invert" because a solution containing the 50–50 mixture and a solution containing sucrose rotate the plane of polarized light in opposite direction. A 50–50 mixture of two sugars, glucose and fructose is used by food manufacturers because it is sweeter, more soluble and crystallizes less readily than sucrose.

invertases. Invertases are enzymes that hydrolyze sucrose to form the monosaccharides, glucose and fructose. The product of invertase action is called *invert sugar*. Invertases are used in the confectionery industry to make invert sugar for the preparation of liquers and ice creams in which the crystalization of sugars from high concentrations is to be avoided. In soft center, chocolate-coated candies, e.g., maraschino cherries, invertase incorporated in the center softens the fondant after it has been coated with chocolate. Invertase is added to sucrose syrups to hydrolyze that sugar and in this way prevent crystallization on standing. It also has been used in the manufacture of artificial honey.

invertase-isomaltase deficiency. A rare disorder in which the individual lacks the enzymes invertase and isomaltase. The latter breaks down one of the intermediate products of starch digestion, *isomaltose**, to form *glucose**.

involution. The change back to a normal condition that certain organs undergo after fulfilling their functional purposes.

iodine (I). Element No. 53. Atom. Wt. 127. Iodine is absorbed in the inorganic form as iodide ions in the upper part of the small intestine. It may be absorbed through the skin. Estimates of the total amount in the body range from 15 to 30 mg, and of this small amount about three-fifths is concentrated in the *thyroid gland*. Iodine serves but one purpose in the body, that is to form an integral part of the thyroid hormones, *thyroxine** and *triiodothyronine*. These hormones are manufactured in the *thyroid gland* from its stored iodide (the iodine anion) and the amino acid *tyrosine**, and they are released in small amounts into the blood. Iodide is supplied to the body by intake of foods or water and represents one of the necessary trace elements. Dietary iodide is absorbed from the alimentary tract, after which approximately 30 percent is removed by the thyroid gland, and the remainder is excreted in the urine.

The following table gives the iodine content of some common food.

Food	Iodine Content μg per 100 gm	Food	Iodine Content μg per 100 gm
Apples	1.6	Halibut	52.0
Beef	2.8	Lettuce	2.6
Bread	5.8	Milk	3.5
Butter	5.6	Oysters	57.7
Cabbage	5.2	Peas	2.3
Carrots	3.8	Pork	4.5
Cheese	5.1	Potatoes	4.5
Cod fish	146.3	Salmon	34.1
Cod liver oil	838.7	Spinach	20.1
Cranberries	2.9	Tomatoes	1.7
Eggs	9.3	Trout, lake	3.1

iodine uptake test. A radioisotope test for diagnosis of thyroid disease; done after administering a dose of radioactive iodide and tracing its uptake by the *thyroid gland*.

iodopsin. (1) A light-sensitive vitamin A protein complex necessary for vision in bright light. (2) Pigment found in cones of the retina; visual violet.

ion. An atom or group of atoms carrying a positive or negative charge, e.g., *cations, anions*.

iron (Fe). Element No. 26. Atom. Wt. 56. About 3 to 5 gm of iron is present in the body, most of which is in the blood as an essential component of the red protein *hemoglobin* of the red blood cells. The body guards its iron stores very carefully and reuses any which is broken down in the body over and over again. Only small amounts of iron lost needs to be replaced, normally about 0.9 mg for males and 1.5 mg for females. The principle loss of iron in females is during *menses* and accounts for a dietary requirement of 30 to 90 percent greater than males. The average menstrual loss of blood is 35 ml which averages to a replacement requirement. The requirements are easily established, but the amount of iron required in the diet is difficult to determine because dietary iron is not quantiatively absorbed. The form of the iron, organic or inorganic, oxidized or reduced, and the presence of other substances greatly influences the amount of iron absorbed. Large amounts of inorganic *phosphates* or oxalates, which occurs in spinach, reduces the absorption of iron by rendering it insoluble. In general, the iron obtained from foods is in organic compounds, a form less favorably absorbed than the inorganic forms. Oxidized iron (the ferric state, Fe^{+3}) is less readily absorbed than reduced iron (the ferrous state Fe^{+2}). The variations in the absorption are not understood. Iron from white bread is more readily absorbed than iron from whole wheat and the iron in beef is readily absorbed even though it is largely in the organic compounds, chiefly in hemoglobin. The presence of reducing agents, such as *ascorbic acid* * (vitamin C) increases iron absorption. Both inorganic and some organic forms can be utilized by the body, however, hemoglobin iron from red meats (veal, beef, lamb) may be absorbed directly into the muscosal cells before the iron is released. Ferric citrate is also a highly available iron source, being converted to the ferrous form before absorption. Iron is distributed throughout the body, being a component of essential enzymes in every call. About 65 to 70 percent, is present in the blood as hemoglobin in the red blood cells. In iron deficiency, the lowered capacity to provide oxygen is largely responsible for the fatigue and apathy characteristics of iron deficiency anemia. Iron-deficiency anemia occurs mainly in young children and women of child-bearing age. There are many types of anemias. Of the nutritional anemias, iron-deficiency anemia is by far the most common. The inorganic forms of iron salts are readily absorbed

Food	Range (mg/100 g)
Beef, mutton, raw, fresh	2.0–4.3
Black (blood) sausage	20
Chocolate, plain	2.8–4.4
Cocoa, powder	2.7–14.3
Corned beef	3.0–11.0
Dried fruit, various	2.0–10.6
Eggs, whole, fresh	2.0–3.0
Fish, raw	0.5–1.0
Fruits, tinned and fresh	0.2–4.0
Greens, leafy vegetables, raw	0.4–18.0
Liver	6.0–14.0
Milk, cow's, fresh whole	0.1–0.4
Millets, various, raw	4.0–5.4
Nuts, various, without shells	1.0–5.0
Oatmeal, raw	3.8–5.1
Potatoes and other root vegetables, raw	0.3–2.0
Pulses, various	1.9–14.0
Treacle	9.2–11.3
Wheat flour, high extraction	3.0–7.0
Wheat flour, low extraction	0.7–1.5

directly into the blood stream where it is transported by the protein transferrin rather than through the *lymphatic system*. Iron absorption occurs chiefly in the upper intestines. Absorption takes place with the iron in the ferrous form (Fe^{+2}), and therapeutically it is usually given this way as ferrous sulfate or *ferrous gluconate* *. Ferric salts are reduced to ferrous salts before absorption. Absorbed iron goes to the bone marrow for red blood cell synthesis, to tissue for cellular oxidation processes, to liver, spleen and bone marrow for storage reserve. The rate of iron absorption varies widely and is conditioned by several factors, which includes the quantity of iron ingested, the body content, the rate of erythropoiesis, and the hemoglobin level. The table on page 250 lists the iron content of some common foods.

iron deficiency anemia. See *anemia*.

irradiation. To treat with ultraviolet rays from sunlight or an artificial source; to treat with x-rays or other radioactive agents.

ischemia. A local deficiency of blood caused chiefly by narrowing of the arteries or the blockage of an artery by a blood clot. See *myocardial infarct*.

isocaloric. Containing an equal number of calories.

isoenzymes. Enzymes from the same source with similar catalytic properties but with slightly different physical or kinetic properties. Some isoenzymes are used in the diagnosis of certain diseases.

isoleucine (Ile). Mol. Wt. 131. One of the *essential amino acids* found in proteins.

$$
CH_3 - CH_2 - \overset{\displaystyle \underset{|}{CH}}{\underset{\displaystyle CH_3}{|}} - \overset{\displaystyle \overset{H}{|}}{\underset{\displaystyle NH_2}{|}}{C} - COOH
$$

Isoleucine

isopropyl citrate. A chelating agent. See *stearylcitrate* *

I.U.—See *International Units*.

J

jaundice. Jaundice is marked by a yellow tint of the skin and whites of the eyes, representing a variety of ailments which may appear at any age. The actual cause is a yellow bile pigment called *bilirubin,* which is normally present in a small quantity in the blood. Excessive quantities of this yellow chemical cause jaundice, a yellow tint of the skin and the whites of the eyes. Bilirubin is a breakdown product of hemoglobin, the oxygen, carrying red pigment in the red blood cells and normally removed from the blood by the liver. Hepatitis is the disorder with which is associated with jaundice. In this disease the liver is inflamed and can no longer perform its work of dealing with the bilirubin produced from the normal destruction of old *red blood cells.* The bilirubin content of blood is normally 0.2 to 0.8 mg/100 ml of plasma. Bilirubin accumulates above normal levels in the bloodstream, and jaundice appears. *Gallstones* may block the bile duct, causing bilirubin to back up, resulting in jaundice. In certain forms of *anemia,* for example hemolytic anemia, red blood cells are destroyed at a rate that exceeds the capacity of the liver to deal with the bilirubin; the result is elevated blood bilirubin and jaundice. In all these conditions jaundice is only a condition, not the underlying cause. Treatment is directed to the cause, not to the symptom.

jejunum. Middle portion of *small intestine,* extending from *duodenum* to *ileum.*

joule. The unit of energy is the joule (J) and is the energy expanded when 1 kilogram (kg) is moved 1 meter (m) by a force of 1 newton (N). Physiologists and nutritionists are concerned with large amounts of energy and the convenient units are the kilojoule ($kJ = 10^3 J$) and the megajourle ($MJ = 10^6 J$). Formerly energy was always expressed quantitatively in units of heat, the unit used being the kilocalorie (kcal). This is defined as the amount of heat required to raise the temperature of 1 kg of water from 14.5 to 15.5°C. Conversion from calories to joules is made by multiplying by 4.184.

K

karaya gum. A complex carbohydrate that manufacturers use as a thickening or stabilizing agent in foods. Manufacturers use karaya gum to prevent oil from separating out of whipped products and salad dressing and to prevent fat from separating from meat and juices in sausages. It improves the texture of manufactured ice cream and sherbert by preventing large crystals from forming.

keratin. A scleroprotein which is the principal constituent of the epidermis—hair, nails, horny tissues, and the organic matrix of the enamel of the teeth.

keratinization. A state in which the epithelial cells become dry and flattened, then gradually harden, forming rough horny scales. The skin and the palms of the hands and the bottoms of the feet are normal keratinized tissues. This process may occur abnormally in the conjunctive cornea, the respiratory tract, the gastrointestinal tract, the genitourinary tract, or the excessive keratinization of the epidermis.

keratomalcia. Dryness and ulceration of the cornea resulting from *retinol* * (vitamin A) deficiency.

keto. A prefix denoting the presence of the carbonyl group attached to two carbons

$$-\overset{|}{\underset{|}{C}}-\overset{O}{\overset{\|}{C}}-\overset{|}{\underset{|}{C}}-$$

bons . See *acetone*.

keto-acid. An organic acid containing a keto group. Alpha (α) keto acid forms when *amino acids* are deaminated or transaminated and is common in intermediary metabolism.

ketogenesis. The formation of *ketone bodies* from *fatty acids* and some amino acids. See *metabolic acidosis*.

ketogenic. Capable of being converted into ketone bodies. Ketogenic substances in metabolism are the fatty acids and the amino acids leucine*. The *amino acids*, *lysine*, *phenylalanine*, and *tryosine* are both ketogenic and glucogenic.

alpha (α) ketoglutaric acid. Mol. Wt. 86. One of the intermediates in the Kreb's (tricarboxylic acid) cycle. It is also a product of deamination of glutamic acid*.

$$HOOC-CH_2-CH_2-\overset{\overset{\displaystyle O}{\|}}{C}-COOH$$

ketone. Any compound containing a keto group. See *acetone* and *fructose*.

ketone bodies. The ketone bodies are substances in the blood that cause a condition called metabolic acidosis or *ketosis*. The ketone bodies are *acetone*, beta (β) *hydroxybutyric acid*. and *acetoacetic acid*. The ketone bodies occur in the blood stream as a result of incomplete oxidation of fatty acids. The condition is called ketosis.

ketosis. A condition in which there is an accumulation in the blood of ketone bodies (beta [β] *hydroxybutyric acid*, *acetoacetic acid*, and *acetone*) as a result of incomplete oxidation of fatty acids. Ketosis occurs when the amount of fat being oxidized is excessive, as with the use of ketogenic diets, in semi-starvation, and uncontrolled *diabetes mellitus*.

kidney. The kidneys are bean-shaped organs about 4½ inches long, 2 inches wide, and 1 inch thick. They lie on each side of the spinal column, against the posterior wall of the abdominal cavity, near the level of the last thoracic vertebra and the first lumber vertebra. The right kidney is usually slightly lower than the left. Near the center of the medial side of each kidney is the central notch or hilum, where blood vessels and nerves enter and leave and from which the ureter leaves. The kidney is composed of an outer shell or cortex, and an inner layer, the medulla. The cortex is made of firm, reddish-brown tissue containing millions of microscopic filtration plants called *nephrons*. Each nephron is a urine-forming unit. The nephron units receive and filter all the body's blood, about once every 12 minutes. Large protein molecules cannot pass through this filtering apparatus. Smaller molecules, small proteins and salts are filtered through but may be actively absorbed by enzymes in the tubules. *Glucose* is an example of a small molecule that is filtered through the filtering apparatus, the *glomerulus*, but is reabsorbed through tubules and glucose does not normally appear in the urine. In diabetes mellitus the concentration of glucose in the blood is so high that it exceeds the ability of tubules of the kidney to reabsorb it all. Glucose therefore appears in the urine during diabetes. During filtration, the nephrons draw off and filter the blood to remove wastes and to return the usable portion of the filtrate to the circulation to maintain the body's fluid balance. The final result is urine which enters the bladder by way of the collecting tubules and the ureter. Below is a diagram of the anatomy of a kidney. See *glomerulus, nephron,* and *urine.*

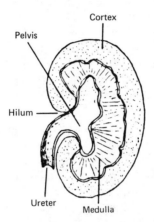

kidney stones. Kidney stones or urinary calculi are formed because the concentration of a particular substance in the urine exceeds its solubility. A low urine volume and the pH of the urine are also factors. About 95 percent of all kidney stones contain calcium. They also may contain magnesium and ammonia combined with phosphate, carbonates, and oxalates. Four percent of renal calculi consist of *uric acid* * and one percent are *cystine* * stones. They vary in size from fine gritty particles to those which fill the pelvis of the kidney, and they may form either in the kidney or the bladder. The presence of mineral deposits in the kidneys may occur in *hyperparathyroidism,* in which oversecretion of the *parathyroid hormone* causes loss of calcium from the bones, resulting in a high blood level of calcium with increased secretion of calcium in the urine. Immobilization for long periods of time, *osteoporosis,* or an abnormally high intake of milk, alkalis, or *vitamin D* *, may also give rise to the formation of calcium phosphate stones.

kilocalorie (kC). The unit of heat used in nutrition. The amount of heat required to raise 1000 gm water 1°C (from 15.5 to 16.5°C); also known as the large calories.

kilogram. One thousand grams. See *gram*.

kinetic energy. The capacity to do work as a result of motion. For example, the kinetic energy of a waterfall can be used to turn a generator to make electricity.

Kola. See *Cola*.

Krebs cycle (tricarboxylic acid cycle, citric acid cycle). The Krebs or tricarboxylic acid cycle is the enzymatic pathway for the oxidation of *fatty acids, carbohydrates,* and *proteins*. The members of the cycle act in a catalytic manner in that they are regenerated and increasing the concentration of any member of the cycle increases the rate of the entire cycle. Central to the oxidation of fatty acids, carbohydrates and proteins is their conversion to *acetyl coenzyme A* * (acetyl-CoA) by catabolic processes. The acetyl—CoA, a two carbon compound, reacts with *oxalacetic acid* * of the Kreb's cycle to form *citric acid* *, a tricarboxylic acid. In the progress of the cycle, oxidation and decarboxylation reactions occur. The result is that oxalacetic acid is regenerated to react with other acetyl—CoA molecules, two CO_2 molecules are produced, and several *coenzymes* are reduced. The reduced coenzymes are oxidized by the *terminal respiratory chain* via the *cytochromes*. The results of these oxidations is the formation of water. Thus in the oxidation of acetyl—CoA, the overall action is Acetyl—CoA + CO_2 ⟶ $2CO_2$ + $2H_2$ + CoA + energy. The CO_2's arise from the reactions of the Krebs cycle and the H_2O and energy arise from the reactions of the terminal respirator chain. (See Fig. p. 257)

These pathways provide for more than 90 percent of the energy in the body. Both the tricarboxylic acid cycle and the terminal respiratory chain are contained within the subcellular particles called *mitochondria*.

kwashiorkor. A nutritional disease described as protein-calorie malnutrition (PCM). The disease is caused by a low and insufficient protein intake, even though the total caloric intake may be adequate. The symptoms are edema, apathy, scaly, and depigmented skin, and depigmented hair. The disease is found in the tropics and subtropics among children 1 to 4 years old. Kwashiorkor is an African word with disputed definition. It is sometimes translated as "red boy" because African children with the disease often have a characteristic

Tricarboxylic Acid Cycle

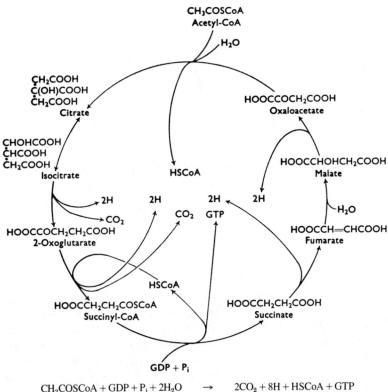

$$CH_3COSCoA + GDP + P_i + 2H_2O \quad \rightarrow \quad 2CO_2 + 8H + HSCoA + GTP$$
Acetyl CoA

Of the 8H, 3 pairs pass through NAD to the cytochrome electron transport chain yielding 3 ATP each. 1 pair passes to FAD and hence to the electron transport system yielding 2 ATP Total—11 ATP.

$$8H + 2O_2 + 11ADP + 11P_i \quad \rightarrow \quad 4H_2O + 11H_2O + 11ATP$$

Sum Total

$$CH_3COSCoA + GDP + 11ADP + 12P_i + 2O_2 \quad \rightarrow \quad 2CO_2 + 13H_2O + GTP + 11ATP + HSCoA$$

red hair color. Kwashiorkor is also translated as "displaced child" since the nutritional disease has its onset when another child is born and the weanling must eat the protein-deficient diet of the community or tribe. See *marasmus*.

L

L. A chemical prefix that denotes a configuration around the asymmetric carbon of a compound. For example, the configuration of the alpha (α) carbon in the L-amino acids found in proteins. The opposite of D-compounds.

labile. Not fixed; unstable; easily destroyed.

lactalbumin. A protein milk.

lactase. An enzyme produced by the muscosal cells that hydrolyzes the *disaccharide lactose** (milk sugar) to yield equal amounts of the *monosaccharides glucose** and *galactose** during the digestive process. If milk is absent or severely restricted in diets after weaning, the enzyme disappears in man somewhere between infancy and adulthood, as it does in most mammals. Once lactase is lost, it cannot be recovered. The absence of lactase produces a condition called lactose intolerance. The symptoms of lactase intolerance are mild and are noticeable only when large amounts of milk are ingested. They include nausea, stomach cramps, and diarrhea. The majority of the adult population of the world is lactose intolerant, with the exception of Caucasians and a few African tribes that keep cow herds and drink milk. The enthusiasm for milk as a major source of protein, worldwide or individually, should be balanced with the possibilities of an intolerance for milk.

lacteal. Tiny vessels in the intestinal wall through which fat is absorbed. It is part of the lymphatic system.

lactic acid. Mol. Wt. 90. Lactic acid is a three-carbon acid produced in milk by bacterial fermentation of lactose. It is also produced during muscle contraction by anaerobic *glycolysis*. For the most part lactic acid is produced industrially by means of homofermentative lactic acid bacteria, or bacteria resembling them. In the food industry lactic acid is used to acidify jams, jellies, confectionery, sherberts, soft drinks, extracts, and other products. It is added to brines for pickles, olives, and horseradish, and to fish to aid in preservation. In addition it makes milk more digestible for infants. Calcium lactate is an important ingredient of some baking powders.

$$CH_3—\overset{\overset{\displaystyle OH}{|}}{CH}—COOH$$

Lactic acid

lactic acid culture. The most commonly used dairy starter is the common butter or lactic starter, which normally consists of a mixture of strains of *Streptococcus lactis* and *S. cremoris* for the production of lactic acid and *Leuconostoc dextranicum* and *L. citrovorum* or *Streptococcus diacetilactis* for the production of flavor and aroma. Leuconostoc strains are often included in cultures for making ripened cheeses. The mixed lactic cultures is used in the manufacture of cultured buttermilk, butter, and most types of cheeses in which the curd is heated at a comparatively low temperature, e.g., cottage, cream, Limburger, cheddar, blue, and brick cheese. The aroma bacteria are especially important in flavor production in cultured buttermilk, butter, and uncured cheeses.

Lactobacillaceae. The very important food bacteria in this family are called the lactic acid bacteria, or "lactics." They ferment sugar chiefly to *lactic acid*,* if they are homofermentative plus small amounts of acetic acid, carbon dioxide, and trace products; or if they are heterofermentative, they produce appreciable amounts of volatile products including alcohol, in addition to lactic acid. The type of lactic acid D or L produced is characteristic of the organism and the medium. The most important characteristics of the lactic acid bacteria is their ability to ferment sugars to lactic acid.

lactogenic hormone. See luteotropic hormone (LTH).

lactose (milk sugar). Mol. Wt. 342. A disaccharide composed of *glucose** and *galactose** the form of carbohydrate in milk. Occurs in the milk of all mammals constituting usually from 6 to 7 percent of the fresh secretions in human milk, and 4.5 to 5 percent in the milk of cows and goats. Lactose is less sweet and much less soluble than *sucrose*,* dissolving only to the extent of about 1 part in 6 parts of water. When hydrolyzed either by heating with acid or by an enzyme such as the lactose of the intestinal juice, each molecule of lactose yields one molecule of glucose and one of galactose. Hence the lactose ingested is absorbed, not as such, but as a mixture of equal parts of glucose and galactose. The enzyme for hydrolyzing lactose is *lactase*. Lactase is often lost in adults and they become intolerant to milk. See *lactase*.

β (1 → 4) D-galactopyranosil-β D-glucopyranose

Lactose

Lactose intolerance. The inability to digest lactose, milk, or milk products. See *lactase*.

laetrile (vitamin B$_{17}$). See *amygdalin*.

lamina propria. Connective tissue structure that supports the epithelial cells of the intestinal mucosa.

lard. The fat rendered from fresh, clean, sound fatty tissues of hogs at the time of slaughter. The tissues do not include bones, detached skin, head fat, ears, tails, organs, windpipes, large blood vessels, scrap fat, skimmings, settlings, pressings, and the like, and are reasonably free from muscle tissue and blood. Lard is used as an ingredient of margarine and cooking fats, and whenever an edible fat is required in baking. Lard contains high concentrations of saturated fatty acids.

lathyrogens. A spastic paralysis of the legs, comes from Lathyrus, the Latin name for certain members of the pea family recognized as having toxic qualities. *Lathyrus sativa,* the chick-pea, *L. cicera,* the flat-podded vetch, and *L. clymenum,* the Spanish vetchling, are three of the more widely eaten species of Lathyrus from which lathyrogens can be isolated. Regular and continued consumption of chick-pea meal results in muscular weakness and spastic paralysis of the legs. It is believed that lathyrogen, beta-N-oxylyl-L-alpha-beta-diaminopropionic acid, a neurotoxic amino acid, is the substance in the chick-peas and vetch responsible for lathyrism.

lauric acid (laurostearic acid). Mol. Wt. 200. A saturated C$_{12}$ fatty acid. Occurs abundantly as *glyceride* in the fat of the seeds of the spice bush, and in smaller proportions in butter, coconut fat, palm oil, and some other vegetable oils.

$$CH_3—CH_2—CH_2—CH_2—CH_2—CH_2—CH_2—CH_2—CH_2—CH_2—CH_2—COOH$$

leaven. Various substances which lighten dough or batter while it is baking and make it more palatable. The word comes from the Latin levare which means "to raise." Though air and steam act as leavening agents to a certain extent, the oldest and best-known ingredient used for leavening is yeast. Leavening agents increase the surface area of dough through the release of gases within the dough. The expansion of these gases during baking increases the size of the finished food, and gives a desirable porous structure. Of the gases created the principal one is carbon dioxide; the others are air and water vapor or steam. Air is a physical means of leavening. It may be incorporated into the batter by means of an egg-white foam or to a lesser degree by creaming fat and sugar. Chiffon, angel food, spongecakes, and souffles are examples of air used as leavening. Steam, another physical leavening, occurs when water is exposed to high temperature. Popovers and cream puffs are leavened by steam. *Baking soda,* also known as *sodium bicarbonate* or bicarbonate of soda is a chemical leavening agent. When the soda is heated in the presence of moisture, carbon dioxide gas is produced. When used by itself, soda leaves a disagreeable taste and produces a yellow color. To prevent this, an acid substance, such as cream of tartar, sour milk, or molasses, is usually used in combination with the soda. *Baking powder,* another chemical leavening agent, is in three forms. The tartrate powders, containing *cream of tartar* and *tartaric acid,* react quickly in batter or dough at room temperature. The phosphate powder, containing calcium acid phosphate, releases two-thirds of its gas at room temperature and the remainder when heat is applied. The double-acting powder contains sodium aluminum sulfate and calcium acid phosphate; it releases a small portion of gas when ingredients are combined, but the greater amount is released in the oven. Yeast is a living plant which can produce carbon dioxide under suitable environmental conditions. It is available in two forms, active dry and compressed. The metabolic processes of the yeast furnish gaseous carbon dioxide, which creates bubbles in the bread and makes it rise. Sourdough is a fermented dough which produces carbon dioxide under suitable environmental conditions. Other actively gas-forming microorganisms, such as wild yeasts, coliform bacteria, saccharolytic clostridium species, heterofermentative bacteria, acid bacteria, and various naturally occurring mixtures of these organisms have been used instead of bread yeasts for leavening.

lecithin. A phospholipid containing *glycerol, fatty acids, phosphoric acid,* and *choline.* Any of a group of fatty substances occurring in animal and plant tissues such as soybeans and corn and egg yolk, composed of units of choline, phosphoric acid, fatty acids and glycerol. Because lecithin is an emulsifying agent, it has become widely used especially by health food adherents on the basis that its presence in the blood may dissolve cholesterol deposits. Lecithin, like cholesterol, also is made within the body. Food manufacturers use lecithin as an antioxidant and emulsifier. Pure lecithin is an important source of choline. The lecithin used as food additives is obtained almost exclusively from the soybean. Used primarily as an emulsifier in margarine, chocolate, ice cream, and baked goods to promote the mixing of oil (or fat) and water. The hydrocarbon chains (R, R′) of the fatty acids varies depending upon the source of the lecithin.

Lecithin

leek. (*Allium porrum*). The first cousin of the onion and garlic has a cylindrical stalk with a small simple bulb, and flat, juicy, compactly rolled-up leaves which are dark green at the top and white towards the bulb. Leeks have a mild onion flavor and are used as a seasoning or a vegetable. The green part has some *carotene* * (vitamin A activity). Raw, 100 gm = 52 calories.

legumes. Food plants which have pods that open along two seams when the seeds are ripe. Legumes are seeds and nuts, although technically they are hard-shelled fruits, similar to seeds in composition. The seeds are usually the edible part of the legume. Peas, chick-peas, beans, lima beans, soybeans, peanuts, and lentils are the best-known food legumes. There are more than 11,000 species of legumes. They are the most important food plants next to cereals. This food group resembles the grains but is characterized by having almost twice as much protein as grains. The dried legumes (beans, peas, lentils, and cowpeas), because of their low moisture content, are as much as 60 percent carbohydrate (starch) and 22 percent protein. Although they are often classed as "meat substitutes" an average serving furnishes probably only about one-third as much protein as an average (100 gm) serving of meat. The quality of their protein is somewhat inferior to that of animal foods, except for the proteins of the peanut and soybean, which are of good *Biological Value* (BV). As a rule most legumes are good sources of *thiamine* * and contribute moderate amounts of *riboflavin* * and *niacin* *. They also contain significant quantities of *phos-*

phorus and *iron* and lesser amounts of calcium. Soybeans (soybean flour) have a high protein content. Soybeans are also a good source of calcium and iron and contain more fat that most other legumes.

lemon (*Citrus limon*). The lemon tree, a member of the citrus family, is a small tree which grows 10 to 20 feet in height. It has a short spine and large, fragrant, white-and-purple flowers. The light yellow fruit is small, oval, and ends in a blunt point. The pulp of the fruit is juice and acid, containing 0.5 percent sugar and 5 percent citric acid. An excellent source of *ascorbic acid** (vitamin C). One lemon provides 40 to 80 percent of one day's need for vitamin C. 1 lemon = 40 calories; lemon juice, 100 gm = 25 calories.

Lemon Balm. See *Balm*.

lentil (*Lens culinaris*). This *legume* is one of the first plants whose seeds were used for food. The lentil seed is small and lens-shaped. It is never used green, but is dried when it is fully ripe. The lentil is extremely nutritious, a good source of carbohydrates and incomplete protein, and is a good meat, milk, cheese, and egg supplement. Lentils also contain some B vitamins and are a good source of iron, with fair amounts of calcium and *carotene** (vitamin A activity). Raw, 100 gm = 340 calories.

lettuce (*Lactuca*). A vegetable whose nutrients are found in the part of the plant that grows above the ground. There are several hundred varieties of lettuce, all originating from a common weed of the roadsides and wastelands of southern Europe and western Asia. The most popular lettuces are: (1) Butterhead, a small, soft, loose-leafed head with its outer leaves light green, and its inner leaves light yellow, with a buttery feel. It is a sweet, succulent lettuce. The most common butterhead varieties are Bibb and Boston. (2) Cos or Romaine. A long, cylindrical head with stiff leaves, dark green on the outside, becoming greenish-white near the center. (3) Crisphead, the most popular type of lettuce. The outer leaves are medium-green in color with flaring, wavy edges. The inner leaves are pale green and folded tightly. Iceberg lettuce is a variety of crisphead. (4) Lamb's tongue or field lettuce. Comes in small clumps of tiny, tongue-shaped leaves on delicate stems. (5) Leaf. A hardy type of lettuce with loose leaves branching from a stalk. It may have a curled or a somewhat smooth leaf of light to dark green. It has a crisp texture. (6) Stem. With an enlarged stem and no head, this lettuce has long, narrow leaves tapering to a point. The flavor is a combination of celery and lettuce. The main variety is celtuce. Lettuce has small amounts of *carotene** (vitamin A activity) and *ascorbic acid** (vitamin C), and minerals, if the outer leaves are eaten. Raw, 100 gm = 13 to 18 calories.

leucine (LEU). Mol. Wt. 131. One of the *essential amino acids* found in protein.

$$CH_3\diagdown \atop CH_3\diagup$$
CH₃\
CH—CH₂—CH—COOH with NH₂

Leucine

leucocytes, polymorphonuclear. *White Blood cells* which are nearly twice as big as the red blood cells and contain both a nucleus divided into several lobes and granules in the protoplasma. They are formed from primitive cells in the lymph glands, spleen, and bone marrow. They are concerned with the reaction of the body to infection by bacteria and to the presence of foreign material in the tissues. They can engulf bacteria and other foreign particles (phagocytosis) and they collect around local areas of infection or damage in very large numbers.

leukemia. A cancer of the white blood cells. White blood cells formed in this disease are abnormal and usually increase in number. They infiltrate various parts of the body. In the bone marrow they "crowd out" the cells that produce red blood cells, normal white cells, and platelets. Since the new cells utilize the available amino acids and vitamins at a prodigious rate, the person with acute leukemia is very likely to suffer from severe debilitation and *avitaminosis*.

levulose. See *fructose* *.

Lichee. See *Litchi*.

licorice (*Glycyrrhiza glabra*). A perennial herb of the pea family. It has long rootstocks, feathery leaves, and flowers of various colors, usually pale violet or blue. Its dried root, or an extract made from it, is used to flavor medicines, tobacco, cigars, cigarettes, soft drinks, candy, and chewing gum.

lignin. A constituent of crude fibers occuring in the cell wall of plants, which is not broken down by intestinal microorganisms to any extent.

lima bean (*Phaseolus*). This round, full, slightly curved bean is an American native. Lima beans were named after Lima, Peru, where the European explorers first came across them. Fresh lima beans are higher in protein than most vegetables, with fair amounts of *carotene* * vitamin A activity) and *Ascorbic acid* * (vitamin C).

Fresh, boiled and drained, 100 gm = 111 calories
Fresh (green), canned, solids and liquids, 100 gm = 71 calories
Fresh (green), canned, solids, drained, 1–10 gm = 96 calories
Fresh baby limas, frozen, boiled and drained, 100 gm = 118 calories
Fresh Fordhook limas, frozen, boiled and drained, 100 gm = 99 calories
Dried Lima beans are a good source of protein, iron, and thiamine and a
good supplement to other protein foods
Dried Lima beans, cooked, 100 gm = 138 calories

lime (Citrus aurantifolia). A small bushy and spiny tropical tree which belongs
to the citrus family. The tree has small white flowers and its fruit, which
measures up to 2½ inches in diameter, is small and compact and resembles the
lemon in shape. The rind of the lime is green, with a very acid and juicy pulp,
which yields a pungent juice. Oil is extracted from the rind. Excellent source of
*ascorbic acid** (vitamin C). Lime juice, fresh or unsweetened, 100 gm = 26
calories; limeade, diluted, 100 gm = 41 calories.

lipid. Applied to any substance that has physical properties similar to fats, that
is, oily or greasy in consistency and most important, soluble in fat solvents. In
addition to true fats and *fatty acids,* lipids include some substances chemically
related to fats plus some others totally unrelated such as cholesterol. The lipids
in blood, for example, include free fatty acids, esterified fatty acids, steroids
such as *cholesterol* and its esters, *triglyceride* and *phospholipids*. Other substances that are classified as lipids are *oils* and *waxes*.

linoleic acid. Mol. Wt. 280. An 18-carbon essential polyunsaturated fatty acid
which contains two double bonds. The body is not able to synthesize linoleic
acid. It has to be obtained in the diet for growth and general well being.
Linoleic acid occurs only in small amounts in food fats. Soybean oil, with 7
percent is the highest. Linoleic acid is of central dietary importance. It is relatively more abundant in foods than *arachidonic acid** (which can be synthesized from linoleic acid) and oleic, and must come from diet. Sources of
linoleic acid include many grain oils and seed oils, which contain 50 percent or
more. Fats and nuts, peanuts and poultry carry 20 to 30 percent. Fats from such
fruits as avocado and olive contain about 10 percent of linoleic acid. Those
from leafy vegetables and legumes run higher, 30 percent or more, but the total
amount of fat in greens is low.

$$CH_3-(CH_2)_4-CH{=}CH-CH_2-CH{=}CH-(CH_2)_7-COOH$$

lipase. Any of a class of enzymes that break down neutral fats or *triglycerides*.
A small quantity of gastric lipase (lipase secreted by the gastric mucosa) acts on

emulsified fats of cream and egg yolk. The major digestive lipase is pancreatic lipase, which acts upon fats in the small intestine. Pancreatic lipase was formerly called steapsin. Enteric lipase acts within the mucosal cells. In order for the digestive lipases to act properly, the fat must be emulsified. Bile salts emulsify fat in the intestine and it is the presence of fat in the intestine that signals the release of bile salts from the gall bladder. Lipases catalyze the following reaction:

$$\text{Triglyceride} \xrightarrow[\text{lipase}]{} 3 \text{ fatty acids} + \text{glycerol}$$

lipase test. An enzyme test on blood, used for the diagnosis of acute *pancreatitis*.

lipids. Lipids vary considerably both in composition and structure. They occur naturally in both animal and plant foods and vary widely in physical and chemical characteristics. When separated from the surrounding tissues with which they usually are associated, most natural fats and oils are found to consist of approximately 98 to 99 percent *triglycerides;* the remaining very small part is composed of monoglycerides, diglycerides, free *fatty-acids,* phospholipids, and an unsaponifiable fraction. Neutral fat or ester of fatty acids and glycerol, is a mixed glyceride containing a variety of fatty acids and glycerol. The physical characteristics of a neutral fat are affected by the size of the fat molecule and by the amount of saturated and unsaturated fatty acids it contains. In general, the more saturated the fat and the higher the molecular weight, the more solid it will be. Glycolipids or cerebrosides are compounds of fatty acids with a carbohydrate and contain nitrogen but no phosphoric acid. Cerebrosides are found in the myelin sheath of nerve fibers in connection with, and possibly in combination with *lecithin.* Phospholipids or phosphatides contain both nitrogen and phosphorus. The best known are the *lecithins,* which are abundant in egg yolk and occur in brain and nerve tissues and in all the cells of the body. Cephalins and spingomyelin are examples. Sterols are complex monohydroxyalcohols of high molecular weight, which are found in nature combined with fatty acids. They contain carbon, hydrogen, and oxygen. The best known is *cholesterol,* which is very widely distributed in the body, being found in the medullary coverings of nerve fibers, in the blood, in all the cells and liquid of the body, in the sebum secreted by the sebaceous glands in the skin, and in the bile. Fat, substances derived from simple and compound lipids by hydrolysis or enzymatic breakdown, are termed derived lipids. Three important members of this group are *fatty acids, glycerides,* and *steroids.* Most digestion of fat takes place in the intestines. Bile emulsifies the fat and puts it into a form which permits more complete hydrolysis by intestinal and pancreatic enzymes. Fats are broken down to fatty acids, glycerol, and monoglycerides. Bile salts and choline help in emulsifying these hydrolynid compounds, producing micelles which are absorbed through the brush border of the intestinal mucosa. During the absorption process the fatty acids, glycerol, and monoglycerides are resynthesized into triglycerides. See *digestive system*.

lipogenesis. The formation of fatty acid through biosynthetic pathways. The precursor of fatty acids is acetyl coenzyme A.

lipoic acid (lipoamide). Mol. Wt. 206. Lipoic acid in the amide form (lipoamide) functions as a cofactor in the oxidative decarboxylation of *pyruvic acid** and *α-ketoglutaric acid**. It functions along with the cofactor form of the B-vitamin *thiamine*, *thiamine pyrophosphate**. Pyruvate, a key product in carbohydrate metabolism is formed in the beginning pathway of glucose oxidation. This key reaction, oxidative decarboxylation, transforms pyruvate to acetyl coenzyme A which ultimately enters the *Krebs cycle** to produce energy. A quantitative requirement for lipoic acid in human nutrition has not been established. It is found in many biological materials, including yeast and liver.

Lipoamide

Lipoic acid (lipoamide)

lipolysis. The breakdown of fat into its component *fatty acids* and *glycerol** by *hydrolysis*.

lipomas. Fatty tumors under the skin, which produce no pain or other symptoms. They may be no larger than a pea, feel soft, move freely under the skin, rarely become malignant.

lipoprotein. A conjugated protein that incorporates *lipids* as a part of its structure. Lipoproteins are associated in a wide variety of complexes that are significant in both the structure and function of cells. Lipoproteins appear to be of two types; those which exist as relatively discrete and identifiable macromolecules are called soluble types. Those that are aggregates of the complex membrane structure are called membrane types or structural lipoproteins. Most soluble lipoproteins circulate in the blood plasma. Some are involved in blood clotting. The ratio of lipid to protein in the serum lipoprotein varies widely and these variations affect their density. Lipoproteins differ in their densities and flotation rates (Sf), depending upon the kind and quantity of lipid associated with the protein. Lipoproteins fall into four general classifications that depend on their density. The table below gives the major classifications of the lipoproteins and their general names.

Percent of Lipoprotein Constituent

Constituent	High Density (HDL, Alpha)*	Low Density (LDL, Beta)*	Very Low Density (VLDL, Prebeta)*	Chylonicrons
Protein	49%	32%	2–13%	0.5%
Triglycerides	7%	7%	64–80%	90%
Cholesterol	17%	35%	8–13%	6%
Phospholipids	27%	25%	6–15%	4%
Density (g/ml) Sf	1.210–1.063	1.063–1.006	1.006	<1.006
Particle size	70–100 Å	100–300 Å	2000 Å	>2000 Å

*Alpha (α), Beta (β) and Prebeta (pre-β) refer to relative migration rates of blood proteins in a separation process called electrophoresis.

The HDL and LDL levels in the serum are a more sensitive index of coronary heart disease than total *cholesterol*. The cholesterol in LDL has a direct relationship to coronary heart disease whereas the cholesterol in HDL has an inverse relationship. In others, it is the distribution of the total cholesterol between the LDL and HDL rather than the total blood cholesterol that better defines the risk of coronary heart disease.

lipotropic. Pertaining to substances that prevent accumulation of fat in the liver.

lipotropic factor. An agent which has an affinity for lipids. It prevents or corrects an excess accumulation of fat in the liver. *Choline** is probably the most important of the lipotropic factors. Protein helps to prevent a fatty liver because it provides amino acids such as *methionine** that contributes to the synthesis of choline.

lithiasis. The formation of stones (calculi) of any kind, for example, *gallstone* and *kidney stone* formations.

lithocholic acid. Mol. Wt. 377. One of the bile acids that form bile salts. A conjugate with *taurine** or *glycine**. See *bile salts, bile acids,* and *bile*.

Lithocholic acid

litchi or lichee nut (*Litchi chinensis*). The fruit of an ornamental tropical tree, the litchi. The litchi is a very distinctive fruit. It is round and 1 to 2 inches in diameter. The rough shell is bright red and leathery. Inside, the shimmery firm white flesh surrounds a single seed. It is juicy and has a pleasant mildly aromatic and slightly acid flavor. Fresh, 100 gm = 64 calories; dried, 100 gm = 277 calories.

liver. The liver is the largest organ in the body. It is located in the upper part of the abdomen with its larger (right) lobe to the right of the midline. It is just under the diaphragm and above the liver end of the stomach. The liver has several important functions. One is the secretion of *bile,* which is stored in the gall bladder and discharged into the small intestines when digestion is in process. The bile contains no *enzymes* but breaks up the fat particles so that enzymes act faster. The liver performs other important functions. It is a storehouse for sugar of the body (*glycogen*), and for *iron* and the B vitamins. It plays a part in the destruction of bacteria and wornout red blood cells. Many chemicals such as poisons or medicines are detoxified by the liver; others are excreted by the liver through the ducts. The liver manufactures part of the proteins of blood plasma. The blood-flow in the liver is of special importance. All the blood returning from the spleen, stomach, intestines, and pancreas is detoured through the liver by the portal vein in the portal circulation, the nepato-portal circulation. Blood drains from the liver by hepatic veins which join a large vein called the inferior vena cava.

lobster (*Homarus*). A member of the family of crustaceans to which shrimps and crabs also belong. They lack spinal columns an have "crusty" outer skeletons or shells with jointed bodies and limbs. Live lobsters are mottled and splotched greenish blue, with touches of orange. The vivid red color, characteristic of lobsters, comes out in cooking. Lobster is a good source of protein and iron. It is low in fat. Cooked and shelled, 100 gm = 95 calories. See *meat* for nutrient content.

locust bean gum. Obtained from the endosperm of the bean of the *carob* tree. Used in food to improve the texture and freeze-melt characteristics of ice cream, to thicken salad dressing, pie filling and barbecue sauce; to make softer, more resilient cakes and biscuits when used as a dough additive; and to increase the palatability of carrageenin gels by decreasing their brittleness and melting temperature. The locust bean gum has a laxative action, indicating that it is not absorbed to any great extent by the body.

loganberry (*Rubus vrsinus logganbaccus*). A berry resembling a blackberry in shape but its color is red and, when fully ripe, it takes on a purple tinge. In flavor it resembles the raspberry, but is more acid. Fresh, 100 gm = 267 calories; canned, in heavy syrup, 100 gm = 404 calories.

loquat (*Eriobotyra japonica*). A tropical evergreen tree and its fruit that is also known as a "Japanese medlar." The loquat tree is a small, ornamental evergreen tree with broad leaves and fragrant white flowers. The fruit is small, round, downy, and yellow-orange in color, with large black seeds. The flesh is pale yellow to orange, very juicy, with a delicious, slightly acid flavor, not as rich and sweet as most tropical fruit.

lovage (*Levisticum officinale*). A perennial herb, also called smellage, a member of the carrot family to which parsley and celery also belong. Lovage is a tall plant, growing 5 to 7 feet with greenish or whitish-yellow flowers. Its large heavy, light-green leaves resemble those of celery, and the greens have a celerylike flavor. The root is strong in taste and smell. Fresh and dried leaves of lovage are used for flavor in cooking; the roots may be blanched and served like celery or candied. The leaves are also used as a potherb.

low-acid. A food that contains low concentrations of *organic acids*. Meat, poultry and most of the common vegetables (except tomatoes) contain little of the *organic acids* and therefore are called low-acid foods. When canning an acid food, such as tomatoes, processing can be in a boiling water bath because the foods acid aids in the destruction of certain spoilage organisms and prevents the growth of *toxins* by other spoilage organisms. To process low-acid foods in a reasonable length of time requires a temperature higher than that of boiling water and requires increased pressure, such as in a pressure cooker to create higher temperatures.

luteinizing hormone (LH). a *gonadotrophic hormone* of the *pituitary* gland that stimulates conversion of a follicle in the ovary into a corpus luteum and secretion of *progesterone* * by the corpus luteum. LH also stimulates secretion of sex hormones by the testes.

luteotropic hormone (LTH). A *gonadotropin* of the pituitary gland, also called the lactogenic hormone or prolactin. Luteotropic hormone activates the corpus luteum in the ovaries and stimulates the production of *progesterone* *. LTH may also be involved in mammary gland development.

lymph. Lymph consists of a fluid plasma containing a variable number of lymphocytes, a few granulocytes, no blood platelets, carbon dioxide and very small quantities of oxygen. In the lymphatics of the intestine, fat content is high during digestion. Lymph is formed from tissue by the physical process of filtration. Colloidal substances from tissue are returned to lymph capillaries rather than to the blood. Water, crystalloids, and other substances also enter the lymph capillaries. Since the process of tissue fluid formation is continuous, lymph formation is also continuous. The lymph system supplements the capillaries and veins in the return of the tissue fluid to the blood. Starting as small blind ducts within the tissues, the lymphatic vessels enlarge to form lymphatic capillaries. These capillaries unite to form large lymphatic vessels, which resemble veins in structure and arrangement. Valves in lymph vessels prevent backflow. Superficial lymph vessels collect lymph from the skin and subcutaneous tissue; deep vessels collect lymph from all other parts of the body. The two largest collecting vessels are the thoracic duct and the right lymphatic duct. The thoracic duct receives lymph from all parts of the body except the upper right side. The lymph from the thoracic duct drains into the left subclavian vein, at the root of the neck on the left side. The right lymphatic duct drains into a correspoinding vein on the right side. Lymph nodes occur in groups up to a dozen or more lying along the course of lymph vessels. Although variable in size they are usually small oval bodies which are composed of lymphoid tis-'sues. Lymph nodes act as filters for removal of infective organisms from the lymph stream. Important groups of those nodes are located in the axilla, the cervical regions, the submaxillary region, the inguinal (groin) region, and the mesentric (abdominal) region.

lymphatic system. The system of lymph vessels and lymph ducts provides for a drainage system for tissue fluid, and is an auxilliary part of the circulatory system, returning an important amount of tissue fluid to the bloodstream through connection with the lymphatic vessels. The spleen belongs in part to the lymphatic system. Unlike the cardiovascular system, the lymphatic system has no pump to move the fluid which it collects, but muscle contractions and breathing movements aid in the movement of lymph through its channels and its return to the blood stream. Following is a diagram of the lymphatic system. The vessels in the shaded area drain into the right lymphatic duct; the rest drain into the thoracic duct. (See diagram p. 272)

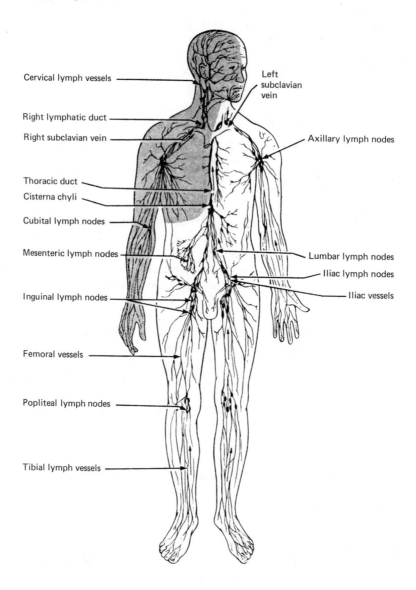

Cervical lymph vessels

Left subclavian vein

Right lymphatic duct

Right subclavian vein

Axillary lymph nodes

Thoracic duct

Cisterna chyli

Cubital lymph nodes

Mesenteric lymph nodes

Lumbar lymph nodes

Iliac lymph nodes

Iliac vessels

Inguinal lymph nodes

Femoral vessels

Popliteal lymph nodes

Tibial lymph vessels

lymphocyte. White blood cells that, upon stimulation by an *antigen*, give rise to *plasma cells,* which produce *antibody.*

lysine. Mol. Wt. 146. One of the *essential amino acids*. It is a basic amino acid. Lysine is one of the essential amino acids that is usually in low concentration in proteins of plant origin.

$$\underset{\underset{\displaystyle H_2N-CH_2-CH_2-CH_2-CH_2CH-COOH}{|}}{NH_2}$$

lysosomes. Structures of cell cytoplasm that contain *digestive enzymes*. Seen as "droplets" within the cell which are of different consistency from the rest of the *cytoplasm*. Separation of these droplets from the cytoplasm and chemical analysis indicates that various digestive enzymes are contained within the lysosomal membrane at the edge of the "droplet." Thus cytoplasm is protected from digestion by enzymes; at the same time ingested nutrients coming into contact with the lysosomes can be acted on. Larger molecules may be broken down to smaller ones which the cell can use. See *cell*.

lysozyme. Lysozyme is an enzyme that hydrolyzes complex polysaccharides. It is found in high concentrations in egg whites and in human tears. In human tears, lysozyme protects the eyes by hydrolyzing the cell walls of air-borne bacteria and thus preventing infection of the cornea. It was the first protein for which the complete three-dimensional structure was determined.

M

macaroni. A food paste made from a mixture of semolina and water, and dried in the form of slender tubes or fancy shapes—elbow macaroni and macaroni shells, for example. The semolina used is the purified middlings (medium-size particles of ground grain) of durum or other hard wheat. Primarily a source of carbohydrate with small quantities of B vitamins. Marcaroni, cooked, 100 gm = 148 calories; macaroni and cheese, 100 gm = 215 calories.

mace. An aromatic spice made from the arillode, or false aril, which covers the seed of the nutmeg. The nutmeg, a tropical evergreen tree, bears a golden pear-shaped fruit which when its external covering is removed, reveals a red arillode over its hard kernel (the nutmeg itself). This arillode is dried, becoming yellowish-orange and, either whole or powdered, is the mace available.

mackerel (*Scomber scombus*). A long, slender, saltwater fish, averaging a length of 1 foot and weighing 1 to 2 pounds. Mackerel scales are small and smooth, its back steely-blue or greenish, its belly silvery-white. The flesh is firm and fatty with a distinctive flavor and a savory taste. A good source of protein. Fresh mackerel, broiled, 100 gm = 236 calories; canned, solids and liquid, 100 gm = 180 calories; salted, 100 gm = 305 calories; smoked, 100 gm = 219 calories. See *meat* for nutrient content.

macrobiotic. A diet based on whole grains.

macrocyte. An abnormally large red blood cell. The vitamin deficiency disease *pernicious anemia* is characterized by the appearance of macrocytes and a condition called *megablastic anemia*. See *pernicious anemia* and *folacin* (folic acid) deficiency.

macromolecules. Large molecules built up from many smaller molecular units or building blocks either of the same or of different types. *Proteins, nucleic acids,* and *polysaccharides* are macromolecules which have amino acids, nucleotides, and monosaccharides as building blocks, respectively. Their spatial structure and function is determined by the number and the sequence of the molecular units of which they are made.

magnesium (Mg). Element No. 12. Atom. Wt. 24. Of the total magnesium, about 0.5 gm/kg fat-free tissue, roughly 60 percent is located in bone. The function of magnesium in hard tissues is not known; one-third of it is in combination with phosphate and the remainder appears to be absorbed loosely on the surface of the mineral structure of bone. A small amount of magnesium is dissolved in the extracellular fluid and is easily exchanged with that absorbed at the bone surface. Within the cells of soft tissue the concentration of magnesium is greater than any other mineral except potassium. Loss of magnesium from the body is usually associated with tissue breakdown and cell destruction. Magnesium is required for cellular respiration, specifically in oxidative phosphorylation leading to formation of *adenosine triphosphate* * (ATP). Magnesium is the activator for many enzymic reactions, and all reactions where ATP is formed. Magnesium is present in foods from both animal and plant sources. Meats, milk, and cereal grains have more magnesium than other foods. In a diet most of the magnesium comes from milk (23 percent), vegetables, including potatoes (20 percent), cereal products and flour (18 percent), meat and eggs (13 percent), coffee and cocoa (9 percent), fruit (6 percent), and dry beans, nuts, and legumes (11 percent). The precise magnesium requirements of man have not been determined, but diets supplying 250 to 300 mg keep healthy adults in balance.

magnesium trisolicate ($2M_gO \cdot 3S:O_3 \cdot 5H_2O$). A compound used as a gastric antacid. See *aluminum hydroxide*.

maize or corn (*Zea mays*). A cereal grain which is also known as Indian corn and corn. The plant is of American origin and was probably first cultivated in Mexico. It is the only native American cereal grain of major importance. See *corn*.

malabsorption syndrome. A term used to grossly describe such conditions as the sprues; *celiac disease, idopathic steatorrhea,* which have in common the failure to absorb various nutrients such as fats, calcium, and other minerals, as well as certain vitamins, notably the fat-soluble ones: *retinol* * (vitamin A), *vitamin D* *, tocopherol* * (vitamin E) and *vitamin K* *.

malic acid (malate). Mol. Wt. 134. Large amounts occur in apples with other fruits containing smaller amounts. The change in flavor that occurs as a fruit ripens is due partly to a decrease in malic acid content and to an increase in sugar content. Malic acid is an important metabolite and is present in all living cells. Used by the food industry as an acidulant and flavoring agent in fruit-flavored drinks, candy, lemon-flavored ice-tea mix, ice cream and preservatives. Two forms of malic acid exists, the D-form and the L-form.

$$HOOC-CH_2-CH-COOH$$
$$|$$
$$OH$$

malignant. Occurring in severe form, frequently fatal; in tumors refers to uncontrolled growth as in cancer.

malnutrition. A condition of the body resulting from an inadequate or excessive supply of food, or impaired utilization of one or more of the essential food constituents.

malonyl coenzyme A. An intermediate compound in the biosynthesis of *fatty acids*.

malt. Malt is a substance made by sprouting or germinating grains, generally barley, but occasionally corn, rye, and oats. After sprouting, the grains are dried and ground. During the process various enzymes, among them *diastase* are formed, partially converting the starch to sugar and changing proteins to amino acids. This makes the formerly hard, raw grain into a mellow, crisp, sweet-tasting malt. When grain is malted, it contributes carbohydrates and proteins to the diet. Malt is used in brewing, distilling, yeast-making, vinegar-making, and as an additive for milk.

malt beverages. Beer and ale are the principal malt beverages, made of malt, hops, yeast, water, and malt adjuncts. The malt is prepared from barley grains which have been germinated and dried, and then the sprouts or germs removed. Hops are the dried flowers of the hop plant. The malt adjuncts are starch- or sugar-containing materials added in addition to the carbohydrates in the malt. Starch adjuncts include corn and corn products, rice, wheat, barley, sorghum grain, soy beans, cassava, potatoes, etc., with corn and rice used most frequently.

maltase. An enzyme in the intestinal juices that splits *maltose* * by hydrolysis into two molecules of *glucose* *. See *digestion* and *maltose*.

maltol, ethyl maltol. Used by food manufacturers to enhance the flavor and aroma of fruit, vanilla, and chocolate flavored foods and beverages. Small amounts of maltol occur naturally in bread crust, coffee, and chicory and as a degradation product in heated milk, cellulose, and starch. Used in gelatin desserts, soft drinks, ice cream and other foods that are high in carbohydrates. Levels used range from 15 to 250 ppm for maltol and 1 to 50 ppm for ethyl maltol. Ethyl maltol can be used in diet foods to mash saccharin's bitter aftertaste and in ordinary foods to permit a lower sugar content.

maltose. Mol Wt. 360. A *disaccharide* resulting from starch hydrolysis maltose yields two molecules glucose on hydrolysis. Formed from *starch* by the action of enzymes (*amylases*) it is therefore an important constituent of germinating cereals, malt and malt products. It is also formed as an intermediate product when starch is digested in the human or other animal body, or hydrolyzed by boiling with dilute mineral acid as in the manufacture of commercial glucose. Maltose is also readily and completely hydrolyzed by boiling with dilute mineral acids or by the enzyme maltase during digestion. In either case each molecule of maltose yields two molecules of *glucose* *

(α1 → 4) Glucopyranosyl-glucopyranose

Maltose

manganese (Mn). Element No. 25. Atom. Wt. 55. Trace element that can be toxic, and cause symptoms of neurological trouble similar to those found in Parkinson's disease. Manganese has many essential functions in each cell of the body. High concentrations are in the pituitary gland, lactating mammary glands, liver, pancreas, kidney, intestinal wall, and bone. The adult human body contains about 20 mg manganese. The highest concentration is in the bone where it is found in both inorganic salts and in the cells of the organic matrix. Absorption of manganese by the body is rather poor and is adversely affected by large amounts of dietary calcium and phosphorus. Excretion is considerable in the feces but urinary losses are very small. The mineral is transported through the body in the plasma, bound to a protein called transmanganin. Manganese is most plentiful in wheat germ, meat, whole buckwheat, barley seed, grapenuts (a cereal), pecans, almonds and Brazil nuts, dry green split peas, fresh turnip greens, fresh spinach, and fresh Brussel sprouts. See *minerals*.

mango (*Mangifera indica*). A tropical fruit of the mango tree. The fruit is oblong in shape and about the size of a large pear. It is green in color, turning orange-yellow when ripe, and has a delicious, pleasantly acid pulp. Mangoes are eaten fresh, may be made into jams or jellies, or such desserts as ice cream. Mangoes are rich in *carotene* * (vitamin A), ascorbic acid* (vitamin C), and vitamin D*. Raw, 100 gm = 66 calories.

manioc (*Manihot*). Tropical plants, also known as cassavas, mandiocs, or yuccas, whose roots yield a tuber which is a staple food in Central and South America. The word comes from the language of the Tupi and Guarani, South American Indian tribes. The manioc or cassava plant is a shrubby perennial that grows to a height of 9 feet, with large parted leaves and roots that end in very large tubers. The tubers produce a flour with an extremely high starch content, which varies from 15 to 30 percent in contrast to 15 to 20 percent for potato flour. The flour, which has very little taste, is used in place of wheat flour. It is either made into nonsweet, thin cakes used like wheat bread, or sprinkled over rice and beans to make them more filling. There are many varieties of manioc, but the two most widely grown for their starchy content are the bitter manioc (*Manioc utilissima* or *esculenta*) and the sweet (*Manioc dulcis,* variety *Aipi*). Tapioca is made from properly treated manioc flour. After the juice has been extracted from the pulp, the pulp is heated over a slow fire until it forms grains which harden in cooking. The roots of the sweet manioc contain no poisonous juices. They are usually roasted under hot ashes and eaten plain or with butter. Their flavor resembles that of the chestnut and they are very high in starch.

manna. The dried sap of certain species of ash, tamarisk, and other trees that grow in the Sinai Desert.

mannitol. Mol. Wt. 182. A versatile substance occurring naturally in the manna ash tree. Obtained by hydrogenation or reduction of *mannose* * and *galactose* * in the same manner as *sorbitol* * from *glucose* *. Commercial quantities are made by synthesis from sugar. A sugar with a variety of industrial uses sometimes employed in the manufacture of foods as improvers. Used as a "dust" in chewing gum, to prevent gum from absorbing moisture and becoming sticky. Mannitol is about two-thirds as sweet as sugar. Since only about 50 percent is used by the body it only generates half as many calories as an equal weight of sugar. Mannitol is frequently used as a sweetening agent in noncaloriogenic chewing gum because bacteria in the mouth have an even harder time digesting it than do humans.

$$
\text{HO—CH}_2\text{—CH—CH—CH—CH—CH}_2\text{OH}
$$

with OH groups on the carbons as shown.

mannose. Mol. Wt. 180. A hexose of more interest to sugar chemists than nutritionists. Small amounts are found in certain foods such as manna from which it takes its name.

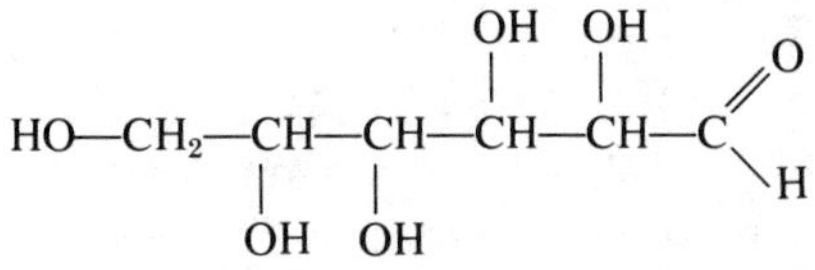

$$HO-CH_2-CH-CH-CH-CH-C\overset{\displaystyle O}{\underset{\displaystyle H}{\diagdown}}$$

with OH groups on the carbons

or

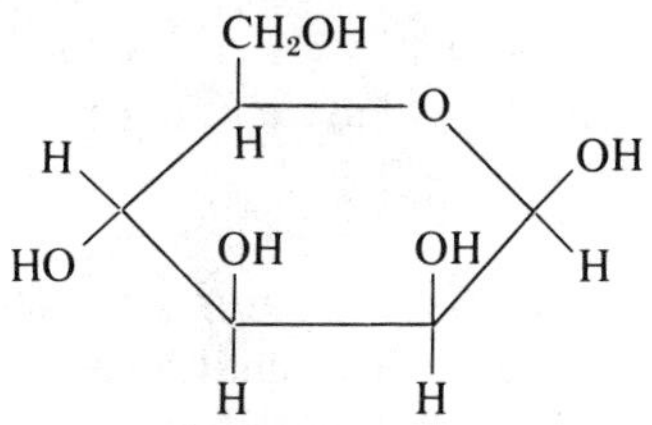

β—D—Mannopyranose

Mannose

maple (*Acer*). A tree native to the north temperate zone. There are 13 species of maple native to the American continent. The sugar, or rock maple (*A. saccharum*) is highly valued as a timber and shade tree, and is the chief source of maple sugar. All maples have a sweet sap, but only the sugar maple and the black maple are tapped to make maple syrup. When the syrup is boiled to the density of strained honey, it is called maple honey. Maple cream or maple butter is syrup boiled to the soft-sugar stage, cooled, and then stirred smooth. Maple sugar is syrup boiled to the hard-sugar stage and then stirred to prevent the individual crystals of sugar from hardening together. Maple syrup can be used on hot cereals, pancakes, waffles, and other quick breads; to sweeten milk, custards, bread puddings, and applesauce and other fruits. A good source of sucrose with some invert sugar and ash. Maple sugar, 100 gm = 348 calories; maple syrup, 100 gm = 252 calories.

marasmus. A protein-calorie malnutrition (PCM) disease. In marasmus both protein and calories are deficient. It is most common in children under 2 years old. There is no edema but there is emaciation, diarrhea is common. There is no depigmentation of the skin or dermacosis. See *Kwashiorkor*.

margarine. A smooth-textured fat used as a spread and in cooking. It may be prepared from animal or vegetable fats or a combination of them in amounts specified by law. The fats may or may not be hydrogenated. The fat ingredients are mixed with pasteurized cream, milk, skim milk, or nonfat dry milk, or any combination of these. When the fat source is vegetable, the fat may be mixed with ground soybeans and water. Optional ingredients such as coloring, flavoring, preservatives, *retinol* * (vitamin A) activity and, *vitamin D* * emulsifiers, butter, and salt may be added. Differences in ingredients affect the flavor, texture, color, spreadability, baking quality, and nutritive value of the finished product. Margarine contributes calories and vitamins A and D. 100 gm = 720 calories.

marjoram (*Majorana hortensis*). A culinary herb, a member of the mint family, known better as sweet marjoram or knotted marjoram. Its downy light-green oval leaves, up to 1 inch long, have a mild sage like flavor, although less strong than sage.

marmalade. A preserve of fruit, usually citrus fruit. The fruits are cut into thin slices with the peel, and cooked in water until tender. Sugar is then added and the mixture is cooked again until the solids are suspended in a clear jellylike mixture. The word marmalade comes from the Portuguese marmelada, derived from the Latin melimelum meaning "honey apple," which in turn can be traced to the Greek melimelon, from meli, "honey," and melon, "apple."

marrow (beef). The fatty filling of beef bones, which is prized for its rich and delicate taste and which is also one of the lightest and most digestible of fats. Marrow is used to enrich dishes, or by itself as a spread, or baked or broiled in the bone. It is very rich in fat with very small amounts of protein. It has the same caloric value as beef fat. Cooked 1 tablespoon = about 100 calories.

marrow (vegetable) (*Cucurbita pepo*). A squashlike edible gourd shaped like a long egg. These gourds can grow to a very large size and it is the smaller marrows which are best for eating. They are peeled, cut into halves, and seeds removed from the center; they are cooked as any firm squash is cooked. Marrow is similar to squash in food and caloric value. See *Squash*.

marshmallow. An American confection made of sugar, unflavored gelatin, corn syrup and flavoring. The mixture is whipped until very light, poured into a pan lined with sugar and cornstarch, and allowed to stand until firm. Then the marshmallows are cut into squares and rolled in additional sugar and cornstarch. 100 gm = 135 calories.

mast cells. Loose connective tissue cells. They are most numerous along blood vessel beds. They form the anticoagulant *heparin*. *Histamine* * is also liberated from those cells in allergic and inflammatory reactions.

mastication. The act of chewing. The function of the mouth, as far as alimentation is concerned is the ingestion of food, the reduction in its size by the action of the teeth, the mixing of particles with saliva, and then the passage of the food into the pharynx in order to be swallowed. Saliva contains an enzyme ptyalin or salivary amylase which initiates the digestion of at least one of the foodstuffs, namely, carbohydrate, however, the mouth is more concerned with ingestion than digestion.

matrix. The groundwork in which something is cast. For example, protein in the bone matrix into which mineral salts are deposited.

mate. A beverage made from the leaves of various species of holly, chiefly *Ilex paraguariensis,* which is also known as yerba mate or Paraguay tea. The plant is an evergreen shrub or small tree. Mate is a relatively inexpensive drink popular in most South American countries. It is greenish in color, has an agreeable aroma, and a slightly bitter taste, which is different from that of tea and less astringent. It is a stimulant, containing up to 5 percent caffeine. Mate is usually drunk as is, but can be flavored in any way. It can be bought in specialty and health food stores, and prepared and served like tea.

mayonnaise. A cold sauce of French origin made with egg yolks, oil, and seasonings, which are blended into an emulsion. It is used as a spread, a sauce for fish, meat and vegetables and as a salad dressing. 100 gm = 718 calories; 1 tablespoon = 110 calories.

mead. An ancient drink made of water and honey, fermented with malt, yeast, and other ingredients. The word is connected with the Greek methy, ''wine,'' and the Sanskrit madhu, ''sweet,'' ''honey,'' or ''mead.''

meat. The meat group includes beef, veal, mutton, lamb, pork, poultry, and fish. It is essentially the flesh of animals, of which more than 100 species are regularly eaten by man. Mammalian lean meat contains about 20 percent protein and 5 percent fat. Lean fish contains about 10 percent protein and less than 1 percent fat. Fat fish contain from 8 to 15 percent fat. Shellfish, lobsters, crayfish, crabs, shrimp, and other crustaceans have very little fat but are rich in cholesterol. Meat ranks as high nutritionally as it does in popularity. It forms the basis for one of the four food groups required for a balanced diet (the others are the milk, bread-cereal, and vegetable-fruit groups). Meat is essentially protein and the word comes from the Greek word meaning ''first'' or ''of primary importance.'' In general, meat contains about 20 to 23 percent protein, a variable amount of fat and lesser constituents, and about 60 percent water. The amount of fat in meats varies with the nutritional state of the animal and the extent of trimming and method of preparation. In addition to protein, muscle meat

Meat and Organ Foods	Wt. Gm.	Approximate Measure	Food Energy cal	Protein gm	Fat gm	Carbohydrate Total gm	Fiber gm	Water gm	Calcium	Phosphorus µg	Iron µg	Vitamin A I.U.	Thiamine µg	Riboflavin µg	Niacin µg	Ascorbic Acid µg
Brains, all kinds, raw	100	3½ ozs.	125	10	9	1	0	79	10	312	2.4	0	0.23	0.26	4.4	18
Crabs, Atlantic and Pacific, hard shell, steamed	100	3½ ozs.	93	17	2	1		79	43	175	0.8	2,170	0.16	0.08	2.8	2
Canned, meat only	100	3½ ozs.	101	17	3	1		77	45	182	0.8		0.08	0.08	1.9	
Duck, domestic raw, flesh only	100	3½ ozs.	165	21	8	0	0	69	12	203	1.3		0.10	0.12	7.7	
Eels, raw, American	100	3½ ozs.	233	16	18	0	0	66	18	202	0.7	1,610	0.22	0.36	1.4	
Fish:																
Bluefish:																
Baked or broiled	100	3½ ozs.	159	26	5	0	0	68	29	287	0.7	50	0.11	0.10	1.9	
Fried	100	3½ ozs.	205	23	10	5	0	61	35	257	0.9		0.11	0.11	1.8	
Cod:																
Broiled	100	3½ ozs.	170	29	5	0	0	65	31	274	1.0	180	0.08	0.11	3.0	
Dried	100	3½ ozs.	375	82	3	0	0	12		891	3.6	0	0.08	0.45	10.9	0
Flounder, baked	100	3½ ozs.	202	30	8	0	0	58	23	344	1.4		0.07	0.08	2.5	
Haddock, fried	100	3½ ozs.	165	20	6	6	0	67	40	247	1.2		0.04	0.07	3.2	2
Halibut, broiled	100	3½ ozs.	171	25	7	0	0	67	16	248	0.8	680	0.05	0.07	8.3	
Herring:																
Atlantic, raw	100	3½ ozs.	176	17	11	0	0	69		256	1.1	110	0.02	0.15	3.6	
Pacific, raw	100	3½ ozs.	98	18	3	0	0	79		225	1.3	100	0.02	0.16	3.5	
Canned in tomato sauce	100	3½ ozs.	176	16	11	4	0	67		243				0.11	3.5	
Smoked, kippered	100	3½ ozs.	211	22	13	0	0	61	66	254	1.4	30		0.28	3.3	
Mackerel:																
Atlantic, broiled	100	3½ ozs.	236	22	16	0	0	62	6	280	1.2	530	0.15	0.27	7.6	
Pacific, canned, solids and liquid	100	3½ ozs.	180	21	10	0	0	66	260	288	2.2	30	0.03	0.33	8.8	

Food	Grams	Measure	Calories	Protein	Fat	Carbohydrate	Water	Calcium	Phosphorus	Iron	Vitamin A	Thiamine	Riboflavin	Niacin	Ascorbic acid
Salmon:															
Cooked, broiled or baked	100	3½ ozs.	182	27	7	0	63		414	1.2	160	0.16	0.06	9.8	
Canned: solid & liquid															
Chinook or King	100	3½ ozs.	210	20	14	0	65	154	289	0.9	230	0.03	0.14	7.3	
Pink or humpback	100	3½ ozs.	141	21	6	0	70	196	286	0.8	70	0.03	0.18	8.0	
Sockeye or red	100	3½ ozs.	171	20	9	0	67	259	344	1.2	230	0.04	0.16	7.3	
Smoked	100	3½ ozs.	176	22	9	0	59	14	245						
Sardines:															
Atlantic type, canned in oil, drained solids	100	3½ ozs.	203	24	11	Tr.	62	437	499	2.9	220	0.03	0.20	5.4	
Pacific type,															
In brine or mustard	100	3½ ozs.	196	19	12	2	64	303	354	5.2	30	0.01	0.30	7.4	
In tomato sauce	100	3½ ozs.	197	19	12	2	64	449	478	4.1	30	0.01	0.27	5.3	
Shad, baked	100	3½ ozs.	201	23	11	0	64	24	313	0.6	30	0.13	0.26	8.6	
Swordfish, broiled	100	3½ ozs.	174	28	7	0	65	27	275	1.3	2,050	0.04	0.05	10.9	
Tuna fish, canned in oil, drained solids	100	3½ ozs.	197	29	8	0	61	8	234	1.9	80	0.05	0.12	11.9	0
Canned in water, solids and liquid	100	3½ ozs.	127	28	1	0	70	16	190	1.6			0.10	13.3	
White fish, cooked, baked, stuffed	100	3½ ozs.	215	15	14	6	63		246	0.5	2,000	0.11	0.11	2.3	
Frog legs, raw	100	3½ ozs.	73	16	Tr.	0	82	18	147	1.5	0	0.14	0.25	1.2	Tr.
Heart:															
Beef, lean, braised	100	3½ ozs.	188	31	6	1	61	6	181	5.9	30	0.25	1.22	7.6	1
Chicken, cooked	100	3½ ozs.	173	25	7	Tr.	67	4	107	3.6	30	0.06	0.92	5.3	4
Pork, cooked	100	3½ ozs.	195	31	7	Tr.	61	4	121	4.9	40	0.20	1.72	6.7	1
Kidneys, raw:															
Beef	100	3½ ozs.	130	15	7	1	76	11	219	7.4	690	0.36	2.55	6.4	15
Lamb	100	3½ ozs.	105	17	3	1	78	13	218	7.6	690	0.51	2.42	7.4	15
Pork	100	3½ ozs.	106	16	4	1	78	11	218	6.7	130	0.58	1.73	9.8	12

Meat and Organ Foods	Wt. Gm.	Approximate Measure	Food Energy cal	Protein gm	Fat gm	Carbohydrate Total gm	Fiber gm	Water gm	Calcium μg	Phosphorus μg	Iron μg	Vitamin A I.U.	Thiamine μg	Riboflavin μg	Niacin μg	Ascorbic Acid μg
Lamb, trimmed to retail basis, cooked:																
Chop, thick, broiled																
Lean and fat	100	3½ ozs.	359	22	29	0	0	47	9	172	1.3		0.12	0.23	5.0	
Lean only (from above serving)	66	2.4 ozs.	125	19	5	0	0	41	8	145	1.3		0.10	0.18	4.1	
Leg, roasted																
Lean and fat	100	3½ ozs.	266	26	17	0	0	55	11	212	1.8		0.15	0.27	5.6	
Lean only (from above serving)	85	3 ozs.	121	19	4	0	0	41	8	157	1.5		0.11	0.20	4.1	
Shoulder, roasted																
Lean and fat	100	3½ ozs.	338	22	27	0	0	50	10	172	1.2		0.13	0.23	4.7	
Lean only (from above serving)	74	2.7 ozs.	150	20	7	0	0	46	9	162	1.4		0.11	0.21	4.3	
Liver:																
Beef:																
Raw	100	3½ ozs.	140	20	4	5	0	70	8	352	6.5	43,900	0.25	3.26	13.6	31
Fried	100	3½ ozs.	229	26	11	5	0	56	11	476	8.8	53,400	0.26	4.19	15.6	27
Calf, fried	100	3½ ozs.	261	30	13	4	0	51	13	537	14.2	32,700	0.24	4.17	16.5	37
Chicken, simmered	100	3½ ozs.	165	27	4	3	0	65	11	159	8.5	12,300	0.17	2.69	11.7	16
Lamb, broiled	100	3½ ozs.	261	32	12	3	0	50	16	572	17.9	74,500	0.49	5.11	24.9	36
Pork, fried	100	3½ ozs.	241	30	12	3	0	54	15	539	29.1	14,900	0.34	4.36	22.3	22
Lobster:																
Raw	100	3½ ozs. meat	91	17	2	1	0	79	29	183	0.6		0.40	0.05	1.5	
Canned or cooked	100	3½ ozs.	95	19	2	Tr.	0	77	65	192	0.8		0.10	0.07		

Luncheon meat:																
Canned, ham or pork	100	3½ oz. slice	294	15	25	1	0	55	9	108	2.2	0	0.31	0.21	3.0	
Oysters, meat only, raw																
Av. Eastern	100	5-8 medium	66	8	2	3		85	94	143	5.5	310	0.14	0.18	2.5	
Oyster stew:																
1 part oysters to 3 parts milk by volume	100	½ c. scant	86	5	5	5		84	117	109	1.4	280	0.06	0.18	0.7	
Pork, fresh, trimmed to retail basis, cooked:																
Chop, thick:																
Lean and fat	100	1 large chop 3½ ozs.	391	25	32	0	0	42	12	268	3.4	0	0.96	0.28	5.6	
Lean only from 1 chop	72	2.6 ozs.	195	22	11	0	0	38	9	248	2.7	0	0.82	0.24	4.9	
Roast, loin or shoulder	100	3½ ozs.	373	23	31	0	0	45	10	232	2.9	0	0.50	0.23	4.9	
Lean only from above serving	77	2.9 ozs.	182	22	10	0	0	44	9	226	2.8	0	0.46	0.22	4.2	
Picnic cut simmered																
Lean and fat	100	3½ ozs.	374	23	31	0	0	46	10	139	3.0	0	0.54	0.25	4.8	
Lean only from above serving	74	2.6 ozs.	157	21	7	0	0	45	9	130	2.7	0	0.49	0.22	4.4	
Pork, smoked ham																
Ham, cooked																
Lean and fat	100	3½ ozs.	289	21	22	0	0	54	9	172	2.6	0	0.47	0.18	3.6	
Lean only from above serving	84	3 ozs.	157	21	7	0	0	52	9	170	2.7	0	0.49	0.19	3.8	
Ham, canned	100	3½ ozs.	193	18	12	1	0	65	11	156	2.7	0	0.53	0.19	3.8	
Pork, fat, salted raw	100	3½ ozs.	783	4	85	0	0	8	Tr.	Tr.	0.6	0	0.18	0.04	0.9	
Shrimp, French fried	100	3½ ozs.	225	20	11	10		57	72	191	2.0		0.04	0.08	2.7	
Canned, dry pack or drained	100	3½ ozs.	116	24	1	1		70	115	263	3.1	60	0.01	0.03	1.8	
Sausage:																
Bologna	100	3½ ozs.	304	12	28	1	0	56	7	128	1.8		0.16	0.22	2.6	0
Frankfurter, cooked	100	2 medium	309	13	28	2	0	56	7	133	1.9		0.16	0.20	2.7	0

Meat and Organ Foods	Wt. Gm.	Approximate Measure	Food Energy cal	Protein gm	Fat gm	Carbohydrate Total gm	Carbohydrate Fiber gm	Water gm	Calcium µg	Phosphorus µg	Iron µg	Vitamin A I.U.	Thiamine µg	Riboflavin µg	Niacin µg	Ascorbic Acid µg
Liver, liverwurst	100	3½ ozs.	307	16	26	2	0	54	9	238	5.4	6,350	0.20	1.30	5.7	
Pork, links or bulk, cooked	100	3½ ozs.	476	18	44	0	0	35	7	162	2.4	0	0.79	0.34	3.7	
Pork, bulk, canned	100	3½ ozs.	381	18	33	0	0	43	11	210	2.8	0	0.20	0.24	3.0	
Vienna sausage, canned	100	3½ ozs.	240	14	20	0	0	63	8	153	2.1	0	0.08	0.13	2.6	
Scallops, cooked, steamed	100	3½ ozs.	112	23	1	Tr.		73	115	338	3.0	0				0
Tongue beef, canned	100	3½ ozs.	267	19	20	0	0	57	10	180	2.5	Tr.	0.05	0.22	2.5	0
Turkey, total edible roasted	100	3½ ozs.	263	27	16	0	0	55					0.09	0.14	8.0	
Flesh only, roasted	100	3½ ozs.	190	32	6	0	0	61	8	251	1.8		0.05	0.18	7.7	0
Veal, cooked:																
Cutlet, broiled	100	3½ ozs.	234	26	13	0	0	59	11	225	3.2		0.07	0.25	5.4	
Roast, medium fat, rib 82 percent lean	100	3½ ozs.	269	27	17	0	0	55	12	248	3.4		0.13	0.31	7.8	
Stew meat without bone medium fat, cooked	100	3½ ozs.	303	26	21	0	0	52	12	138	3.3		0.05	0.24	4.6	

contributes moderate amounts of *thiamine* * and *riboflavin* *, moderate amounts of iron, and generous quantities of *niacin* * and phosphorus. The organ meats, particularly liver and kidney, furnish proteins of a very high quality, generous quantities of practically all the B-complex vitamins, iron, phosphorus, copper, and other trace minerals, and moderate amounts of *ascorbic acid* (vitamin C); in addition liver contains very large quantities of *retinol* * (vitamin A). Besides the muscle of animals, almost any part of the animal organs are a good source of high quality protein. Liver and kidney have been mentioned, but heart, tongue, brain, thymus and pancreas (sweetbreads), tripe (ox or sheep stomach), calves and pig feet, maws (pig stomach), and chitterlings (pigs intestines) are a few examples of organs that are used as food. It is all of good nutritional value. The table on pp. 282–286 gives the nutritional content of some of the common meats and organ foods.

megaloblast. Primitive red blood cells of large size with large nucleus; present in blood when there is a deficiency of *cobalamin* * (vitamin B_{12}) and/or *folacin* *. See *pernicious anemia.*

megaloblastic anemia. Anemia marked by the presence of oversize nucleated red blood cells (megaloblasts).

megavitamin doses. The ingestion of vitamins at levels many times the *Recommended Daily Allowances* (RDA). Except when recommended by a physician as a specific therapy, there is no evidence that any of the vitamins taken in excess of the RDA has an added beneficial effect. High ingestion levels of *retinol* * (vitamin A) and *vitamin D* * has in fact lead to *vitamin toxicity* (hypervitaminosis). Even the water-soluble vitamins, though not generally considered as toxic can develop toxic symptoms in some individuals when taken for prolonged periods at high levels. The toxicity level for vitamins appears to vary considerably among individuals, and may vary by factors as high as 100. See *vitamin toxicity.*

meiosis. (1) The process whereby a germ cell, with two of each chromosome, gives rise to sperms, or eggs, each with only one of every pair of chromosomes. (2) The physiological mechanism underlying Mendel's laws, the process that produces sex cells. As for genetics the most important consequences of meiosis is that it results in cells that contain only one complete set of alleles. Since genes are located on chromosomes, this means that cells produced by meiosis contain only half the chromosome number that other cells have, the haploid number as compared with the diploid number. *Mitosis* is the cellular effect that results in two cells identical to one another and to the parent cell that divided to produce them. All have the diploid number of chromosomes. In human beings, meiosis produces cells with 23 chromosomes in the nucleus, and mitosis produces cells with 46.

melanin. The dark amorphous pigment of the skin, hair, and certain other tissues. The amino acid *tyrosine* * is a *precursor* to melanin. An inborn error of tyrosine metabolism called *albinism* causes a generalized lack of pigment in the skin, eyes, and hair.

melanocyte-stimulating hormone (MSH). The smallest part of the pituitary gland is the median lobe which produces just one hormone, melanocyte-stimulating hormone (MSH). Melanocytes are cells in the skin which contain the dark pigment melanin. In the presence of MSH these cells become more prominent and so make the skin darker. There are also indications that MSH can effect the excitability of the central nervous system. Like all pituitary hormones MSH is made up of amino acids joined together. Compared with other hormones MSH is really quite a small peptide.

melatonin. A hormone of the *pineal gland* that inhibits output of sex hormones by the gonads.

melon. A fruit of a number of annual trailing plants which grow from seed and belong to the gourd family, Cucurbitaceae. The word melon comes from the Greek meleopepon, a combination of melon meaning "apple" and pepon, a kind of edible gourd. The two best known groups of edible melons are *Cucumis melo,* the muskmelons, and *Citrullus vulgaris,* the watermelons. Muskmelons are divided into two principal varieties; the net-skinned, *C. melo cantalupensis,* of which cantaloupes and Persian melons are the most familiar; and the smooth-skinned, *C. melo inodorus,* to which group honeydews and casabas belong. There are many variations of these two types of muskmelons, including Crenshaw, honeyball, and Christmas melons.

Cantaloupe, 100 gm = 30 calories
Casaba, 100 gm = 27 calories
Honeydew, 100 gm = 33 calories
Watermelon, 100 gm = 26 calories

membrane. A thin layer of cells forming a pliable tissue that serves as a covering or envelope of a part, a lining of a cavity, a partition (septum) or a connection between structures. Certain membranes are combined layers of tissues that form partitions, lining envelopes or capsules. They reinforce and support body organ and cavities. Others are a combination of connective tissue only (examples: mucous, pleural, pericardial, and peritoneal membranes). Connective tissue membranes are combinations of connective tissue only (examples: meninges, fascia, periosteum, and synovia). Different kinds of membranes are associated with different body systems (examples: plueral membranes with the respiratory system; pericardial membranes with the circulatory system; peritoneal membranes with the digestive system; meningeal membranes with the nervous system; fascial membranes with the muscular system; and periosteal and synovial membranes with the skeletal system).

membrane, mucous. A mucous membrane is usually composed of three layers of tissue; the epithelium, a supporting lamina propria, and a thin, usually double layer of smooth muscle. The mucous membranes are attached to the parts beneath them by loose connective tissue, called submucous connective tissue. The functions of the mucous membranes are protection, support of blood vessels and lymphatics, and provision of a large surface for secretion and absorption.

membrane, serous. Thin, transparent, strong, and elastic membranes whose surfaces are moistened by a self-secreted serous fluid. They consist of simple squamous epithelium and a layer of areolar connective tissues which serve as a base. Serous membranes are found lining the body cavities and covering the organs which lie in them, and forming the fascia bulbi and part of the membranous labyrinth of the ear. The function of the membranes is mainly protective, such as secreting serum which covers its surface, supplying the lubrication for organs as they move over each other.

membrane, synovial. Membranes associated with the bones and muscles. They consist of an outer layer of fibrous tissue and an inner layer of areolar connective tissue with loosely arranged collagenous and elastic fibers, connective tissue cells, and fat cells. Synovial membranes secrete synovid, a viscid fluid that resembles the white of egg, and contains hyaluronic acid. They are divided into three classes, articular, mucous sheaths, and bursae mucosae. The function of synovial membrane is mainly protective, such as secretory serum which covers its surface, supplying the lubrication for organs as they move over each other.

menadione. Mol. Wt. 172. A synthetic compound, having greater *vitamin K**** activity than the naturally occurring vitamin; used as a reference standard for biological assays of vitamin K. In large doses, synthetic vitamin K has produced toxic effects; consequently a dose in excess of 5 mg should be avoided. See *vitamin K****.

Mendel's Laws. Mendel laid the foundation for the science of genetics, his experiments led to the conclusion that, (1) inheritance is particulate; (2) the particles, i.e., the genes, are present in pairs which separate in the formation of sex cells (first law); (3) the segregation of one pair of alleles is independent of that of any other pair (second law). Mendel not only discovered what later were called genes, but also two basic laws regulating the manner in which they are passed on from one generation to the next.

menhaden oil (*Brevoortia tyrannus*). The menhaden a food fish found in very large quantities off the eastern coasts of North America. The flesh of the fish contains about 14 percent of oil. The color varies with the quality of the oil and the care and speed that have been secured in its production.

Menkes' syndrome. A rare genetically determined failure of copper (Cu) absorption, leading to progressive mental retardation, failure to keratinize hair, which becomes kinky, hypothermia, low concentrations of Cu in plasma and liver, skeletal changes and degenerative changes in the elastic membrane.

menopause. A permanent cessation of menses.

menses. A physiologic hemorrhage in females that occurs at approximately 4-week intervals. The source of the hemorrhage is the uterine membrane. Under normal circumstances hemorrhage is preceded by ovulation.

menstrual. Pertaining to the menses.

mercury (Hg). Element No. 80. Atom Wt. 201. A silver-white, heavy liquid metal, slightly volatile. Though naturally occurring in small amounts, mercury has increased in concentration because of industrial wastes. It has been found to be close to toxic levels in some samples of seafoods. The highest permissible level in American foods is 0.5 parts per million. Mercury is readily absorbed by intact skin and the respiratory and gastrointestinal tracts.

metabolic acidosis. A result of faulty intake or output of acids. Metabolic acidosis occurs in various circumstances, such as *ketosis,* resulting from uncontrolled diabetes or starvation; chronic renal failure; or the loss of bicarbonate in severe diarrhea. See *ketosis.*

metabolic alkalosis. A result of faulty intake or output of bases. Metabolic alkalosis occurs where there is an abnormally high loss of *hydrochloric acid* (HCl). Loss of HCl occurs as a result of vomiting. Metabolic alkalosis can also occur by the ingestion of large amounts of alkaline salts such as bicarbonates.

metabolic pool. The assortment of nutrients available within the body at any given moment for the metabolic activities of the body, e.g., amino acid pool, calcium pool.

metabolism. The word metabolism is a general term used to cover all the chemical changes that go on in the tissues of the body. It includes both synthetic (anabolic) and degradative (catabolic) pathways. Metabolism = *Anabolism + Catabolism*. Under energy metabolism included are the chemical changes by which fat, carbohydrate, and protein (and alcohol) are broken down and gradually oxidized to release energy or by which they may be synthesized into compounds such as *adenosine triphosphate* * (ATP) in which unneeded energy may be stored. Metabolism includes only chemical changes within tissue cells, it does not include those that occur in digestion of foods. The diagram below greatly simplifies the metabolism of the foodstuffs, protein, fat, and carbohydrate.

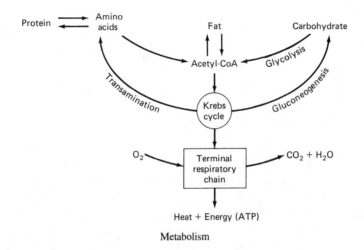

Metabolism

methemoglobin. When the iron in hemoglobin becomes oxidized to the ferric (F^{+3}) state the result is methemoglobin, which lacks the ability to combine with oxygen. Methemoglobin formation can be caused by phenacetin, nitrites, nitriates, and acetanilid.

methanol (wood alcohol). Mol. Wt. 32. CH_3OH. An alcohol derived from wood. It is poisonous and cannot be treated to make it nonpoisonous. It is not to be confused with *ethanol* *.

methionine (MET). Mol. Wt. 149. An *essential amino acid*. The body can make *cysteine* * from methionine but not vice versa, so that methionine is the dietary essential. Methionine is concerned with the important process of trans-methylation. The chief dietary sources of methyl (-CH₃) groups appear to be methione and *betaine* * (a quaternary amine) which are called methyl donors. Methionine gives up the -CH₃ group attached to its sulphur atoms. See *betaine*.

$$CH_3—S—CH_2—CH_2—\overset{\overset{\displaystyle NH_2}{|}}{CH}—COOH$$

methyl malonic acid. Mol. Wt. 118. As a *Coenzyme A* derivative, it is an intermediate in the synthesis of *fatty acids*. A derivative of *folacin* *, Coenzyme B_{12}, is required to convert methyl malonate to succinate. In certain genetic diseases relating to *folacin* * (vitamin B_{12}) methyl-malonuria results because it cannot be converted to succinate, hence its measurement in urine can be used to determine folacin status.

$$HOOC—\overset{\overset{\displaystyle CH_3}{|}}{CH}—COOH$$

milligram (mg). One thousandth of a gram or 1/28000 of an ounce.

milliliter. One thousandth of a liter or about 1/30 of an ounce (volume). See *liter*.

micelle. A dispersion of particles to form an emulsion of a two-phase lipid water complex of macromolecular dimensions by the detergent action or soap effect of a dispersing agent. Common dispersing agents (emulsifiers) in the body are *phospholipids*, such as *lecithin* *, and the *bile salts* *. The dispersing agents have two distinct solubility properties in a single molecule. One part of the molecule is fat soluble (hydrophobic) and the other part is water soluble (hydrophilic). The center of micelles contain lipid material dissolved or held together by the hydrophobic part of the molecule. The hydrophilic part of the molecule is either positively (+) or negatively (−) charged and is on the surface of the micelle. The hydrophilic part interacts with water and holds the particles in suspension in water to form an emulsion. Micelle formation is important in the digestion of *fats* and *lipids*, and in the transport of fat as chylomicrons. See *emulsification* and *emulsifiers*.

microbiological. Pertaining to microorganisms (microscopic plants or animals). Refers usually to a method by which certain microorganisms are used to determine the amounts of a particular nutrient, like a vitamin or an *amino acid,* in a food. Such assays or analysis are possible because these microorganisms must have these vitamins and amino acids in order to grow.

microgram. A microgram is 1/1000 of a milligram or a millionth of a gram.

micronutrients. Nutrients present in very small amounts in food. As applied to mineral elements, the term usually refers to those present in the body in amounts less than that or iron. See *minerals*.

milk. Distinguished by the high quality of its proteins and its high content of *calcium* and *phosphorus*. It is a good source of *riboflavin** and *retinol** (vitamin A) and supplies generous quantities of *lactose* and readily digested milk fat. The major protein of milk is casein; lesser amounts of lactalbumin and lactoglobulin are also present. Milk is a fluid secreted by female mammals as food for their young. Human milk is the sole natural food for the human infant. Cow's milk is the usual substitute for human milk but milk from other mammals is substituted in many parts of the world. Cow's milk is much higher in protein, 35 gm/liter, than human milk, 15 gm/liter of protein. Human milk is usually richer in *retinol** (vitamin A) and *ascorbic acid** (vitamin C) than cow's milk. All milks are a poor source of iron and of *vitamin D**. Cow's milk cannot be fed to human infants directly. It must be processed first by diluting to reduce the protein concentration, then adding sugar is to bring the carbohydrate level up to that of human milk; and finally the milk is pasturized to protect it from *pathogens*. An infant's normal requirement for milk is about 160 ml/Kg/day (2.5 oz/lb/day). Milk is a valuable food for children. From age 1 to 5 about 500 ml (about 6 oz) of milk per day and about half that amount until growth ceases, are ample amounts. Casein is the major protein of milk and has a high biological value. The major carbohydrate is *lactose** (milk sugar). The casein found in milk of most warm-blooded animals is similar, the lactalbumin and lactoglobulin are, however, species-specific and differ in the composition and immunologic properties. Cow's milk is poor in iron and *ascorbic acid** (vitamin C). The *retinol** (vitamin A) content of milk varies with the feed of the cow; the vitamin D content of nonenriched milk varies with the availability of sunlight and is greater in the summer months. Much of the nutritional excellence of fresh, whole fluid milk is also found in evaporated and powdered milk. Fat-free skimmed milk is as desirable, and skimmed milk powder is the most economical source of good protein, calcium, and phosphorus. Cheese contains all the casein and some of the albumin and minerals of the whole milk from which it is derived. When made from whole milk it also contains the original butterfat.

milk products. Many products derive from milk and are stables in many diets, countries and cultures. Some of the more important of these milk products are listed below:

Pasteurized milk: Milk which has been heated to kill any harmful bacteria and then cooled immediately to 50°F or lower.

Homogenized milk: Pasteurized milk in which the particles have been broken down and evenly distributed throughout the milk by a mechanical process. In homogenized milk the cream does not rise to the top of the container as it does in nonhomogenized milk. Homogenized milk forms a softer curd in the stomach and is more easily digested.

Fortified milk: Pasteurized milk containing added amounts of one or more of the essential nutrients present in milk. The most common addition is vitamin D.

Low-sodium milk: Milk used for special diets. It is milk from which 90 percent of the sodium has been removed and replaced with potassium. Part of the B vitamins and calcium are lost in the process. Low sodium milk is also in powdered form.

Chocolate milk: Pasteurized milk to which chocolate syrup or cocoa is added. Vanilla, salt, sugar, and a stabilizer may also be added to keep the drink well mixed.

Evaporated milk: Homogenized whole milk from which about 60 percent of the water has been removed by heating. Vitamin D is added to provide 400 International Units per pint of evaporated milk. When diluted with an equal amount of water, it has about the same food value as a fresh whole milk.

Condensed milk: Milk made by evaporating a mixture of whole milk and sugar. It differs from the unsweetened evaporated milk only in the addition of the sugar which accounts for 40 to 45 percent of the final product.

Skim milk: Fresh milk from which some fat has been removed; available as fluid skim milk, buttermilk, fortified skim milk, and flavored milk drinks.

Fluid skim milk: Made of whole milk from which some fat has been removed. The milk fat remaining usually varies from 1 to 2 percent.

Buttermilk: Milk to which a lactic-acid producing culture is added. (Generally the milk used is skim, although buttermilk may occasionally be produced from whole milk, concentrated fluid milk, or reconstituted nonfat dry milk). Butter granules may be added to enhance the flavor. Acidophilus milk is a form of buttermilk used for special diets and available in fluid form.

Fortified skim milk: Skim milk to which vitamins, including vitamin C and minerals are added. Each quart usually contains the minimum daily vitamins and mineral requirements for health.

Cream: The milk fat that separates from whole milk. It contains almost all of the fat, about one-third the concentration of protein, and about one-third the concentration of lactose in milk.

Butter: An An emulsion of milk-fat globules, air, and water produced by churning cream or whole milk. The liquid that remains after the churning is called buttermilk.

Rennet: Commercial preparation of rennin which causes milk protein to precipitate. It is the first step in cheese making.

Whey: The fluid from the precipitated protein in the formation of curds. It contains lactose, little protein, and little fat.

Cheese: Cheese is made from clotted milk. The clotting of the milk is effected by adding rennet. The clot or curd is separated from the liquid (whey), salted, and pressed to form a cake. Bacteria and molds then ferment and ripen the cheese cake. The characteristic flavor, color, and texture of cheese depends upon the source of milk (cow, sheep, goat, etc.), the kind and combination of bacteria and mold, and the conditions of the ripening process. Cheeses are very nutritious foods containing 25 to 35 percent of a protein of high biological value, rich in *calcium, retinol** (vitamin A) and *riboflavin**. The fat content varies widely from 16 to 40 percent, depending upon the type of cheese. Cheeses should be avoided when certain antidepressant drugs are prescribed. Some antidepressants inhibit an enzyme, monoamine oxidase, which ordinary destroys *tyramine**, a product of the amino acid *tyrosine**. Tyramine stimulates the sympathetic nervous system and may cause headaches, nausea, dizziness, and a rise in blood pressure. This caution applies to any other food, drink, or medicine which contains *amines*.

Fermented milk sources: Various bacteria are used to sour or curdle milk. All of these bacteria breakdown *lactose** to *glucose** and *galactose** which are eventually converted to *lactic acid**, which may be as high as 3 percent. Sour or fermented milks are usually hygenically safe when there may be doubt about dairy hygiene because the initial steps involve boiling the milk to reduce the volume. After cooling, the boiled milk is usually inoculated with a small quantity of sour milk and allowed to stand for 24 hours. (a) Acidophilus milk is obtained by inoculating milk with *Lactobacillus acidophilus* which will grow so profusely in milk that growth of a pathogenic contaminant is greatly diminished. *L. acidolphilus* is also found naturally in the alimentary tract of human adults. (b) Yogurt is milk that has been greatly concentrated by boiling various bacteria which are inoculated for the souring (lactic acid) and in some countries yeast fermentation produces alcohol in addition. Soured and fermented milks contain all fat, protein, calcium, and vitamins that occur in the original milk. These milk products are therefore nutritious foods but there is no evidence that they possess any special properties beyond that. The table on pages 296–303 gives the nutrient values of some milks and milk products.

millet (*Panicum miliaceum*). Any of a large number of small seeded *cereal grains* and forage grasses, or the grain or seed of these grasses. It is generally grown as a cereal in Asia and Africa, providing a diet staple for one-third of the

Table of Food Composition*

Milk, Cheese, Cream, Imitation Cream; Related Products		Water	Food Energy	Protein	Fat
		Grams	*Per-cent*	*Calo-ries*	*Grams*	*Grams*

Milk, Cheese, Cream, Imitation Cream; Related Products		Grams	Percent	Calories	Grams	Grams
Milk:						
Fluid:						
Whole, 3.5% fat	1 cup	244	87	160	9	9
Nonfat (skim)	1 cup	245	90	90	9	Trace
Partly skimmed, 2% nonfat milk solids added.	1 cup	246	87	145	10	5
Canned, concentrated, undiluted:						
Evaporated, unsweetened.	1 cup	252	74	345	18	20
Condensed, sweetened.	1 cup	306	27	980	25	27
Dry, nonfat instant:						
Low-density (1⅓ cups needed for reconstitution to 1 qt.).	1 cup	68	4	245	24	Trace
High-density (⅞ cup needed for reconstitution to 1 qt.).	1 cup	104	4	375	37	1
Buttermilk:						
Fluid, cultured, made from skim milk.	1 cup	245	90	90	9	Trace
Dried, packaged	1 cup	120	3	465	41	6
Cheese:						
Natural:						
Blue or Roquefort type:						
Ounce	1 oz.	28	40	105	6	9
Cubic inch	1 cu. in.	17	40	65	4	5
Camembert, packaged in 4-oz. pkg. with 3 wedges per pkg.	1 wedge	38	52	115	7	9
Cheddar:						
Ounce	1 oz.	28	37	115	7	9
Cubic inch	1 cu. in.	17	37	70	4	6
Cottage, large or small curd:						
Creamed:						
Package of 12-oz., net wt.	1 pkg.	340	78	360	46	14
Cup, curd pressed down.	1 cup	245	78	260	33	10
Uncreamed:						
Package of 12-oz., net wt.	1 pkg.	340	79	290	58	1

	Fatty Acids									
	Unsaturated									
Satu-rated (total)	Oleic	Lin-oleic	Carbo-hy-drate	Cal-cium	Iron	Vita-min A Value	Thia-mine	Ribo-flavin	Niacin	Ascor-bic Acid
Grams	Grams	Grams	Grams	Milli-grams	Milli-grams	Inter-national units	Milli-grams	Milli-grams	Milli-grams	Milli-grams
5	3	Trace	12	288	0.1	350	0.07	0.41	0.2	2
—	—	—	12	296	.1	10	.09	.44	.2	2
3	2	Trace	15	352	.1	200	.10	.52	.2	2
11	7	1	24	635	.3	810	.10	.86	.5	3
15	9	1	166	802	.3	1,100	.24	1.16	6	3
—	—	—	35	879	.4	1 20	.24	1.21	.6	5
—	—	—	54	1,345	.6	1 30	.36	1.85	.9	7
—	—	—	12	296	.1	10	.10	.44	.2	2
3	2	Trace	60	1,498	.7	260	.31	2.06	1.1	—
5	3	Trace	1	89	.1	350	.01	.17	.3	0
3	2	Trace	Trace	54	.1	210	.01	.11	.2	0
5	3	Trace	1	40	0.2	380	0.02	0.29	0.3	0
5	3	Trace	1	213	.3	370	.01	.13	Trace	0
3	2	Trace	Trace	129	.2	230	.01	.08	Trace	0
8	5	Trace	10	320	1.0	580	.10	.85	.3	0
6	3	Trace	7	230	.7	420	.07	.61	.2	0
1	Trace	Trace	9	306	1.4	30	.10	.95	.3	0

Table of Food Composition (*Continued*)

Milk, Cheese, Cream, Imitation Cream; Related Products		Grams	Water Per-cent	Food Energy Calo-ries	Protein Grams	Fat Grams
Cup, curd pressed down.	1 cup	200	79	170	34	1
Cream:						
Package of 8-oz., net wt.	1 pkg.	227	51	850	18	86
Package of 3-oz., net wt.	1 pkg.	85	51	320	7	32
Cubic inch	1 cu. in.	16	51	60	1	6
Parmesan, grated:						
Cup, pressed down	1 cup	140	17	655	60	43
Tablespoon	1 tbsp.	5	17	25	2	2
Ounce	1 oz.	28	17	130	12	9
Swiss:						
Ounce	1 oz.	28	39	105	8	8
Cubic inch	1 cu. in.	15	39	55	4	4
Pasteurized processed cheese:						
American:						
Ounce	1 oz.	28	40	105	7	9
Cubic inch	1 cu. in.	18	40	65	4	5
Swiss:						
Ounce	1 oz.	28	40	100	8	8
Cubic inch	1 cu. in.	18	40	65	5	5
Pasteurized process cheese food, American:						
Tablespoon	1 tbsp.	14	43	45	3	3
Cubic inch	1 cu. in.	18	43	60	4	4
Pasteurized process cheese spread, American.	1 oz.	28	49	80	5	6
Cream:						
Half-and-half (cream and milk).	1 cup	242	80	325	8	28
	1 tbsp.	15	80	20	1	2
Light, coffee or table	1 cup	240	72	505	7	49
	1 tbsp.	15	72	30	1	3
Sour	1 cup	230	72	485	7	47
	1 tbsp.	12	72	25	Trace	2
Whipped topping (pressurized).	1 cup	60	62	155	2	14
	1 tbsp.	3	62	10	Trace	1

Fatty Acids										
Saturated (total)	Unsaturated		Carbohydrate	Calcium	Iron	Vitamin A Value	Thiamine	Riboflavin	Niacin	Ascorbic Acid
	Oleic	Linoleic								
Grams	Grams	Grams	Grams	Milligrams	Milligrams	International units	Milligrams	Milligrams	Milligrams	Milligrams
Trace	Trace	Trace	5	180	.8	20	06	.56	.2	0
48	28	3	5	141	.5	3,500	.05	.54	.2	0
18	11	1	2	53	.2	1,310	.02	.20	.1	0
3	2	Trace	Trace	10	Trace	250	Trace	.04	Trace	0
24	14	1	5	1,893	.7	1,760	.03	1.22	.3	0
1	Trace	Trace	Trace	68	Trace	60	Trace	.04	Trace	0
5	3	Trace	1	383	.1	360	.01	.25	.1	0
4	3	Trace	1	262	.3	320	Trace	.11	Trace	0
2	1	Trace	Trace	139	.1	170	Trace	.06	Trace	0
5	3	Trace	1	198	.3	350	.01	.12	Trace	0
3	2	Trace	Trace	122	.2	210	Trace	.07	Trace	0
4	3	Trace	1	251	.3	310	Trace	.11	Trace	0
3	2	Trace	Trace	159	.2	200	Trace	.07	Trace	0
2	1	Trace	1	80	.1	140	Trace	.08	Trace	0
2	1	Trace	1	100	.1	170	Trace	.10	Trace	0
3	2	Trace	2	160	.2	250	Trace	.15	Trace	0
15	9	1	11	261	.1	1,160	.07	.39	.1	2
1	1	Trace	1	16	Trace	70	Trace	.02	Trace	Trace
27	16	1	10	245	.1	2,020	.07	.36	.1	2
2	1	Trace	1	15	Trace	130	Trace	.02	Trace	Trace
26	16	1	10	235	.1	1,930	.07	.35	.1	2
1	1	Trace	1	12	Trace	100	Trace	.02	Trace	Trace
8	5	Trace	6	67	—	570	—	.04	—	—
Trace	Trace	Trace	Trace	3	—	30	—	Trace	—	—

Table of Food Composition (*Continued*)

Milk, Cheese, Cream, Imitation Cream; Related Products		Water	Food Energy	Protein	Fat
	Grams	*Per-cent*	*Calo-ries*	*Grams*	*Grams*
Whipping, unwhipped (volume about double when whipped):					
Light	1 cup	239	62	715	6	75
	1 tbsp.	15	62	45	Trace	5
Heavy	1 cup	238	57	840	5	90
	1 tbsp.	15	57	55	Trace	6
Imitation cream products (made with vegetable fat):					
Creamers:					
Powdered	1 cup	94	2	505	4	33
	1 tsp.	2	2	10	Trace	1
Liquid (frozen)	1 cup	245	77	345	3	27
	1 tbsp.	15	77	20	Trace	2
Sour dressing (imitation sour cream) made with nonfat dry milk.	1 cup	235	72	440	9	38
	1 tbsp.	12	72	20	Trace	2
Whipped topping:					
Pressurized	1 cup	70	61	190	1	17
	1 tbsp.	4	61	10	Trace	1
Frozen	1 cup	75	52	230	1	20
	1 tbsp.	4	52	10	Trace	1
Powdered, made with whole milk.	1 cup	75	58	175	3	12
	1 tbsp.	4	58	10	Trace	1
Milk beverages:					
Cocoa, homemade	1 cup	250	79	245	10	12
Chocolate-flavored drink made with skim milk and 2% added butterfat.	1 cup	250	83	190	8	6
Malted milk:					
Dry powder, approx. 3 heaping teaspoons per ounce.	1 oz.	28	3	115	4	2
Beverage	1 cup	235	78	245	11	10
Milk desserts:					
Custard, baked	1 cup	265	77	305	14	15
Ice cream:					
Regular (approx. 10% fat).	½ gal.	1,064	63	2,055	48	113

Fatty Acids										
Saturated (total)	Unsaturated		Carbohydrate	Calcium	Iron	Vitamin A Value	Thiamine	Riboflavin	Niacin	Ascorbic Acid
	Oleic	Linoleic								
Grams	Grams	Grams	Grams	Milligrams	Milligrams	International units	Milligrams	Milligrams	Milligrams	Milligrams
41	25	2	9	203	.1	3,060	.05	.29	.1	2
3	2	Trace	1	13	Trace	190	Trace	.02	Trace	Trace
50	30	3	7	179	.1	3,670	.05	.26	.1	2
3	2	Trace	1	11	Trace	230	Trace	.02	Trace	Trace
31	1	0	52	21	.6	[2]200	—	—	Trace	—
Trace	Trace	0	1	1	Trace	[2]Trace	—	—	—	—
25	1	0	25	29	—	[2]100	0	0	—	—
1	Trace	0	2	2	—	[2]10	0	0	—	—
35	1	Trace	17	277	.1	10	.07	.38	.2	1
2	Trace	Trace	1	14	Trace	Trace	Trace	Trace	Trace	Trace
15	1	0	9	5	—	[2]340	—	0	—	—
1	Trace	0	Trace	Trace	—	[2]20	—	0	—	—
18	Trace	0	15	5	—	[2]560	—	0	—	—
1	Trace	0	1	Trace	—	[2]30	—	0	—	—
10	1	Trace	15	62	Trace	[2]330	.02	.08	.1	Trace
1	Trace	Trace	1	3	Trace	[2]20	Trace	Trace	Trace	Trace
7	4	Trace	27	295	1.0	400	.10	.45	.5	3
3	2	Trace	27	270	.5	210	.10	.40	.3	3
—	—	—	20	82	.6	290	.09	.15	.1	0
—	—	—	28	317	.7	590	.14	.49	.2	2
7	5	1	29	297	1.1	930	.11	.50	.3	1
62	37	3	221	1,553	.5	4,680	.43	2.23	1.1	11

Table of Food Composition (*Continued*)

Milk, Cheese, Cream, Imitation Cream; Related Products		Water	Food Energy	Protein	Fat
		Per-cent	*Calo-ries*	*Grams*	*Grams*
		Grams			
	1 cup	133	63	255	6	14
	3 fl. oz. cup	50	63	95	2	5
Rich (approx. 16% fat).	½ gal.	1,188	63	2,635	31	191
	1 cup	148	63	330	4	24
Ice milk:						
Hardened	½ gal.	1,048	67	1,595	50	53
	1 cup	131	67	200	6	7
Soft-serve	1 cup	175	67	265	8	9
Yoghurt:						
Made from partially skimmed milk.	1 cup	245	89	125	8	4
Made from while milk	1 cup	245	88	150	7	8

Dashes in the columns for nutrients show that no suitable value could be found although there is reason to believe that a measurable amount of the nutrient may be present.

[1] Value applies to unfortified product; value for frotified low-density product would be 1500 I.U., and the fortified high-density product would be 2290 I.U.

worlds's population. In North America it is used mostly as forage. High in carbohydrates and proteins. Whole grain, uncooked, 100 gm = 327 calories.

minchin. Fermented minchin is made from wheat gluten from which the starch has been removed. The moist, raw gluten is placed in a closed jar and allowed to ferment for 2 to 3 weeks, after which it is salted. The final product is cut into strips to be boiled, baked, or fried.

minerals. "Inorganic elements." The following are known to be present in body tissue; calcium, cobalt, chlorine, flourine, iodine, iron, magnesium, manganese, molybdenum, phosphorus, potassium, selenium, silicon, sodium, sulfur, zinc. Although mineral elements constitute but a small proportion (4 percent by weight) of the body tissue, they are essential as structural components and in many vital processes. Mineral constituents obtained from food, aid in the regulation of the acid-base balance of body fluids and of osmotic pressure, in addition to the specific functions of individual elements in the body.

	Fatty Acids									
	Unsaturated									
Satu-rated (total)	Oleic	Lin-oleic	Carbo-hy-drate	Cal-cium	Iron	Vita-min A Value	Thia-mine	Ribo-flavin	Niacin	Ascor-bic Acid
Grams	Grams	Grams	Grams	Milli-grams	Milli-grams	Inter-national units	Milli-grams	Milli-grams	Milli-grams	Milli-grams
8	5	Trace	28	194	.1	590	.05	.28	.1	1
3	2	Trace	10	73	Trace	220	.02	.11	.1	1
105	63	6	214	927	.2	7,840	.24	1.31	1.2	12
13	8	1	27	115	Trace	980	.03	.16	.1	1
29	17	2	235	1,635	1.0	2,200	.52	2.31	1.0	10
4	2	Trace	29	204	.1	280	.07	.29	.1	1
5	3	Trace	—	—	—	—	—	—	—	—
2	1	Trace	13	294	.1	170	.10	.44	.2	2
5	3	Trace	12	272	.1	340	.07	.39	.2	2

*Table 2, Nutritive Values of the Edible Parts of Foods, in *Nutritive Value of Foods,* Home and Garden Bulletin No. 72. United States Department of Agriculture, United States Government Printing Office, Washington, D.C., 1971.

[2] Contributed largely from beta-carotene used for coloring.

Some minerals are present in the body largely in organic combinations, as *iron* in *hemoglobin* and *iodine* in *thyroxin**; others occur in the body in inorganic form, as calcium salts in bone and sodium chloride in blood. The terms "minerals" and "inorganic elements" do not imply that the element occurs in inorganic form in food or body tissue. Minerals that are electropositive are known as *cations* and those include the metallic element minerals such as calcium, magnesium, potassium, and sodium ions. The electronegative minerals are known as *anions* and include chlorine, fluorine, iodine and in their ionic forms, phosphorus as phosphate and sulfur as sulfate. Combinations of these positive and negative elements lead to formation of salts such as sodium chloride, calcium phosphate and potassium sulfate. In body fluids, the salts dissociate completely in their respective anion and cation forms. In foods, minerals are present in various forms mixed or combined with proteins, fats and carbohydrates. Some processed or refined foods, such as fats, oils, sugar, and cornstarch, contain almost no minerals. The total mineral content of a food is determined by burning the organic or combustible part of a known amount of food and

Group I Major Minerals

Minerals	Functions in the Body	Metabolism	Food Sources	Daily Allowances
Calcium	Hardness of bones, teeth Transmission of nerve impulse Muscle contraction Normal heart rhythm Activate enzymes Increase cell permeability Catalyze thrombin formation	*Absorption:* about 40 percent; according to body need; aided by gastric acidity, vitamin D, lactose; excess phosphate, fat, phytate, oxalic acid interfere *Storage:* trabeculae of bones; easily mobilized *Utilization:* needs parathyroid hormone, vitamin D *Excretion:* 60–85 percent of diet intake in feces; small urinary excretion; high protein intake increases urinary excretion *Deficiency:* retarded bone mineralization; fragile bones; stunted growth; rickets; osteomalacia; osteoporosis	Milk, hard cheese Ice cream, cottage cheese Greens: turnip, collards, kale, mustard, broccoli Oysters, shrimp, salmon, clams	Infants: 360–540 mg Children: 800 mg Teen-agers: 1200 mg Adults: 800 mg Pregnancy: 1200 mg Lactation: 1200 mg
Phosphorus	Structure of bones, teeth Cell permeability Metabolism of fats and carbohydrates: storage and release of ATP Sugar-phosphate linkage in DNA and RNA Phospholipids in transport of fats Buffer salts in acid-base balance	*Absorption:* about 70 percent; aided by vitamin D *Utilization:* about 85 percent in bones; controlled by vitamin D, parathormone *Excretion:* about one third of diet in feces; metabolic products chiefly in urine *Deficiency:* poor bone mineralization; poor growth; rickets	Milk, cheese Eggs, meat, fish, poultry Legumes, nuts Whole-grain cereals	Infants: 200 to 400 mg Children: 800 mg Adults: 800 mg Pregnancy: 1200 mg Lactation: 1200 mg
Magnesium	Constituents of bones, teeth Activates enzymes in carbohydrate metabolism Muscle and nerve irritability	*Absorption:* parallels that of calcium; competes with calcium for carriers *Utilization:* slowly mobilized from bone	Whole-grain cereals Nuts; legumes Meat Milk Green leafy vegetables	Infants: 60 to 70 mg Children: 150 to 250 mg Women: 300 mg Men: 350 mg

Mineral	Functions	Metabolism	Food Sources	Requirement
				Pregnancy and lactation: 450 mg
Sulfur	Constituent of proteins, especially cartilage, hair, nails Constituent of melanin, glutathione, thiamin, biotin, coenzyme A, insulin High-energy sulfur bonds Detoxication reactions	*Excretion:* chiefly by kidney *Deficiency:* seen in alcoholism, severe renal disease; hypomagnesemia, tremor Absorbed chiefly as sulfur-containing amino acids Excreted as inorganic sulfate in urine in proportion to nitrogen loss	Protein foods rich in sulfur-amino acids Eggs Meat Milk, cheese Nuts, legumes	Not established Diet adequate in protein meets need
Sodium	Principal cation of extracellular fluid Osmotic pressure; water balance Acid-base balance Regulate nerve irritability and muscle contraction "Pump" for glucose transport	*Absorption:* rapid and almost complete *Excretion:* chiefly in urine; some by skin and in feces; parallels intake; controlled by aldosterone *Deficiency:* rare; occurs with excessive perspiration and poor diet intake; nausea, diarrhea, abdominal cramps, muscle cramps	Table salt Milk Meat, fish, poultry Egg white	Not established Probably about 500 mg except with excessive perspiration Diets supply substantial excess
Potassium	Principal cation of intracellular fluid Osmotic pressure; water balance; acid-base balance Nerve irritability and muscle contraction, regular heart rhythm Synthesis of protein Glycogenesis	*Absorption:* readily absorbed *Excretion:* chiefly in urine; increased with aldosterone secretion *Deficiency:* following starvation, correction of diabetic acidosis, adrenal tumors; muscle weakness, nausea, tachycardia, glycogen depletion, heart failure	Widely distributed in foods Meat, fish, fowl Cereals Fruits, vegetables	Not established Diet adequate in calories supplies ample amounts
Chlorine	Chief anion of extracellular fluid Constituent of gastric juice Acid-base balance; chloride-bicarbonate shift in red cells	*Absorption:* rapid, almost complete *Excretion:* chiefly in urine; parallels intake *Deficiency:* with prolonged vomiting, drainage from fistula, diarrhea	Table salt	Not established Daily diet contains 3 to 9 gm, far in excess of need

Group II Trace Minerals

Minerals	Functions in the Body	Metabolism	Food Sources	Daily Allowances
Iron	Constituent of hemoglobin, myoglobin, and oxidative enzymes: catalase, cytochrome, xanthine oxidase	*Absorption:* about 5 to 10 percent; regulated according to body need; aided by gastric acidity, ascorbic acid *Transport:* bound to protein, transferrin *Storage:* as ferritin in liver, bone marrow, spleen *Utilization:* chiefly in hemoglobin; daily turnover about 27 to 28 mg; iron used over and over again *Excretion:* men, about 1 mg; women, 1 to 2 mg; in urine, perspiration, menstrual flow; fecal excretion is from unabsorbed diet *Deficiency:* anemia; frequent in infants, preschool children, teenage girls, pregnant women	Liver, organ meats Meat, poultry Egg yolk Enriched and whole-grain breads, cereals Dark-green vegetables Legumes Molasses, dark Peaches, apricots, prunes, raisins Diets supply about 6 mg per 1000 kcal	Infants: 10 to 15 mg Children: 10 to 15 mg Teen-agers: 18 mg Men: 10 mg Women: 18 mg Pregnancy: 18+ mg Lactation: 18 mg
Manganese	Activation of many enzymes: oxidation of carbohydrates, urea formation, protein hydrolysis Bone formation	*Absorption:* limited *Excretion:* chiefly in feces *Deficiency:* not known	Legumes, nuts Whole-grain cereals	Not established
Copper	Aids absorption and use of iron in synthesis of hemoglobin Electron transport Melanin formation Myelin sheath of nerves Purine metabolism Metabolism of ascorbic acid	*Transport:* chiefly as protein, ceruloplasmin *Storage:* liver, central nervous system *Excretion:* bile into intestine *Deficiency:* rare; occurs in severe malnutrition Abnormal storage in Wilson's disease	Liver, shellfish Meats Nuts, legumes Whole-grain cereals Typical diet provides 2 to 5 mg	Infants and children: 0.08 mg per kg Adults: 2 mg

306

	Function	Metabolism	Food Sources	Daily Allowances
Cobalt	A constituent of cobalamin no other role known.	*Absorption:* as a cobalamin-protein (intrinsic factor) complex; about 2–3 μg daily. Maximum about 5 to 10 percent. *Transport:* bound to a protein, transcobalamin. *Storage:* liver mainly; small amount in bone marrow. *Utilization:* as a constituent of cobalamin; 2–5 μg is enough for 3–5 years. *Excretion:* almost completely reabsorbed. *Deficiency:* megaloblastic anemia; pernicious anemia; rare.	Meats, poultry Fish, eggs. Not present in plants. Typical diet provides about 10 μg.	Infants: 0.3 μg Children: 1–2 μg Adults: 2–3 μg
Iodine	Constituent of diiodotyrosine, triiodothyronine, thyroxine; regulate rate of energy metabolism	*Absorption:* controlled by blood level of protein-bound iodine *Storage:* thyroid gland; activity regulated by thyroid-stimulating hormone *Excretion:* in urine *Deficiency:* simple goiter; if severe, cretinism—rarely seen in U.S.	Iodized salt is most reliable source Seafood Foods grown in non-goitrous coastal areas	Infants: 35–45 mcg Children: 60–110 mcg Teen-agers: 115–150 mcg Men: 130 mcg Women: 100 mcg Pregnancy: 125 mcg Lactation: 150 mcg
Zinc	Constituent of enzymes: carbonic anhydrase, carboxypeptidase, lactic dehydrogenase	*Absorption:* limited; competes with calcium for absorption sites *Storage:* liver, muscles, bones, organs *Excretion:* chiefly by intestine *Deficiency:* only in severe malnutrition	Seafoods Liver and other organ meats Meats, fish Wheat germ Yeast Plant foods are generally low Usual diet supplies 10 to 15 mg	Infants: 3–5 mg Children: 10 mg Teen-agers: 15 mg Adults: 15 mg Pregnancy: 20 mg Lactation: 25 mg

Group II Trace Minerals (Continued)

Minerals	Functions in the Body	Metabolism	Food Sources	Daily Allowances
Fluorine	Increases resistance of teeth to decay; most effective in young children Moderate levels in bone may reduce osteoporosis	*Storage:* bones and teeth *Excretion:* urine Excess leads to mottling of teeth	Fluoridated water; 1 ppm	Not established
Molybdenum	Cofactor for flavoprotein enzymes; present in xanthine oxidase	Absorbed as molybdate Stored in liver, adrenal, kidney Related to metabolism of copper and sulfur	Organ meats Legumes Whole-grain cereals	Not established
Selenium	Antioxidant Constituent of glutathione oxidase	Stored especially in liver, kidney Spares vitamin E	Meat and seafoods Cereal foods	Not established
Chromium	Efficient use of insulin in glucose uptake; conversion of glucose to fat, glucose oxidation, protein synthesis Activation of enzymes	Usable form in organic compound: glucose tolerance factor	Liver, meat Cheese Whole-grain cereals	Not established

There is an additional group of trace minerals that occurs in food for which no functions are known. These minerals are as follows: cadmium; lithium; lead; mercury; boron; aluminum; arsenic; tin; nickel; and silicon.

weighing the resulting ash. The ash is then analyzed for individual mineral elements. Most foods have been analyzed for 10 or more minerals, but in dietary practice the figures most commonly used are those for calcium, phosphorus, and iron, and for therapeutic purposes, sodium, potassium, and magnesium. The elements concerned in the mineral metabolism may exist in the body and take part in its functions in at least three kinds of ways. (1) As a constituent of the bones and teeth giving rigidity and relative permanence to the skeletal tissues. (2) As essential elements of the organic compounds which are the chief solid constituents of the soft tissues (muscles, blood cells, enzymes, etc.). (3) As soluble salts (electrolytes) held in solution in the fluid of the body, giving these fluids their characteristic influence upon the elasticity and irritability of muscle and nerve, supplying the material for the acidity or alkalinity of the *digestive juices* and other secretions, and yet maintaining the approximate neutrality of the body's fluids as well as their osmotic pressure and solvent power. Minerals found in the human body may be grouped according to whether they are present in large amounts (major minerals) or are present in small amounts and have a known function (trace minerals), or are present in small amounts but their function is not understood. There are seven minerals contributing from 60 to 80 percent of all the inorganic material in the body. The tables on the preceeding pages show the minerals, their functions, their sources in foods, and the *Recommended Daily Allowances* (RDA) of each.

mint (*Mentha*). A fragrant herb of which there are over 30 species. Among the most popular varieties of this upright plant with red-veined stems and sharply aromatic leaves are the peppermint and spearmint, as well as American apple mint, bergamot mint, curly mint, and red mint. The names indicate the difference either in flavor or in shape of the mint leaves.

miscible. A liquid capable of being dissolved in another liquid at any ratio.

mitochondrion. The "powerhouse of the cell" responsible for transforming chemical bond energy of nutrients into higher energy phosphate bonds of *adenosine triphosphate* * (ATP). There may be 50 to 2500 of these organs of respiration in a single cell, each containing 500 to 10,000 complete sets of oxidative enzymes. Each enzyme assembly contains 15 or more active molecules in a highly ordered arrangement which is an integral part of the organelle structure. The mitochondria contain the *Krebs* (tricarboxylic acid) *cycle* * and the *terminal respiratory chain*. The mitochondria are, in general, about the size of bacteria, but size and shape can vary markedly depending on the cell type and its physiological state. A schematic presentation of a mitochondrion is given on p. 310.

Most of the activity of the cell which is necessary for survival is completely dependent upon the ability of the mitochondria to release the energy in a nu-

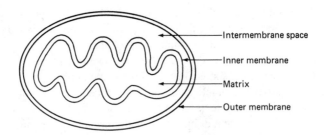

Outer Membrane	Intermembrane Space	Inner Membrane	Matrix
Monoamine oxidase;	Adentlate kinase	NADH dehydrogenase	*Kreb's* (tricarboxylic
Phospholipase A₂;		*Terminal respiratory chain*	acid) *cycle*
Kynurenine 3-monoxy-		Carnitine acyltransferase	Aspartate trans-
aminase			
genase;		ATPase	Glutamate dehydro-
NADH dehydrogenase;		β-hydroxybutyrate	genase
Nucleoside diphospho-		Dehydrogenase	*Fatty acid oxidation*
kinase		Carnitine acyltransferase	*enzymes*

trient molecule and transduce that energy into a form of cellular work; osmotic, mechanical, electrical, chemical. The major source of chemical energy for cellular processes is the compound ATP. The major source of ATP comes from the mitochondria. The mitochondria contain the *Krebs cycle* * and terminal respiratory chain which are instrumental in the oxidation of foodstuffs to carbon dioxide (CO_2), water (H_2O), and energy (ATP + heat). More than 90 pervent percent the oxygen (O_2) used by the cells can be accounted for by the oxidation processes in mitochondria. Mitochondria also produce *citric acid* * which provides *acetyl coenzyme A* *, the building block for the synthesis of fatty acids in the cytoplasm. The major function of mitochondria are oxidative, and in that sense degradative processes, but mitochondria are also involved in the elongation of fatty acids, a process also performed by the microsomes in the cytoplasm. See *terminal respiratory chain*.

mitosis. The process whereby cells divide and multiply, each cell forming two daughter cells which contain replicas of all the original chromosomes.

molasses. The thick brown syrup that is separated from raw sugar during the various stages of refinement. The sugar cane is cut close to the ground because the lowest ends are the richest in sugar. The stalks are torn into small pieces and passed through three sets of rollers and extract a dark-grayish, sweet juice. The juice is boiled down to a thick syrupy mass which includes crystals of sugar. This heavy syrup is then put into containers with holes through which the liquid drips, leaving the crystalized sugar behind. The liquid is molasses. The best grade of molasses is obtained by crude milling processes, as the syrup contains more sugar at this point. If the syrup is boiled more than once, the first boiling produces a darker, thicker, less-sweet product which is used in cakes and candies. Blackstrap molasses, a cattle food and industrial product as well as a popular health food, is the result of a third boiling. The word "molasses" comes from the Portuguese melaco derived from the Latin root mel, which means "honey," and aceus, which means "resembling." Sorghum molasses is the syrup from the stalk of a group of grains which look much like corn. This syrup is a pure product from which no sugar is extracted. It has the consistency, color and taste of molasses. A fair source of iron and calcium. Light, 100 gm = 252 calories; dark, 100 gm = 232 calories; blackstrap, 100 gm = 213 calories.

molecule. A group of atoms held together by chemical bonds. The identifiable units of chemical structure. A chemical combination of two or more atoms that form a specific substance. For example, the combination of an atom of sodium and an atom of chlorine make a molecule of sodium chloride, or table salt. There are also large, complex molecules such as hemoglobin. Proteins and starches are examples of even larger and very complex molecules containing many atoms.

molybdenum (Mo). Element No. 42. Atom. Wt. 96. The molybdenum content of tissues of all animal species is very low. In adult man, the liver contains about 3.2 ppm and kidney about 1.6 ppm. Molybdenum content of muscle, brain, lung and spleen ranges from 0.14 to 0.20 ppm. Molybdenum is a component of the enzymes xanthine oxidase and aldehyde oxidase. Both enzymes contain *flavin adenine dinucleotide* * (FAD) as well as molybdenum, and both function in terminal respiratory chain. There is little concrete evidence establishing the quantitative requirement for molybdenum in humans. Among the food sources of available or enzyme-producing molybdenum, those containing 0.6 ppm weight include legumes, cereal grains, some of the dark green leafy vegetables, and animal organs. Fruits and most root and stem vegetables contain less than 0.1 ppm. The element plays a role in the activity of several flavoproteins and is thought to facilitate the linkage of flavin nucleotide to protein. Xanthine oxidase contains one atom of molybdenum. Parts of the body containing comparatively large amounts of the element are the liver, kidneys, and bones.

monocytes. Monocytes are twice as big as the polymorphonuclear leucocytes but they have a single large nucleus and no granules. They have similar functions to the polymorphonuclear leucocytes but they can engulf many more bacteria and a greater amount of dead tissue. They contain enzymes which attack the fatty walls of certain bacteria like the tuberculosis bacillus. In general monocytes are more prominent in the reaction to chronic infections and in the later stages of acute infections.

monoglyceride. The *glycerol* molecule with a single *fatty acid* attached through an ester bond.

monilial vaginitis. An inflammation of the vagina caused by *Candida alibcans,* a member of the yeast family that thrives in warm moist places. The condition is often seen in uncontrolled *diabetes mellitus* because the sugar from urine provides an excellent medium for the growth of the *yeast.*

monosaccharides. Simple sugars, containing one sugar group, expressable by the general formula $C_n(H_2O)_n$. Monosaccharides are polyhydric, that is they contain several —OH groups, which accounts for their sweet taste and their solubility. Monosaccharides are classified according to the number of carbons in the molecule. For example, *glucose* * has six carbons and is therefore a hexose, and according to whether the molecule contains an aldehyde group, an aldose, or a keto-group, a ketose. Glucose is an aldose, and fructose is a ketose. The classifications of several naturally occurring are given below. Monosaccharides are soluble and can be absorbed into the body fluids without further change. They are the units from which the more complex carbohydrates are formed. Glucose or dextrose, found in fruits, especially the grape and in body fluids; fructose or levulose, found with glucose in fruits; *galactose* * obtained by hydrolysis of *lactose* * (milk sugar) and certain gums. The monosaccharides are important in nutrition because they are the units of complex lipids and proteins in addition to their use as a source of energy. The monosaccharides in honey arise largely from the breakdown of sucrose, which contains one glucose and one fructose unit. Fruits and certain fresh vegetables are the richest sources of monosaccharides eaten.

Classification	-Aldoses	Ketoses
Trioses	*Glyceraldehyde*	Dihydroxyacetone
Tetroses	Erythrose	Erythrulose
	Threose	
Pentose	Xylose	Xylulose
	Ribose	Ribulose
	Arabinose	
Hexoses	*Glucose* (dextrose)	*Fructose* (levulose)
	Galactose	
	Mannose	Sorbose
Heptoses		Sedoheptulose

monosodium glutamate (MSG). Mol. Wt. 159. A sodium salt of *glutamic acid**. A widely used flavor enhancer. Monosodium glutamate imparts no flavor of its own in the concentration allowed in foods. The detailed chemical and biological action of flavor enhancers is only partially understood. In 1908 a Japanese chemist, Dr. Kidunae Ikeda, discovered the flavor enhancing properties. He discovered that the ingredient in the seaweed *Laminaria japonica* had an unusual ability to enhance or intensify the flavor of many high protein foods was monosodium glutamate. Monosodium glutamate is added to meats and fish and their products, sauces, soups and other foods to acclerate their flavor. Other flavor enhancers are *disodium guanylate and disodium inosinate.*

$$\overset{\displaystyle NH_2}{\underset{\displaystyle |}{HOOC-CH_2-CH_2CH-COO^- \; Na^+}}$$

monosomic. The presence in a diploid cell of only one member of a given chromosome pair.

monounsaturated. Having a single double bond as in a fatty acid, e.g., *oleic acid.**

mucin. A substance containing *mucopolysaccharides* secreted by goblet cells of the intestine and other glandular cells. Mucin has a protective lubricating action.

mucopolysaccharides. The mucopolysaccharides are heteropolysaccharides and occur in combination with protein in both body secretions and structures. Many tend to be highly viscous and are responsible for the viscosity of body mucous secretions. They are generally components of the extracellular, amorphous ground substances that surround the collagen and elastin fibers and the cells of connective tissue, and may be involved in the induction of calcification, control of metabolities, ions and water, and the healing of wounds. Mucopolysaccharides, along with *glycoproteins* and *glycolipids,* also form the cell coat that is present in most animal cells. Mucopolysaccharides contain amino sugars, either D-glucosamine or D-galactosamine together with uronic acids, either D-glucuronic acid or L-induronic acid; in addition they may contain acetyl or sulfate groups.

mucoprotein. A conjugated protein containing a carbohydrate group such as chondroitin sulfuric acid.

mucosa. The cells that make up the mucous membrane lining of passages and cavities, as in the gastrointestinal, respiratory, and genitourinary tracts.

mucous membrane. See *membranes, mucous.*

mulberry (*Morus*). A tree and its edible berrylike fruit. There are three principal varieties; black red, and white. The leaves of the white mulberry, *Morus alba,* are used in silkworm cultivation. Mulberries resemble blackberries in shape and structure, ranging in color from white through red to black. The fruit is soft and bland in taste and can be eaten raw. Cooked it is used in making desserts, preserves, and wine. Raw, 100 gm = 62 calories.

mullet. The name is used to describe several families of important food fish. The best known are the gray mullets of the family Muglidae, which include the genera known as striped and white mullets; and the red mullets, including striped red mullet, surmullet, and goatfish, of the family Mullidae. Mullets are of moderate size, from a half to five pounds in weight. Their flesh is tender, white, and firm-textured with a sweet, delicate taste. The flesh contains a clear yellow oil with a mild nutlike flabor. Striped mullet, raw, 100 gm = 146 calories.

mung beans. Small green beans grown mainly in India. Popular with health food devotees for cultivating sprouts.

muscat, muscatel (*Vinifera*). Muscat is the name of several varieties of grapes, cultivated especially for making raisins and wine. The muscat is a white or black grape with a sweet and musty flavor. Muscatel, the wine made from the muscat grape is a sweet desert wine which can vary in color from golden or russet-amber to light red. It is a sweet, rich, and fruity wine with the typical aroma and flavor of the grape.

muscle. The muscles of the body include three types; the smooth muscle in the walls of internal organs; the cardiac muscle in the walls of the heart; and the skeletal muscle attached to and causing movements of bones. The cells of muscles have the ability to contract, and it is this power of muscle contraction that produces body movement. Muscle tissue is made up of cells that are specialized for changing shape, which they accomplish by shortening their elongated form. When muscle cells are attached to one another and to other tissues of the body, they are organized into muscles. Muscles are made up of muscle cells (for contraction), connective tissue (to hold the cells together), vascular or blood vessel tissue (to nourish the other cells) etc. Muscles are therefore organs made up of several kinds of specialized tissue. The major protein component of skeletal muscle filaments is *myosin*. Myosin and another protein, actin, interact with one another during the process of contraction. *Calcium* is intimately involved in the complex contraction mechanism also. The energy for the contraction derives its energy from *adenosine triphosphate* * (ATP) by a mechanism that is not definitively understood, although mechanisms have been proposed that accommodate what is known about the details of contraction. Contractions result in the hydrolysis of ATP to *adenosine diphosphate* * (ADP),

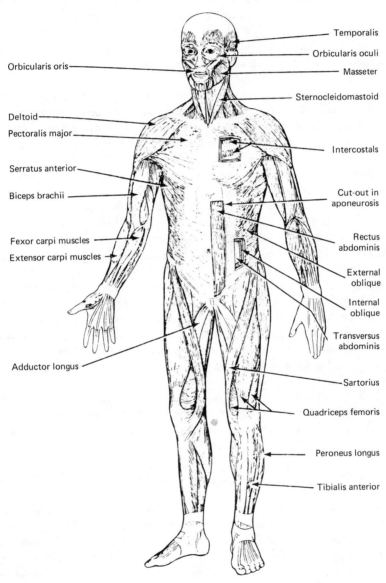

Temporalis

Orbicularis oculi

Orbicularis oris

Masseter

Sternocleidomastoid

Deltoid

Pectoralis major

Intercostals

Serratus anterior

Biceps brachii

Cut-out in aponeurosis

Fexor carpi muscles

Rectus abdominis

Extensor carpi muscles

External oblique

Internal oblique

Transversus abdominis

Adductor longus

Sartorius

Quadriceps femoris

Peroneus longus

Tibialis anterior

Principal muscles (anterior view).

inorganic phosphate salt, and heat. Since the muscle requires sustained levels of energy for work, the ATP is supplied by *glycolysis* and by enzymes that will convert ADP back to ATP. One of these enzymes is adenylate kinase (2 ADP$\rightleftharpoons$ATP + AMP) and another is *creatine phosphokinase* (CPK). The CPK uses a storage form of chemical energy that is almost exclusively in muscle, *creatine phosphate* * (CP). The conversion of CP to ATP by CPK is as follows: CP + ADP$\longrightarrow$ creatine + ATP. *Creatine* * can either be rephosphorylated at some later time during rest or it is converted into *creatinine* * and excreted in the *urine*. The major skeletal muscles in man are shown on page 315.

mucus. A viscous fluid secreted by mucous membranes and glands, consisting mainly of mucin (a *glycoprotein*), inorganic salts and water. Mucus serves to lubricate the gastrointerestinal mucosa and thus helps move food along the digestive tract, and protects linings and cavities generally.

mushroom. Mushrooms are fungi, members of the enormous and varied group of living things which are responsible for decay. They belong to the Basidiomycetes class, together with such organisms as smuts and rusts. Like most other fungi, mushrooms lack chlorophyll, which means that, unlike green plants, they cannot manufacture their own food but must obtain nourishment from others, living or dead. When the mycelium is mature enough to reproduce, a sudden rain or a damp night provides the needed stimulus and the fruit springs up. Mushrooms can be bland or peppery, nutty or sweet, resemble veal cutlet, breast of chicken, steak, sweet breads, kidneys, or oysters. The aroma runs the gamut from delightful to a stink like rotten fish. Although about 50 of the species growing wild in America are edible, experts urge those interested to concentrate on the few that are easy to identify. First is the morel, then the shaggymane, the sulphur shell, and the puffball.

muskellunge or musky. A freshwater fish of the pike family. The fish is greenish brown in color, spotted with black. In weight it can vary from 7 to 40 pounds. The flesh is lean, white, firm, and delicious. It can be broiled, baked, or panfried. Raw, 100 gm = 109 calories.

muskmelon. See *melon*.

mustard (*Brassica*). Any of several herbs cultivated for its pungent seeds and/or leaves. The seeds are used to make the various forms of mustard seasonings, the leaves are used as a vegetable and known as mustard greens. The mustard plant belongs to a large family which includes many well known vegetables; broccoli, Brussel sprouts, Chinese cabbage, collards, kale, kohlrabi, red cabbage, rutabaga and turnips. The word mustard is derived from the Old

French mostarde or moustard, which meant a condiment made from mustard seed and must, the juice of grapes or other fruit before and during fermentation. Excellent source of *carotene* * (vitamin A, activity) *thiamine* *, *riboflavin* *, and *ascorbic acid* * (vitamin C). Raw, 100 gm = 31 calories; Cooked and drained 100 gm = 23 calories.

mutagens. (1) Agents inducing mutation, for example, short-wave radiation and certain chemicals. (2) Any force or influence, radiation, a chemical or other factor, which can cause mutation to occur in genes. Most mutagens are also *carcinogens*.

mutation. A change in the genetic material, the DNA of the organism, which involves changes in the sequence (change of type of number) of the DNA building blocks, the *deoxyribonucleotides*. This may result in proteins or ribonucleic acids with altered structures and/or functions. Many mutations occur spontaneously in the normal cause of events. It has been found possible to increase the frequency of mutations by exposing organisms to radiation and to chemical agents called *mutagens*.

mycoses. Infections caused by *fungi*. Members of the vegetable kingdom, of which molds that grow on bread or cheese are representative. Fungi contain no chlorophyll. There are many varieties including yeastlike forms and molds that produce penicillin.

myocardial infarction. A syndrome caused by permanent damage to a portion of the heart musculature due to sudden, overwhelming myocardial ischemia, a secondary to insufficient blood supply. It usually results from the thrombotic occlusion of one of the larger branches of an atherosclerotic coronary, accompanied by severe pain, shock, cardiac dysfunction, and often abrupt death. Thrombus occurs most commonly in an atherosclerotic vessel with a narrowed lumen. The clot often starts on a roughened calcified plaque or ulcerated atheroma and may form gradually or rapidly.

myocardium. The heart muscle.

myoglobin. An iron-protein complex in muscles that transports oxygen. Myoglobin combines with oxygen more firmly than hemoglobin. Myoglobin is a major protein component of red muscle.

myosin. A protein in muscle; the contractile element in muscle that combines with *actin* to form actomyosin, an enzyme that catalyzes the dephosphorylation of *adenosine triphosphate* * (ATP) during muscle contraction. See *muscle*.

myristic acid. Mol. Wt. 228. $CH_3(CH_2)_{12}COOH$. A long chain *fatty acid* obtained from nutmeg butter, coconut oil, butter, lard, and many other *fats,* as well as from spermaceti and wool *wax.*

myxedema. A condition which results from a deficiency of *thyroxin* * secretion in an adult. Myxedema is characterized by a low basal metabolism and decreased heat production. Myxedema in adults presents a picture almost the exact opposite of *hyperthyroidism.* All functions are markedly reduced. Inertia, exhaustion, apathy, and lack of initiative are the outstanding traits. The individual in advanced cases thinks slowly and inefficiently. As the condition progresses, the intellectual deterioration becomes more marked together with a notable lack of imagination. The general picture is that of an advanced schizoid state. While psychosis is rare in this condition, a syndrome resembling the depressed phase of the manic-depressive phychosis or of paranoid schizophrenia may occur. These states may be characterized by a great variety of illusions, hallucinations, confusion, and delirium.

N

NAD (NADH). See *nicotinamide adenine dinucleotide**.

NADP (NADPH). See *nicotinamide adenine dinucleotide phosphate**.

natto. Boiled soybeans wrapped in rice straw and fermented from one to two days. The package becomes slimy on the outside. *Bacillus natto,* probably identical with *B. subtilis,* grows in the natto, releasing the trypsinlike enzymes that are supposed to be important in the ripening process.

natural foods. A vaguely used term, usually taken to mean foods that have a minimum of refining (e.g., whole-grain cereals), and no additives or preservatives, but sometimes used to include foods grown without chemical fertilizers, hormones, or pesticides. The so-called *organic foods*.

natural vitamins. Refers to vitamins derived from natural foods in contrast to synthetic vitamins.

necrosis. Death of a cell or cells or of a portion of an organ or tissue.

nectarine. A delicate variety of peach, smaller in size, roundish, and with a smooth skin that ranges in color from orange-yellow to red, sometimes mixed with green. The flesh is very juicy and may be red, yellow, or white in color. The fruit contains a pit. Fair source of *carotene** (vitamin A activity) and, *ascorbic acid** (vitamin C). Raw, 100 gm = 64 calories.

negative nitrogen balance. See *nitrogen balance*.

neonatal. Pertaining to the newborn.

neoplasm. Any new or abnormal growth, usually rapid, such as a tumor.

nephritis. Sometimes called "Bright's disease," refers to a general inflammation and resulting degeneration of the cells of the kidney. Classified as a noninfectious disease. Two specific diseases are classified under the general heading, *glomerulonephritis* and *nephrosclerosis*. Glomerulonephritis may be acute or chronic.

nephron. The functional unit of the kidney consisting of a tuft of capillaries known as the glomerulus attached to the renal tubule. Blood flows through afferent arterioles into the glomerulus, where the filtration of blood occurs and leaves by way of efferent arterioles. The filtered blood, containing low molecular weight substances only passes from the glomerulus to the tubules. About 1.2 liters of blood is filtered each minute. The tubules have three functions: (1) One function is the selective reabsorption of small molecules and ions in the filtrate such as water, sodium ion, bicarbonate, *amino acids,* and *glucose.* If the materials and others were not reabsorbed, within half an hour the body would have lost all of the substances. (2) The other function of the tubules is secretion. The secretion of substances concerns primarily the *acid-base balance* maintenance. This balance, the maintenance of the pH at 7.4, is accomplished as positive ions such as sodium (Na^+) are absorbed from the filtrate by the cells lining the tubule, hydrogen ion (H^+) replaces Na^+ in the filtrate. The H^+ is then neutralized by ammonia (NH_3) to form ammonium ion (NH_4^+). The kidney thus excretes ammonia to balance the charge and the acid in the exchange of the Na^+ from the filtrate into the cells. The NH_3 is generated from the amino

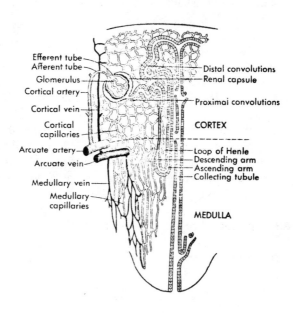

acid *glutamine**. After the selective absorption and secretion functions are complete, what remains is *urine*. (3) The third function is the conversion of *vitamin D** derivative, l-hydroxy-cholecalciferol (formed in the liver) to the very active vitamin D form 1,25-dihydroxycholecalciferol. (See *vitamin D**). The diagram shows the nephron within the kidney. See *kidney, glomerulus, urine*.

nephrosclerosis. A kidney disease that occurs among older people, usually the result of atherosclerosis and essential hypertension of long standing. The blood supply to the kidney decreases gradually because of the thickening of the wall and the narrowing of the lumen of the blood vessels. Usually this is accompanied by increased blood pressure and is characterized by urea nitrogen retention in the blood. Disorder may run a prolonged benign course or an acute malignant one.

nephrotic syndrome. Term applies to those cases of renal disease which regardless of underlying etiology, exhibit albuminuria, hypoalbuminemia, and massive edema. There is no concomitant hypertension or nitrogen retention. This syndrome may be seen during the nephrotic stage of chronic *glomerulonephritis,* in syphilitic nephritis, lipoid nephrosis, renal amyloidosis, and other disorders. In this condition large amounts of protein may be lost daily in the urine. The kidney is able to retain plasma globulins to some extent, but plasma albumins leak out passively. The total blood proteins may be reduced from 7 to 4.5 grams per 100 ml or less because of the massive albumin loss. In the nephrotic syndrome the kidney is also often unable to excrete salt normally and salt retention and consequently *edema* compounds the effects of the prevailing *hypoalbuminemia*.

nervous system. Consists of the brain, spinal cord, ganglia, nerve fibers, and their sensory and motor terminals (e.g., motor endplates on striated muscle). These are grouped into the integrated systems, the somatic and the visceral systems. Main function is to correlate the afferent nerve impulses in the sensory centers and to coordinate the nerve impulses in the motor centers. The nervous system contains centers for sensation, emotion, thinking, and many other functions. On page 322 there is a diagram of the nervous system.

net dietary protein calories percent (NDp Cal %). The NDp Cal % is a value denoting the quality and quantity of a protein in a given diet, but also accounts for the percent of the total calories that derive from protein. A given diet may be of high-quality protein but of an insufficient percentage of the diet, a condition which might lead to *marasmus,* a disease of *protein calorie malnutrition* (PCM). The NDp Cal % is defined as

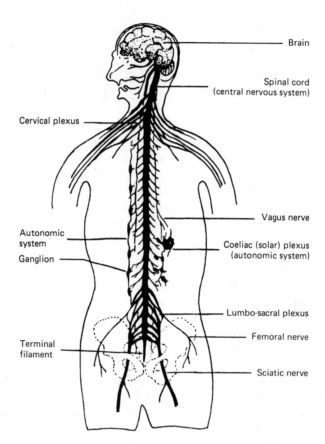

	Brain
	Spinal cord (central nervous system)
Cervical plexus	
	Vagus nerve
Autonomic system	
Ganglion	Coeliac (solar) plexus (autonomic system)
	Lumbo-sacral plexus
	Femoral nerve
Terminal filament	Sciatic nerve

$$\text{NDp Cal } \% = \frac{\text{Protein calories}}{\text{Net dietary calories}} \times \text{NPUop} \times 100$$

The NDp Cal % allows comparisons of the qualities of various types of diets, particularly among the different cultures. See *biological value, chemical score, net dietary protein value,* and *net protein utilization.*

net dietary protein value (NDpV). The NDpV is a value denoting the quantity and the quality of proteins in diets. If is defined as

$$\text{NDpV} = \text{Dietary Nitrogen Intake} \times 6.25 \times \text{NPUop}.$$
where NPUop is *net protein utilization,* operative.

The NDpV permits comparisons of the qualities of various types of diets, particularly among different cultures. See *biological value, chemical score, net protein utilization,* and *net dietary protein calories per cent.*

net protein utilization (NPU). A biologically determined value to indicate the quality of proteins. The value is defined as

$$\text{NPU} = \frac{\text{Dietary Nitrogen Retained}}{\text{Dietary Nitrogen Intake}} \times 100$$

It differs from the *biological value* (BV) in that the losses due to the process of digestion are taken into account in the NPU value, since only the retained nitrogen is considered in the determination. The method for determining the NPU may vary, but in general most proteins are tested by either their ability to promote growth in young animals or their ability to maintain *nitrogen balance.* The NPU is usually measured at or slightly below the maintenance level required of proteins. Values determined for all other conditions are called operative and are designated as NPUop. The NPUop is a frequently used value in comparisons of diets. See *biological value, net dietary value, net dietary protein calories percent,* and *chemical score.*

neuritic. Pertaining to inflammation of a nerve.

neurons. Cells specialized to carry on the rapid communications required for coordinated function both within the organism and between the organism and its environment. The exploitation of two characteristics of protoplasm, irritability, and conductivity permit these cells to react to various stimuli in a fraction of a second and to transmit the excitation to another location. A typical neuron consists of a nucleated cell body with protoplasmic branches of processes. The size and distribution of these processes vary greatly at different sites and in cells with different functions, but two main kinds are found, the axon and the dendrite. The dendrites normally conduct impulses towards the cell body and the axones conduct away from it. The overall size of the neuron structure varies from a millimeter or so in the spinal cord to over a yard in length in the leg. The neurons which carry nerve impulses from the tissues of the body into the central nervous system are called afferent. The diagram on page 324 depicts a neuron.

neuropathy. Disease of the nervous system.

neutral fats. Esters of *fatty acids* with *glycerol,* in the ratio of three fatty acids to each glycerol base. They are therefore called *triglycerides.* See *fat.*

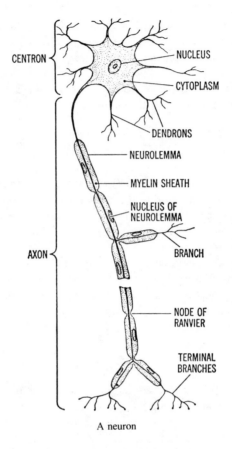

A neuron

niacin (nicotinic acid, nicotinamide). Mol. Wt. 123. A water-soluble, heat-stable vitamin of the B complex. Functionally active as the niacinamide coenzymes, *nicotinamide adenine dinucleotide* * (NAD) and *nicotinamide adenine dinucleotide phosphate* * (NADP). These coenzymes are essential to cell respiration, carbohydrate and protein metabolism, and lipid synthesis. Deficiency results in skin lesions, gastrointestinal, and cerebral manifestations which characterize the neural disease *pellagra*. Dietary sources include preformed niacin and the *precursor* to niacin equivalents (*tryptophan* *) and are related to caloric consumption. The actual requirement for niacin varies with the nature of the diet, approximately 1 mg of niacin may be expected to be formed for each 60 mg of tryptophan in the diet. Because niacin can be formed in the body if tryptophan is furnished, the amount of preformed niacin in foods that comprise the diet is not necessarily a measure of the total quantity available to the body. Milk, for example, is much more effective in preventing pellagra than would be expected from its niacin content, because milk proteins have a very high tryptophan content. It is not entirely clear whether man himself or bacterial flora convert tryptophan to niacin. In general, animal products contain the vitamin as nicotinamide, while in plants most of it is present as nicotinic acid. Both the acid and the amide are equally effective. Most foods that are good sources of the B vitamins *thiamine** and *riboflavin** are also high in niacin content, such as liver, lean meats whole grains, nuts, yeast, and legumes.

The tables below show the niacin content of several common foods and the

Natural Sources of Nicotinic Acid

Food	Range (mg/100 gm edible portion)
Good sources	
Beef, mutton, pork	3.0–6.0
Bemax	5.7
Brewer's yeast	30.0–100.0
Fish, fresh and cured	2.0–6.0
Liver and kidney	7.0–17.0
Marmite	60.0
Meat extract	38.0–103.0
Millets, various	1.2–3.2
Rice, lightly milled	4.0–4.5
Sorghum	2.5–3.5
Wheat bran, outer bran only	25.0–46
Wheat flour, wholemeal	4.0–5.5
Wheat-germ meal, germ fraction finely ground	3.0–7.0
Moderate Sources	
Cashew nuts	2.0
Chocolate, plain	1.0
Cocoa powder	1.0–1.5
Fruit, dried	1.0
Maize, whole	1.5–2.0
Oatmeal	0.9–1.3
Pulses	1.5–3.0
Rice, highly milled	1.0–1.6
Wheat flour, British (1956) regulation	1.5
Wheat flour, 70% extraction	1.0
Poor sources	
Cheese	0.03
Eggs, fresh	0.1
Fruits, fresh tropical and temperate	0.2–1.5
Green leafy vegetables	0.2–1.5
Maize, meal	0.2–1.5
Milk	0.1
Potato	1.0
Vegetables, assorted, 30% green	0.5

Nicotinic acid   Nicotinamide

The Nicotinic Acid Equivalent In Some Common Foods
(All values in mg/1000 kcal)

Food	Nicotinic Acid	Tryptophan	Nicotinic Acid Equivalent
Beef	24.7	1280	46.0
Eggs	0.6	1150	19.8
Maize	5.0	106	6.7
Maize grits	1.8	70	3.0
Milk—cows	1.2	673	12.4
human	2.5	443	9.9
Wheat, white flour	2.5	297	7.4

nicotinic acid (niacin) equivalents in foods with high concentrations of tryptophan but sometimes low concentrations of niacin itself.

Niacin functions in glycolysis and tissue respiration. The coenzyme forms of niacin, *nicotinamide adenine dinucleotide* * (NAD), and *nicotinamide adenine dinucleotide phosphate* * (NADP) function in many important enzyme systems which are necessary for cell respiration. Along with flavine coenzyme, *flavine adenine dinucleotide* * (FAD) they act as hydrogen acceptors and donors in a series of oxidation-reduction reactions, concerned with the release of energy from food. Niacin, *riboflavin* * (the vitamin precursor of FAD) and other members of the vitamin B complex are also involved in the oxidation of *glucose* * and synthesis and oxidation of the *fatty acids*.

niacin equivalent. The total niacin available from the diet including preformed niacin plus that derived from the metabolism of tryptophan; 60 mg tryptophan = 1 mg niacin.

niacinamide (nicotinamide). See *niacin*.

nickel (Ni). Element No. 28. Atom. Wt. 59. Nickel is known to activate several enzyme systems, although whether this is a specific function is not known. It is present in high levels in ribonucleic acids for reasons that are not yet clear. Nickel is widely distributed in foods, especially plant foods. A normal diet would supply about 0.3 to 0.6 mg per day.

nicotinamide. See *niacin**.

nicotinamide adenine dinucleotide (NAD, NADH). Mol. Wt. 663. A coenzyme form of the vitamin *niacin** used for a number of enzymes, chiefly the dehydrogenases. Exchanges hydrogen atoms with substrate molecules. It is also called disphosphopyridine nucleotide (DPN). NAD is necessary for tissue respiration, through its association with the dehydrogenases. Lactate dehydrogenase, malate dehydrogenase, and beta (β)-hydroxybutyrate dehydrogenase are examples of enzymes that require NAD/NADH as a coenzyme. Oxidation-reduction reactions are also associated with the reactions in which NAD participates. It is the oxidation of NADH by the *terminal respiratory chain* that accounts for the major conversion of oxidation energy to chemical energy, *adenosine triphosphate** (ATP). See *nicotinamide adenine dinucleotide phosphate* (NADP, NADPH)*.

Nicotinamide adenine dinucleotide (NAD, NADH)

nicotinamide adenine dinucleotide phosphate (NADP, NADPH). Mol. Wt. 743. A coenzyme form of the vitamin *niacin** used for a number of enzymes, chiefly the dehydrogenases. The oxidized (NADP) and reduced (NADPH) forms are equivalent structurally to the oxidized and reduced forms of NAD and NADH. (See *nicotinamide adenine dinucleotide*). The NADP and NADPH also function with dehydrogenases and are associated with oxidation and reduction reactions. As a broad generalization, it can be stated that oxidation-reduction reactions that involve NADP/NADPH are generally anabolic (synthetic) and those reactions that involve NAD/NADH are generally catabolic (degradative). An example of these separate roles for the niacin derivatives is fatty acid synthesis and fatty acid oxidation (degradation). The fatty acid synthetic pathway uses NADPH oxidation-reduction reactions, while the fatty acid oxidation pathway uses NAD.

NADP

nicotinic acid. See *niacin*.

ninhydrin. A chemical compound that gives color with peptides and amino acids. It is used to quantify amino acids and to identify peptides.

nitrite. Commonly used to refer to sodium nitrite ($NaNO_2$). Nitrites are food additives used to prevent bacterial growth, e.g., in bacon. At high temperatures, nitrate combines with secondary amines to produce nitrosamines. Nitrosamines have caused tumors and genetic mutations in tests on laboratory animals. Under certain conditions nitrites have also been found to be toxic.

nitrogen (N). Element No. 7. Atom. Wt. 14. A chemical element essential to life. Plants can use nitrogen compound direct from the soil, and nitrogen-fixing bacteria can use nitrogen directly from the air, and ultimately reduce nitrogen supplied as amino acids by protein foods.

nitrogen balance. Nitrogen balance means that the amount of nitrogen ingested is equal to the amount of nitrogen excreted. To determine the extent of protein metabolism, the nitrogen balance is studied. The amount of nitrogen is an accurate index of the amount of protein involved. If the amount of nitrogen that goes into the body in food and the amount that leaves the body in the excreta are determined, what has been used by the body can be calculated. If the nitrogen intake and nitrogen output are equal, the individual is in nitrogen balance or equilibrium. Should the intake of nitrogen be greater than the amount excreted in the urine and feces, the individual is in a state of positive balance. That is, the build-up (anabolism) or synthesis of tissue proteins is greater than the breakdown (*catabolism*) activities. An example of a positive nitrogen balance would be the case of a growing child or animal where the nitrogen goes into new tissue and material during growth. Should the intake of nitrogen, however, be less than the amount excreted, a negative balance exists. A negative nitrogen balance inevitably occurs when the protein intake is reduced below the amount required for maintenance of body tissues. Negative nitrogen balance may occur temporarily when the levels of protein intake are decreased. Negative nitrogen balance may occur at levels of protein intake that are above the minimum requirement, if the body is forced to burn protein because the diet furnishes too little carbohydrate and fat to meet the energy requirement.

nitrogenous. A substance containing nitrogen is referred to as nitrogenous. Proteins contain nitrogen, as do the chemical components of protein, amino acids. Protein decomposition products containing nitrogen are called nitrogenous extractives. They are found in well-ripened meat and contribute to the flavor of meat.

nondisjunction. The failure of a pair of homologous chromosomes to separate normally during the reduction division of *meiosis;* both members of the pair are carried to the same daughter nucleus and the other daughter cell is lacking in that particular chromosome.

normal saline. See *physiologic saline.*

nuclease. A nucleic acid splitting enzyme which results in the production of *nucleotides,* the subunits which form *nucleic acids.*

nucleic acid. Nucleic acids are complex, high molecular weight molecules containing nitrogenous bases (*purines* and *pyrimidines*), five carbon sugars (*ribose* * or *deoxyribose* *) and phosphate. The nucleic acids are divided into two major groups that relate to their structure, the *deoxyribonucleic acids* * (DNA) and the ribose nucleic acids (RNA). The DNA molecule contains as major constituents *cytosine, thymine, adenine* and *guanine* as nitrogenous bases, and deoxyribose as the five carbon sugar. The RNA molecule contains as major constituents *cytosine, uracil, adenine,* and *guanine* as the nitrogenous bases and ribose as the *pentose.* Nucleic acids are found in all living cells, with the exception of the red blood cells of humans, and the structures of these compounds are believed to be directly related to the characteristics not only of the individual cell but of the organism itself. The almost infinite variety of possible structures for nucleic acids allow information in coded form to be recorded in giant molecules and in somewhat similar fashion to the complex language symbols used to convey ideas. Such stored information controls the inherited characteristics of the next generation, as well as many of the ongoing life processes of the organism. DNA is found primarily in the nucleus of the cell and is identified as the genetic material. RNA is found mainly in the cytoplasm outside the nucleus and functions prominently in protein synthesis.

nucleolus. A spherical body found within the cell nucleus, it is rich in robonucleic acid and believed to be the site of synthesis of *nucleoproteins.*

nucleoprotein. A conjugated protein found in cell nuclei that results from the combination of a protein with nucleic acid. Nucleoproteins are essential for cell division and reproduction.

nucleotide. A molecule composed of a phosphate group, a five-carbon sugar-ribose or deoxyribose and a nitrogenous base, a flavin, *purine, pyrimidine,* or *pyridine. Flavin adenine dinucleotide* *, *adenosine triphosphate* *, *cytosine triphosphate,* * and *nicotinamide adenine diphosphate* * are respective examples of nucleotides.

nutmeg (*Myristica fragrans*). The hard kernel of the apricot-like fruit of the different varieties of the nutmeg tree. The tree, is a tropical evergreen, growing to a height of 20 to 40 feet. In appearance it resembles the pear tree. The fruit is intermingled with the flowers, and carefully split in half to expose the hard seed, which is the nutmeg proper, covered by a false aril which is carefully removed, dried, and used to make mace, sister spice of nutmeg. The nutmeg itself is also dried in the sun or over charcoal fires. It is oval in shape, gray-brown in color, and contains fat, volatile oil, acid and starch. It is an aromatic spice, used a great deal in cooking.

nutrient. A general term for any substance which can be used in the metabolic processes of the body. Scientists have identified over 50 different elements or chemical substances in food. These substances are grouped into six major classes called "nutrients." The Basic Six are *proteins, carbohydrates, vitamins, minerals, fats,* and *water.* The real bulk of all foods are proteins, carbohydrates, fats, and water. Many of the minerals and vitamins are only needed in minute amounts in a balanced diet. In digestion nutrients are reduced to their simplest forms in preparation for absorption.

nutrient density. Term relates the concentration of important nutrients in a food (vitamins, minerals, proteins) to the caloric value of that food. The enrichment and fortification of selected foods (e.g., cereals, flour, bread and milk) represent efforts to provide a good nutrient density in popular foods. In the case of packaged foods, including convenience packaged meals, and liquid meals, the responsibility falls directly on the producer to provide appropriate nutrient densities.

nutrition. The combination of processes by which the living organisms receives and utilizes the materials necessary for the maintenance of its functions and for the growth and renewal of its components. Normal nutrition is a condition of the body resulting from the efficient utilization of sufficient amounts of the essential nutrients provided in the food intake.

nutritional anemia. See *anemia.*

nutritional antagonist. A compound whose structure is so similar to a specific nutrient (an *antimetabolite*) that it can substitute for the nutrient in certain enzyme systems for which the specific nutrient is necessary, thus leading to at least partial inactivity of these systems. Hence, an effect similar to a deficiency is produced in a short time. (See *antivitamins*) True nutritional antagonism, or inhibition can always be overcome by high enough levels of the nutrient in question.

nutriture. The condition of well-being of the body as related to the consumption and utilization of food for growth, maintenance, and repair. Nutriture, or nutritional status, may be appraised by such methods as clinical examinations of the condition of the skin, eyes, mouth, tongue, gums, and muscles; determination of overweight or underweight; often by measurement of blood pressure and pulse rate; biochemical tests on the blood for various constituents associated with health; and urinalysis.

nuts. The word is used to describe a large number of dry fruits which generally consist of a single kernel enclosed in a woody shell. Acorns, filberts, and hazelnuts are examples of true nuts. The Brazil nut represents another type of dry fruit popularly classed as a nut; some nuts are, botanically speaking legumes. The peanut, for instance, is the pod of a vine of the pea family. Some fruits whose kernels are not dry are called nuts because of their nutlike shells. The litchi nut for example, is a fleshy raisinlike fruit enclosed in a shell. But not all the shells of true nuts are hard. The almond and pecan, for instance, come in more than one variety. Some have hard shells, some have soft ones, and some have paper-thin shells. The edible portion is the kernel. Most edible nuts contain less carbohydrate than legumes and are rich in protein and very rich in fat. They contain fair to generous amounts of *thiamine**, *riboflavin**, and *niacin** and represent good sources of iron and phosphorus. The proteins of nuts have a biologic value similar to the legumes (soybeans excepted). The digestibility of nuts is rather low, primarily because of their compact physical state.

nyctalopia. Night blindness due to a vitamin A deficiency. See retinal*, retinol*, rhodopsin, and *rod vision*.

O

oat, oatmeal (*Avena*). Oats are the grains of a cereal-grass plants, or the plant itself. Like the rest of the grains, oats consist of a soft inner part surrounded by a husk which is removed before being eaten by humans. Some varieties of oats, however, are hulless. The grain is used to make rolled oats and oatmeal and as feed for livestock. Most cultivated varieties of oats have a smooth-surfaced hull, although some varieties are hairy. To produce rolled oats, the husked sterilized grains are flattened by heated rolls, into the flakes. To make oatmeal, the groats (edible portion of the oats with the hull removed) are steel-cut in three sizes and ground in grades from coarse to extra-fine. Oats are the most nutritious of cereals, containing a good amount of fat, proteins, and minerals. Good source of *niacin*,* fair source of *thiamine** and *tocopherol** (vitamin E). The caloric values for 100 gm of the various oat products are:

Oatmeal or rolled oats, cooked = 55 calories
Oat and wheat cereal, cooked = 65 calories
Oat granules, maple-flavored, quick-cooking, cooked = 60 calories
Oat flakes, maple-flavored, instant cooking, cooked = 69 calories
Oat cereal with toasted wheat germ and soy grits, cooked = 62 calories
Shredded oats with added nutrients = 379 calories
Puffed oats (with or without corn or wheat) with added nutrients = 397 calories
Flaked oats (with soy flour and rice) with added nutrients = 197 calories

obesity. Obesity is the accumulation of excess fat. Obesity is usually determined by comparing an individual's weight to tables of standard weights. Overweight is then determined by the percent above the norm for a given height. Sometimes a body frame may not fit the norm and a person with a large frame and a large musculature can be more than 20 percent above the standard weight and not be obese. For a normal young man about 12 percent body weight is standard, and for young women the value is about 25 percent. Measurement of body fat is difficult, but a simple, reasonable reflection of obesity can be obtained by the skinfold test. An instrument called skin calipers, measures the thickness of skin folds at four sites, the biceps and triceps muscles, over the iliac crest bone and under the scapula bone (see the muscle and skeleton diagrams). Obesity arises only when the intake of food or calories is in excess of the physiological caloric need. While genetics may play a role in obesity, the influence of heredity is a difficult one to separate from the environment. Occasionally, individuals are obese because of some glandular disorders, *hypothyrodism, Cushing's syndrome, hypopituitarism,* and *hypogonadism,* but such instances are very rare and are not an essential feature of these conditions. The overwhelming majority of obese individuals show no clinical evidence of glandular disorders. The basal metabolic rates of obese individuals are within normal limits. The obese individual appears to have biochemical patterns with respect to fat and carbohydrate metabolism that differ from the nonobese person. The obese person does not develop *ketosis* readily and *glucose* appears to be oxidized at a slower rate. These observations appear to be a consequence of obesity and not the cause since all of the biochemical patterns become normal when the obese individual reaches normal weight. Many complications appear to accompany obesity. They include an association with high levels of *cholesterol* *; an increased incidence of *diabetes mellitus;* increased tendency towards heart disease; increased incidence of varicose veins; and a decrease life expectancy.

oedema. See *edema*.

offal. The word derives from "off-fall," the parts of an animal removed in the dressing process; offal includes the brains, sweetbreads, stomach, and intestines of an animal as well as the organ meats. See *meats* for nutrient contents.

oil. (1) A liquid digestible *triglyceride*. An oil differs from a fat by its liquid state at ordinary temperatures. Chemically oils differ from fats in that they contain a great number of unsaturated bonds in the *fatty acids* esterified to the *glycerols* *. Fat and oils belong to the same class of food, neutral fats. (2) Oil is also used to describe a class of nondigestible, hydrocarbon chemicals unrelated to nutrition. Processed fatty oils are hydrogenated oils, stearines, oleines, segregated oils, interesterified oils, products of fractional crystallization (e.g., certain cocoa butter substitutes), margarines, butter, cooking fats. Refined fatty oils are products prepared from the crude fatty oils by neutralization, bleaching, and deodorization.

okra (*Hibiscus esculentus*). A tall annual plant, of the mallow family which yields an edible pod with a gooey, mucilaginous quality. Okra should be eaten when very tender. Okra is used to flavor and thicken gumbos or soup-stews. Fair source of vitamins A and C. Boiled and drained, 100 gm = 29 calories.

oleic acid (oleate). Mol. Wt. 282. An unsaturated fatty acid. Oleic acid is a liquid at room temperature, a property of most unsaturated fatty acids. (See *oil*). The trans isomer of oleic acid, *elaidic acid* is a solid at room temperature. The difference in the physical properties is related to the ease of association of molecules in the trans isomer.

$$CH_3(CH_2)_7 \overset{H}{-}C \overset{H}{=}C-(CH_2)_7COOH$$

oleomargarine. A smooth-textured fat used as a spread and in cooking. The name comes from elo-, a combining form meaning "oil" and from margaric acid, a constituent of animal fat.

olfactory nerve. The olfactory nerve receives and transmits impulses associated with the sense of smell. Cell bodies of the bipolar neurons of this nerve are located in the olfactory mucosa of the superior most portion of the nasal cavity. The sense of smell is a necessity for a discriminating sense of taste.

oligosaccharides. A general term to express the linkage of several *monosaccharides* in a single molecule. The general class of oligosaccharides includes sugars containing any number, from 3 to as many as 10 monosaccharide units joined together. More than 10 monosaccharide units is generally classified as a *polysaccharide,* but there is no definite division between the classifications. This bonding is the glycoside linkage common to the *disaccharides,* oligosaccharides, and polysaccharides. See *polysaccharides.*

olive (*Olea europea*). The fruit of a 25- to 40-foot subtropical evergreen tree. Olives, as they grow on the tree, are pale green. When they begin to turn straw-colored, they are picked and prepared in various ways for eating. Fresh olives are very bitter. The bitterness is removed in the preparation. Green fermented olives, the well-known Spanish-style olives, are soaked in lye for a short time, washed, and then kept in barrels of salt solution for 6 to 12 months. This causes a lactic-acid fermentation and gives them their astringent taste. Sugar is added from time to time to keep fermentation going. When the olives are properly fermented, they are packed in a weak salt brine and bottled. As the olive becomes riper it develops more oil. Ripe olives are either green or black. The "black" color of the "ripe" olive is developed during the lye treatments. Between treatments they are exposed to the air to develop the characteristic dark color. Green, 1 large = 7 calories; ripe, 1 large = 11 calories; dried and salt-cured, 1 large = 20 calories.

olive oil. A product obtained by crushing tree-ripened olives, then extracting the liquid by pressing the pulp or by centrifugal separators. The first "crude olive oil'' is obtained from this liquid by settling and skimming or by "washing" by a continuous flow of clear water. Refining produces the clear oil used for salads and cooking.

onion (*Allium cepa*). The underground bulb. There are many kinds of onions with different-colored skins and in size they vary from the very small bulbets of the spring or green onions, also known as scallions, to the huge round red Italian onions. A pungent, volatile oil, rich in sulphur is the cause of the onion's strong smell and flavor. Onions are a member of the lily family which includes such flowers as the tulip, hyacinth, and lily-of-the-valley as well as the edible leek, garlic, chive, and shallot. All have a bulb growing under the ground and a stalk, leaves, and flowers above. The word "onion" comes through French from Latin, probably from the Latin word unus, meaning "one," perhaps because the onion is a single bulb with a spherical shape. Onions contain some *ascorbic acid* * (vitamin C) with small amounts of other vitamins and minerals. Green parts of the onion yield some *carotene* * (vitamin A activity).

Dry, raw, 100 gm = 38 calories
Dry, boiled and drained, 100 gm = 29 calories
Green, raw, bulb and entire top, 100 gm = 36 calories
Green, raw, bulb and white portion of top, 100 gm = 45 calories
Green, green portion of tops only, 100 gm = 27 calories

opsin. Protein compound which combines with *cis*-11 *retinal,* vitamin A aldehyde, to form *rhodopsin,* visual purple. Visual purple is necessary for night vision via the rods in the retina. A vitamin A deficiency will lead to night blindness because rhodopsin is not formed at normal levels. See *retinal* *, *retinol* * and *rhodopsin.*

orange (*Citrus*). There are many varieties of oranges, but the three principal species are the sweet, common, or China orange, *C. sinensis;* the loose-skinned orange, *C. mobilis;* and the sour, bitter, Seville orange, *C. aurantium.* The best-known sweet oranges are the golden-yellow Valencia, or Spanish, heavy and juicy, with large coarse-grained fruit; Mediterranean oranges which have a fine grained fruit; blood oranges with a red, or red and white streaked pulp; and the seedless navel or Washington navel oranges. Oranges are excellent sources of ascorbic acid (vitamin C) and some *carotene* * (vitamine A activity). Once juices are squeezed or canned juices are opened, vitamin C combines with air and forms a new compound which has no vitamin value. After 24 hours in refrigerator; 20 percent vitamin C loss; after 24 hours at room temperature; 60 percent vitamin C loss. 100 gm has the following caloric value:

Peeled raw oranges = 49 calories
Orange juice, fresh or frozen = 45 calories

Orange juice, canned, unsweetened = 48 calories
Orange juice, canned, sweetened = 52 caalories
Candied orange peel = 316 calories

oregano (*Origanum vulgare*). Also called wild marjoram, a beautiful plant which grows in clumps with purplish, pink, lilac, or white flowers. It is the dark-green leaf, shaped like a roundish egg, that is used as a culinary herb. Leaves may be used fresh or dried. The tops of the plant may also be used. The flavor is similar to that of sweet marjoram or thyme, all belonging to the mint family. Oregano is considerably more bitter and pungent and should be used with discretion. Vegetable-juice cocktails and bean, beef, game, or tomato soups may be flavored with oregano. Oregano is often used as a seasoning in Mexican and Italian dishes.

organ. A member of a system, composed of tissues associated in performing some special function for which it is especially adapted. Systems are made up of organs with a corresponding division of labor and special adaptation of the organ to its particular share of the work of the system.

organelles. The various structures with the cell. Some examples of the formed elements of the cell are the *mitochondria,* the *Golgi complex* or apparatus, *endoplasmic reticulum, ribosomes,* and *lysosomes.* See *cell.*

organic. A large group of chemical compounds that contain carbon.

organic acids. Acids containing only carbon, hydrogen, and oxygen, and the carboxylic acid group (—COOH). Among the best known are *citric acid** (which occurs in high concentrations in citrus fruits) and *acetic acid** (the major acid in vinegar). Aerobically the organic acids may be oxidized completely to carbon dioxide and water. Saturated fatty acid derivatives are degraded to acetic acid, two carbons at a time.

organic foods. A somewhat loosely used term most generally taken to mean foods grown by ''organic gardening'' methods, with no chemical fertilizers or pesticides used. Sometimes the term is used more broadly and interchangeably with ''natural foods,'' to include foods not only ''organically'' grown but containing no chemical additives, such as preservatives, hormones, dyes, and antibiotics, and which have undergone only a minimum of refining to preserve original nutrients.

orgeat. A syrup used in France, Spain, Italy, and other Latin-American countries as a refreshing drink when mixed with water, or as a flavoring for frostings and fillings. The syrup is usually made from an emulsion of almonds and sugar with a little rosewater or orange-flower water added.

ornithine. Mol. Wt. 132. A nonessential amino acid of the *urea cycle* formed from *arginine* * when urea is split off. Ornithine and one other, *citrulline* * are the two amino acids that do not occur in proteins.

$$NH_2-CH_2-CH_2-CH_2-\underset{\underset{NH_2}{|}}{CH}-COOH$$

osmosis. The word osmosis comes from the Greek word osmos meaning "to push" or "to thrust." The passage of solvent molecules from the lesser to the greater concentration of solute when two solutions are separated by a membrane which selectively prevents the passage of solute molecules but is permeable to the solvent.

osmotic pressure. The force that a dissolved substance exerts on a membrane that allows solvent to pass through but not the solute (semipermeable membrane), when solutions of differing solute concentrations are separated by a semipermeable membrane. The tendency is for solvent to pass over to the higher concentration until the concentrations of solute on both sides of the semipermeable membrane are equal. Osmotic pressure is a measure of the force of that tendency for water to pass across the semipermeable membrane from the less concentrated to the more concentrated solution, until the concentration of dissolved particles on both sides are equal. Therefore net exchanges of water between the various fluid compartments of the body occur as a result of osmotic pressure, due chiefly to differences in the concentration of electrolytes. Osmotic pressure in the cellular fluid is regulated mainly by the concentration of *potassium ions* and in the extracellular fluid by the concentration of *sodium ions*. Plasma protein also plays an important role in maintaining osmotic equilibrium in the extracellular fluid compartments by remaining in the plasma, because they are not permeable to cell membrane, the plasma proteins prevent the net exchange of water from plasma into the interstitial space. An excess of fluid in the interstitial space is known as *edema* and results from lowered osmotic pressure in the plasma relative to the interstial space.

ossification. The process of forming bone. Cartilage is made into bone by the process of ossification. The minerals, calcium and phosphorus are deposited in the cartilage, changing into bone.

osteoarthritis. A common type of arthritis in which there is a gradual "wearing out" or degeneration of the joint rather than an acute inflammatory type of process. Rarely leads to crippling, with most persons suffering from this disease being over 40 years of age, having only mild pain and stiffness of the joints. The joints of the fingers are often affected.

osteoblasts. Bone-forming cells.

osteoclasts. Giant multinuclear cell found in depressions on bone surfaces, which cause resorption of bone tissue and the formation of canals.

osteomalacia. A nutritional disease. Prolonged deficiency of dietary calcium and *vitamin D* * or sunlight may result in osteomalacia, sometimes called adult rickets. This condition is characterized by poor calcification of the bones with increasing softness, so that they become flexible, leading to deformities in the spine, thorax or pelvis. These bone changes may be accompanied by rheumatic pains and exhaustion. See *vitamin D* *.

osteoporosis. A condition of abnormal porousness or "thinning" of bone due to insufficient production of the protein matrix in which calcium salts are deposited. Occurring principally in women after middle age. The remaining bone is normally mineralized.

ovaries. Described as two almond-shaped glands, one on either side of the abdomino-pelvic cavity. They produce female germ cells, ova, and female hormones, *estrogen* * and *progresterone* *. These hormones maintain the normal menstrual cycle. An ovum is expelled from the surface of an ovary in a process called ovulation which generally occurs about halfway between each menstrual period. An expelled ovum is picked up by the free end of a fallopian tube for transportation to the uterus.

oxalacetic acid (oxalacetate). Mol. Wt. 132. An intermediate in the *Krebs* (tricarboxylic acid) *cycle* *. The reaction of oxalacetate with *acetyl-Coenzyme-A* * to form *citric acid* * is considered the first step in the Kreb's cycle. Oxalacetate is the alpha (α) ketoacid equivalent of the nonessential amino acid *aspartic acid* * which can be formed by *transamination*.

$$\underset{\displaystyle \text{HOOC—CH}_2\text{—C—COOH}}{\overset{\displaystyle \text{O}}{\overset{\displaystyle \|}{}}}$$

oxalic acid (oxalate). Mol. Wt. 90. HOOC—COOH. A dicarboxylic acid which occurs as a result of metabolic processes in the body, and which is found in certain foods, especially cocoa, rhubarb, spinach, and some other greens.

Oxalic acid forms insoluble salts with calcium, mangnesium, and iron, and acts to prevent these minerals from being absorbed during digestion.

oxidation. Oxidation may be interpreted in several ways. The addition of oxygen to a molecule is one form of oxidation. For example, $2H_2 + O_2 \longrightarrow 2H_2O$. In this example hydrogen has been oxi-
      (hydrogen) (oxygen) (water)
idized. Every oxidation must also be accompanied by the opposite reaction, a *reduction,* and in this example oxygen was reduced. In the oxidation of food, the over-all products are CO_2, H_2O and energy. The carbons and hydrogens of food are oxidized and the oxygen is reduced. Oxidations do not need to involve oxygen and may be interpreted as a removal of hydrogens. For example, the oxidation of a saturated fatty acid, $R-CH_2-CH_2CH_2CH_2COOH$, to an unsaturated fatty acid results when hydrogens are removed.

$$R-CH_2-CH_2COOH + FAD \longrightarrow R-CH=CH-CH-COOH + FADH_2$$

This reaction takes place during the oxidation of fatty acids (except that the fatty acid is a *coenzyme A* * derivative). The fatty acid is oxidized by the removal of two hydrogens and the FAD (*flavin-adenine dinucleotide*) undergoes reduction by the addition of hydrogens. A more general interpretation of oxidation and reduction reacts is based on the removal of electrons (oxidation) and the addition of electrons to atoms in the molecule. This interpretation of oxidation-reduction reactions covers all cases and types of oxidation, but it is often not so clear or so graphic as the interpretations above. Oxidations and reduction are essential in utilization of food to provide energy. The oxidation of foodstuffs, *fats, carbohydrates,* and *proteins* takes place in a stepwise manner with one carbon being oxidized to CO_2 at a time. The oxidation of the carbons occurs mainly through the *Kreb's cycle* *, the oxidation of hydrogen mainly through *oxidative phosphorylation* in the *terminal respiratory chain* *, where chemical energy, *adenosine triphosphate* * (ATP) is produced. Both the Kreb's cycle and oxidative phosphorylation occur in the organelles called *mitochrondria*. Mitochondria account for more than 90 percent of the oxygen we use to oxidize foods to carbon dioxide, water, and energy. See *Kreb's cycle* and *terminal respiratory chain.*

oxidative phosphorylation. The cellular process responsible for the conversion of the energy in foods into chemical energy. The process is called "oxidative" because the hydrogens of foods (metabolites) are oxidized to water (see *oxidation*), and "phosphorylation" because the addition of phosphate to *adenosine diphosphate* * (ADP) is coupled to the oxidation process. The result is the formation of the principal form of chemical energy in the cell *adenosine* *triphosphate** (ATP). The enzymatic complex involved with oxidative phosphorylation reactions is called the *"terminal respiratory chain."* The terminal respiratory chain is contained within the mitochondria. The process of oxidative-phosphorylation has a theoretical efficiency of about 42 percent. That means that in the oxidation of foodstuffs about 58 percent of the energy is converted to heat and the remainder is converted to ATP. The ATP can then be used for work or converted to other forms of energy, e.g., muscular work or electrical energy. The conversion of ATP to other forms of energy is again accompanied by a conversion of a part of the energy to heat. Overall, the efficiency of extracting the energy in foods into chemical, osmotic, electrical, and kinetic end products is about 25 to 30 percent. The remainder of the energy is converted to heat, a necessary energy form for the environment (body). See *oxidation* and *terminal respiratory chain*.

oxycalorimeter. In the indirect measurement of heat in an oxycalorimeter the amount of oxygen required to burn a weighed sample of food is measured. The energy yield of the food is then obtained using standard factors established with the bomb calorimeter to convert the known volume of oxygen to calories. The dried sample, a single food or a mixture of foods, is ignited and burned in a stream of nearly pure oxygen in a closed circuit.

oxygen (O). Element No. 8. Atom. Wt. 16. Oxygen is the final acceptor of electrons in aerobic life systems. The result of the reduction of oxygen to O^{-2} is the immediate formation of water (H_2O). The details of the mechanism of reduction of oxygen are not known. In the passage of electrons to oxygen, several *oxidation-reduction* processes occur, and in some processes the energy of oxidation is conserved as chemical energy (see *oxidative phosphorylation* and the *terminal respiratory chain*). Thus in the maintainance of aerobic life, electrons flow from foodstuffs to oxygen. This flow of electrons and conservations of energy occurs in each cell, the oxygen being carried to the cells by the *hemoglobin* in the *red blood cell*. In anaerobic life systems the processes are similar except that the final electron acceptor is not oxygen.

oxygen debt. A term that accounts for the continued hyperventilation and the increased metabolic and physiologic rates that follows the cessation of exercise, particularly vigorous exercise. An explanation for the phenomenon is related to *glycolysis* and the accumulation of *lactic acid**. During vigorous exercise, energy is required. The immediate source of energy is the metabolism of *glucose** which is increased to accommodate the sudden demand. Glucose via glycolysis is degraded to *pyruvic acid** at a rate faster than the pyruvate can be oxidized. During glycolysis, *adenosine triphosphate** (ATP), a form of chemical energy required for muscle contraction, is produced. The accumulating pyruvate is converted to a reduced form, lactic acid, which accumulates as muscle activity continues. In other words, the muscle has received a part of its energy under anaerobic conditions. When muscle activity ceases, the lactic acid can now be oxidized back to pyruvate since the pyruvate formation from glycolysis diminishes. However, the store of lactic acid means that the oxidation mechanisms are still being flooded with pyruvate. The demand to oxidize the pyruvate at above resting rates to carbon dioxide, water, and energy continues until lactic acid concentrations are at resting levels.

oxystearin. A modified *fatty acid* that manufacturers add in amounts up to 0.125 percent of vegetable oils to prevent them from clouding up in the refrigerator.

oxytocin. A hormone that stimulates uterine contractions and lactation in females. A polypeptide with eight amino acids: *tyrosine*, proline*, glutamic acid*, aspartic acid*, glycine*, cystine*, leucine*,* and *isoleucine**. It is formed mostly in the paraventricular nuclei of the hypothalmus. The term oxytocin also refers to rapid childbirth. It is so named because it causes vigorous contractions of the uterus, thus expelling the fetus. Oxytocin also causes contraction of the myoepithelial cells arranged around the mammary ducts in such a way that contraction forces the milk out.

P

PABA. See *Para-Amino Benzoic Acid.*

palatability. The quality characteristic (such as color, flavor, and texture) of a food product that makes an impression on the organs of touch, taste, smell, or sight and has significance in determining the acceptability of the food produced to the user.

palmitic acid. Mol. Wt. 254. A 16-carbon saturated *fatty acid* widespread in foods. The difference in consistency of various fats at room temperature is due to differences in the kinds and amounts of fatty acids that enter into their composition. Palmitic and *stearic acids* which enter largely into the compounds of solid fats. They are called saturated fatty acids because they cannot take up any more hydrogen.

$$
\begin{array}{c}
\quad\; H \; H \; H \; H \; H \; H \; H \; H \; H \; H \; H \; H \; H \; H \; H \\
\quad\; | \; \; | \; \; | \; \; | \; \; | \; \; | \; \; | \; \; | \; \; | \; \; | \; \; | \; \; | \; \; | \; \; | \; \; | \\
H - C^{16}C^{15}C^{14}C^{13}C^{12}C^{11}C^{10}C^{9}\,C^{8}\,C^{7}\,C^{6}\,C^{5}\,C^{4}\,C^{3}\,C^{2}\,C^{1}OOH \\
\quad\; | \; \; | \; \; | \; \; | \; \; | \; \; | \; \; | \; \; | \; \; | \; \; | \; \; | \; \; | \; \; | \; \; | \; \; | \\
\quad\; H \; H \; H \; H \; H \; H \; H \; H \; H \; H \; H \; H \; H \; H \; H
\end{array}
$$

palm oil. The oil palm bears a great number of nutlike fruits and oil and is expressed from both the pulp and the kernel. The oil from the kernel is palm oil, an important source of margarine, and is used in the cooking in many parts of the tropics.

pancreas. A long, tapering organ lying behind the stomach. The head of the gland lies in the curve of the small intestine near the pyloric valve. The body of the pancreas extends to the left toward the spleen. The pancreas secretes a digestive juice which acts on all types of foods. Several enzymes in pancreatic juice digest proteins. Other enzymes digest starches into sugars and other enzymes digest fats into their simplest forms. The pancreas has another important function, the production of the hormones *insulin* and *glucagon*. See *digestion, digestive system.*

pancreatic juice. Pancreatic juice contains at least four classes of enzymes: (1) *proteases,* (2) *amylases,* (3) *lipases,* and (4) *nucleases.* In addition, the pancreatic secretion contains a considerable quantity of bicarbonate ion, which makes it alkaline and which functions to neutralize the highly acid *gastric juice.* Sodium, potassium, calcium, and magnesium concentrations in pancreatic juice reflect the concentrations of these cations in the plasma. The pancreas secretes trypsinogen. When trypsinogen reaches the intestinal tract it is converted into trypsin by trypsin already present and by enterokinase. Trypsin is a proteolytic enzyme. Pancreatic amylases are enzymes that speeds the conversion of carbohydrates to the simple sugars. *Ptyalin* is the salivary amylase that initiates this process. The pancreatic amylases continues the work so that intermediary sugars, *maltose** and *isomaltose*,* are formed. The pancreatic juice also contains amylases which act specifically on these intermediary sugars, maltose, sucrose, and lactose, to convert them to the simple sugars glucose, fructose, and galactose. Pancreatic lipase catalyzes the conversion of the fat molecule into its component fatty acids and glycerol. The bile salts make it possible for the lipase to act on fat and to bring about this conversion. *Nucleases* break down *nucleic acids* to component parts. See *digestive system.*

pancreatitis. An inflammation of the *pancreas.* It may be acute or chronic in nature and frequently accompanies obstruction of the pancreatic duct due to *gallstones* or the back flow of *bile* into the pancreatic duct.

pancreozymin. Hormone produced in mucosa of the *duodenum* (small intestine) that stimulates secretion of enzymes from the *pancreas.*

pangamic acid (vitamin B_{15}). Mol. Wt. 281. Isolated from apricot kernels, rice bran, seeds, brewer's yeast, oxblood, and liver. Appears to be found wherever the *B-complex vitamins* are found. There is no clear evidence of its effectiveness or function in man, but it was proposed for treatment of cardiovascular and rheumatic diseases in the past.

D-Gluconic acid 6-[bis (methylethyl)] amino acetate

panocha. A candy made of brown sugar, milk, butter, and nuts. Also a coarse sugar made in Mexico.

pantothenic acid. Mol. Wt. 291. The biochemical role of pantothenic acid is involved primarily as a part of *coenzyme A **, one of the most important substances in body metabolism. As part of coenzyme A, pantothenic acid is essential for the intermediary metabolism of carbohydrates, fats, and proteins for their synthesis, breakdown, and release of energy. It functions primarily by affecting the removal or acceptance of important chemical groups with two, three, four (or more) carbon atoms at a time. Coenzyme A is also needed for the formation of such important sterols as cholesterol and the adrenocortical hormones. Pantothenic acid functions also as a component of the enzyme *fatty*

$$\begin{array}{c} \quad\quad\; \text{CH}_3 \;\; \text{OH} \quad \text{O} \;\; \text{H} \\ \quad\quad\;\; | \quad\quad | \quad\quad \| \quad | \\ \text{HO--CH}_2\text{--C--CH--C--N--CH}_2\text{--CH}_2\text{--COOH} \\ \quad\quad\;\; | \\ \quad\quad\; \text{CH}_3 \end{array}$$

The following are the levels of pantothenic acids in foods:

portion

Food	μg/100 gm	Food	μg/100 gm
Bananas	300	Oysters	490
Beans, dried lima	830	Peaches	140
Beef, brain	2100–2900	Peanuts, roasted	2500
Beef, heart	2100–2500	Pears	70
Beef, kidney	3400	Peas, fresh	600–1040
Beef, liver	5700–8200	Peas, dried	2800
Beef, muscle	1100	Pineapple	170
Bread, whole wheat	570	Pork, bacon	280–980
Bread, white	400	Pork, ham	340–660
Broccoli	1400	Pork, kidney	3100
Cauliflower	920	Pork, liver	5900–7300
Cheese	350–960	Pork, muscle	470–1500
Chicken	530–900	Potatoes, Irish	400–650
Eggs	2700	Potatoes, sweet	940
Lamb	600	Salmon	660–1100
Lamb, kidney	4300	Soybeans	1800
Milk, whole	290	Tomatoes	310
Mushrooms	1700	Veal chop	110–260
Oats	1300	Wheat, whole	1300
Onions	140	Wheat, germ	2000
Oranges	340	Wheat, bran	2400

acid synthase involved in fatty acid synthesis in the body. Pantothenic acid exists in all cells of living tissues and therefore is present in all natural foods. Foods especially rich are yeast, heart, salmon, liver, eggs, wheat and rice germ or bran, peanuts, and peas. Moderate to good amounts are contained in such foods as milk, poultry, whole grains, broccoli, mushrooms, and sweet potatoes. Most vegetables and fruits and refined foods contain lesser amounts. Losses up to 50 percent can occur in frozen vegetables and meat, and in many canned food products. The quantitative requirement for pantothenic acid in man has not been established. In animals, pantothenic acid supplements have been shown to increase fertility and longevity. Pantothenic acid is fairly stable in neutral solutions but is destroyed by acid and alkali and by prolonged dry heat. The calcium salt of the vitamin is the form in which it is used generally. Calcium pantothenate is odorless and slightly bitter in taste. Pantothenic acid in pure form is a pale yellow viscous oil.

papain. A *proteolytic enzyme* from *papaya*. It is used in medicine and in meat tenderizers. Papain is used medically as an aid for stomach disorders and sold in health food stores as a digestant.

papaw or paw paw (*Asimina triloba*). A North American fruit of the custard family, varying from 2 to 6 inches in length and shaped like a short fat banana, dark brown to blackish in color, with a soft creamy flesh in which many seeds are embedded. It is sweet, rich, custardlike and slightly aromatic.

papaya (*Carica papaya*). A small tropical tree with a large, fleshy fruit which grows on the stalk from the trunk, just below the leaves. The fruit, which resembles a melon, has a rind and a juicy flesh that is orange in color. It has a delicious, sweet-tart musky taste. The fruit is the source of the enzyme *papain,* a *protease*.

paprika. The Hungarian name given to a spice or condiment made by grinding the ripe dried pods of red capsicum or bell peppers.

para-aminobenzoic acid. Mol. Wt. 137. A part of pteroylglutamic acid, one of the forms of the vitamin *folacin* *. Para-aminobenzoic acid is growth factor for bacteria, and *glutamic acid* is an amino acid commonly found in proteins of

$$NH_2$$

$$CO_2H$$

foods and body tissues. The fact that para-aminobenzoic acid (PABA) is a unit in the structure of folacin may be a reason for its tentative status as a vitamin. It is no longer considered as such for human beings, since it is now known to be a component of pteroylglutamic acid. It also is not a necessary constituent in the human diet. Clincally PABA has been used to treat some ricketsial (bacteriae) diseases. It is effective because it acts as an *antimetabolite* to a material essential to the growth of the ricketsiae.

parabens. Nickname for methyl, propyl, and heptyl esters of parahydrobenzoic acid. Used as a preservative, closely related to *sodium benzoate*. Parabens can prevent bacteria and mold from growing in almost all foods.

parasitic worms. Some parasitic worms can be seen with the unaided eye, but others have to be identified only with a microscope. The smallest are roughly the size of pinheads, while a tapeworm can grow to a 30-foot length. Many parasites including the flukes (one of two types of flatworms), are more prevalent in the tropics. The other type of flatworm, the tapeworm, is found in the U.S. and is acquired by eating beef, pork, or fish containing the parasite. Inside the intestine, the tapeworm attaches itself to the intestinal wall and proceeds to grow. Some roundworms common in this country include the pinworm, intestinal roundworm, and hookworm. Another roundworm, found in pork, causes trichinosis, a disease in which the parasites eventually penetrate muscles.

parasympathetic nervous system. The autonomic nerve fibers which originate from cell bodies lying in the brain stem and in the sacral part of the spinal cord forming the parasympathic nervous system. Preganglionic nerve fibers arising from cells in the midbrain travel out with the third nerve fibers to the ciliary ganglion, which gives rise to postganglionic fibers supplying the pupil, iris, and ciliary muscles. Other preganglionic fibers arise from nerve cells in the medulla and travel with the nerve fibers of the seventh and ninth cranial nerves to innervate the salivary and other glands of the head and neck. Other cell bodies in the medulla give rise to the largest autonomic nerve in the body, the vagus nerve (tenth nerve), which contains all the preganglionic fibers to the many ganglia lying in or near the viscera of the chest or upper abdomen. Short postganglionic nerve fibers run from these ganglia to supply the heart, intestines, pancreas, and spleen. Ninety percent of all the parasympathetic nerve fibers in the body travel in the vagus nerve. The remainder of the parasympathetic nervous system consists of preganglionic fibers arising in the sacral region of the spinal cord and eventually terminating in pelvic ganglia, from which postganglionic fibers travel to the smooth muscle of the bladder, rectum, and genitalia.

parathormone (parathyroid hormone, PTH). A hormone of the *parathyroid* glands which control calcium and phosphorus metabolism in three ways: (1) It stimulates the intestinal mucosa to increase calcium absorption; (2) it mobilizes calcium rapidly from bone; and (3) it causes renal excretion of phosphate. All of these responses act together and are needed to regulate the circulating amounts of calcium and phosphorus to maintain them within normal levels.

parathyroid glands. The parathyroid glands, usually four in number are located in the posterior surfaces of the lobe of the *thyroid gland*. These glands produce the hormone, *parathormone,* which helps to regulate the amount of *calcium* and *phosphorous* in the blood. Calcium normally stored in the bones is released into the blood as required for normal nerve and muscle tissue function. When there is too little calcium in the blood, a type of muscle twitching called *tetany* develops. Because of the location of the parathyroid gland in relation to the thyroid, special observation for tetany may be required in the immediate postoperative period following thyroid surgery. Calcium is given by intravenous infusion to relieve the symptoms of tetany.

parboiled rice (converted rice). Rice that has been especially treated with heat and water before the husks are removed so that the nutrients in the outer layers of the kernel are driven inward to the kernel. This reduces the loss of nutrients when the outer layers are removed in milling. See *rice.*

parenchyma. Functional tissue of an organ or gland as distinct from its supporting framework.

parenteral. The entrance of a substance into the body by means other than through the gastrointestinal tract. For example, the introduction of nutrients by way of veins or into subcutaneous tissues.

parfait. French parfait is an ice made of a single flavor frozen in a plain mold. American parfait consists of ice cream served with whipped cream in a tall narrow glass called a parfait glass. The ice cream is layered into the glass with the cream (or fruit or sauce).

parietal cells. Cells of the gastric glands in the fundus of the stomach which produce hydrochloric acid for the purpose of digestion. See *gastric juice.*

parsley (*Petroselinum crispum*). A hardy biennial herb plant widely used for flavoring and as a garnish. The pasley family, or Umbelliferae, includes many herbs and spices such as anise, dill, angelica, chervil, caraway, coriander, cumin, fennel, lovage, sweet cicely, and the common vegetables celery and carrots. Parsley is a small green plant of which there are more than 30 varieties, distinguished by the shape of their foliage; curled, moss-curled, double-curled, or fern leafed, for example; and plain or common parsley. Bunches of parsley leaves are used whole as a garnish or in a bouquet garni. Chopped, either fresh or dried, parsley is used to flavor soups, meat dishes, fish stuffings, cream or cheese sauces, eggs, breads, flavored butter, marinades, and most vegetables and salads. Nutritive values (1 cup); *carotene* * (vitamin A) 8230 I.U. per 100 gm; *thiamine* * 0.11 mg; *riboflavin* * 0.28 mg; *niacin* * 1.4 mg; *ascorbic acid* * (vitamin C) 193 mg; protein, 3.7 gm; calories 50; fat 1.0 gm; carbohydrates 9.0 gm; calcium 193 mg; iron 4.3 mg; phosphorus 84 mg; potassium 80 mg.

parsnip *(Pastinaca sativa)*. The edible underground root of a biennial plant, of the carrot family. The sweet flavor of the parsnip develops only after the first frost, as cold weather changes the starch to sugar. Nutritive values (1 cup): *thiamine* * 0.08 mg; *riboflavin* * 0.12 mg; *niacin* * 0.2 mg; *ascorbic acid* * (vitamin C) 18 mg; protein 1.5 gm; calories 78; fat .5 gm; carbohydrates 18.2 gm; calcium 57 gm; iron .7 mg; phosphorus 80 mg; potassium 570 mg.

part per million (ppm). A way of expressing amounts, especially of trace minerals or contaminants in diets or foods. Examples of how small a part per million is, it is equal to 1 pound in 500 tons, 1 inch in about 16 miles, or 1 cent in $10,000.

passion fruit *(Passiflora)*. The edible fruit of the passion flower, a vine with solitary spectacular flowers which is a native of tropical Brazil. The fruit is also known as granadilla. It has a sweet-acid flavor, and is used as a table fruit, as well as for making sherberts, candy, and refreshing beverages. Nutritive values (1 cup): *carotene* * (vitamin A) 700 I.U. per 100 gm; *thiamine* * trace; *riboflavin* * 0.13 mg, *niacin* * 1.5 mg; *ascorbic acid* * (vitamin C) 30 mg; protein 2.2 gm; calories 90; fat .7 gm; carbohydrates 21.2 gm; calcium 13 mg; iron 1.6 mg; phosphorus 64 mg.

pasta. The Italian word for "paste" which in culinary usage describes an alimentary paste made from semolina and water. Semolina is the purified middlings of hard wheat. There are over 100 varieties, some shaped like lasagna, others in small decorative shapes such as stars, hearts, animals, and letters.

pasteurization. A heat treatment that kills part but not all the microorganisms present in a substance and usually involves the application of temperatures below 100°C (212°F). The heating may be by means of steam, hot water, dry heat, or electric currents, and the products are cooled promptly after the heat treatment. Pasteurization is used, (1) when more rigorous heat treatment would harm the quality of the product, as with milk; (2) when one aim is to kill pathogens; (3) when the main spoilage organisms are not very heat-resistant, like the yeasts in fruit juices; (4) when any surviving spoilage organisms will be taken care of by additional preservative methods, as is done in the chilling of market milk; and (5) when competing organisms are to be killed, allowing a desired fermentation by specific microorganisms, usually by added starter organisms, as in cheese making for example.

pastrami. A preserved meat of eastern European origin, made from plate brisket or round of beef dry-cured with salt and saltpeter, *sodium nitrate**. The beef is then rinsed and rubbed with a paste or garlic powder, ground cuminseed and pepper, cinnamon cloves, and allspice, smoked and cooked.

paté. A meat or fish paste, or a pie or patty with a filling such as meat or fish paste. The most famous is the paté de foie gras, or goose liver paté.

pathogen. A microorganism that causes a disease or pathological condition.

pauchouse. A French name for a bouillabaisse made of freshwater fish. It is made with five kinds of fish, almost always including eel and pike.

pavlova. A dessert of Australian origin which consists of a meringue topped with whipped cream and berries, or whipped cream, passion fruit, and banana slices.

pawpaw. See *papaw*.

PBI. See *protein bound iodine*.

pea (*Pisum sativum*). The seed and plant of a cool-season hardy annual. Chief among the many varieties are the garden, or green pea and the field, or stock pea, *P. Sativum* var. *arvense*. The seeds of garden peas can be classified as smooth-skinned or wrinkled. Field peas, which have a small hard seed, are used chiefly for making yellow split peas and as livestock fodder. See *pea, immature* and *pea, mature* for nutrient content.

pea, immature. Nutritive value (1 cup); *carotene** (vitamin A) 680 I.U. per gm; *thiamine** (vitamin B$_1$) 0.34 mg; *riboflavin** .16 mg; *niacin** 2.7 mg; *ascorbic acid** (vitamin C) 26 mg; protein 6.7 mg; calories 98; fat 0.4 gm; carbohydrates 17.7 gm; calcium 22 mg; iron 1.9 mg; phosphorus 122 mg; potassium 200 mg.

pea, mature. Nutritive values (1 cup): *carotene** (vitamin A), 370 I.U. per 100 gm; *thiamine** 0.77 mg; *riboflavin** 0.28 mg; *niacin** 3.1 mg; *ascorbic* acid* (vitamin C) 2 mg; protein 23.8 gm; calories 339; fat 1.4 gm; carbohydrates 60.2 gm; calcium 57 mg; iron 4.7 mg; phosphorus 388 mg; potassium 200 mg.

peach (Prunus or Amygdalus persica). The peach is a rounded fruit with a fuzzy velvety skin, creamy yellow when ripe. The flesh may be white or yellow with a pitted or furrowed stone of the free or cling type. Nutritive values (1 cup); *carotene* * (vitamin A), 880 I.U. per 100 gm; *thiamine* * .02 mg; *riboflavin* * 0.05 mg; niacin .9 mg; *ascorbic acid* * (vitamin C), 8 mg; protein 0.5 gm; calories 46; fat 1 gm; carbohydrates 12 gm; calcium 8 mg; iron 0.6 mg; phosphorus 22 mg; potassium 310 mg.

peanut (Arachis hypogaea). A spreading annual plant related to peas and beans. Peanuts are often called groundnuts, monkey nuts and earthnuts. The pods of the peanut vary. They may grow from 1 to 2 inches in length, with one, two or three seeds. The seed has a thin papery coat which may be any color from white to purple. The most common colors are mahogany, red, rose, and salmon. Nutritive values (1 cup): *thiamine* * 0.30 mg; *riboflavin* * 0.13 mg, *niacin* * 16.2 mg; protein 26.9 gm; calories 559; fat 44.2 gm; *carbohydrates* 23.6 gm; *calcium* 74 mg; *iron* 1.9 mg; *phosphorus* 393 mg; *potassium,* 337 mg.

peanut butter. A blend of peanuts which have been shelled, roasted, blanched, and then ground. Small amounts of salt and hydrogenated vegetable oil are added.

peanut flour. Flour made from ground peanuts from which the greatest part of the oil has been extracted.

peanut oil. Oil obtained by the cold pressing of peanuts. When filtered it is sweet, nearly colorless, and used both for table use and in cooking.

pear (Pyrus). A tree and its fruit cultivated in temperature zones. The pear tree belongs to the rose family, whose varieties include apples, plums, apricots, raspberries, and strawberries. Fruit may be roundish or bell-shaped, symmetrical or uneven. It may have a long or short neck. The stem is attached to the fruit. The skin ranges in color from green to yellow with red tinge to russet. Flesh is fine-grained and juicy. Taste may be sweet buttery, spicy to acid. Nutritive values (1 cup): *carotene* * (vitamin A), 880 I.U. per 100 gm; *thiamine* * .02 mg; *riboflavin* * .05 mg; *niacin* * 9 mg; *ascorbic acid* * (vitamin C) 8 mg; protein 0.5 gm; calories 46; fat 0.1 gm; carbohydrates 12 gm; calcium, 8 mg; iron 0.6 mg; phosphorus 22 mg; potassium 310 mg.

pecan (*Carya illinoensis*). A native American nut of the pecan tree. Pecans have very thin shells and the meat has a fat content of over 70 percent, which is higher than that of any other vegetable product. Nutritive values (1 cup): *carotene** (vitamin A) 50 I.U. per 100 gm; *thiamine** .72 mg; *riboflavin** 0.11 mg; *niacin** 0.9 mg; *ascorbic acid** (vitamin C) 2 mg; protein 9.4 gm; calories, 696; fat 73 gm; carbohydrates 13 gm; calcium 74 mg; iron 2.4 mg; phosphorus 324 mg; potassium 300 mg.

pectic substances. A class of polymers of galaturonic acid, a derivative of *galactose**, found in fruit. See *pectins*.

pectinases. Enzymes that hydrolyze pectin, a carbohydrate in fruits that causes the juice to jell. See *pectin*.

pectins. Nondigestible *polysaccharides* that are polymers of galacturonic methyl esters (oxidized forms of *galactose**). Pectins occur in vegetables but are found mostly in fruits. Pectins are often used as a base for fruits and jellies because they gel or solidify in the presence of the sugar and acid in fruit juices. This property of solidifying into a gel also makes them useful in cosmetics and drugs.

pectolytic bacteria. Some bacterial species of *Erwinia, Bacillus* and *Clostridium* contain pectolytic *enzymes* which are responsible for the softening of plant tissue and the loss of the jelling power of fruit juices. Most authorities agree that two enzymes, pectinesterase and polygalacturonase, are chiefly involved in the *hydrolysis* of *pectin* which prevents gel formation. The pectolytic enzymes or pectinases are used in the food industry for clarification of fruit juices, wines, vinegars, syrups and jellies that contain suspended particles of pectin. Pectinases also help prevent the jelling of fruit juice concentrates. Pectinases are extracted from bacteria or plant materials for these uses.

pellagra. A vitamin deficiency disease caused by a lack of *niacin** (nicotinic acid, nictotinamide) in the diet. The disease is rare in Europe and North America, although several decades ago high incidences occurred among the poor in the southern United States. The earliest symptom of pellagra is *glossitis,* a burning sensation of the tongue. Advanced stages of the disease are characterized by the 4 D's, diarrhea, dermatitis, dementia, and death. The dermatitis is precipitated by exposure to the sun, heat, or friction and appears only on areas of the body subjected to those conditions. The disease is closely associated with cultures or conditions that are nutritionally poor but have a high consumption of corn. Corn or maize is not deficient in niacin, but it appears to be bound in some form that makes niacin unavailable. Corn is also very low in

the amino acid *tryptophan* * which has niacin activity. Pellagra is almost unknown in Mexico, which has a corn culture. However, during the preparation
of tortillas, the maize (corn) is treated with lime water and the bound form of
niacin is apparently released by treatment with alkali. See *niacin.*

pemmican. North American Indian cake made of dried and powdered meat
mixed with melted fat, and various berries, and herb seasoning.

pentose. A class of simple sugar (*monosaccharide*) containing five carbon
atoms, as for example, *ribose* *, arabinose, *xylose* *. Pentoses are synthesized
by all types of animals as well as man from *glucose* * and a.e not essential in
the diet. Pentose sugars most commonly present in human foods are L-
arabinose and D-xylose which are widely distributed in fruits and root vegetables. The pentoses, *deoxyribose* * and ribose, are components of *deoxyribonucleic acid* * (DNA) and *ribonucleic acid* (RNA). The pentoses are
normally found in human urine in small amounts, related to the dietary intake.

penuche. A candy made from brown sugar which is cooked to a soft ball stage,
cooled to lukewarm, and then beaten until smooth and creamy.

pepper, red. The ground product derived from cayenne peppers and large long
peppers of the Cayenne groups such as the Long Red Cayenne. Cayenne and
red peppers are used to add flavor to meat, fish, and egg dishes, sauces, etc.

peppergrass (*Lepidium*). Garden cress and shepherd's purse are other names
for this annual spring herb. The flavor is similar to watercress, and like watercress it is used as a garnish or in salads.

peppermint (*Mentha piperita*). An aromatic perennial herb, with a cool refreshing flavor. Its leaves are used for flavoring and oil. The oil is made by
steam distillation after the crop, in full blossom, is dried, and it is used widely
for gum, candy, dentifrices, and other pharmaceutical preparations.

pepperone. A highly spiced dry sausage of Italian origin. It is made from
coarsely ground beef and pork mixed with salt, coarsely ground black pepper,
cayenne, and garlic. The mixture is cured and stuffed into casings and linked in
pieces 10 to 12 inches long. The sausage is then air-dried at moderate room
temperatures for 3 to 4 weeks.

pepsin. Formed in the *pyloric glands* and the *chief cells* of the gastric glands in
the stomach. It is present in these cells in the form of a *zymogen,* an anteced-
ent inactive substance called propepsin, or pepsinogen, which is quickly

changed to active pepsin by the action of hydrochloric acid. Pepsin (gastric protease) is a proteolytic enzyme requiring an acid medium in which to function. It has the property of hydrolyzing proteins through several stages into polypeptides with hydrolysis taking place preferentially at the amino acid residues *tryptophan*, phenylalanine*, tyrosine*, methionine** and *leucine**.

peptic ulcer. An ulcer is a circumscribed defect of varying depth in the lining of the stomach or duodenum. If deep enough, it may extend through the wall of the digestive tract and perforate, causing *peritonitis;* or it may erode into a blood vessel, producing bleeding. The cause of peptic ulcer is not known completely but hydrocholoric acid plays an important role in its development. Hydrochloric acid also is important in the production of ulcer pain. The continuous neutralization of acid promotes the healing of ulcers. The term ''peptic'' ulcer relates to the enzyme pepsin which together with the hydrochloric acid, contributes to the digestive action of the stomach content upon the surface of the stomach or duodenum, presumably impairing the integrity of localized areas and thus leading to the formation of peptic ulcer.

peptide. The linkage of amino acids together by *peptide linkage* or amide bonds in a chainlike molecule is a peptide. Prefixes indicate the number of amino acid units involved, e.g., a dipeptide consists of two amino acids joined together, and a polypeptide contains a large but unspecified number of amino acids. Peptides are intermediate products of the enzymatic hydrolysis of protein.

peptide linkage (peptide bond). The amide linkage of two amino acids by condensation of the amino group of one amino acid with the *carboxyl* group of another amino acid.

$$
\begin{array}{ccc}
& H & H \\
& | & | & R \\
& C & N & | \\
H_2N \diagup \; | \; \diagdown \diagup \; \diagdown \diagup C \diagup COOH \\
& R & C & | \\
& \| & H \\
& O
\end{array}
$$

Peptide linkage

peptization. Colloidal dispersions are sometimes prepared by adding a third substance to the system. This substance acts upon the particles and reduces them to colloidal dimensions. Such a substance is called a peptizing agent and the process is known as peptization. Certain of the digestive processes of animals involve peptization.

peptones. An intermediate product of enzymatic hydrolysis of protein. The term is seldom used today, polypeptide is used in its stead. One of the soluble forms that results from the action of gastric juice upon proteins. Peptones are a stage in protein digestion prior to the formation of amino acid. Soluble in water, not coagulable by heat, and not precipitated by saturating their solutions with ammonium sulfate or zinc sulfate. These represent an advanced stage of cleavage to small polypeptides.

perch (*Perca fluviatilis*). A widely distributed, spiny-finned freshwater food fish. Known also as the yellow, barred, or ring perch, they are carnivorous, voracious, and prolific. Perch grow to a large size in still brackish waters of bays and inlets. They are distinctively colored with an olive back lightening along the sides to golden yellow. The pike-perch is a genus closely related to the perch family, but showing some resemblance to the pike in the elongated body shape. One of the best-known species of this group is the wall-eyed pike, a famous game fish. The name perch is also widely applied to many other spiny-finned fish, including some salt water varieties. Among the latter are the so-called "ocean perch" which belong to the sea bass and rockfish family. Perch is a mild fish, with firm white coarse flesh and a delicate flavor. Perch are a good source of protein.

Yellow perch, Raw, 100 gm = 91 calories
Pike perch, Raw, 100 gm = 93 calories
Ocean perch, Atlantic, Raw, 100 gm = 88 calories
Ocean perch, Pacific, Raw, 100 gm = 95 calories

percomorph. Refers to fish of the perch family. Percomorph oil, prepared from the livers of such fish, is a concentrated source of *vitamin D* *.

periosteum. The membrane covering bone surfaces. See *bone*.

peristalsis. The esophagus is composed chiefly of muscles which contract in wavelike fashion along the length of the tube, and the entire digestive tract. These are called peristaltic waves or movements. The term peristalsis means "clasping and compressing" and describes the contraction of one part of the tube, then contraction below it and relaxation of the originally constricted segment, and etc. Many tubes composed of smooth muscle exhibit peristalis.

peritoneum. A membrane covering the intestinal organs.

peritonitis. An inflammation of the peritoneum, the membrane covering the intestine. It usually occurs when one of the organs it encloses ruptures or is per-

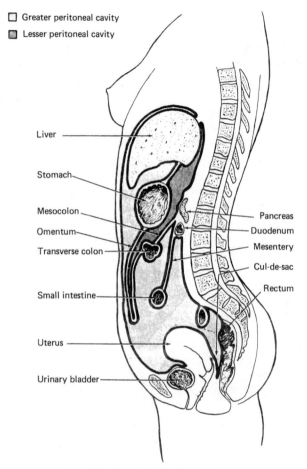

☐ Greater peritoneal cavity
▦ Lesser peritoneal cavity

Liver

Stomach

Mesocolon

Omentum

Transverse colon

Small intestine

Uterus

Urinary bladder

Pancreas

Duodenum

Mesentery

Cul-de-sac

Rectum

Abdominal cavity showing peritoneum.

forated so that the organ's contents (including bacteria) are spilled into the abdominal cavity. The most common cause is rupture of the appendix following appendicitis. Symptoms are nausea, vomiting, and severe abdominal pain. The abdominal muscles become very rigid and are tender to pressure.

peroxidase. An enzyme that catalizes the oxidation of certain organic compounds with hydrogen peroxide. The general reaction is $RCH_2CH_2OH + H_2O_2 \xrightarrow{\text{peroxidase}} RCH_2COOH + H_2O$. The enzyme is very active in plant tissue and a small amount of this activity is found in kidney, liver, milk, and leucocytes. The enzyme contains iron. See *catalase*. peroxidase

peroxisomes. An organelle within the cytoplasm that contains several oxidative enzymes. Among its contents are *catalase* and D-amino acid oxidase. The organelle is about 0.5 microns in diameter.

persimmon (*Diospyros*). A warm-weather fruit of which there are two species of importance. One of them is the common or American persimmon, *D. virginiana*. This species produces a small, pulpy fruit which can vary in size from a half to two inches in diameter, is yellow or orange with a reddish cheek and has large seeds embedded in its soft flesh. The second species, *D. Kaki,* is known as the Oriental or Japanese persimmon. The tree can reach 40 or more feet in height; its fruit grows to some three inches in diameter. Some varieties have large seeds in the semitransparent pulp; other varieties are seedless. When ripe the fruit somewhat resemble a tomato in size and surface texture, and are reddish-orange in color. The taste is deliciously sweet, with a faint acid tinge, but persimmons must be ripe to be edible. Persimmons are eaten out-of-hand and used in salads and puddings. Persimmons contain fair quantities of *ascorbic acid* * (vitamin C) and *carotene* * (vitamin A). American, raw, 100 gm = 127 calories; Japanese, raw 100 gm = 77 calories.

pH. The pH is an expression of the *hydrogen ion* (H^+) concentration in water solutions. The generally used scale is from 0 to 14 where 0 is equivalent to a concentration of 1 molar hydrogen ion and 14 is 10^{-14} (0.00000000000001 molar). The pH scale has an expotential function. The "p" comes from the German word "potenz" which means power in the sense of an exponent, e.g., a^2 is "a" to the second power. The pH is exactly neutral with the equal quantities of H^+ and OH^- ions in solutions, as in water. A deviation from 7 to 14 indicates increasing alkalinity, whereas a deviation from 7 toward 1 indicates increasing acidity. Blood at pH 7.4 is slightly alkaline. Urine varies from strongly acid, pH 5, to strongly alkaline pH 8. Very small changes in the numerical value of pH represents large changes in acidity or alkalinity, e.g., a change in pH 7 to 6 represents a tenfold increase in acidity. The acidity or alkalinity of a solution is referred to as its reaction, and in physiology the reaction of body fluids is usually expressed in terms of pH. The reaction of blood, for example is pH 7.4 which is slightly alkaline. See *acids, acids and bases.*

phagocyte. A cell capable of ingesting bacteria or other foreign material. It is a defense mechanism performed by *macrophages* (leucocytes) in the blood and in the lymph nodes and other organs. See *phagocytosis.*

phagocytosis. The engulfing of microorganisms and cells by phagocytes, usually white blood cells (leucocytes) or other related cells. Phagocytes are present in the blood and lymph and also in the lungs, liver, and spleen.

pharmacology. The science of drugs, especially the actions of drugs on the body. No drug can introduce a new action in the body. Drugs modify actions which are already there and can either increase or decrease the actions or functions of the cell.

pharynx. The pharynx, or throat, connects the nose and mouth with the lower air passages and esophagus. It is divided into three parts; the nasopharynx, the oropharynx, and the laryngopharynx. It is continued as the esophagus. Both air and food pass through the pharynx. It carries air from the nose to the larynx, food from the mouth to the *esophagus*. The walls of the pharynx contains masses of lymphoid tissues called adenoids and tonsils.

phenformin. An oral *hypoglycemic* agent used in the treatment of *diabetes*.

phenotype. The outward expression of gene action in a given environment.

phenylalanine (PHE). Mol. Wt. 165. An essential amino acid. The nonessential amino acids tryosine and cystine are an intermediate class, between amino acids that can easily be formed from a number of precursors and those that cannot be made at all. Tyrosine can be made only from the essential amino acid phenylalanine by addition of one hydroxyl (OH) group, and the reverse reaction (removal of the OH from tyrosine* to form phenylalanine) does not take place. Part of the need for phenylalanine in the body is to form tyrosine if the latter is not included in the diet. Thus the presence of tyrosine will reduce or spare the amount of phenylalanine required in the diet. Phenylalanine is a precursor to several important metabolites in addition to tyrosine. They include the skin pigment *melanin* and the hormones *epinephrine*, *norepinephrine*, and *thyroxine*.

$$\text{C}_6\text{H}_5 - \text{CH}_2 - \overset{\overset{\text{H}}{|}}{\underset{\underset{\text{NH}_2}{|}}{\text{C}}} - \text{COOH}$$

phenylketonuria (PKU). The excretion of phenylpyruvic acid and other phenyl compounds in the urine, resulting from the hereditary lack of an enzyme necessary for the conversion of the amino acid phenylalanine to tyrosine. Phenylalanine derivatives accumulate in blood and tissues, and mental retardation occurs in infants.

phenylpyruvic acid. Mol. Wt. 164. An intermediate metabolic product of the essential amino acid *phenylalanine* *.

$$\text{CH}_2\text{C—COOH}$$
$$\underset{O}{\overset{\|}{}}$$

phloem. A vascular tissue in which material can move up and down, and functions, particularly in the transport of organic materials such as carbohydrates and amino acids. Phloem is a complex tissue and contains both parenchyma and sclerenchyma cells in addition to cells unique to it; sieve cells and companion cells. The sieve cells are the vertical transport unit.

phosphates. *Salts* of *phosporic acid,* H_3PO_4.

phosphocreatine (creatine phosphate). Mol. Wt. 211. A chemical form of energy stored primarily in muscle tissues. It is the energetic equivalent of adenosine triphosphate (ATP) and acts to provide energy for muscle contraction. Phosphocreatine is a metabolic derivative of acetic acid. The end product of phosphocreatine is creatinine which is excreted in the urine.

$$\overset{NH}{\overset{\|}{H_2O_3P\text{—NH—C—N—CH}_2\text{COOH}}}$$
$$\underset{CH_3}{\overset{|}{}}$$

phospholipids. Compounds consisting of glycerol, two fatty acids, and a phosphate group. Phospholipids have the useful property of attracting both water soluble and fat soluble substances due to the hydrophilic (water-attracting) phosphoryl grouping and the hydrophobic (water-repelling) fatty acids in the molecule. They act as emulsifiers in the body and during digestion. In combination with protein, they are constituents of cell membranes and membranes of subcellular particles where they serve as a liaison between fat-soluble and water-soluble materials that must penetrate the membrane and interact once they have gained entry. Examples of phospholipids are *lecithin* * and *phosphatidic acid* which is the precursor to other phospholipids.

phosphoprotein. A conjugated protein that contains phosphorus, e.g., *nucleoprotein, casein.*

phosphoric acid. Mol. Wt. 101. A strong acid capable of dissociating three hydrogen ions (H^+). The *sodium* * and *potassium* * salts of phosphoric acid serve as important *buffers* within and outside of the cell. The three dissociation constants of phosphoric acid are 7.25×10^{-3} M, 6.31×10^{-8} M, and 3.98×10^{-13} M, corresponding to pK' values of 2.14, 7.20, and 12.4, respectively. It is the second pK' value, 7.20 which is important in maintaining the neutrality of the blood and cells.

$$
\begin{array}{c}
O \\
\parallel \\
HO-P-OH \\
\vert \\
OH
\end{array}
$$

phosphorus (P). Element number 15. Mol. Wt. 31. The human body contains roughly 12 gm/kg fat-free tissue; of this amount about 85 percent is contained in the inorganic phase of skeletal structures. The phosphorus content of plasma is about 3.5 mg/100 ml plasma. Organic phosphates are a part of the structure of all body cells and are intimately involved in cellular functions and phosphate salts act as important *buffers*. Phosphorus is a constituent of the high energy compound ATP and thus is necessary for energy transductions, which are necessary for all cellular activity. Rich sources of phosphorus in the diet are meats (especially organs), fish and poultry, cheeses and milk, eggs, nuts, legumes, and all foods made from grains. Fruits (especially dried ones) and vegetables contribute lesser amounts of phosphorus to the diet. In general, edible roots, stems, and flowerlets of plants contain similar amounts of both calcium and phosphorous. The intake of phosphorous is considered sufficient if the diet is adequate in calcium.

phosphorus absorption. Normally about 70 percent of the phosphorus ingested in foods is absorbed. Most favorable absorption takes place when *calcium* and phosphorous are ingested in approximate equal amounts. As with calcium, the presence of *vitamin D* * increases absorption. Simple phosphates such as calcium phosphate or potassium sodium phosphate are absorbed as such in the small intestine.

phosphorus test. A chemical test on blood; used in diagnosis of certain diseases of the kidney and metabolism.

phosphorylation. The addition of phosphate to an organic compound. The process of phosphorylation is essential for life since many biosynthetic pathways depend on the additions of phosphate to metabolites. The oxidation of the sugars to carbon dioxide and water and energy commences with the formation of sugar phosphates. The major form of chemical energy is *adenosine triphosphate* (ATP) which derives its important biosynthetic role by transferring phosphate to other metabolites. The process whereby the energy of oxidation is conserved as chemical energy is called *oxidative phosphorylation* and relates to the synthesis of ATP.

photolyisis. The splitting of a molecule under the action of light; e.g., the cleavage of water in photosynthesis by the radiant energy absorbed by chlorophyll.

photosyntheis. The metabolic process that makes possible the capture and utilization of the energy in sunlight. The process by which plants containing chlorophyll are able to manufacture carbohydrates by combining carbon dioxide from the air and water from the soil. Sunlight is used as energy and chlorophyll is a catalyst. See *photolysis*.

phylloquinone. Compound used as a prothrombogenic agent. See *vitamin K* *.

physiologic saline. A solution of sodium chloride isotonic (having the same osmotic pressure) as blood. The isotonic concentration of physiologic saline, also called normal saline, is 0.154 normal or about a 0.9 percent solution.

phytic acid. Mol. Wt. 660. Inositol hexaphosphonic acid; a phosphoric acid ester of *inositol* *; occurs in nuts, legumes, and outer layers of cereal grains; the insoluble calcium magnesium salt is called phytin. Because phytic acid forms insoluble salts with calcium, iron and magnesium, it interferes with the intestinal absorption of these minerals.

Phytic acid

piccalilli. A pickle relish made with chopped green tomatoes, red and green peppers, onions, sugar, vinegar, pickling spices, and often cabbage. It originated in the East Indies.

pigeon pea (*Cajanus cajan*). A tropical legume, widely grown in India where it is known as red gram; also popular in the West Indies.

pigment. Any of the coloring materials in the cells and tissues of plants and animals. In fruit and vegetables, the green pigment is chlorophyll; orange to red pigments are carotenoids; red to blue colors are anthocyanins; light-yellow pigments are flavones and flavonols. In man, the dark skin pigment is melanin, a derivative of the essential amino acid *phenylalanine**. In meat the chief pigment producing the pink or red color is myoglobin.

pignolia. The edible seed of the cones of a nut pine (*Pineus*). Nutritive values (1 cup): *carotene** (vitamin A) 230 I.U. per 100 gram; *thiamine** 0.67 mg; *niacin** 1.4 mg; proteins 31.1 gm; calories 552; fat 47.4 gm; carbohydrates 11.6 gm.

pike (*Esox lucius*). An important family of American freshwater food and game fish which includes the pike, the smaller pickerel, and the larger muskellunge. All have long bodies, heads with sharp points, jaws that look like a duck's bill, and vicious teeth. The common or Great Lakes pike is grayish-blue or green in color with many whitish or yellowish spots. Their average weight is about 10 pounds. Pickerels average 2 to 3 pounds, and the muskellunge, average 5 to 6 feet in length and often weighs over 60 pounds. Pike have a good texture and flavor, and are a good source of protein.

Muskellunge, Raw, 100 gm = 109 calories
Pickerel, Raw, 100 gm = 84 calories
Pike, Raw, 100 gm = 90 calories

pilaf. A rice dish basic to the cuisines of Greece and the Near East and southern Asia. The dish is usually made of well-seasoned long-grained rice sauteed in oil or butter, then boiled in bouillon or broth. A pilaf can contain meats, fish, seafood, vegetables, and any herbs or spices.

pilchards. Fully grown sardines, smaller than herrings; usually canned in oil, brine, or tomato sauce.

pilnut. (*Canarium ovatum*). An edible seed of the Philippine burseraceous tree. The seed tastes like a sweet almond. Nutritive values (1 cup): *carotene** (vitamin A) 40 I.U. per 100 gm; *thiamine** .88 mg; *riboflavin** 0.09 mg; *niacin** 0.5 mg; protein 11.4 gm; calories 669; fat 71.1 gm; carbohydrates 8.4 gm; calcium 140 mg; iron 3.4 mg; phosphorus 554 mg.

pimento. Refers to the sweet red pepper, the kind from which paprika is made.

pineal gland. Shaped somewhat like a pine cone (hence the name) it is connected to the thalmus of the brain by a hollow stalk. The pineal gland excretes the hormone *melantonin stimulating hormone* (MSH).

pineapple (*Ananas comosus*). A hardy perennial herbaceous plant, native to northern South America. The plant grows abut knee-high, has a short stem and a round head of stiff grayish striped leaves, with spiny tips and prickly edges. The lavender-blue flowers grow in these heads, and the golden yellow fruit emerges from the leaves. Pineapples weigh from 1 to 20 pounds; the average weight is between 3 and 6 pounds. Pineapple is a fair source of *ascorbic acid**** (vitamin C), and has small amounts of *carotene**** (vitamin A).

Raw, 100 gm = 52 calories
Canned, water pack, solids and liquids, 100 gm, = 39 calories
Canned, light syrup pack, solids and liquid 100 gm, = 59 calories
Canned, heavy syrup pack, solids and liquid, 100 gm, = 74 calories
Frozen chunks, 100 gm = 85 calories
Canned juice, unsweetened, 100 gm = 55 calories
Frozen concentrate, unsweetened and undiluted, 100 gm = 179 calories
Frozen concentrate, sweetened and diluted with 3 parts water 100 gm = 52 calories
Candied, 100 gm = 316 calories

pine nut (*Pinus*). The edible seed of several varieties of pines; the seed develops in the pine cone which is heated in order to spread its scales and make the seed easy to dislodge. Some pine nuts come from native American trees and are known as Indian nuts, pignons, or piñons. Others comes from the Mediterranean stone pine. Pine nuts are the size of a small bean, with a thin, light brown shell. The meat is white or cream-colored. The texture is soft and the flavor mild. Pine nuts contain some protein, and are high in fat. Imported, 100 gm = 552 calories; domestic, 100 gm = 635 calories.

pinkil. A sausage made of beef, oats, and pork fat.

pinto beans. A speckled, pink bean related to the kidney bean and common in Mexico and the southwest United States. It is used dried.

pinocytosis. Proteins and fats sometimes enter cells by the process of pinocytosis. The word means "cell drinking." It does not mean the cell itself is engulfed. Rather, as these large molecules become attached to the cell's outer surface, the cell membrane forms a pocket and encircles them. This creates an invagination, or incupping on the cell surface from which the engulfed material is eventually released into the cell cytoplasm. Apparently this is the mechanism by which fat, for example, is absorbed from the small intestine.

piperade. A combination of tomatoes, sweet peppers, and onions, or any two of them, which is cooked until very tender. To this combination eggs are added.

pirogi. A Russian dish of savory and plump turnovers made from dough filled with a meat, fish, or vegetable mixture. Served with borscht or a meat broth.

pistachio (*Pistacia vera*). The edible seed of a small evergreen tree. Cashew and sumac trees are members of the same family. The fruits of the pistachio tree grow in clusters. Each fruit is about the size of an olive, about one-half to one-inch long with a thin, hard, brownish-red shell. Within it is found a seed, the pistachio nut, which is pale green to creamy white in color, a single solid piece. It has a fine texture and a mild pleasing flavor. The nutmeats are used for coloring and flavoring ice cream, cakes, and confectionery. They are also eaten out of the shell as is, or salted. The color of the nut is so distinctive that its name has been given to a special shade of light green. Pistachios contain some protein and niacin and are rich in calcium, phosphorus, iron, *carotene* * (vitamin A), and *thiamine* *. Shelled, 100 gm = 594 calories.

pituitary gland. The pituitary gland, located deep within the skull, is also called the hypophysis. This small gland has the two lobes, the adenohypophysis (the anterior lobe) and the neurohypophysis (the posterior lobe), each producing distinctive hormones. The hormones produced by the adenohypophysis of the pituitary have names with the suffix "trophin," meaning nourishing. (1) *Somatotrophin* (STH) means body nourishing. This hormone influences skeletal and soft tissue growth. (2) *Adrenocorticotrophic hormone* (ACTHO) stimulates the cortex of the *adrenal gland* to produce its hormone, *thyroxine* *, an *iodine* * *derivative* of the amino acid *tyrosine* *. The posterior lobe, the neurohypophysis of the pituitary gland produces the hormone oxytocin that stimulates the contraction of the smooth muscle of the uterus, so it is important in childbirth. Another posterior lobe hormone which helps prevent excessive water excretion from the kidney is called the *antidiuretic hormone* (ADH).

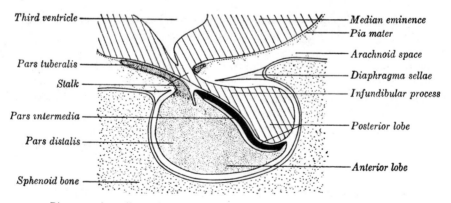

Diagrammatic median sagittal section of the hypophysis cerebri or pituitary gland.

Anterior lobe hormonal secretions:
  Growth hormone (STH, Somatotrophic hormone)
  Thyroid-Stimulating hormone (TSH, Thyrotrophic hormone)
  Follicle stimulating hormone (FSH)
  Luteinizing hormone (LH)
  Lactogenic hormone (Prolactin)
  ACTH (Adrenocorticotrophic hormone)
Posterior lobe hormonal secretions.
  Vasopressin (Pitressin) *ADH* (Antidiuretic hormone)
  Oxytocin

pizza. A savory open pie of Italian origin. The word pizza in Italian means "pie" any kind of pie, and the particular pie known in the United States as pizza is pizza alla Napoletana, a dish typical of Naples. A pizza consists of a thin layer of yeast dough, rolled or patted to fit a large cookie sheet or special pizza pan, topped with tomatoes, tomato paste, herbs, and slices of Mozzarella cheese. The variations are endless, anchovies, sausages, vegetables, olives, anything can go into the sauce. The pizza is then baked until the cheese is bubbly and the crust edge is golden brown. Caloric value: Home recipe, cheese topping, baked, 100 gm = 236 calories, frozen baked, 100 gm = 245 calories.

placenta. An organ within the uterus of the mother which connects to the developing fetus. The fetus obtains food and oxygen from the mother through the placenta. The blood vessels of the mother are in close contact with the blood vessels of the fetus so that interchanges of fetal blood substances and oxygen diffuse from maternal blood vessels into fetal blood vessels. Waste products and carbon dioxide diffuse fetal blood vessels into maternal blood vessels. The fetus is connected to the placenta by the umbilical cord. The health status and development of the fetus depends upon the condition of the placenta.

plantain (*Musa paradisciaca*). The fruit of a large treelike tropical herb. The plantain belongs to the same family as the common eating banana, but plantains are larger, starchier, and less sweet; they must be cooked to be palatable. When boiled, baked, or fried, or made into flour they are excellent and very digestible. Plantain is an important food plant in the tropics, occupying the same position of an essential staple as does the potato in the temperate zones. Plantain is high in carbohydrates and a fair source of *carotene* * (vitamin A) and vitamin B. Raw 100 gm = 119 calories.

plaque. Patches of unnatural formations on tissues such as tooth surfaces and inner arterial walls. The plaque on teeth surfaces are mineral deposits and predispose to tooth decay. The plaques found in walls of arteries, called atheroma, contain *cholesterol*, oleic acid*, neutral fat,* and some connective or scar tissue of protein origin. Their formation is related to abnormal fat metabolism. They contribute to stiffening of blood vessel walls, closing of arteries, choking circulation, and rupturing arteries. See *atherosclerosis.*

plasma. Making up more than one-half of the total volume of blood, plasma is the liquid carrier for blood cells, carbon dioxide, dissolved wastes, and nutrients. It brings hormones and antibodies (protective substances) to the tissues. Other components of plasma are water, oxygen, nitrogen, fat, carbohydrates, and proteins. Fibrogen, one of the plasma protein, helps blood clotting. When blood clots, the liquid portion that remains is *serum.* Blood serum contains no blood cells.

plasma cells. Round or irregular-shaped white blood cells found in greatest numbers in all connective tissues but especially in the connective tissue of the alimentary mucous membrane and great omentum. Plasma cells derive from lymphocytes and are the actual formers of circulating *antibodies.*

plasma proteins. Plasma protein consists mainly of the proteins albumin and globulin which influence the shift of water from one compartment to another. Proteins are colloids and form colloidal solutions. Such a solution is a mixture of large, gelatinous particles or molecules which do not readily pass through separating membranes. Therefore they normally remain in the blood vessels, where they exert a collodial *osmotic pressure* (COP), which maintains the integrity of the blood volume in the vascular compartment.

Plasma Proteins	g/liter Range
Total Protein	58–78
Albumin	35–56
Globulins	16–31
Fibrinogen	2–4

platelets. One type of *white blood cell.* Tiny, granular corpuscles about 2μ in diameter which are formed from special bone-marrow cells called *megakaryocytes* and are concerned in the control of bleeding after injury. There are usually 250,000–750,000 in every ml of blood and their presence is essential for the normal retraction of blood clots which expresses the serum. The platelets break up in areas of damage to the blood vessels and liberate a compound called *serotonin** which causes small blood vessels to contract strongly, tending to reduce bleeding after the injury.

platelet count. A microscopy test on blood; used in the diagnosis of persons having a tendency to hemorrhage.

plum (*Prunus*). The tree and edible fruit of many species. A large family which also includes almonds, apricots, cherries, and peaches. The fruits grow in clusters, have a smooth skin, and a flattened pit. Plums may be round or oval; with a skin in various shades of purple, red, blue, yellow, or green. The flesh is thick and juicy and it may be sweet or tart. They are delicious in the natural state, stewed, or made into sauce. Most important among the many plum varieties are the common, or European plum, *domestica;* the oriental, or Japanese plum, *salicina;* the native American wild plums including *P. americana, P. nigra,* and *P. mexicana;* and the beach plum, *P. maritima.*

Fresh prune-plums, raw, 100 gm = 75 calories;
Fresh damson, raw, 100 gm = 66 calories;
Fresh Japanese and hybrid, raw, 100 gm = 48 calories;
Canned prune-plums, solids and liquid, water pack, 100 gm = 46 calories;
Canned prune-plums, solids and liquid, light syrup pack, 100 gm = 64 calories;
Canned prune-plums, solids and liquid, heavy syrup pack, 100 gm = 83 calories;
Canned prune-plums, solids and liquid, extra heavy syrup pack, 100 gm = 102 calories
Canned greenage, solids and liquid, waterpack, 100 gm = 33 calories.

plumcot. A cross between an apricot and a Japanese plum. The fruits are characteristically large, resembling the apricot externally. The color may range from bright yellow to mottled red, with the flesh having similar variations.

plum pudding. A sweet pudding made with currants, raisins, citrus peel, and spices, either steamed or boiled. Served for dessert with hard sauces or other preferred sauces.

poi. A staple food in the Pacific Islands, made from the edible root of the *taro.* The taro is a plant of the subtropics and tropics, grown for its large underground tuber which has a high starch content and is extremely digestible. The taro root is too acrid to eat raw. To make poi, the root is cooked, pounded, and kneaded until smooth, then mixed with water. It is either strained and served immediately, or more commonly allowed to ferment for a few days.

poisons. A poison is any substance which may cause death, serious illness, or some other harmful effect when it is introduced into the body in a relatively small quantity. The effects of poisons may be local or remote, some poisons have both effects. Local effect means direct action on the part to which the poison is applied, such as corrosion or irritation of the skin. Remote effect means that the action of the poison is in some organ remote from the seat of application or point of introduction. Acute poisoning is the condition brought about by taking an overdose of poison. Chronic poisoning is the condition brought on by taking repeated doses of a poison or as a result of the absorption of poison over a longer period. Some occupational groups are subject to chronic poisoning such as phosphorus, mercury, lead arsenic, etc. See *food poisoning* and *food toxins*.

pollack or pollock (*Pollachius virens*). A saltwater fish which resembles the cod. Also known as the coalfish, found in the Atlantic from Norway to the Mediterranean. A closely related species, the Alaska pollack is plentiful in the Bering Sea and north Pacific waters. The flesh is white, firm, and lean, with a pleasant, delicate flavor. A good source of protein. Raw, 100 gm = 95 calories; cooked and creamed, 100 gm = 128 calories.

polycythemia. A condition characterized by the presence of excess red blood cells that contain a high concentration of hemoglobin. There are several types of polycythemia. One type may be caused by an excess of cobalt. Cobalt is the core of *cobalamin* * (vitamin B_{12}), which is an essential factor in *red blood cell* formation.

polyhydric alcohols. Organic chemists classify as polyhydric alcohols such substances as glycerine (glycerol), mannitol, sorbitol, and propylene glycol, which have one thing in common; they have more than one hydroxyl or OH group. All polyhydric alcohols have in common the ability to readily absorb and retain water (in chemical terms they are hydroscopic) and thus are sometimes added to foods to keep them moist. They are sweet to the taste. Polyhydric alcohols are allowed in foods as *humectants* (water retainers), sweetness controllers, dietary agents, and softening agents. Their chemical action is based on their multiplying of hydroxyl groups that hydrogen-bond to water. This holds water in the food, softens it, and keeps it from drying out. An added feature of polyhydric alcohol is their sweetness. Effective polyalcohols added to sweeten sugarless chewing gum are *mannitol**, *sorbitol**, and *xylitol**.

polymorphism. The existence in a population of multiple genetic forms of a given characteristic.

polyneuritis. A term applied to any condition in which there is symmetrical involvement of the peripheral nerves and is usually believed to be the result of some nutritional, toxic, or metabolic disturbance, but may be inflammatory in nature. Polyneuropathy may result from a deficiency of any one of three B vitamins; *thiamine**, *pyridoxine** (vitamin B_6), or *pantothenic acid**. This vitamin deficiency is exhibited occasionally by alcoholics, and may be associated with stomach and liver symptoms. There has been considerable evidence to indicate that polyneuritis is due to disturbances in the enzyme system of the peripheral nerves.

polyneuropathy. A disease which involves many nerves and affects the peripheral nerves. Symptoms similar to *beriberi,* usually relieved by thiamin* or vitamin-B complex therapy. Chief symptoms are weaknesses, numbness, partial paralysis, and pain in the legs. Motor, reflex, and sensory reactions are lost in most cases. Recovery is a slow process involving weeks or months, and a year may pass before an individual is able to walk unaided. See *polyneuritis.*

polypeptide. A compound consisting of more than three amino acids joined together by *peptide* bonds. See *protein.*

polypeptide chains. Macromolecules consisting of amino acids joined by *peptide* linkage. The term polypeptide is often used in the same sense as the term *protein,* but the concept of protein includes additional characteristics. See *protein.*

polysaccharides. (1) The prefix poly means many and polysaccharides are complex carbohydrates composed of many simple sugar building blocks (*monosaccharides*) bonded together in long chains. They are synthesized by exactly the same kind of condensation reactions as the *disaccharides* and like disaccharides they can be broken down to their constituent monosaccharides by hydrolyses. *Starches* are polysaccharides and are the principal carbohydrate storage products of higher plants; they are composed of many glucose units bonded together. *Glycogen** is a polysaccharide and is the principle carbohydrate storage product in animals. Glycogen is sometimes called "animal starch." *Cellulose** is a highly insoluble polysaccharide occurring widely in plants. Cellulose is the most abundant product of life in the world. (2) The polysaccharides are complex compounds of high molecular weight composed of varying numbers of monosaccharide molecules linked together in long chains. The characteristics of a polysaccharide are determined by the number and kind of monosaccharide units it contains and their arrangement within the polysaccharide molecule. Polysaccharides tend to be insoluble in water and are major constituents of cell membranes. See *starch**, *glycogen** and *dextrin**.

polyunsaturated. An organic compound, such as a *fatty acid,* in which there is more than one double-bond carbon group. The essential fatty acids are among the more highly unsaturated fatty acids (*linoleic**, *linolenic**, and *arachidon-*

ic* acids) and have two, three and four double bonds (respectively) per molecule, hence they are said to be polyunsaturated. Polyunsaturated fats occur in all liquid vegetable oils (corn, cottonseed, safflower, soybeans); in margarines containing substantial amounts of the above oils in liquid form; in fish, mayonnaise, salad dressing and in nuts, walnuts, filberts, pecans, almonds, peanuts, peanut butter.

polyuria. Excessive urination. One symptom of diabetes mellitus.

pomegranate (*Prunica granatum*). The fruit of a bush or small tree with bright green leaves and orange-red flowers. Pomegranates are one of nature's most interesting fruits, about the size of a large orange, with a vaguely six-sided shape, and a hard, leathery skin which can range in color from light yellow to deep purplish-red, but is most often a pinkish- or brownish-yellow. The flesh is a brilliant red, enveloping a large quantity of little seeds. The little flesh there is has a delicious sweet, pleasantly acid taste. Pomegranate is eaten as a fruit, in salads, and sprinkled over desserts. Raw pulp 100 gm = 63 calories.

pompano (*Trachinotus carolinus* and *Palometa Simillima*). An important salt water food fish. The pompano, related to the mackerel, reaches a length of about 18 inches and has a silvery blue skin that is highly polished with gold reflections, and touches of orange on the fins. Its rich yet delicate flavor makes it loved by gourments. A good source of protein and fat. Raw, 100 gm = 166 calories.

popover. A quick bread made from an egg-rich batter. A well-made popover is large, light, puffed up on top, with firm crisp brown walls. The center cavity is moist and yellow. Baked, 100 gm = 224 calories.

poppy seed (*Papaver somniferum*). The minute seeds of an annual species of the large Poppy family. The seeds make an excellent food flavoring in cooking and baking.

porgy. The name applied to various marine food and game fish of the sea bream family. One genus, *Pagerus,* is crimson with blue spots, and is called the red porgy. The variety familiar in Atlantic Coastal waters from Cape Cod to South Carolina belongs to the *Stentotomus genus* and is more commonly known as the scup. The fish is tender, flaky, and of good flavor. Good source of protein. Raw, 100 gm = 112 calories.

pork. The flesh of domestic swine is called pork. Although all flesh of domestic swine may properly be called pork, once pigs or hogs (the older swine) are butchered, the word "ham" is used to describe the rear-leg cuts, particularly when they are cured and/or smoked; and the word "bacon" is used to describe the side of meat, with spareribs removed, when it is cured and smoked. A very good to excellent source of high-quality protein, fair to good in *iron*, fair to good in *niacin**, fair in *riboflavin**, and very good to excellent in *thiamine**.

Boston butt, edible portion, 100 gm = 389 calories
Picnic shoulder, edible portion, 100 gm = 420 calories
Loin roast, edible portion, 100 gm = 387 calories
Spareribs, edible portion, 100 gm = 467 calories

porphyrin. A class of pigmented compounds containing pyrrole nuclei joined in a ring structure. The *heme** of *hemoglobin* belongs to this class of compounds. See *protoporphyrin**.

portal. Usually refers to a portal circulation of blood through the liver. Blood is brought into the liver by the portal vein and out by the hepatic vein.

positive nitrogen balance. See *nitrogen balance.*

porridge. A dish made by boiling a grain or vegetable in water or milk to make a thickened soup to be eaten with a spoon. Today the word is used chiefly in connection with boiled grains, and although a porridge can be made from any grain, the word now is associated mostly with oatmeal.

posset. A beverage made from hot milk, curdled, with wine and lemon juice. It is sweetened with sugar or molasses and sometimes thickened with flour or bread.

posterior. Situated towards the back or at the back.

postprandial. After a meal. For example, many physiological or chemical analyses must be done 12 to 18 hours postprandially, which indicates essentially overnight without food.

potassium (K). Element No. 19. Mol. Wt. 39. Potassium content of the body is about 125 gm, as the potassium ion, K^+, found primarily inside the cells where it functions in association with various enzymes. It is intimately concerned with transmission of the nerve impulse, with skeletal muscle contraction, and with cardiac contraction. Excess or lack of the normal amount of potassium causes immediate malfunctioning of the heart. Daily requirements are estimated at 2 to 4 gm per day. The average diet will readily supply this amount since potassium is widespread in vegetables, fruit, and meat. Meats and other lean muscle tissues, milk, many fruits, especially dried dates, bananas, cantaloupes, apricots, and citrus fruits are good sources of potassium. Tomato juice and the dark green leafy vegetables are also high in nutrient. The following is the potassium content of foods which may contribute substantially to the potassium intake.

Food	mg/100 g Food
All bran	100
Beef, mutton, and poultry	225–400
Biscuits	110–170
Bread, white, and brown	110–225
Breakfast cereal, various brands	110–425
Cheese	100–200
Chocolate milk	350
Coffee, instant, teaspoonful in cup of hot water	138
Dried fruit, various raw	700–1880
Eggs, fresh, whole	150
Fish, various types	225–425
Fresh fruit	120–370
Fruit juices, pure	130–225
Milk, fresh, whole	160
Nuts	400–900
Potato chips	1020
Rice, polished	110
Soya flour	1660
Syrup, golden	225
Treacle	1500
Vegetables, boiled	80–500
Vegetables, raw and salad	200–300

potassium bromate ($KBrO_3$). Mol. Wt. 167. Used to artificially age and improve baking properties of flour. Bromate is used at levels of 5 to 75 ppm. Baking converts bromate (BrO_3^-) to bromide (Br^-) which is absorbed by the body when bread is digested. Bromide circulates harmlessly in the blood and is gradually excreted in the urine.

potato (*Solanum tuberosum*). The white potato is a starchy white tuber of the nightshade family. The common white potato, like corn and tomatoes originated in the Americas and is now the most important starchy food in the temperature regions of America and Europe. Potatoes contain 75 to 80 percent of water and yield from 290 to 380 KJ (70 to 90 kcal)/100g. Of the energy 7.6 percent comes from protein, a negligible amount from fat and most from starch. The protein content is low, about 2 g/100 g, but has a high biological value when fed to man. Potatoes are a useful source of protein tuberin, and contains small but not very important amounts of minerals and the B-group of vitamins. They are a good source of potassium, but variable in *ascorbic acid* * (vitamin C). The ascorbic acid content will vary from 5–50 mg/100 g since there are losses due to storage. (See *vegetables* for nutrient content.) One medium-size potato is a fair source of *ascorbic acid* * (vitamin C). This can be significant when eaten in quantities. Potatoes are a fair source of *thiamine* * and *niacin* *.

Baked in skin, 100 gm = 93 calories
Boiled in skin, 100 gm = 76 calories
Boiled, pared before cooking = 65 calories
French-fried, 100 gm = 274 calories
Mashed, milk and table fat added, 100gm = 94 calories
Frozen, hash-browned, 100 gm = 224 calories
Frozen, French-fried, heated, 100 gm = 220 calories
Frozen, mashed, heated, 100 gm = 93 calories
Potato chips, 100 gm = 568 calories

potato flour or starch. A very fine flour made from potatoes ground to a pulp and freed from their fibers. The residue is flour. Potato flour is used, both for cooking, as in gravies, and sauces, and stewed fruits thickened with potato flour to make a pudding, and for baking, where it gives a dry texture to cakes. Contains some protein, *calcium* *, *phosphorus* *, *riboflavin* *, *thiamine* *, *niacin* *, and *ascorbic acid* * (vitamin C). 100 gm = 351 calories.

pot herb. Any herb whose leaves, stems, or blossoms are cooked like a vegetable. Some of the commonest ones are: borage, chervil, chicory, lovage, sorrel, sweet cicely, and rampion. When cooking pot herbs the leaves are cooked in similar fashion to spinach.

pot liquor. The liquid left in the pot after cooking vegetables.

pot pie. A meat or poultry pie, usually made with vegetables and potatoes and baked in an uncovered casserole with a single or double crust of pastry or biscuit dough.

pot roast. A term applied to larger cuts of meat which are cooked or braised, that is cooked slowly in a small amount of liquid or in steam. The meat may or may not be browned in a little fat before it is braised. See *meat* for nutrient content.

poultry. A word describing all domesticated birds bred and raised for use as human food. The most common are chickens, Rock Cornish hens, ducks, turkeys, geese, guinea fowls, and pigeons, the last marketed as squabs. Other birds occasionally domesticated for the same purpose are peafowl (peacocks), quail, pheasants, and swans. Wild ducks and wild turkeys are considered game birds and not poultry. Poultry ranks as high nutritionally as any food. Since poultry contains many essential nutrients, protein being chief among them, it is recognized as one of the important members of the meat group, one of the four food groups essential for a balanced diet. (The other three are the milk, bread-cereal, and vegetable-fruit groups). In addition to its excellent qualifications as a protein food, poultry is a good source of calcium, phosphorus and iron minerals. Important vitamins present in poultry are *riboflavin*, thiamine*,* and *niacin*.*

powdered sugar. Made from granular sugar by simply grinding the sugar into extremely fine particles and then mixing this sugar with cornstarch to prevent caking.

ppm. See parts per million.

prawn (*Peneus setiferus*). A shrimp-like crustacean ranging in length from 1 inch to 6 inches, and in the tropics may grow to a length of 2 feet. Prawns are sold as shrimp, the only distinction between them is that prawns are considered the large shrimp and the small shrimp are called "shrimps."

pre-beta (β) lipoproteins. The very low-density lipoproteins (VLDL), still carrying large lipid content but including about 8–13 percent *cholesterol,* formed in the liver from endogenous fat sources. See *lipoproteins.*

precipitate. When a chemical comes out of solution due to chemical or physical forces, it is said to precipitate. The curdling of milk (precipitation of casein) that occurs when it is treated with acid (mixing milk with vinegar or grapefruit juice) is a familiar example of precipitation.

precursors. Chemical compound or metabolites may be or are ultimately converted in the body to form another chemical or metabolite. The amino acid *phenylalanine** is converted to the hormone *epinepherine** by a series of biochemical reactions. Phenylalanine, then, is a precursor to epinepherine.

preservative. Any chemical used to increase the safety, shelf life, or pallability of foods. There are two broad classes of preservatives, *antimicrobials* which in-

Poultry
Table 1. Composition of Foods—Edible Portion

Food and Description	Wt. Gm.	Approximate Measure	Food Energy cal	Protein gm	Fat gm	Carbohydrate Total gm	Carbohydrate Fiber gm	Water gm	Calcium μg	Phosphorus μg	Iron μg	Vitamin A I.U.	Thiamin μg	Riboflavin μg	Niacin μg	Ascorbic Acid μg
Chicken, cooked																
Light meat	100	3½ ozs.	166	32	3	0	0	64	11	265	1.3	60	0.04	0.10	11.6	0
no skin, roasted, fried	100	3½ ozs.	197	32	6	1	0	60	12	280	1.3	50	0.05	0.25	12.9	0
Dark meat	100	3½ ozs.	176	28	6	0	0	64	13	229	1.7	150	0.07	0.23	5.6	0
no skin, roasted, fried	100	3½ ozs.	220	30	9	2	0	58	14	225	1.8	130	0.07	0.45	6.8	0
Canned, boneless	100	3½ ozs.	198	22	12	0	0	65	21	247	1.5	230	0.04	0.12	4.4	4
Livers, fried	100	3½ ozs.	140	22	14	2.3	0		16	240	7.4	32,200			11.8	20
Duck, domestic, flesh only	100	3½ ozs.	165	21	8	0	0	69	12	203	1.3		0.10	0.12	7.7	
Turkey, total edible roasted	100	3½ ozs.	263	27	16	0	0	55				Tr.	0.09	0.14	8.0	0
Flesh only, roasted	100	3½ ozs.	190	32	6	0	0	61	8	251	1.8		0.05	0.18	7.7	0

hibit the growth of microorganisms, and antioxidants which prevent rancidity and discoloration due to oxidation.

pressor amines. Amines that promote the rapid constriction of blood vessels and thus elevate the blood pressure dramatically. *Tyramine* * and *histamine* * are pressor amines that occur naturally in such foods as bananas and cheese. See *cheese*.

pretzel. A long roll of dough traditionally twisted into the shape of a loose knot or the letter B. There are two kinds of pretzels, hard and soft, and either salted or unsalted. Hard salted pretzels are also made in the form of sticks and bite-size balls. Small amounts of potassium, calcium, phosphorus, and vitamins, such as *ascorbic acid* * (vitamin C) and *carotene* (vitamin A). Raw, 100 gm = 42 calories.

prickly pear (*Opuntia*). A name given to a cactus and its fruit. Some species of prickly pear have edible fruit. Among them are *O. vulgaris*, or barberry fig, and *O. tuna* or tuna, common in the southwestern United States. The tuna, varies from pearshape to round and is yellowish-rose in color when ripe. Sweet, flavorsome and juicy, it may be peeled, sliced, chilled, and served with lemon juice. Small amounts of potassium, calcium, and phosphorus, and *ascorbic acid* * (vitamin C) and *carotene* * (vitamin A).

primary structure. The sequential order of the building blocks or structural units in macromolecules without taking their spatial structure into consideration. For example, the sequence of *nucleotides* in *nucleic acids* or the sequential order of the *amino acids* in porteins.

principal food constituents. There are three principal constituents of foods. The first is *protein*, the second is the *carbohydrates*, a general term including sugars and *starches*. The third is the fats or *lipids*. Lipids is actually a general term that includes the proper fats and other fat-like substances, such as *cholesterol* *.

proenzyme. Inactive form of enzyme, e.g., pepsinogen. Proenzyme is a genetical term which includes *zymogens*.

progesterone. Mol. wt. 314. The hormone produced in the corpus luteum of the ovary and in the placenta. It acts with estradiol to regulate estrous and menstrual cycles and to maintain pregnancy. Progesterone is also a precursor to *corticosterone* * and *aldosterone* *.

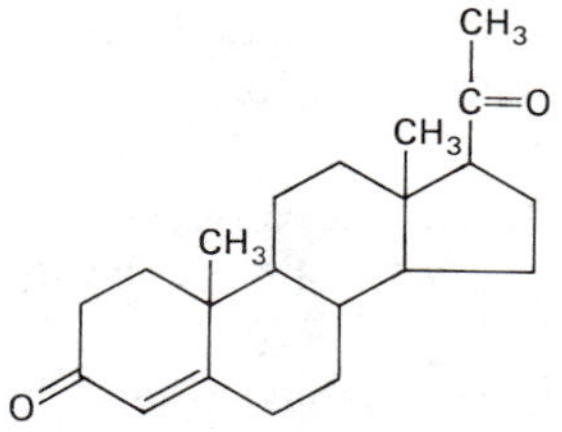

Progesterone

prolactin. See *luteotropic hormone* (LTH).

prolamines. Major plant proteins that are insoluble in neutral solutions, but soluble in weak acids and alkali, and present in cereals. Prolamines are insoluble in water but dissolve in alcoholic solution. On hydrolysis they give large quantities of *proline** and ammonia. Typical prolamines are gliadin from wheat, and zein from maize.

proline. Mol. Wt. 115. Proline is not a true *amino acid* since its nitrogen in the ring structure is an imino group. Because of the structure of proline, it has a special significance in amino acid structure. The presence of proline in an amino acid sequence prevents the formation of the alpha (α) helix at that point. Proline often occurs at points in the *polypeptide* chain sequency of amino acids where bends or changes of direction of chain occur. Proline and glycine* occur in very high concentrations in collagen and give collagen its special structural features. See *collagen*.

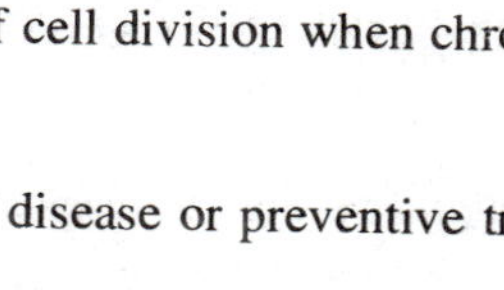

Proline

prophase. The beginning of cell division when chromosomes are first visible in the nucleus.

prophylaxis. Prevention of disease or preventive treatments.

Propionibacteriaceae. Bacteria of the genus *Propionibacterium* are found in foods which ferment *lactic acid**, *carbohydrates*, and *polyalcohols* to *propionic* and *acetic acids**, and carbon dioxide. In Swiss cheese certain species ferment the lactates to produce the gas that aids in the formation of the holes, or "eyes," and also contributes to the flavor.

propylgallate. Mol. Wt. 170. An antioxidant added to foods to retard spoilage of fats and oils. It may also increase slightly the shelf life of foods. Propylgallate is used at levels up to 0.02 percent (of the fat or oil content) in animal fat, vegetable oil, meat products, potato sticks, and chicken soup base, and up to 0.1 percent in chewing gum.

$$\underset{\text{HO}\text{OH}}{\underset{\text{OH}}{\overset{\overset{\displaystyle O}{\overset{\|}{C}}-OCH_2CH_2CH_2CH_3}{\bigcirc}}}$$

propylene glycol. Mol. Wt. 76. A humectant and one of several additions (*glycerol* * and *sorbitol* * are the two others) that are used in foods to help maintain the desired moisture content and texture. Manufacturers add between 0.03 and 5 percent propylene glycol to candy, baked goods, icings, shredded coconut, and moist pet foods. Propylene glycol also serves as a carrier for oily flavoring and helps them dissolve in soft drinks and other water-based foods.

$$\begin{array}{c} \text{OH} \quad \text{OH} \\ | \qquad | \\ CH_3-C-C-H \\ | \qquad | \\ \text{H} \quad \ \text{H} \end{array}$$

Propylene glycol alginate. See *alginate*

prostaglandins. Fatty acids which are thought to be formed in the çell membrane. They are extremely potent substances which produce a variety of physiological effects in small doses. They have a very wide spectrum of actions including behavioral and central nervous system effects as well as actions which appear to mimic or inhibit many of the known hormones. It is believed that prostaglandins serve as regulators of hormonal action by modulating cyclic formations. The essential fatty acid, *arachidonic acid* * is a *precursor* to the prostaglandins. There are several classes of prostaglandins that depend on the hydrocarbon chain structures and the positions of the hydroxyl groups. As examples some of the structures and classifications are given below.

$$
\begin{array}{ccc}
 & R & R' \\
E_1 & -(CH_2)_5CO_2H & -(CH_2)_3CH_3 \\
E_2 & -CH=CH(CH_2)_3CO_2H & -(CH_2)_3CH_3 \\
E_3 & -CH=CH(CH_2)_3CO_2H & -CH=CHCH_2CH_3
\end{array}
$$

PGF (α or β)

etc.

prosthetic group. A small organic chemical group (nonprotein) attached to an *apoenzyme* (protein) and required for enzyme activity. A prosthetic group differs from a *coenzyme* only by the higher affinity for the apoenzyme. Coenzymes are more readily removed from the apoenzyme while prosthetic groups often require chemical treatment or extreme conditions for removal. Functionally prosthetic groups and coenzymes are similar.

protamines. A basic polypeptide that is simpler than *histones, albuminoids,* or *globulins*. Protamins are soluble in water, not coagulable by heat, possess strong basic properties, and on hydrolysis yield a few amino acids, among which the basic amino acids greatly predominate.

proteolytic enzymes. See *protease*.

protease. A protein-splitting enzyme. An enzyme that digests protein. Enzymes are usually named to indicate the substance in which they act. Proteolytic enzyme proteases include the proteinases, which catalyze the hydrolysis of the protein molecule into large polypeptides and the peptidases, which hydrolyze these *polypeptide* fragments as far down as amino acids. The preparation of proteases from microorganisms are mixtures of proteinases and peptidases with varying specificities. Proteases from microorganisms are used primarily for their proteinase activity. Bacteria proteases have been applied to fish livers to liberate fish oil, to meat for tenderization and to malt beverages for clarification and maturation. Fungal proteases are active in the manufacture of soy sauce and other oriental mold fermented foods. Proteases are sometimes added to bread dough, where along with amylases they help improve the consistency of the dough; they are added for thinning egg white so that it can be filtered before drying, and for the hydrolyses of gelatinous protein material in fish waste. Example of proteases are *pepsin, trypsin, chymotrypsin,* and *dipeptidases* all of which aid in the digestion of protein.

protein. Proteins are high molecular weight *polypeptides*. The unit structure or building block of proteins are the *amino acids* and the linear linkage of these amino acids is an amide linkage called the *peptide linkage (bond)*. The peptide bonds are formed through linkage of the alpha-amino group of one amino acid with the alpha-carboxyl group of another. There are 22 amino acids which may participate in the formation of a protein and the kind, number, and sequence of the amino acids determines the physical and chemical characteristics of a protein. The variations are enormous and in nature the extent of that variety is evident. Some proteins are biological catalysts called enzymes; some proteins are a part of cell membranes; some proteins, such as collagen, are for structural purposes outside the cell and others are for structural purposes within the cell, such as the microtubules; some proteins act as carriers of vitamins, metals, oxygens, and a variety of metabolites. Within each of the possible activities of protein are large numbers of different proteins involved in the same general type function. For example, there is an estimated 2 to 4000 individual biochemical reactions going on with each cell, each different and each catalyzed by a different enzyme. Proteins are classified in several ways and some of the classifications overlap one another. The most general classification is to separate proteins into simple proteins and conjugated proteins. Simple proteins contain only amino acids. Conjugated proteins have additional nonprotein molecules as an integral part of their structure. Examples of a simple protein are serum albumin and *collagen*. Examples of conjugated proteins are *hemoglobin* which contains a *heme* group, and *casein* which contains phosphate groups. Proteins are also classified according to the nonprotein components. Another classification of proteins is based upon its three-dimensional structure. Thus globular proteins have a generally round shape, albumins are more elliptical; scleroproteins are fibrous in structure; and *keratins,* which also have one very long dimension with complex intra- and intermolecular bondings. In addition to the primary structure of proteins, the peptide bonds, and the sequence of amino acids, there are three other levels of protein structure. The secondary level of structure relates to the twists and turns that the amino acids make relative to one another along the chain. The secondary structure is determined by the sequence of the amino acids and *hydrogen bonds*. The *alpha* (α) *helix* is an example. The tertiary or third level of structure is the twists and turns one part of the chain of amino acid makes with respect to other part of the chain. The pleated sheet is an example. The tertiary structure determines the overall shape of the molecule. Sometimes separate polypeptide chains associate with one another as a defined unit. The resulting structure is called the quartenary level of structure and each polypeptide chain is called a subunit. Hemoglobin is an example of a protein which requires a quaternary level of structure to be functional. Hemoglobin is composed of four subunits, two alpha (α) subunits, plus two beta (β) subunits. Many enzymes require a quartenary level of structure to be functional. Listed below are examples of proteins in the several different classifications mentioned, with their names, functions, and sources.

Simple Proteins

Name		Source	Function
Globular			
Albumins	Serum albumin Lactalbumin Ovalbumin	Blood Milk Eggs	The albumins function as carrier proteins, and osmotic regulators
Globulins	Myosin	Muscle	A part of the contractile element of muscle
Fribrous			
Collagens	Collagen	Connective tissue, tendons. Elastic tissues.	Structural support
Keratins	Alpha keratin	Hair	Structural support

Congugated Proteins

Name	Nonprotein Component	Source	Function
Nucleoprotein	Nucleic acid	Chromosomes	A part of the genetic apparatus
Mucoproteins	More than 4% carbohydrate	Blood, stomach, mucous linings (intrinsic factor)	Carrier proteins; protects cells
Glycoproteins	Less than 4% carbohydrate	Blood (alpha, beta, and gamma globulins)	Antibodies Enzymes
Lipoproteins	Phospholipids	Membrane	Enzymes; protection; permeability control
Chromoproteins	Heme	Blood (chemoglobin)	Carries oxygen
Metaloprotein	Iron	Blood (transferrin)	Carries iron
Phosphoprotein	Phosphate	Milk (casein)	Nutrient for offspring

Nutritionally proteins are important with respect to amount and with respect to the quality of the protein, i.e., its biologic value. About 1 gm of good-quality protein per kilogram of body weight, as a rule of thumb is sufficient to meet all but the most stringent activity required for a *nitrogen balance*. There is evidence to show that less than half of that value is consistent with good health. A protein uptake that is too low will result in a protein-calorie malnutrition known as *marasmus*. The preferred method for determining the amount of protein intake needed is based upon the individual energy expenditure or caloric requirements per day. The table below gives some examples amples of protein intakes recommended as adequate, based on sex, age, caloric requirements, weight, and the percent of the total caloric intake that should be protein. The quality of the protein is taken as 75 out of a possible 100 (see discussion below) which represents a good protein quality that is found in a well balanced meal.

Recommended Protein Intakes

	Age Years	Calorie Requirements kcal/day	Weight kg	Protein gm/kg	Protein gm/day	Protein Calories as Percent of Total Calories
		(a)	(b)	(c)	(d)	(e)
Both sexes	1–3	1300	12.0	2.4	29	9.0
	4–6	1700	18.0	2.0	36	8.5
	7–9	2100	24.0	1.8	42	8.0
	10–12	2500	30.0	1.6	48	7.75
Females	13–15	2600	46.0	1.0	48	7.5
	16–19	2400	55.0	0.80	44	7.25
	adults	2300	55.0	0.75	41	7.0
Addition for pregnancy	—	—	—	—	8	—
Addition for lactation	—	—	—	—	20	—
Males	13–15	3100	44.0	1.3	58	7.5
	16–19	3600	62.5	1.0	65	7.25
	adults	3200	65.0	0.85	55	7.0

The quality of a protein, its *biological value,* depends upon the correct proportions of the essential amino acids to meet the demands of the body. In this regard, hen's eggs are the best. Hen's eggs are the standard to which all other proteins are compared. It means that the addition of one or more, or a combination of essential amino acids does not increase the ability of the protein from hen's eggs to support growth and repair of tissues at a low level of intake and still maintain *nitrogen balance.* The table on page 383 gives the essential amino acid composition of some proteins.

The comparative quality of the proteins of several foods is given below. Given is the essential amino acid that is lacking in maximum proportion, the limiting amino acid, and which therefore lowers its value below that of hen's egg. Given for comparison is the *chemical score,* based on amino acid analysis of the food, and biological assessment, based on the *net protein utilization* (NPU) in an animal.

Essential Amino Acid Composition of Egg, Milk, Beef, and Wheat
(mg of amino acid per gm of total N)

	Hen's Egg	Cow's Milk	Beef Muscle	Wheat Flour
Isoleucine	415	407	332	262·
Leucine	553	630	515	442
Lysine	403	496	540	126
Phenylalanine	365	311	256	322
Tyrosine	262	323	212	174
Sulphur-containing amino acids	346	211	237	192
Threonine	317	292	275	174
Tryptophan	100	90	75	69
Valine	454	440	345	262

The Limiting Amino Acid, Chemical Score and NPU of Some Common Food Proteins

Food	Limiting Amino Acid	Chemical Score	Biological Assessment (NPU)
Beans	S	42	47
Beef	S	80	80
Cow's milk	S	60	75
Egg	—	100	100
Fish	Tryptophan	75	83
Maize	Tryptophan	45	56
Pork	S*	80	84
Potato	S	70	71
Rice	Lysine	75	67
Wheat flour	Lysine	50	52

* Sulphur-containing amino acids (methionine + cysteine)

What also must be considered in the estimate of whether or not a given food is a good source of protein is the percent of the total calories in that food that is from protein.

The metabolism of protein is the metabolism of its building blocks, the amino acids. Internally, the protein breaks down to amino acids and the body reuses them to build other proteins, or oxidizes them as a source of energy. Protein as an energy source is limited to less than 20 percent of the total caloric need even under conditions of starvation to death. Under normal circumstances about 10 percent or less of protein (dietary plus endogenous) is oxidized for energy. Proteins (amino acids) supply about 4 calories per gram of protein. The amount of

Protein Content of Various Foods, Expressed as gm/100 Kcal and as Their Contribution (percent) to the Total Calories Provided by Each Food

Value of Foods as a Source of Protein	Protein Content g./100 Kcal	Percent Kcal Provided by Protein
Poor		
Cassava	0.83	3.3
Cooked bananas (plantains)	1.0	4.0
Sweet potatoes (*Ipomoea batatas*)	1.1	4.4
Taros	1.7	6.8
Adequate		
Maize (whole meal)	2.6	10.4
Millet (*Pennisetum glaucuam*)	3.4	13.6
Millet (*Setaria italica*)	2.9	11.6
Potatoes	1.9	7.6
Rice (home-pounded)	2.0	8.0
Sorghum (*Sorghum vulgare*)	2.9	11.6
Wheat flour (medium extraction)	3.3	13.2
Good		
Beans and peas	6.4	25.6
Beef (thin)	9.6	38.4
Cow's milk (e.5 percent fat)	5.4	21.6
Cow's milk, skimmed	10.0	40.0
Fish, dried	15.3	61.6
Fish, fatty	11.4	45.6
Groundnuts (peanuts)	4.7	18.8
Soya bean	11.3	45.2

urea in the urine is a direct reflection of the number of grams of protein (as amino acids) that have been oxidized by the body. Proteins from vegetables and from animals may or may not be of similar quality (NPU value). Most grains and vegetable proteins on an individual basis have a lower biological value than meat proteins since one or more of the essential amino acids is not contained in a high enough proportion. However, a mixture of several vegetable proteins can raise the biological value of the mixture to the equivalent of meat or animal proteins and some vegetable proteins, such as in rice, potatoes, and soya beans have an NPU value almost equivalent to meat proteins. Proteins that contain all the essential amino acids in sufficient quantity and in the right combination to maintain nitrogen equilibrium are known as "complete proteins." Proteins that do not supply all the essential amino acids, so are unable to support nitrogen equilibrium are incomplete proteins. This deficiency may be partial or complete. A partially incomplete protein will sustain life, but will not support growth.

Protein functions: Dietary proteins furnish the amino acids for synthesis of tissue protein and other special metabolic functions. (1) Proteins as *enzymes* are used in repairing (*anabolism*) worn-out body tissue proteins resulting from the continual "wear and tear" (catabolism) going on in the body. (2) Proteins are used to build new tissue (anabolism) during growth by supplying the necessary amino acid building blocks. (3) Proteins are a source of heat and energy. They supply 4 calories per gram of protein. (4) Proteins contribute to numerous essential body secretions and fluids. Many hormones have amino acid components. (5) Proteins are important in the maintenance of normal osmotic pressure relationships among the various body fluids. The plasma proteins of the blood play a vital role in these relations. (6) Proteins play a large role in the resistance of the body to disease. *Antibodies* to specific disease are found in part of the plasma globulin, specifically in what is known as the gamma globulin fraction of plasma. (7) Dietary proteins furnish the amino acids for a variety of other metabolic and structural functions.

Protein synthesis: Proteins are all synthesized from their building blocks, the amino acids. There is no storage of proteins or amino acids equivalent to the fat deposits for lipids or the *glycogen** reserves for carbohydrates. The synthesis of proteins requires a high expenditure of energy and involves the genes *deoxyribonucleic acid** (DNA), for genetic direction (translation) to a *ribonucleic acid* (RNA) called messenger-RNA (m-RNA) that transcribes the "message" in conjunction with the *ribosomes* and selects the amino acid proper for the particular *genetic code*. The amino acids are brought to the messenger-RNA-Ribosome complex by another ribonucleic acid called transfer-RNA. Each amino acid has a specific transfer-RNA and it is required to transfer the amino acid to the growing polypeptide chain in proper sequence. Each of these complex reactions requires an energy expenditure. It is estimated that each cell has between 2000 to 4000 different proteins.

Protein oxidation: Protein breakdown, its oxidation and formation of urea, is the total of the catabolism of its individual amino acids. Cells contain *cathepsins, proteases*, which digest proteins in a manner similar to those in the digestive system. The resulting individual amino acids are then oxidized by several different pathways. The oxidation of amino acids is incomplete. All of the carbons are not excreted as carbon dioxide. One carbon from each amino acid is excreted as *urea**, which also contains nitrogen and oxygen. Urea is excreted into the urine and is proportional to the amount of protein that was oxidized. Protein oxidation usually accounts for 7 to 10 percent of the total energy expenditure.

protein-bound iodine of serum (PBI). A blood test which measures the levels of protein bound iodine in the serum. The normal range is 4 to 8μg per 100 cc of serum. The PBI is an index of thyroid function and a test for hypo- or *hyper-thyroidism*.

protein-calorie malnutrition (PCM). A term used to describe several different types of deficiency conditions related to diets low in protein but with varying levels of calories from carbohydrate. The terms used to describe PCM are *kwashiorkor* and *marasmus*. Kwashiorkor results from a diet very low in protein but generally adequate in calories mainly from carbohydrates, while marasmus results from a diet inadequate in protein and calories. See *kwashiorkor* and *marasmus*.

protein hydrolysate. A mixture of amino acids and *polypeptides* prepared by the digestion of protein by acids, alkalies, or proteases. Properly prepared hydrolysates may be used for either oral or *parenteral* administration. Some methods of hydrolysis lead to the destruction of certain *essential amino acids*.

proteinuria. Excretion of protein in the *urine*. It is an abnormal condition.

proteolytic. Effecting the hydrolysis of protein. See *proteases*.

prothrombin. A *proenzyme* of *thrombin* (factor II) produced in the liver. Thrombin is a blood-clotting factor that requires *vitamin K* * for its formation. The function of vitamin K is needed to carboxylate the *prothrombin* so that it can be converted to thrombin by another enzyme. See *vitamin K* * and *thrombin*.

protoplasm. The material within the cell membrane and of the formed elements except the *nucleus*. The essential protein substances of living cells upon which all the vital functions of nutrition, secretion, growth, and reproduction depend. The viscid, translucent gluelike material containing fine granules and composed mainly of proteins, which makes up the essential material of plant and animal cells and has the properties of life. The chemical composition is as follows:

Oxygen	76%	Magnesium	0.02%
Carbon	10.5%	Iron	0.01%
Hydrogen	10.0%	Calcium	0.02%
Nitrogen	2.5%	Sodium	0.05%
Phosphorus	0.3%	Chlorine	0.01%
Potassium	0.3%		
Sulfur	0.02%		

protoplast. A type or model of organism, all the living contents of a cell; or a bacterial or plant cell without its rigid cell wall, which depends on an isotonic or hypertonic medium to hold it together.

protoporphyrin. A class of porphyrin compounds. Protoporphyrin IX combined with iron forms the *heme** in *hemoglobin*.

protovitamins. See *provitamins*.

protozoa. One-celled animals, a few of which cause illness in man. Important diseases caused by protozoa include systemic infections such as malaria and amebic dysentery, and local infections such as trichomoniasis which affects the external genitalia.

provitamins (protovitamin). Substances occurring in foods which are not themselves vitamins but are capable of conversion into vitamins in the body. Thus carotenes are provitamins of vitamin A. *Beta (β) carotene** is a provitamin of vitamin A (*retinol**) since it can be converted to the vitamin.

proximate composition. As applied to food, the term usually includes the percentage of protein fat, total carbohydrate, ash, and water; caloric values may also be included.

prune. A *plum* dried without fermentation. Prunes are made from several varieties of cultivated plums, most often blue-purple freestone prune-plums. Good source of iron and a concentrated source of energy.

Uncooked, 100 gm = 225 calories
Cooked, fruit and liquid without added sugar, 100 gm = 119 calories
Juice, canned or bottled, 100 gm = 77 calories

PSP test. Initials stand for phenolsulfonaphthalein, which is a dye administered directly into the vein. The purpose of the test is to estimate the ability of the kidneys to excrete the dye in a given number of hours. It is therefore a measure of kidney function.

psychic secretion. Small amounts of saliva and gastric juice are secreted all the time, but their flow is stimulated when food is present. Factors that stimulate the flow of saliva are chewing, taste, sight, smell or even the thought of food. The latter type of stimulus causes what is known as psychic secretion.

pteroylglutamic acid. A part of the vitamin *folacin**.

ptyalin. The amylase or starch-digestive enzyme that occurs in the saliva.

pulse. A characteristic associated with the heartbeat and the subsequent wave of expansion and recoil set up in the wall of an artery. Pulse is defined as the alternate expansion and recoil of an artery. With each heartbeat, blood is forced into the arteries causing them to dilate (expand). The arteries contract (recoil) as the blood moves further along in the circulatory system. The pulse can be felt at certain points in the body where an artery lies close to the surface. The most common location for feeling the pulse is at the wrist, proximal to the thumb (radial artery) on the palm side of the hand. Alternate locations are in front of the ear (temporal artery), at the side of the neck (carotid artery), and on the top (dorsum) of the foot (dorsalis pedis).

pulses (legumes). The nutrition properties of pulses resemble the whole cereal grains. All pulses have a higher protein content than cereals. Most contain about 20 gm of protein/100 gm dry weight. Pulses are rich in lysine, are good sources of the B group vitamins (except *riboflavin* *). Pulses are devoid of any *ascorbic acid* * (vitamin C) although large amounts of ascorbic acid are formed on germination. See *legumes*.

pumpkin (*Cucurbita pepo*). The name of a gourd belonging to the Cucurbitaceae family which also includes the melons, cucumbers, and squash. The pumpkin's flesh is orange colored and has a distinctive sweet flavor. The word comes from the Old French pompion, in its turn derived from the Greek word pepon meaning "cooked by the sun." A good source of vitamin A, fair source of iron. Raw, 100 gm = 26 calories; canned, 100 gm = 33 calories; pumpkin seeds, dry, shelled, 100 gm = 553 calories.

pumpkin spice. A blend of cinnamon, cloves, and ginger, ground together to weld the flavors permanently.

purines. Purine bases are compounds which contain heterocyclic nitrogenous ring structures. The purine derivatives in the body catabolize to *uric acid* *. Purines are supplied in the diet by meats and are synthesized also in the body. The following are the major purines and their corresponding *nucleosides* and *nucleotides*.

Purine	Nucleoside	Nucleotide
Adenine	Adenosine	Adenosine monophosphate (AMP) or adenylic acid
Guanine	Guanosine	Guanosine monophosphate (GMP) or gyanylic acid
Hypoxanthine	Inosine	Inosine monophosphate (IMP) or inosinic acid

The purine structure is a part of the coenzyme *nicotinamide adenine dinucleo-tide* * (NAD). Meat and foods containing high concentrations of purines are to be avoided under certain conditions, as for example with *gout*. The purine and *pyrimidine* bases derive from the *nucleic acids* in foods. See *pyrimidines*.

Purine Content in Foods
per 100 gm

Group I (0–15 mg)	Group II (50–150 mg)	Group III (150–800 mg)
Vegetables	Meats, poultry	Sweetbreads
Fruits	Fish	Anchovies
Milk	Seafood	Sardines
Cheese	Beans, dry	Liver
Eggs	Peas, dry	Kidney
Cereals, bread	Lentils	Meat extracts
Sugar, fats	Spinach	Brains

Adapted from Turner, D.: Handbook of Diet Therapy, Ed. 5, Chicago: University of Chicago Press, 1971.

For the structures see *adenosine triphosphate* *, *guanosine triposphate* *, *inosine triphosphate* *, and *ribonucleotides* *.

purpura. Refers to small hemorrhages in the skin and mucous membranes; they occur as a result of leakage from the capillaries into the tissue spaces of the subcutaneous tissues. If the hemorrhages are small, pinpoint in size, they are called petechiae; the larger ones which resemble bruises are called echymoses. Purpura is a symptom and may be secondary to a number of diseases including scurvy, liver disease with failure to utilize *vitamin K,* and allergy to certain drugs.

putrefaction. The decomposition of proteins by microörganisms under anaerobic conditions, resulting in the production of incompletely oxidized compounds some of which are foul smelling.

pyelonephritis. An infection of the kidney caused by bacterial invasion of the kidney and urinary tract.

pyloric stenosis. A condition in which the muscular tissue of the pylorus thickens and hardens, constricting the size of the opening from the stomach to the *duodenum*. As it progresses, partial or complete obstruction may occur. The primary symptom is projectile vomiting with no sign of nausea. See *digestive system*.

pyorrhea. If *gingivitis* is not treated, the gum tissue may gradually separate from the tooth and a pocket may form between the soft gum tissues and the hard tooth surface. Bacteria, saliva, and food debris collect in the pockets and intensify the destructive process. Pus usually forms (pyorrhea means "pus flowing"). The bone adjacent to the area disappears, more attaching tissue is lost and the pocket deepens and widens. Eventually the tooth loosens and its movement in chewing sets up additional irritation.

pyridine. Mol. Wt. 79. A six-membered heterocylic nitrogenous base. It is obtained commercially from coal tar. The pyridine ring structure is found in the vitamin *niacin* * or *nicotinamide* *; in the cofactors *nicotinamide adenine dinucleotide* * (NAD) and *nicotinamide adenine dinucleotide phosphate* * (NADP); and in *pyridoxal phosphate* * (vitamin B_6).

Pyridine

pyridoxal phosphate. Mol. Wt. 247. The cofactor form of *pyridoxine* (vitamin B_6). Pyridoxal phosphate and pyridoxamine phosphate are readily interchangeable and equivalent in the body. They act as coenzymes in reactions involving the *transamination* of amino acids and function as the agent of the transfer of amino groups from an amino acid to an *alpha-keto acid*. In general pyridoxal phosphate serves as a cofactor for a variety of enzymes involving the amino acids, decarboxylases (the removal of CO_2); dehydrases (the removal of water); sulfhydrase (the addition of sulfhydryl groups), and many other reactions. More than 50 specific reactions of amino acids requiring pyridoxal phosphate are known. See *pyridoxine* (vitamin B_6).

Pyridoxal Phosphate   Pyridoxamine Phosphate

pyrimidines. Pyrimidines are compounds which contain a heterocyclic nitrogenous ring structure. The pyrimidine derivatives in the body are catabolized to CO_2 and water or to beta (β)-amino isobutyric acid which is excreted. Pyrimidines are supplied in the diet by meats and are also synthesized in the body. The following are the major purines and their corresponding *nucleosides* and *nucleotides*.

Pyrimidine	Nucleoside	Nucleotide
Thymine (5-methyl uracil)	Thymidine	Thymidine monophosphate (TMP), or thymidylic acid
Pyrimidines Uracil	Uridine	Uridine monophosphate (UMP), or uridylic acid
Cystosine	Cytidine	Cytidine monophosphate (CMP), or cytidylic acid

See *ribonucleotides* for structures.

pyridoxine (vitamin B₆). A generic name. Three forms of vitamin B₆ occur in nature, pyridoxine, pyridoxal, and pyridoxamine. In the body the forms undergo conversion to *pyridoxal phosphate* *. The most potent and active forms in body metabolism are the derivatives *pyridoxal phosphate* and *pyridoxamine phosphate*. The term pyridoxine or simply vitamin B₆ is used to designate the entire group, as well as one of its components. Pyridoxine is a water-soluble, heat-stable vitamin that is sensitive to light and alkalis. It is absorbed in the upper portion of the small intestine, and is found throughout the body tissues. In its active phosphate forms of vitamin B₆ pyridoxal phosphate is an active coenzyme in many types of reactions in amino metabolism: (1) Pyridoxal phosphate is active in decarboxylation; (2) pyridoxal phosphate also aids in deamination; (3) in transamination reactions (transfer of amino groups), pyridoxal phosphate acts as a coenzyme which splite off NH_2 and transfers it to a new carbon skeleton which forms a new amino acid or other compound; (4) in transulfuration (transfer of sulfur) pyridoxal phosphate aids reactions of the sulfur-containing amino acids, as in the transfer of sulfur from methionine to another amino acid (serine) to form the derivative cysteine. Pyridoxal phosphate plays a

Pyridoxine   Pyridoxal   Pyridoxamine

role in hemoglobin synthesis as a cofactor in the synthetic pathway to porphyrin. Vitamin B_6, pyridoxine, is also involved in metabolic processes of the central nervous system (CNS). In severe vitamin B_6 deficiency, convulsive seizures occur. Vitamin B_6 appears to prevent uncontrolled excitation of the CNS. Vitamin B_6 deficiency is extremely rare in man. Some years ago an infant formula was deficient in vitamin B_6 because of a heat process in its preparation, resulting in symptoms of vitamin B_6 deficiency. Occasionally, a vitamin

Food	μgm 100 gm Food	Food	μgm 100 gm Food
Apple	26	Milk, human	3.5–22
Asparagus, canned	30	Milk, evaporated	25–41
Banana	320	Milk, dry	330–820
Barley	320–560	Milk, dry skim	550
Beans, green, canned	32	Molasses, blackstrap	2000–2490
Beef	230–320	Oats, rolled	93–150
Beer	50–60	Onions	63
Beet greens	37	Orange juice, canned	16–31
Brains, beef	160	Orange juice, fresh	18–56
Cabbage	120–290	Peaches, canned	16
Cantaloupe	36	Peanuts	300
Cauliflower	20	Peas, fresh	50–190
Carrots, raw	120–220	Peas, canned	46
Cheese	98	Peas, dry	160–330
Cod	340	Pork	330–680
Corn, canned	68	Potato	160–250
Corn, yellow	360–570	Raisins	94
Corn grits	200–250	Rice, whole	1030
Cottonseed meal	1310	Rice, white	340–450
Eggs, fresh	22–48	Rye	300–370
Flounder	100	Salmon, canned	450
Frankfurter	130	Salmon, fresh	590
Grapefruit juice	8–18	Sardines, canned	280
Grapefruit sections	17–24	Soybeans	710–1200
Halibut	110	Spinach, canned	60
Ham	330–580	Strawberries	44
Heart, beef	200–290	Tomatoes, canned	710
Honey	4–27	Tuna, canned	440
Kidney, beef	350–990	Turnips	100
Lamb	250–370	Veal	280–410
Lemon juice	35	Watermelon	33
Lettuce	71	Wheat, bran	1380–1570
Liver, beef	600–710	Wheat germ	850–1600
Liver, calf's	300	White flour	380–600
Liver, pork	290–590	Yams	320
Malt extract	540	Yeast, baker's	620–700
Milk, whole	54–110	Yeast, brewer's dry	4000–5700

B_6 deficiency is seen in chronic alcoholics. Vitamin B_6 deficiency can be prevented by 2–3 mg of vitamin B_6 daily in adults. On p. 392 is a list of the pyridoxine (vitamin B_6) content in some common foods.

Best Sources of Vitamin B
(Pyridoxine Compound)

	Food Sources	Total B Content mg per 100 gm
Grain	Barley	0.39
	Brown rice	0.53
	Buckwheat flour	0.58
	Corn	0.48
	Oatmeal	0.12
	Popcorn	0.37
	Rice cereal, dry	0.14
	Soya flour	0.57
	Wheat	0.41
	Wheat bran	0.82
	Wheat germ	1.31
	Whole-wheat bread	0.20
	Whole-wheat cereal	0.40
Milk	Canned, evaporated	7.50
	Cow's fluid	0.10
Meat	Beef, ground, cooked	0.10
	Frankfurter, cooked	0.16
	Ham (cured and fully cooked)	0.70
	Liver	1.42
	Salmon, canned	0.28
Vegetables & Fruits	Bananas	0.32
	Carrots	0.21
	Frozen peas	0.11
	Lima beans	0.60

pyrophosphate. A pyrophosphate is the salt of pyrophosphoric acid. The pyrophosphoryl group is formed by the condensation of two phosphate groups:

$$2 \begin{bmatrix} & O & \\ & \| & \\ O-&P&-O \\ & | & \\ & O & \end{bmatrix}^{-3} \xrightarrow[-H_2O]{} \begin{bmatrix} O & & O \\ \| & & \| \\ O-P-&O&-P-O \\ \| & & \| \\ O & & O \end{bmatrix}^{-4} + H^+$$

Phosphate   Pyrophosphoryl group or bond

Pyrophosphate bonds are very important in the energetics of the cell. One storage form of chemical energy in the body, *adenosine triphosphate** (ATP), has pyrophosphate bonds. The "breaking" of pyrophosphate bonds is accompanied by a large release of energy which can be used by the body for work or synthetic reactions. Often compounds containing pyrophosphate bonds are said to contain "high energy" phosphate bonds. It is by the synthesis of the pyrophosphate bonds in ATP, using the oxidation energies from foods, that the energy of oxidation is conserved. The process is called *oxidative phosphorylation.*

pyruvic acid. Mol. Wt. 88. Pyruvic acid or pyruvate (the salt form) is the end product of glycolysis (the degradation of glucose). Pyruvate is formed in the cytosol and enters the mitochondria where it is oxidized completely to CO_2, water, and energy to complete the oxidation of glucose via the *Kreb's cycle** and *oxidative phosphorylation.*

$$
\begin{array}{c}
CH_3 \\
| \\
C=O \\
| \\
COOH
\end{array}
$$

Q

quince. The round to pear-shaped fruit of the *Cydonia cydonia* tree. When ripe the fruit is rich yellow or greenish-yellow with a strong odor and hard flesh. Its taste is so tart and astringent that it cannot be eaten raw. Quinces are full of natural pectin and are used for making marmalades, jellies, jams, fruit paste, butters, preserves, and syrups. Raw, 100 gm = 57 calories.

quinones. An aromatic ring structure that contains two carbonyl (C=O) groups as a part of the ring. Quinones can undergo *oxidation-reduction* reactions.

Semi-quinone

The oxidation reduction reactions involve an intermediate stage called a semiquinone in which only one electron is transferred. Quinones are important in the body because the vitamin K and coenzyme Q (ubiquinone), a member of the oxidative phosphorylation chain, are quinone derivatives.

R

rachitis. See rickets.

radiostol. A substance produced by the action of ultraviolet light upon *ergosterol* *; it contains a large amount of *vitamin D* *.

radish (*Raphanus sativus*). The pungent fleshy root of a hardy annual plant widely used as a salad vegetable. The name radish is derived from the Latin word for "root," radix. Radishes come in many shapes and colors, round, long, or oblong, and white, pink, red, yellow, purple, or black. Their taste varies from mild to peppery. Depending upon the variety, they can be from one inch to two or more feet long and weigh up to several pounds apiece. Common radish, raw, 100 gm = 17 calories.

raffinose. A trisaccharide of galactose, glucose, and fructose, found in molasses.

α-D-galactosyl (1→6)-α-D-glucosyl (1→2) .β-D-fructoside

Raffinose

raisin. The name given to several varieties of grapes when they are dried, either naturally in the sun or by artificial heat. When grapes are dried, their skins wrinkle, they have a higher sugar content, and a flavor quite different from that of fresh grapes. The word raisin comes from the Latin word racemus meaning "a cluster of grapes or berries." Varieties of grapes dried to make raisins run from dark bluish-brown to golden. The two most popular varieties are muscats and sultans. When the fruit is ripe it is picked and spread out on trays to dry in the sun, and dehydrated indoors and given a sulfur treatment. This preserves the golden color. Raisins contain a variety of vitamins and minerals, especially iron. Their natural sugar content makes them an excellent sweet for children. Uncooked, 100 gm = 289 calories; cooked, with sugar added, fruit and liquid, 100 gm = 213 calories.

rancid. Having a disagreeable odor of flavor. Rancid usually describes foods with a high content of fat when oxidation of unsaturated fatty acids to aldehydes or hydrolysis has occurred.

rancidity. The process of becoming rancid. Rancid fats have typical rank odors and flavors, changed baking properties and other properties different from those of the original fat. The fats that contain fatty acids are very susceptible to oxidative (oxygen and light) attack and the essential fatty acids are the chief substances that are affected by rancidity. In the process of rancidification, the oxidation going on also destroys the *retinol*, carotene** (vitamin A), and *vitamin E** which may be present; thus a rancid fat has diminished quality.

raspberry (Rubus). The fruit of a bush which is a member of the rose family. Raspberries grow wild in woods and are also cultivated. The berry is made up of many small drupelets. In contrast to blackberries, which retain their stems or receptacles when the fruit is picked, the stem of a raspberry separates from the berry and remains on the plant. Raspberries may be red, purple, black, or amber in color. They are a delicately flavored fruit and can be eaten raw or used for jellies, jams, puddings, pies, etc. A fair source of iron and *ascorbic acid** (vitamin C). Fresh, red, raw, 100 gm = 57 calories. Fresh, black, raw, 100 gm = 73 calories.

ravioli. Shells or cases of noodle dough filled with meat, chicken, cheese, or spinach. Although the word is Italian, this type of food preparation is by no means a uniquely Italian dish. It occurs under different names in many lands. The Chinese know ravioli as won ton, the Jews as kreplach, and the Russians as pelmeni.

RDA. See Recommended Daily Allowances and Appendix 8.

receptors. Receptors are free nerve endings distributed to the tongue, nasapharynx, orbit, and other mucous surfaces. Like other pain endings their threshold is relatively high, but the response fatigues slowly, and the receptors adapt little under most conditions of chemical stimulation.

Recommended Daily Allowances. The RDA are usually several times greater than the minimum daily requirement which is the quantity of nutrient which will reverse or prevent a nutritional disease or deficiency symptom.

reconstitute. To restore to the normal state, usually by adding water, such as reconstituting dry milk by adding water to make it fluid milk.

red blood cell (erythrocyte, red corpuscles). The red blood cell is the major cell in the blood. Men normally have about 5 million red corpuscles per milliliter (0.000034 ounce), and women have about 4.5 million per milliliter. The average person has 35 trillion (35,000,000,000,000) cells. The erythrocyte is shaped like a solid doughnut and is about 7 microns (0.0003 inch) in diameter. The red blood cells make up about 45 percent of the total volume in men and about 40 percent in women (see *hematocrit*). The average life span of red blood cells is about 120 days after they have been discharged from the bone marrow where as they mature they form various stages, proerythroblasts, erythroblasts, normoblasts, and reticulocytes. The mature red blood cell has no *nucleus* or *mitochondria*. The red blood cell therefore does not divide nor does it consume much oxygen. The most important constituent in the erythrocyte is the protein *hemoglobin* which accounts for its red color. The *heme* * moiety of hemoglobin is red and contains the reduced iron (Fe^{+2}). The blood of the average male contains 16 gm of hemoglobin in 100 ml of blood and the blood of the average female has 14 gm per 100 milliliters. The primary function of hemoglobin and the erythrocyte is the transport of oxygen from the lungs to other tissues. The oxygen combines with heme and does not oxidize the iron which remains in reduced (ferrous) state. The oxygen carrying capacity of hemoglobin is 1.34 ml of oxygen per gram. The hemoglobin also acts as one of the major *buffers* of blood in maintaining the pH and is important in carrying some of the carbon dioxide (carbohemoglobin) away from the tissues to the lungs. Occasionally, the iron in the hemoglobin becomes oxidized to *methemoglobin* (ferrihemoglobin). The oxidized iron (Fe^{+3}) can be reduced via the enzymes called methemoglobin reductases.

About 20 million erythrocytes are destroyed every minute. *Bile pigments,* biliverdin and bilirubin, green and red in color, respectively, form from the breakdown of heme and are responsible for the color of *bile.* The bile pigments are converted to stercobilin by bacterial action in the intestines, which is responsible for the brown color of feces.

In order for erythrocytes to be produced and maintained at normal levels, several vitamins and iron are required. The vitamins *folacin, pyridoxine,* and *cobalamin* * (vitamin B_{12}) are intimately involved in erythrocyte maintenance. A deficiency of any of these nutritional factors results in nutritional anemia. Some anemias are genetic diseases that result in abnormal hemoglobins that may vary in shape, ability to transport oxygen, and have a shortened erythrocyte life span, as for example sickle cell anemia.

red blood cell count. A count of blood cells to determine or test for anemias. See *hematocrit*.

red dye number 2 (Amaranth). Widely used food coloring accounting for about one-third of all coloring. The dye is used in soft drinks, ice cream, pistachio nuts, candy, baked goods, pet foods, sausage, breakfast cereals, and other foods. Red No. 2 was banned by the Food and Drug Administration in 1976.

red dye number 3 (Erythrosine). A food dye used in color cherries in canned fruit cocktail, because it is insoluble in acidic solutions and therefore does not stain other fruit.

red pepper. See pepper, red.

reduction. Reduction is the opposite of *oxidation* and like oxidation can be interpreted in several ways. The addition of a hydrogen to a molecule is a reduction.

$$2H_2 \;+\; O_2 \;\longrightarrow\; 2H_2O$$
$$\text{hydrogen} \quad \text{oxygen} \qquad \text{water}$$

In this example, oxygen is reduced. Every reduction must also be accompanied by the opposite reaction, an oxidation, and in this example hydrogen is oxidized. In biological oxidations of food, the carbons and hydrogens are oxidized and oxygen is reduced. A more general interpretation is the addition of electrons to a molecule. Thus the oxidation of the irons in the cytochromes of the terminal respiratory chain undergoes reductions and oxidations based on the addition and removal of electrons, respectively.

$$e \;+\; Fe^{+3} \underset{\text{oxidation}}{\overset{\text{reduction}}{\rightleftharpoons}} Fe^{+2}$$
$$\text{electron} \quad \text{ferric} \qquad\qquad \text{ferrous}$$
$$\text{iron} \qquad\qquad\qquad \text{iron}$$
$$\text{(oxidized)} \qquad\qquad \text{(reduced)}$$

reducing sugar. A sugar that can undergo oxidation and in turn reduces some reagents or metals. The ions of silver, bismuth, or copper are frequently used in various tests and are reduced as they oxidize the sugar. The changes in color or precipitation of the metal (reduced) indicates a positive test. A positive reducing sugar indicates a free aldehyde ($>C=O$) group in the sugar. The aldehyde group is oxidized to a carboxylic acid (—COOH) group. *Glucose* is reducing sugar because the aldehyde group is free. The glucose in *sucrose* is not a reducing sugar because the aldehyde group is not free, but involved in a chemical bonding with *fructose.* *

refuse. That portion of foods which is inedible (as bones, pits, shells), or usually discarded in preparation of food for the table (as potato parings and tough outer leaves of vegetables). In food values expressed on the "as purchased" basis, the nutrients in refuse have been disregarded.

regional enteritis. An inflammatory disease which involves the small bowel and is manifested by diarrhea, abdominal cramping, pain, fever, anemia, and weight loss. Usually the inflammation begins in the terminal ileum and spreads towards the *jejunum*. The inflammation frequently leads to narrowing of the bowel or stricture formation.

regurgitation. The backward flow of food; casting up of undigested food. Regurgitation also describes the backward flow of blood through the valves in the heart, that do not close properly.

rehydration. Soaking or cooking or using other procedures to make dehydrated foods take up the water they lost during drying.

remission. A lessening of the severity or temporary abatement of symptoms.

renal. Pertaining to the kidney.

renal threshold. That concentration of a given substance in the blood above which the excess will be eliminated in the urine. For example, when the blood glucose level exceeds about 180 mg per 100 ml of blood, the kidneys cannot reabsorb the excess, the renal threshold has been exceeded, and glucose enters the urine. This is what occurs in untreated diabetes mellitus.

renal tubules. See *nephron*.

renin. An enzyme produced in the kidney in response to a drop in blood pressure. Renin, a *protease,* acts on angiotensinogen in the plasma to form *angiotensin* I which in turn is converted to angiotensin II by another plasma enzyme. The angiotensinogen comes from the liver. Angiotensin increases the blood pressure and stimulates the *adrenal glands* to produce *aldosterone* *, which in turn increases water and sodium ion reabsorption in the renal tubules. Do not confuse renin with *rennin,* an enzyme that curdles milk in the gastric juice. See *water balance.*

rennet. A combination of two enzymes or ferments, rennin and pepsin, obtained from the membranes of the stomachs of young mammals. The best quality is that from an animal so young that it has received no other food than milk, the most desirable coming from a calf's stomach. Rennet's chief importance from a food standpoint is its property of coagulating milk and its widest food use is in the manufacture of cheese.

rennin. An enzyme contained in the gastric juice which precipitates milk in solid form (curds). Heat-treated cow's milk and human milk make for a finer, more easily digested curd than ordinary cow's milk. Rennin is especially abundant in gastric juice of babies and young animals fed on milk; it is less important in adults when the hydrochloric acid content of the gastric juice is sufficient alone to coagulate milk. Do not confuse this enzyme rennin with *renin,* an enzyme from the kidney.

repressor. A substance which prevents the formation of one or more enzymes in cells.

reproductive system. Consists of the testes, seminal vesicles, penis, urethra, prostate, and bulbourethal glands in the male; the ovaries, uterine tubes, uterous, vagina, and vulva in the female. All these systems are closely interrelated and dependent on each other.

requirements. Although the average minimal requirements for various nutrients cannot be stated with accuracy, certain "minimum daily requirements" for food-labeling purposes have been designated in regulations for enforcement of the Federal Food Drug and Cosmetic Act. Should not be confused with the *Recommended Dietary Allowance.*

residue. (1) Remainder; the contents remaining in the intestinal tract after digestion of food; includes fiber and other unabsorbed products. (2) That portion of a molecule included in another larger molecule, as "a number of amino acid residues are contained in a polypeptide."

resorption. A loss of substance, e.g., loss of mineral salts from bone.

respiration. In breathing, respiration is composed of two basic movements, the inspiration (intake, inhalation) of air into the lung, and expiration (exhalation) of the contents of the lung to the outside. Respiration also means the uptake or utilization of oxygen by a living system and the discharge of carbon dioxide. A cell or tissue is thus considered to respire. The oxygen is taken up by cells from the blood which carries oxygen from the lungs. The cells use the oxygen to oxidize the nutrients that have also been delivered to the cells by blood. The oxidation of the nutrients, *fats, carbohydrates,* and *amino acids* (proteins) results in the formation of carbon dioxide CO_2, water, and energy. The water and CO_2 enter the blood and are expired through the lungs. The energy, largely chemical energy in the form of *adenosine triphosphate,* is retained by the cell for work, biosynthesis, and other functions.

respiratory acidosis. A condition when the pH of the blood is below 7.4 because of the high concentration of carbon dioxide (CO_2) in the blood, which forms *carbonic acid* (H_2CO_3). In certain diseases, such as *emphysema,* when CO_2 cannot be properly expelled, respiratory acidosis results.

respiration alkalosis. A condition when the pH of the blood is greater than 7.4. The primary cause of respiratory alkalosis is hyperventilation (excessively rapid breathing) which removes the carbon dioxide CO_2 from the blood. Hyperventilation may result from a number of causes among which are fever, hysteria, and heart failure.

respiratory chain. See terminal respiratory chain.

respiratory quotient (R.Q.). The respiratory quotient is the ratio of the volume of carbon dioxide expired to the volume of oxygen utilized. The respiratory quotient differs for carbohydrates, fats, and proteins because the amount of oxygen atoms and the completeness of combustion varies with each foodstuff. The R.Q. reflects the generalized equation; foodstuff + oxygen $\longrightarrow$

$$CO_2 + H_2O$$

carbon dioxide + water + energy. As an example, glucose oxidation is as follows: $C_6H_{12}O_6 + 6\ CO_2 \longrightarrow 6\ O_2 + 6H_2O + 268$ kcal.

$$\frac{6 \text{ volumes of } CO_2}{6 \text{ volumes of } O_2} = \text{R.Q.} = 1.0$$

The R.Q. of the major food classes are:

Food	R.Q.
Carbohydrate	1.0
Protein	0.80
Fat	0.71
Average mixed diet	0.82

respiratory system. Consists of the nose, pharynx, larynx, trachea, bronchi, and lungs. The main function is to provide oxygen for body tissues and to remove carbon dioxide. See *respiration*.

reticular tissue. Fibrous connective tissues which form the supporting framework of *lymph glands, liver, spleen, bone, marrow,* and *lungs*.

reticulocyte. A young red blood cell occurring during active blood regeneration.

reticuloendothelium. A system of *macrophages* concerned with *phagocytosis*, present in *spleen, liver, bone marrow, connective tissue,* and *lymph nodes*.

retina (eye). The back of the eye is lined by the retina which consists of three main layers: (1) The innermost layer which the light first penetrates is a complex network of nerve cells and fibers which finally run together and leave the eye to form the optic nerves. (2) Behind the nerve network there is a layer of light sensitive cells of two different types, the rods and the cones. (3) The hindmost layer, forming a backing to the rods and cones, consisting of a black pigment called melanin. This absorbs any excess light and prevents reflection across the eye. There are about 7 million cones and 120 million rods in each eye. Most of the cones are massed together at one tiny spot, the macula, at the back of the eye, which is the central focusing point of the whole optical system of the eye. The cones are color sensitive, with three different kinds of cone, each sensitive to either red, green, or blue. The rods contain a pigment called visual purple (rhodopsin) which is bleached by light at the green-violet end of the spectrum. Rodopsin contains a vitamin A (retinol) derivative called 11-cis retinal. A deficiency of vitamin A is first manifested by a nutritional disease called night-blindness (*nyctalopia*) resulting from a deficiency of the visual purple content of the rods. See *retinol** and *rhodopsin*.

retinal. The aldehyde form of vitamin A which is necessary for the synthesis of rhodopsin (visual purple). Light ($\gamma\nu$) causes a change in the structure of 11-*cis* retinal, after going through a series of changes. See *retinol* and *retinene*.

retinene. One of a series of derivatives of vitamin A aldehyde formed as an intermediate step in bleaching or *rhodopsin* in the rods of the retina. See *retinal** and *retinol**

retinoic acid. A derivative of vitamin A (*retinol**). The acid form of vitamin A. The exact function of this form of the vitamin A is not definitely established, but it is believed that retinoic acid is involved in maintaining the health and integrity of epithelial tissue. See *retinal* and *retinol*.

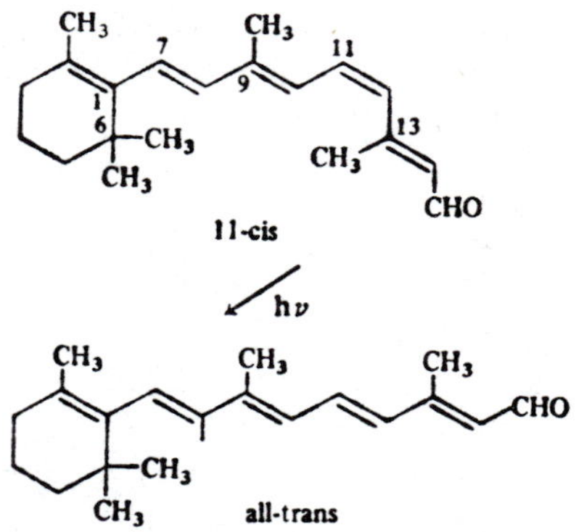

11-cis

hν

all-trans

Retinal

retinol (vitamin A). Retinol is the form of vitamin A that occurs in the livers of animals, which are a good source of the vitamin. Retinol is the storage form of vitamin A and occurs chiefly as the retinyl ester. The principal fatty acid associated with retinyl derivative is *palmitic acid**. *Retinoic acid**, *retinal** and retinol are various oxidation states of vitamin A. The conversion of retinol to retinoic acid and retinal occurs readily. *Rhodopsin* when treated with light releases all-trans retinal which is an inactive form of the vitamin A (11-*cis* retinal). Conversion of all-*trans* retinal to 11-*cis* retinal can occur two ways: (1) In the retina where there is an enzyme to convert it directly or, (2) the all-*trans* retinal is reduced to a retinol which is first converted to an 11-*cis* retinal in the liver and subsequently reoxidized to 11-*cis* retinal for the formation of rhodopsin in the *retina*. Vitamin A (retinol) at high levels is toxic. High levels (500,000 units per day) can cause headaches, nausea, nosebleed, anorexia, and dermatitis within a few days. The Recommended Daily Allowance (RDA) for vitamin A of 5000 units is liberal. While it is possible to receive toxic levels of vitamin A (*retinol**) in fish oils from shark or halibut because they contain such high concentrations (2,000 to 100,000 units), it is doubtful that it is possible to reach toxic levels from plant sources of the vitamin, such as carrots. In plants the vitamin A activity is derived from *carotene** which must be converted to retinol. The conversion of carotene to retinol is attended with losses due to ab-

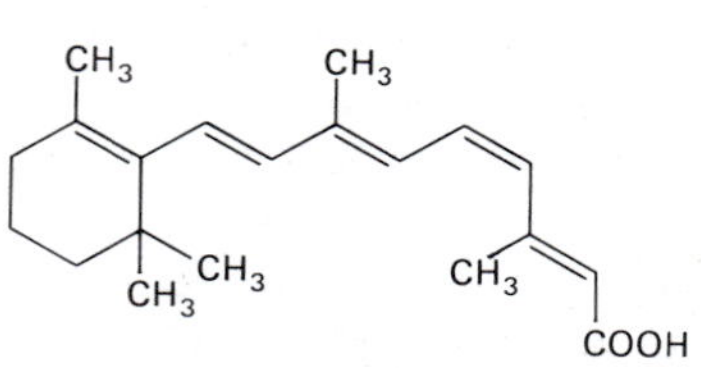

Retinoic acid

sorption and losses occurring during the chemical conversion. As a result carotene has ¹/₆ the vitamin A activity of retinol. See *vitamin toxicity, retinoic acid*,* and *retinal*.*

11-*cis* Retinol

A different form of the vitamin occurs in fish liver oils, vitamin A₂.

Vitamin A₂: predominant form in fish liver oils

The table on page 406 shows the vitamin A content or activity of various foods.

rhodopsin (visual purple). Rhodopsin is formed from the combination of protein opsin and ll-*cis* retinal, a derivative of vitamin A (*retinol**). When rhodopsin is exposed to light, the retinal undergoes configurational changes to the all-trans retinal and separates from opsin, which will only combine with the ll-*cis retinal**. These changes due to light are complex and only partly understood. It is known that there are several configurational changes that occur, but the structures are not known. These reactions occur in the retina and are accompanied by nerve impulses that translate in the brain to what we know as sight. Rhodopsin is in the rods of the retina and therefore is associated with weak light (scoptopic) vision. Color vision is associated with the cones in the retina, requiring more light to cause a nerve impulse, and is not so well understood as scoptopic vision.

rhodotorula. Red, pink, or yellow yeasts which may cause discoloration in foods, e.g., colored spots on meats or pink areas in saurkraut.

rhubarb (*Rheum*). A hardy perennial plant grown for its thick succulent leafy stalks. The plant has large clumps of broad green leaves, up to two feet across,

Dietary Sources of Vitamin A Activity

Source	Range (μg. retinol equivalents/ 100 gm edible portion)
Fatty fish and their oils	
Cod-liver oil	12,000–120,000
Halbut-liver oil	600,000–10,800,000
Herring, fresh	27
Salmon, canned	24–75
Sardine, canned	40–90
Shark-liver oil	13,500–180,000
Tuna, canned	20–60
Dairy produce	
Butter	720–1,200
Cheese, whole, fatty type	360–520
Eggs, fresh, whole	300–340
Margarine, vitaminized	900
Milk, fresh, whole	20–70
Meats	
Beef	0–15
Liver	1,200–13,500
Mutton	0–15
Fruit and vegetables*	
Apricots	70–280
Bananas	10–30
Carrots	600–1,500
Leafy vegetables	8–1,200
Orange juice	19–25
Red palm oil	4,000–10,000
Sweet potatoes, colorless	80
Sweet potatoes, red and yellow	360–770
Tomatoes	110–300
Negligible sources	
Bacon and pork	trace only
Cereals (except maize)	trace only
Lard and vegetable oils	trace only
Potatoes	trace only
Sugar, jams and syrups	trace only
White fish	trace only

*Figure calculated on the assumption that 1 μg β-carotene in the diet is taken to have the same biological value as 0–167 μg retinol.

growing on thick fleshy red and green leaf stalks which average 12 to 18 inches in length, but can be much longer. There are many varieties of rhubarb, but the only important distinction in the edible types is between forced or hothouse rhubarb and field rhubarb. The first usually has slender pink to light red stalks with yellow-green leaves, and the second deep red stalks and green leaves.

Only the leaf stalks of the rhubarb are edible. Leaves and root contain a substance that can sometimes be poisonous. Rhubarb is used in pies, desserts, jam, and wine. Fair source of *carotene** (vitamin A). Fresh, cooked, with added sugar, 100 gm, = 141 calories.

riboflavin. Mol. Wt. 376. Riboflavin is a vitamin of the B complex; sparingly soluble in water, decomposed by exposure to light, heat-labile in alkaline solutions but otherwise thermostable. The name "riboflavin" was adopted since the factor contains the pigment flavus and the pentose sugar D-*ribose* and is nitrogenous in nature. In pure form, it exists as fine orange-yellow crystals which are practically odorless and bitter-tasting. In water solutions riboflavin shows a characteristic yellow-green fluorescence. Riboflavin functions biologically as the coenzymes *flavin mononucleotide** (FMN), and *flavin adenine dinucleotide** (FAD), which are components of the flavoproteins, essential to protein and energy metabolism; participates in biological oxidations. The deficiency disease, ariboflavinosis, is frequently associated with deficiencies of other B vitamins. Human requirements are now considered to be more closely related to energy expenditure than to protein intake; recommended daily allowances have been computed on the basis of caloric intake. Riboflavin is widely distributed in both plant and animal tissues. It is formed by all high plants, chiefly in the green leaves. Riboflavin is involved in cell respiration. In tissues where respiration is taking place, riboflavin occurs in combination with phosphoric acid as flavin mononucleotide (FMN), and with phosphoric acid and adenine as flavin adenine dinucleotide (FAD). These combined with specific proteins, make up a number of different flavoprotein enzyme systems in which the riboflavin-containing nucleotides are the *coenzymes*. These flavoproteins function in oxidative processes in living cells. They play a major role with thiamine- and niacin-containing enzymes in a long chain of oxidation-reduction reactions by which hydrogen is released and finally combines with oxygen to form water. It is one of the factors essential for successful reproduction, and is essential for general health because it is the active constituent of several coenzymes that are essential to oxidation processes in the various body tissues. It is essential for the health of tissues of ectodermal origin such as the skin, eyes and nerves.

Riboflavin

Free riboflavin, such as is found in some foods, must be phosphorylated in the intestinal tract before it can be absorbed. Once it enters the blood, it is distributed to all cells of the body. Free riboflavin is excreted as such in the urine and feces. The amount of riboflavin needed is related to body size, metabolic rate, and rate of growth. Liver, milk, cheese, eggs, leafy vegetables, enriched bread, lean meat, and legumes are the foods among the richest in riboflavin. Dried yeast is a still richer source.

Natural Sources of Riboflavin

Food	Range (mg/100 gm edible portion)
Good and moderate sources	
Beef, mutton and pork, raw	0.10–0.3
Brewer's yeast	1.3–4.0
Cheese	0.3–0.5
Chocolate, plain	0.2
Cocoa, powder	0.3–0.4
Eggs, fresh	0.3–0.5
Fish, various, fresh and cured	0.2–0.4
Fruit, dried	0.1
Green leafy vegetables	0.05–0.30
Liver and kidney	2.0–3.3
Maize, whole	0.1
Milk, fresh cow's	0.15
Millets	0.10–0.15
Nuts	0.2
Oatmeal	0.15
Pulses, various, fresh	0.1–0.3
Wheat and barley, whole grain	0.12–0.25
Wheat bran, bran layer only	0.5
Wheat flour, wholemeal	0.10–0.15
Wheat germ, e.g., Bemax	0.67
Wheat germ, germ fraction steam-heated and finely ground	0.25
Poor sources	
Fruits, fresh, tropical and temperate	0.01–0.1
Maize, meal	0.02–0.1
Potatoes, all seasons	0.05
Rice, highly milled	0.03–0.05
Rice, lightly milled	0.05–0.1

ribonuclease. An enzyme that hydrolyzes *ribonucleic acid* (RNA) to *mononucleotides*.

ribonucleic acid (RNA). A *polynucleotide,* composed of the pyrimidine bases, cytosine and uracil; the purine bases, adenine and guanine; the sugar *ribose**; and phosphate. There are different types of RNA that have distinct structure,

functions, and subcellular distributions. Messenger RNA (mRNA) with specific enzymes copies the message from the *deoxyribonucleic acid* * (DNA)
genetic triplet code in the nucleus of the cell. The mRNA then enter the cytoplasm where it combines with ribosomal RNA (rRNA) in the *ribosomes*. The
ribosome-mRNA complex then complexes with transfer RNAs (tRNA) which
bring amino acids to form peptide bonds. The mRNA determines the sequence
and length of the *polypeptide chains*. The constituents of the nucleic acid can
be formed by the body from small compounds and there is no specific requirement in the diet for the biosynthetic incorporation into RNA or DNA. The
nucleotides of the ribosomal chain consist of components like those in a chain
of deoxynucleic acid (DNA), a phosphoric acid molecule, a distinctive sugar
known as ribose, and one purine or pyrimidine. The purines are identical to
those found in DNA, adenine and guanine. The pyrimidines, include cytosine,
but instead of thymine, the ribosomal polynucleotide chains of RNA contain
the pyrimidine uracil. Together DNA and these forms of RNA constitute the
basic tools the cells employ in making a protein according to genetic information.

ribonucleic acid polymerase (RNA-polymerase). An enzyme which catalyses
the formation of ribonucleic acids. Under the influence of RNA-polymerase,
the *ribonucleotides* attached to the DNA by base pairings are linked together to
form polynucleotides such as *messenger, ribosomal,* or *transfer-RNA. See
deoxyribonucleic acid* (DNA).

ribonucleotides. Building blocks of the ribonucleic acids (RNA) each consists
of the sugar, ribose, a phosphate group and a base. The dominant ribonucleo-

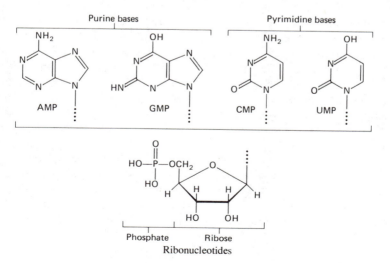

Ribonucleotides

tides adenylic acid (AMP); guanylic acid (GMP); cytidylic acid (CMP); and uridylic acid (UMP). The structures are as follows:

ribose. A five-carbon sugar; a constituent of nucleic acid. Mol. Wt. 150.

Ribose

ribosomes. Dense particles in cell cytoplasm that are the site of protein synthesis. Cell particles composed of ribosomal ribonucleic acid (RNA) and various proteins. During protein synthesis, messenger-RNA is bound to the ribosomes and this is where the translation of the nucleotide sequence of m-RNA to the amino acid sequence of the proteins takes place. See *ribonucleic acid.*

rice (*Oryza sativa*). A cereal grain. Rice is a major foodstuff of Asia and common in the western world. About 8 percent of the total energy provided by rice is protein of good quality, with a net dietary protein (NPU) value of about 65. The limiting *essential amino acids* in rice are *lysine** and *threonine**. All of the cereal grains, wheat, rice, millet, oats and rye, as whole grains, have similar nutritive value and chemical constitution. They have no *ascorbic acid** (vitamin C) and little or no *retinol** (vitamin A) or *carotene**. Rice, like other grains, has high concentrations of calcium and iron which are not totally available as nutrients because of the presence of *phytic acid**. The *thiamine** content of rice varies according to the degree of milling. Rice that has only the husk removed contains about 250 mg of thiamine per 100 grains; hand milling, or one polishing of the rice, removes half of the thiamine; and rice polished three times and ready for the market contains 70 mg of thiamine or about one-third of the original content. Washing and boiling causes further losses of the B-complex vitamins up to 50 percent. Parboiled rice is steamed by special process so that the thiamine and other vitamins and minerals are distributed throughout the kernel with only a slight loss taking place in washing and cooking. In cultures where the staple diet is rice, outbreaks of beri-beri, a disease due to a thiamine deficiency have occurred when highly polished rice was substituted for hand-milled rice. In modern times, beri-beri is not common but not unknown in Asia. *Niacin** (4 mg per 100 g) and *riboflavin** (120 mg per 100 g) are the other B-complex vitamins present in unpolished rice. See *cereal grains.*

Brown rice, cooked, 100 gm = 119 calories
White rice, all types, cooked, 100 gm = 109 calories
Parboiled white rice, cooked, 100 gm = 106 calories
Rice, granulated, breakfast cereal, cooked, 100 gm = 50 calories
Rice flakes, 100 gm = 390 calories
Rice, puffed, 100 gm = 399 calories

rice, brown. The grain or seed of the grass *Oryza sativa;* an aquatic plant widely cultivated in warm climates on wet land. Brown rice is rich in the vitamins of the B complex, *thiamine*, niacin** and *riboflavin**, and in *iron* and *calcium*. It is higher in many of these vitamins and minerals than enriched, parboiled, or other processed rice.

rice flour. Ground rice made principally from the rice broken during milling. It cannot be used in breadmaking but is used commercially for making ice creams and confections. Another use is by persons on allergy diets.

rickets (rachitis). A nutritional disease resulting from a deficiency of *vitamin D** in the young. Vitamin D is a precursor to 1,25-dihydrocholecalciferol* which promotes the absorption of *calcium* from the intestine and the deposition of calcium and *phosphate* into bone. In the young, a vitamin D deficiency results in "soft" bones that grow in a distorted manner depending on the stresses and forces placed on the growing bones by muscles or weight. Once the bone deformity has occurred it cannot be reversed, even though vitamin D will strengthen and harden additional bone growth. Vitamin D can be biosynthesized in the body but requires sunlight. A vitamin D deficiency in an adult results in *osteomalacia*. The deposition of calcium into bone is also under the hormonal control of *calcitonin* and *parathormone*. An intake of 300–400 I.U. per day of vitamin D is the Recommended Daily Allowance and is about three times the intake need for satisfactory growth and calcium absorption from the intestine. Levels about three times higher than the RDA may be toxic in some individuals. Vitamin D is probably the most toxic of the vitamins. See *bone, vitamin D*, osteomalacia,* and *vitamin toxicity.*

rocamble (*Allium scordoprasum*). A European leek, used like garlic but milder in flavor.

rock candy. Large, hard, clear crystals of sugar, made by pouring sugar syrup cooked to a certain density into deep pans that have been laced with heavy thread on which the crystals deposit while being formed.

Rock Cornish hen. A small fowl with small bones and all white meat. It was developed from the Cornish hen, an English breed of domestic fowl with a pea comb, very close feathering, and a compact, sturdy body. Rock Cornish hens weigh from one-half to one and a quarter pounds and are broiled or roasted.

rockfish (Sebastodes). A saltwater food fish. The fish is sometimes mistakenly called the rock cod. Among the best known and most valuable rockfish are the black fish, bocaccio, rasher, red rockfish, Spanish flag, yellow-backed rockfish, and the yellowtail rockfish. The skin varies in color from dark gray to bright orange and the meat from almost a pure white to a deep pink. The texture and flavor of the meat of all the species seem to be the same; texture is firm and when cooked, it is white and flaky, resembling crabmeat; flavor also resembles crabmeat and the fish is often steamed and used for salads. Oven-steamed, 100 gm = 107 calories.

roe. Fish eggs still enclosed in the thin natural membrane in which they are found in the female fish are called roe or hard roe. Roe is taken from many species of fish. Shad roe is perhaps the most popular and best known. However, many different varieties are marketed including alewife, herring, cod, mackerel, mullet, salmon, shad, and whitefish. The size of the roe varies with the fish. Shad roe is usually from 5 to 6 inches long, about 3 inches wide, and an inch or more thick. Soft roe or milt is the male fish's reproductive gland and filled with secretion or the secretion itself. It has a soft creamy consistency and the vein must be removed before cooking. A source of protein. Cod and shad, cooked, 100 gm = 126 calories; canned cod, haddock, or herring, solids and liquid, 100 gm = 118 calories.

rod vision. Rod vision depends on the presence of *rhodopsin* (vision purple) which in turn requires a derivative of *retinol* * (vitamin A), 11-*cis retinal* *. Rod vision is responsible for the ability to see in dim light. The cones, a different type of nerve cell, are responsible for the ability to see color and require an intense light to see compared to the rods. A *retinol* * (vitamin A) deficiency produces night-blindness (nyctalopia), an inability to see in dim light. Some individuals with nyctalopia require as much as 100 times more light than normal to see. Nyctalopia is reversed by *retinol* * (vitamin A).

romaine (Lactuca). One of the principal types of lettuce, also known as Cos lettuce. Romaine has a long narrow cylindrical head with stiff leaves and a broad rib. The leaves are dark green on the outside, becoming greenish-white near the center. Romaine is flavorful and crisp and lends itself to tossed salads of mixed greens. See *Lettuce*

rope. A condition in bread characterized by gelatinous threads that form in the center spore-forming bacteria (*Bacillus mesentericus, B. subtilis*) that may contaminate dough and survive the baking process. As the bacteria multiply they digest the bread.

rosefish (*Sebastes marinus*). Also known as redfish, this is a saltwater food fish. When mature it reaches a length of about 11 inches, weighs about 1 pound, and is bright rose-red or orange-red in color. It may be marketed as an ocean perch. The fish is fatty, with firm flesh, and bland flavor. Fresh, pan-fried, 100 gm = 227 calories; frozen, breaded fried, reheated, 100 gm = 319 calories.

rose hip (*Rosa*). The fleshy swollen red seed capsule of any of various roses, but especially wild rose. The capsules are rich in *ascorbic acid* * (vitamin C) and are used commercially in making an ascorbic acid (vitamin C) concentrate. They are also sold dried whole, cut, or powdered. Rose hips are an excellent source of *carotene* * (vitamin A activity), the B-complex, *tocopherol* * (vitamin E), *vitamin K* *, and is frequently used together with rose hips to make organic ascorbic acid (vitamin C) supplements.

rosemary (*Rosemarinus officinalis*). A perennial evergreen shrub which grows wild in southern Europe and is cultivated throughout the rest of Europe and the United States. It reaches a height of from 4 to 5 feet, and has branching stems which bear long thin dark green leaves with grayish undersides and a strontly aromatic smell. The leaves, fresh or dried, are used as an herb seasoning.

rum. Rum is an alcoholic beverage distilled from the fermented products of sugar cane. There are three chief kinds of rum. The oldest type is Jamaican rum, heavy, dark, full-bodied and usually aged in wood. Cuban rum, which is dry and light bodied is a relatively modern refinement. Rums more aromatic than either the Jamaican and Cuban are produced throughout the Caribbean area.

rutabaga (*Brassica napobrassica*). A root vegetable which belongs to the Mustard family and is closely related to cabbage, cauliflower, Brussel sprouts, kale, kohlrabi, mustard, and turnips. Rutabaga is larger than the turnip, has smooth yellowish skin and flesh, and smooth leaves. The flesh has a typical sweet flavor. There are white varieties of rutabaga, but the yellow is the best known. Some vitamin A and a small amount of *ascorbic acid* * (vitamin C). Boiled and drained, 100 gm = 35 calories.

rye (*Secale cereale*). One of the cereal grains. Rye is similar to rice in composition. *Lysine* * is the limiting essential *amino acid* in rye and it contains about 11 grams of protein per 100 grams of rye. The *thiamine* *, *niacin* *, and *riboflavin* * content is similar to that of rice. Rye also contains no *ascorbic acid* * (vitamin C) or *carotene* * (vitamin A activity). The iron content is similar to that of rice, but rye is a better source of calcium. Rye also contains a small amount of the protein complex called *gluten,* which allows it to form a dough similar to that of wheat. Rye and wheat can be used to make breads because of their gluten content. The other cereal grains do not contain significant amounts of gluten. See *cereal grains*.

Whole grain, 100 gm = 334 calories
Light flour, 100 gm = 357 calories
Medium flour, 100 gm = 330 calories
Dark flour, 100 gm = 327 calories
Wafers, whole-grain, 100 gm = 344 calories

S

saccharin (ortho-benzosulfimide). A sugar substitute that is more than 400 times sweeter than *sucrose**. It has no nutritive value and is used as a substitute for sugar. Recently, saccharin has been suspected as a cancer-causing agent. It is usually marketed as the sodium or calcium salt.

Saccharin (ortho-benzosulfimide)

Saccharomyces. A class of fungi known as yeast cells of which there are several species. In the food industry, the yeast is used under anaerobic and aerobic conditions, depending upon the intended use. *S. cerevisiae* or baker's yeast is used in baking under aerobic conditions. Its popular use in breads derives both from its ability to produce carbon dioxide (CO_2) and cause bread to rise, and the general taste it imparts. Strains of *S. cerevisiae* are also used under anaerobic conditions to promote the production of *ethanol** in beers and ales. In this regard, yeasts are subdivided into the "top" and "bottom" yeast. The top yeast, buoyed to the surface of the fermenting liquids by CO_2 is generally involved in making beers, and the bottom yeast which remains at the bottom of fermenting liquids generally is involved in making light ales and lager. The maintenance of a yeast culture is one of the great secrets of brewing because the yeasts make unpredictable genetic changes (mutate) in its characteristics. The wine industry depends on fermentation of grape juices, by added yeasts and those who grow naturally on the skins of grapes.

safflower oil. An edible oil from the seeds of the safflower plant, *Carthamus tinctorius*. Safflower oil is high in *linoleic acid**, an *essential fatty acid*.

Safflower oil is light, flavorless and colorless. It does not solidify under refrigeration and is good for salad dressings and marinades, as well as for frying.

saffron (*Crocus saturis*). A small crocus, with purple flowers. There are three deep orange-yellow stigmas, or filaments, in the center of each tiny blossom. These are aromatic when dried, with a pungent taste, and are used to add flavor and color in cooking. The name saffron is an adaptation of the Arabic word za'faran, "yellow". The different varieties of saffron have varying degrees of pungency. Saffron gives distinctive color to breads and cakes and is also used with rice dishes, enhances cream soups, sauces, potatoes, and veal and chicken dishes.

sage (*Salivia officinalis*). There are over 500 varieties of this herb growing in temperature zones. The fresh or dried leaves are used in cooking for their aromatic bitter taste. Dalmation sage, grown in Yugoslavia is one of the best varieties of the plant. In addition there are the common garden sage (*S. officinalis*), other varieties are white sage, Cyprus sage, *S. horminum*, meadow sage, pineapple sage, and clary sage. The name "sage" comes through French from the Latin salvus, meaning "safe, whole, or healthy."

sago. A starch extracted from the pithy trunks of various tropical palms, among them the sago palm. It is basic food in the southwest Pacific, where sago meal is used for making thick soups, biscuits and puddings. To make sago, the palm trees are felled and the trunk is cut into pieces. The bark is taken off and the inner portion is soaked in water to remove the starch. The pulpy paste that results is dried and used as sago meal. When the paste is rubbed through a sieve, pearl sago results. Sago flour is also made from the sago meal.

sake. The national alcoholic drink of Japan. Made by fermenting rice. It is yellowish-white and is often drunk warm. Its flavor lies somewhere between western beers and wines.

salami. One of a variety of sausages of Italian origin that can be eaten without being cooked. There are Italian, German, Hungarian, French, and kosher salamis. The word is Italian and implies "salted" meaning that the meat is preserved. Salamis differ from each other by their composition of meats, their spicing, and their salting and curing, and their shape. Salami most often contains pork and some beef although there are pure pork and pure beef salamis. Salamis are divided into two major groupings, hard and soft. Excellent source of protein, good source of iron, *thiamine**, *riboflavin** and *niacin**. Hard salami, 100 gm = 450 calories; soft salami, 100 gm = 311 calories.

saliva. Secreted by the salivary glands, parotid, submaxillary, and sublingual, and by the numerous minute buccal glands of the mucosa of the mouth. The volume of saliva is about 1 liter per day. It consists of a large amount of water containing some glycoprotein material, mucin, inorganic salts, and salivary amylase, (ptyalin). It has a specific gravity of about 1.005 and is nearly neutral in reaction (pH about 6.4 to 7.0). Substances in saliva include inorganic salts in solution, chlorides, carbonates, and phosphates of sodium, calcium, and potassium. The function of saliva are to soften and moisten the food, assisting in *mastication* and *deglutition;* to coat the food with mucin, lubricating it and ensuring a smooth passage along the esophagus; to moisten or liquefy solid food, providing a necessary step in the process of stimulating the taste buds.

salivary amylase (ptyalin). Salivary amylase is formed in the *salivary glands* and initiates starch into *dextrins* and *maltose* * in the mouth. The process of reducing starch to maltose is a gradual one, consisting of a series of changes which take place in successive stages and result in a number of intermediate compounds. The change due to salivary amylases are best effected at the temperature of the body, in a neutral solution, and requires the presence of calcium. The time food spends in the mouth and the general bulk of food does not allow much degradation of starch by salivary amylase. In the stomach, the acid conditions denatures salivary amylase and the further degradation of starches occurs in the small intestines where several amylases reduce starches to *glucose* *, for absorption by the intestinal mucosa. See *digestive system.*

salivary glands (parotid glands). Salivary glands lie in the sides of the face in front of and slightly below the ears. *Saliva* from these glands reaches the mouth through parotid ducts, which open on the inner surfaces of the cheeks opposite the second molar teeth. There are also a pair of submaxillary glands in the angles of the lower jaws and a pair of sublingual glands under the tongue. Ducts from these glands open into the floor of the mouth beneath the tongue. Saliva from the six glands mixes with food in the mouth and softens and lubricates it. Saliva contains a digestive enzyme, *salivary amylase* (ptyalin), which acts to convert starch to sugar. In Asia and Africa, a nutritional disease associated with inadequate protein intake in children has been observed which causes the salivary glands to swell.

salivation. The issue of saliva into the mouth. Saliva can be stimulated to flow by a complex of physical, chemical, and psychological stimuli.

salmon (*Oncorhynchus*). Considered among the greatest of sport and food fishes. The name comes from Romans, from salmo, which comes from the verb "to leap." There is only one variety of Atlantic salmon, and five varieties of Pacific sockeye (*O. nerka*), spring (*O. tschawytscha*), coho (*O. kitsutch*), pink (*O. gorbuscha*), and chum (*O. keta*). In addition there is the steelhead, which is more closely related to the Atlantic than to the other Pacific salmon, and the blueblack, which is really a coho with darker markings. Salmon contain large amounts of phosphorus, potassium, some sodium, *thiamine**, *riboflavin**, and *niacin**, and some *carotene** (vitamin A). Canned salmon contains some calcium if the bones are eaten. Fresh, baked steak, 100 gm = 140 calories; canned, 100 gm = 164 calories.

Salmonella. Infections by certain species of this bacteria are sometimes called "food poisoning" because the symptoms in general resemble those of staphylococcus poisoning and the outbreak is commonly explosive. The *Salmonellae* are gram-negative, nonspore-forming rods that ferment *glucose**, usually with gas but do not ferment *lactose**, or *sucrose**. They are typed on the basis of their antigen content. Humans and animals are directly or indirectly the source of the contamination of foods with *Salmonellae*. The organisms may come from actual cases of the disease or from carriers. The organisms also may come from cats, dogs, swine, and cattle. Chickens, turkeys, ducks, and geese may be infected with any of a large number of types of *Salmonella* which are found in the fecal matter, in hen's eggs, and flesh of dressed fowl. Meat products such as meat pies, hash, sausages, cured meats (ham, bacon, and tongue), sandwiches, chili, etc. when allowed to stand at room temperature over a period of time will permit growth of Salmonellae.

Salmonellosis (food infection). About 1300 serotypes of the *Salmonella* genus have been identified, each being capable of causing infection in man. The typhoid and paratyphoid bacilli which infect man, belong collectively to the genus *Salmonella*. They produce various infections of the intestinal tract. The types of *Salmonella* that are chiefly responsible for human disease are *S. typhi* and *S. paratyphi*. They are rod-shaped bacteria that resist cold and survive for long periods in soil, ice, water, milk, and foods. Since they do not form spores they are easily killed by being boiled for 5 minutes or by pasteurization. Drying and direct sunlight also kill them. These organisms grow easily in simple common foods such as milk, custards, egg dishes, salad dressings, and sandwich fillings. Meat, poultry, fish, eggs, and dairy products that are eaten raw or have been inadequately heated are most frequently implicated in Salmonellosis. Contaminated cake mixes, bakery foods, ·coloring agents, powdered yeast, and chocolate candy have also caused outbreaks of the infection. Animals including cattle, swine poultry, fish, dogs and birds, harbor the organism. They are usually infected by contact of one animal with another or by animal feeds. Flies and rodents coming in contact with feces of animals or man are responsible for contamination of food.

salsify (*Tragopogan porrifolius*). Another name for oyster plant. An elongated root eaten as a winter vegetable, boiled, baked, or in soups; the young leaves may be eaten for salad.

salt. One of a class of compounds found when the hydrogen atom of an acid radical is replaced by a metal or metal-like radical. The most common salt is sodium chloride (NaC1), the sodium salt of *hydrochloric acid**. Other metal or metal-like salts in food may include calcium, potassium, sodium magnesium, sulfur, manganese, iron, cobalt, zinc, and other metals. They may be chlorides, sulfates, phosphates lactates, citrates, or in combination with proteins, as in calcium caseinate. See *sodium chloride*.

salt, iodized. Table salt (*sodium chloride**) to which has been added 1 part per 10,000 of iodine as potassium iodide (KI).

saltpeter. The potassium salt of nitric acid. See *sodium nitrate*.

salt pork. The side of a hog, cured; it is a fattier portion with less lean than bacon. The fat is cured by the dry-salt method and is not smoked. Salt pork is used for larding and barding. It is also used for flavoring and for adding fat to many dishes such as baked beans, clam chowder, stew, etc. Contains *niacin**, *thiamine**, and *riboflavin**, some calcium and potassium, and a trace of iron. 100 raw, gm = 783 calories. Fried, 100 gm = 341 calories.

salting out. Separation of proteins from solution by addition of high concentrations of inorganic salts, usually sodium sulfate or ammonium sulfate.

sand dab. A lean, saltwater fish belonging to the flounder family. A small fish, its flesh has a delicate subtle flavor. Raw, 100 gm = 79 calories.

saponification. The splitting of fat by an alkali, yielding *glycerol* and *soap*. This may occur during the digestion of fat. See *soap*.

saprophytic nutrition. A type of heterotrophic nutrition in which organisms absorb their required nutrients through the cell membrane following the extracellular digestion of nonliving organic material. Saprophytes differ from parasites in that the latter derive their nutrients from other living cells or tissues, sometimes at the expense of the life of the host.

saprophytic plants or animals. A saprophytic plant or animal (yeasts, molds, and most bacteria) is one that absorbs food materials from dead or decaying matter or from the dead parts of living plants or animals. These food materials cannot be absorbed into the body or the organism without first being digested. For this reason saprophytes secrete extracellular digestive enzymes.

sardine. The name used to describe various small saltwater food fish with weak bones which can be preserved in oil. It is not the name of a specific kind of fish. Sardines include the pilchard, alewife, herring, and sprat. It is probably the French sardine, found in abundance around the island of Sardinia, from which the overall name is derived. Sardines are fatty fish. They differ according to kind, depending on locality. Sardines are an excellent source of protein and good source of calcium, iron, and niacin. Atlantic, canned in oil, solids and liquids, 100 gm = 311 calories. Canned in tomato sauce, solids and liquid, 100 gm = 197 calories.

sardine oils. Obtained from fish caught in Japanese waters and off the French and Spanish coasts. Japanese and/or Korean sardine oil is manufactured from the Japanese sardine, *Clupanodon melanosticta,* and the European oil from *Clupea sardinus, L.* The oils have high iodine values and have been used to a limited extent as drying oils for the manufacture of paints. They are also used in the leather industry and have been hydrogenated for edible use.

sassafras (*Sassafras albidum* or *variifolium*). A tree of the laurel family, one variety of which, is a native of North America. The bark is rough and gray, and the bright green leaves are of three shapes, all on the same tree. These leaves, when dried and ground, are the prime ingredients of file, a thickening and seasoning agent which forms the base of gumbo.

satiety value. That quality of food contributing to satisfaction and resulting in a sustained sense of comfort or well being, fullness, or gratification of appetite.

saturated fats. *Fat* which contains a large number of *saturated fatty acids* as a part of the fat molecule. *Unsaturated fats* (oils) contain unsaturated fatty acids. Saturated fat occurs in most animal fat and animal products, for example, meat—beef, veal, lamb, pork, products such as cold meats, sausages, eggs, whole milk, lard, cheese, cream, sweet and sour; ice cream and butter. Saturated fat also occurs in some plant products, for example, coconut, coconut oil, and *chocolate*. Oils may be converted to an unsaturated fat by reducing the unsaturated fatty acid by a chemical process called hydrogenation.

saturated fatty acids. An organic acid in which the carbons contain the maximum permissible numbers of hydrogens is a saturated fatty acid. As a class of compounds, they have the general formula $C_nH_{2n}O_2$. *Acetic acid* * (vinegar), *butyric acid* *, and *stearic acid* * are examples of saturated fatty acids. The following are some naturally occurring fatty acids.

Common Name	Chemical Name	Chemical Formula
Butyric	*n*-Butanoic	$C_4H_8O_2$
Caproic	*n*-Hexanoic	$C_6H_{12}O_2$
Caprylic	*n*-Octanoic	$C_8H_{16}O_2$
Capric	*n*-Decanoic	$C_{10}H_{20}O_2$
Lauric	*n*-Dodecanoic	$C_{12}H_{24}O_2$
Myristic	*n*-Tetradecanoic	$C_{14}H_{28}O_2$
Palmitic	*n*-Hexadecanoic	$C_{16}H_{32}O_2$
Stearic	*n*-Octadecanoic	$C_{18}H_{36}O_2$
Arachidic	*n*-Eiocosanoic	$C_{20}H_{40}O_2$

saturation. To cause to unite with the greatest possible amount of another substance, through solution, chemical combination, or the like. A *saturated fat,* for example, is one in which the component fatty acids are completely filled or saturated with hydrogen atoms. A fatty acid is said to be saturated if all available chemical bonds of its carbon chain are filled with hydrogen. If one bond remains unfilled, it is a monounsaturated fatty acid. If two or more bonds remain unfilled, it is a polyunsaturated fatty aicd. Fats of animal sources are generally more saturated than fats from plant sources.

saurekraut. Pickled cabbage made from cabbage which has been cut fine and allowed to ferment in a brine made of its own juice, salt, and occasionally other spices. U.S. Grade A sauerkraut is white or cream-colored with long uniform shreds, crisp firm texture, and a good flavor. Canned, solids and liquid, 100 gm = 18 calories; canned juice, 100 gm = 10 calories.

sausage. A preparation of minced or ground meat, usually seasoned with salt and spices and stuffed into a casing. Sausages may be made of all pork, all beef, or a combination of two or more meats. They may be fresh or smoked, dry or semidry and they may be uncooked, partially cooked or fully cooked. The name sausage is derived from the Latin word for salt. Sausage is high in fat good amounts of protein, iron and the B vitamins. The caloric values which follow are given for an edible portion of 100 gms.

Blood sausage = 394 calories
Bockwurst = 264 calories
Bologna, all meat = 277 calories
Bologna, with cereal filler = 262 calories
Braunschweiger = 319 calories

Cappicola = 499 calories
Cervelat, dry = 451 calories
Frankfurter, all meat, raw = 296 calories
Frankfurter, with cereal filler, raw = 248 calories
Headcheese = 268 calories
Kielbasa = 304 calories
Knockwurst = 278 calories
Liverwurst, fresh = 307 calories
Liverwurst, smoked = 319 calories
Mortadella = 315 calories
Pork sausage, links or bulk, cooked = 476 calories
Pork sausage, links, smoked (country style) = 375 calories
Salami, dry = 450 calories
Salami, cooked = 311 calories
Souse = 181 calories
Thuringer, cervelat = 307 calories
Vienna sausage, canned = 240 calories
See *meats* for nutrient content.

savory (*Satureia hortensis and S. montana*). Two closely related herbs which belong to the mint family. The aromatic leaves of both plants are widely used for seasoning.

scallion (*Allium*). The name is given without much exactitude to several plants of the onion family; the green onion, the shallot, and the leek. The word scallion, like *shallot,* comes from the Latin name of the shallot, *A. ascalon,* which relates to the ancient city of Ascalon where it is probable that this vegetable was developed near the Mediterranean coast of Palestine and Syria. After trimming, the entire scallion is used, usually chopped or minced as a seasoning vegetable. Raw, 100 gm = 46 calories.

scallop. A group of bivalve mollusks with ribbed rounded shells. Only the muscle which opens and closes the shell is used for eating. A good source of protein. Low in fat, scallops have some calcium, a large amount of phosphorus, traces of riboflavin and niacin. Fresh, raw, 100 gm = 81 calories; fresh, steamed, 100 gm = 112 calories; frozen, breaded, friend, reheated, 100 gm = 194 calories. See *Fish* for nutrient content.

Schizosaccharomyces. Yeasts which produce asexually by fission and form four or eight ascospores per ascus after isogamic conjugation, have been found in tropical fruit, molasses, soil, honey, and elsewhere. A common species is *S. pombe.*

scrapple. A very solid mush made from the by-products of hog butchering; the mush is sliced and fried for a breakfast or supper dish. The basis for the making of scrapple is a broth produced by the cooking of the hog's head, liver, tongue, meaty bones, and other scraps. The meat that remains in the broth is ground, and other ground pork meat may be added. Meat and broth are then combined and seasoned, and the mixture is boiled. The mixture is normally thickened with cornmeal. Unfried, 100 gm = 366 calories.

scrod (*Gadus* and *Melanogrammus*). A young *cod* or young *haddock* weighing from 1½ to 2½ pounds. A scrod is also a whole small cod split and boned for cooking.

scurvy. A nutritional disease caused by a lack of *ascorbic acid* * (vitamin C). "A Treatise on Scurvy," written in 1773 by James Lind recounts a classic nutritional experiment in the prevention of a nutritional disease. About 40 years later limes, which were shown to be antiscorbutic, were routinely issued to British sailors to prevent scurvy, hence the nickname "limey" for British sailors. The antiscorbutic substance in food was named vitamin C in 1920 to distinguish it from two other vitamin fractions isolated from foods, the fat soluble *vitamin A* * and the water soluble *vitamin B* *. Both vitamins A and B were later shown to consist of more than one factor. The chemical name *ascorbic acid* * was suggested by Szent-Gjorgi in 1933 who also isolated sufficient quantities of the antiscorbutic substance to permit chemical analysis and synthesis by others in 1933. Besides man and other primates, only the guinea pig, and a species of fruit bat require ascorbic acid in the diet, other animals synthesize ascorbic acid from *glucose* *.

sebum. The secretion of the sebaceous glands, which contain *fats, soaps, cholesterol* *, protein, remnants of epithelial cells, and inorganic salts. It serves to protect the hairs from becoming too dry and brittle, as well as from becoming too easily saturated with moisture. Upon the surface of the skin it forms a thin protective layer, which serves to prevent undue absorption or evaporation of water from the skin. This secretion keeps the skin soft and pliable. However, this retained secretion often becomes discolored, giving rise to the condition commonly known as blackheads.

secretin. A hormone secreted by the mucosa of the small intestine, duodenum, and *jejunum,* by interaction with substances present in the acid *chyme* discharged from the stomach into the duodenum. Carried by the blood to the various organs, secretin stimulates the flow of *pancreatic juice,* the secretion of bile, and gastric enzyme *pepsin,* but inhibits *gastric acid* secretion.

sedatives (drugs). Drugs which have a calming, quieting effect and in large doses, induce sleep. An example is phenobarbital.

selenium (Se). Element number 34. Atomic weight 79. An essential micronutrient that is toxic at high concentrations. In terms of abundance in the earth, selenium occurs with frequency comparable to gold. Certain plants have the capability of concentrating selenium (woody aster, golden weed, gray's vetch) and are responsible for alkali disease and the blind staggers in horses that graze on these plants. On the other hand, the judicious addition of selenium to the feed of lambs and calves markedly improves their health. No instances of selenium toxicity is known or has been described in man. The amount of selenium in human blood varies greatly throughout the world from 1 to 10 micromoles per liter. The amount of selenium in water varies from 0.01 to 4 micromoles per liter of water. The content in animals also varies, therefore it is impossible to establish normal ranges of selenium in man. Selenium is required for the activity of the enzyme glutathione peroxidase which protects *unsaturated fatty acids* from oxidation of unsaturated bonds (peroxidation). It is through its protection of fatty acids from peroxidation that an associative relationship *vitamin E* (tocopherol) occurs. Vitamin E also protects unsaturated fatty acids from peroxidation. Selenium can also replace sulfur in some amino acid and proteins.

semolina. The purified middlings (medium-size particles of ground grain) of wheat. The word is derived from the diminutive of the Italian semola, "bran." The best semolina, the type used in the manufacture of macaroni, spaghetti, and other pastas is obtained in the milling of durum wheat.

sequestrant (sequestering agent). Compound capable of combining with metal ions in solution with an affinity that prevents their dissociation into free ions. A sequestrant is the same as a *chelator*. Sequestrants or chelators are often used in soft drinks to maintain clarity and color; in food containing unsaturated fats to prevent or slow peroxidations catalyzed by heavy metals; and to prevent heavy metals from making antioxidants ineffective by their combination with them. *Citric acid** is a naturally occurring compound that is used as an additive sequestrant in shortenings, lard, mayonnaise, soup, salad dressing, margarine, cheese, vegetable oils, pudding mixes, vinegar and confectionary.

serine. Mol. Wt. 105. A nonessential amino acid found in proteins.

$$HO-CH_2-\overset{\displaystyle NH_2}{\underset{\displaystyle H}{C}}-COOH$$

serosa. The membranes lining the cavities that contain the heart, intestines, and lungs, and covering their contents.

serum. The fluid portion of the blood that separates from the blood cells after clotting. It differs from *plasma* in that serum lacks the fibrinogen separated with the clot.

sesame (*Sesamum indicum*). An annual tropical and subtropical herbaceous plant. Sesame is grown for its tiny grayish-white or black seeds which have a sweet nutty flavor and which yield a bland oil when pressed. The cake left after the oil has been expressed from the seeds has also been used for food and fodder. Caloric values: Sesame seed, dry, whole, 100 gm = 563 calories; sesame seed, dry, decorticated, 100 gm = 582 calories; sesame oil, 100 gm = 884 calories.

sex glands or gonads. The gonads (derived from the Greek word meaning seed) consist of the testes in men and the ovaries in women. In addition to producing sperm and ova, the glands elaborate hormones that are responsible for the special male and female characteristics. The male sex glands are the two testes, which lie enclosed in the scrotal sac of the skin just below the penis, and secrete semen containing the male reproductive element, the sperm. They also contain the important male sex hormone, testosterone. In the female sex glands, like the testes, the two ovaries have more than one function. They produce the ova, or eggs; they also secrete hormones needed for both reproduction and feminine characteristics. The ovaries lie in the front part of the abdomen, below the navel, and each is connected with the uterus by a fallopian tube. The ovarian hormones are estrogen and progesterone. They are produced in small amounts before puberty and after menopause, and in abundance during the childbearing years, the period when a woman has her regular monthly cycles. Menstruation involves the discharge of the extra, unusued blood and tissue built up in preparation for conception.

serum albumin. The predominant carbohydrate-free protein is albumin, which constitutes more than 50 percent of the total serum protein. Since serum alumbin has a high affinity for free fatty acids and other anions it binds these anions very effectively and therefore serves as a transport or carrier protein. In this manner, free fatty acids which are toxic in the free form, hemolytic and insoluble, are solubilized, removed and transported to the liver as a soluble, nontoxic fatty acid albumin complex. Serum albumin also serves to control the osmotic pressure of the blood as well as maintain the buffering capacity of the blood pH. Serum albumin is approximately 69,000 in molecular weight and is a typical globular protein with a low α-helical configuration.

shad (*Alosa*). An important food fish of the family Clupeidae which also includes herrings. They differ from herrings chiefly in being larger and in the fact that they enter rivers to spawn. The common American shad, *A. sapidissima,* can reach a weight of 14 pounds, but the average weight ranges from 1½ to 8 pounds, with 4 or 5 pounds most common. The fish has a compressed body with a rounded bluish back, silvery sides and undersurface. It is excessively bony, but the dark-pink flesh is delicious and its roe is prized.

Fresh, raw 100 gm = 170 calories
Fresh, baked, 100 gm = 201 calories
Canned, solids and liquid 100 gm = 157 calories
Roe, raw, 100 gm = 130 calories
Roe, baked or broiled, 100 gm = 126 calories

shaddock or pummelo (*Citris grandis*). A citrus fruit native to the East Indies. It is similar to the grapefruit and may be its ancestor. It grows to the size of a watermelon, weighs up to 20 pounds, has a coarse thick rind and reddish, aromatic, but bitter flesh.

shallot (*Allium ascalonium*). A mild-flavored cousin of the onion, chive, garlic, and leek, which belongs to the Liliaceae or Lily family. The shallot, *A. ascalonium,* derives its name from the ancient Palestinian city, Ascalon, where it was probably first grown. The shallot has a thick outer skin shading from reddish to gray, the bulb underneath greenish at the base and violet on the upper portion. It grows in clove form, with several cloves attached to a common disc. The Jersey, or "false" shallot, is of various shapes, often larger than the "true" shallot, with thin red skin, and bulb sometimes white but usually all violet. The edible part of the shallot is the bulb, which after maturity and dry storage is used just as the garlic onion is used. The green tops are sometimes marketed as *scallions.* Fresh shallots are rich in *carotene* * (vitamin A), *ascorbic acid* * (vitamin C), and in iron. Dried shallots contain less vitamin C than fresh ones. Fresh, tops only, 100 gm = 27 calories; dry bulbs, raw, 100 gm = 72 calories.

sheepshead. A saltwater fish, a cousin of porgies and scups. The sheepshead has large broad incisor teeth, much like a sheep. The flesh of all sheepshead is white, tender, and pleasant. They can be fried, sauteed, baked. Saltwater, raw, 100 gm = 113 calories; freshwater, raw, 100 gm = 121 calories.

shellfish. Shellfish belong to two very large classes, the mollusks and the crustaceans, and are found in salt and fresh water. The mollusks have a soft structure and are partially or wholly enclosed in a one- or two-part shell. The former, called "univalve" mollusks, include the abalone, conch, and periwinkle. The latter, called "bivalve," include the clam, cockle, mussel, oyster, and scallop. Crustaceans are covered with a crustlike shell and have segmented bodies. Among them are the crab, crayfish, lobster, prawn, and shrimp. Shellfish are good sources of protein and iodine, and contain some amounts of the B vitamins. The crustaceans are higher in protein content than the mollusks. See *fish* for nutrient contents.

sherbert. A frozen dessert made of a fruit juice or puree, a sweetener, and water, to which milk, beaten egg white, gelatin, or marshmallow is added.

sherry. A Spanish aperitif or dessert wine, the color varying from pale amber to dark brown and the taste from very dry to very sweet. Sherry is made differently from other wines. After the sweet juice from the pressed grapes has fermented in its own way, it is blended with many similar wines from different years. Brandy is added to the mixture and the beverage is allowed to age in special casks. Sherry improves with aging.

shigellosis. Bacillary dysentery is caused by rod-shaped bacteria of the genus Shigella. The Shigella organisms grow easily in foods, especially in milk. The boiling of food and water or pasteurization of milk kills the organisms. Several species that may cause Shigellosis are spread by feces, fingers, flies, milk and food, and by articles handled by unsanitray carriers.

shish kebab. A dish of meat, usually lamb, broiled or skewered. The name comes from the Turkish, shish, meaning skewer, and kebap, roast meat. Today it has come to mean as well a skewered combination of meat, fruits, and vegetables which may or may not have been marinated and seasoned with herbs and spices before broiling.

shrimp. A 10-legged (decapod) crustacean, whose comparatively small size is responsible for its name; the Middle English shrimpe meant "puny person" and the name is akin to the Swedish skrympa, meaning "to shrink." Shrimps vary considerably in size, ranging from the great Mexican and Gulf shrimps to the tiny half-inch creatures found in the cold waters off Scandinavia. The color of shrimps also varies but is some pale shade, usually brownish red or grayish green. The bright-pink color of the shell of cooked shrimps is due to a chemical change that takes place through exposure to heat. Most shrimps available in markets are actually the abdomens and tails of shrimps, with the stalked eyes, heads and feelers removed. The line of demarcation between shrimps, scampi, and prawns is not clearly defined. Shrimp are high in protein, low in fat.

Fresh, raw, 100 gm = 91 calories
Fresh, fried, 100 gm = 225 calories
Frozen, breaded, raw, 100 gm = 139 calories
Canned, wet pack, solids, and liquids, 100 gm = 80 calories
Canned, dry pack or drained solids of wet pack, 100 gm = 116 calories
Shrimp paste, 100 gm = 180 calories

siderophilin. See *Transferin*

Siderosis. Term used to describe the presence of excess iron in the body, as demonstrated by the presence of an iron storage protein, *hemosiderin* in the tissues. Siderosis may occur because of (1) an excessive iron intake, (2) excessive destruction of red cells in hemolytic conditions and after multiple blood transfusions, and (3) failure to regulate absorption. It is not clear whether a minor degree of siderosis affects health. Siderosis is one of the factors which may cause cirrohosis of liver.

simple sugar. See *monosaccharide.*

skeletal muscle or striated muscle. It is skeletal muscle that consitutes what is often called flesh or meat. There are about 400 skeletal muscles made up of about 250 million individual cells called muscle fibers. They form about 30 percent of the total body weight. Muscle fibers are elongated structures, 1–50 millimeters long but only 0.010–0.1 millimeter in diameter, which are attached at both ends to either connective tissue or bone. The cell membrane around each muscle fiber is called the *sarcolemma* and the fiber is full of minute protein threads (myofibrils), 1 micron in diameter. The myofibrils run along the whole length of the muscle fiber and are made up of many longitudinal strands of a protein called *myosin.* Each muscle fiber is connected to the central nervous system by a branch of a motor nerve fiber which ends in a specialized termination called the motor end-plate. Of the three muscle types, skeletal, cardiac, and smooth, skeletal muscle acts most rapidly, completing a single contraction and relaxation in less than 0.1 second. Cardiac muscle contracts and relaxes in 1–5 seconds and smooth muscle contracts and relaxes in periods as long as 2 minutes. Skeletal muscle is generally under voluntary control, among the exceptions is the upper third of the esophagus. All muscle attached to bones is striated muscle. Striated muscle is also attached to tongue, the soft palate, the scalp, the pharynx, and the extrinsic eye muscles. See *meat, cardiac muscle,* and *smooth muscle.*

skeleton. The bone framework of animals in the phylum chordata and the subphylum vertebrata (vertebrates). The human skeleton contains 206 bones held together by *muscle* and *tendons, Cartilage* also functions as part of the framework, but is not composed of bone and is not a part of the skeleton.

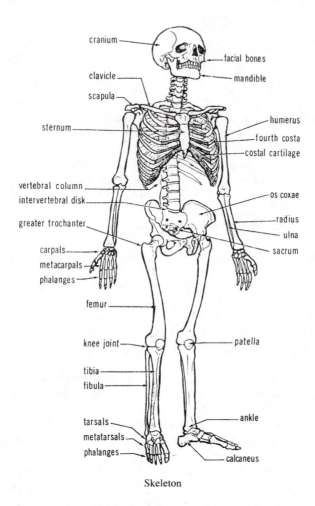

cranium

facial bones

clavicle

mandible

scapula

sternum

humerus

fourth costa

costal cartilage

vertebral column

os coxae

intervertebral disk

greater trochanter

radius

ulna

carpals

sacrum

metacarpals

phalanges

femur

knee joint

patella

tibia

fibula

tarsals

ankle

metatarsals

phalanges

calcaneus

Skeleton

skin. The skin is called the integumentary or covering body system and serves the body in many important ways. The most obvious feature of the skin is its outward appearance. Four functions of skin are protective: as a mechanical barrier to the entrance of bacteria; regulation of body temperature, through control of heat loss; sensory perception, through nerve endings that transmit sensations of touch, heat, cold, and pain; an excretion of body wastes through sweat. The skin has two principal layers, the epidermis or outer layer and the dermis, the inner layer or true skin. The epidermis and dermis are supported by a subcutaneous (under-the-skin) layer which connects the skin to underlying muscles.

skull. The skull forms the bone framework of the head, and has 29 bones; 8 cranial, 14 facial, 6 ossicles (3 tiny bones in each ear) and 1 hyoid (a single bone between the skull and neck area). The cranial bones support and protect the brain. At birth there is an opening, the fontenella, at the top of the skull. These bones fuse together after birth in firmly united joints called sutures. The 8 cranial bones include 1 frontal, 2 parietal, 1 occipital, 2 temporal, 1 ethmoid, and 1 sphenoid. The frontal bone forms the forehead, part of the eye socket, and part of the nose. The parietal bones form the dome of the skull and the upper side walls. The occipital bone forms the back and base of the skull. The temporal bones form the lowest part of each side of the skull and contain the essential organs of hearing and of balance in the middle and inner parts of the ear. The ethmoid and sphenoid bones complete the floor of the cranium, the ethmoid toward the front and the sphenoid toward the center. The air spaces in the frontal, ethmoid, and sphenoid bones are sinuses.

sloe (*Prunus*). The fruit of the blackthorn, (*P. spinosa*) which grows wild in woods and hedges in most parts of the British Isles. The sloe, in French is called prunelle, is edible but not usually picked to be eaten. Its chief use is to flavor sloe gin. In the United States the name sloe is also given to the fruit of the native plum tree (*P. americana*) which is occasionally used for jams, jellies, and conserves. The fruit of the American tree is small and bitter and generally yellow or reddish-yellow in color.

smell. Sensory endings for the sense of smell are located in the olfactory membrane over the surface of the superior nasal conchae (chamber) and the upper part of the septum. These sensory nerve endings are the least specialized of the special senses. To smell anything well, air is sniffed into the higher nasal chambers and thus brings the odoriferous particles in great numbers into contact with the olfactory hairs. Odors can also reach the nose by way of the mouth. Many flavors of food are really odors rather than gustatory (taste) sensations, and one becomes aware of them just after swallowing. Each substance smelled causes its own particular sensation, and one is able not only to recognize a multitude of distinct odors but also to distinguish individual odors in a mixed smell. The taste of any substance is usually a combination of taste and smell.

smelt (*Omerus*). Any of several small fish belonging to the family Osmeridae. Their backs are greenish and translucent, sides and belly are silvery. The name is also used for various silversides of the family Atherinidae, which resemble the true smelt. Their flesh is delicate, rich, and oily, Smelt contain some calcium, large amounts of phosphorus, some *thiamine*, riboflavin, retinol** (vitamin A), and a small amount of *niacin**. Fresh, raw, 100 gm = 91 calories. Canned, solids and liquid, 100 gm = 200 calories.

smooth muscle (visceral muscle). In smooth muscle, each fiber appears as a single spindle-shaped cell containing many *nuclei*. The individual muscle fibers seen in skeletal muscle are fused into a single syncytium. Smooth muscle also contains myofibril elements for contraction. The transverse striations seen in *cardiac muscle* and skeletal muscle are absent in smooth muscle, which accounts for the names "nonstriated muscle" or "plain muscle." Smooth muscles are not usually subject to voluntary (conscious) control. Contractions are slow, sustained, and sometimes rhythmical. Smooth muscle is found in the walls along the *digestive tract,* the *trachea* and bronchi, the *urinary bladder,* the gall bladder, the urinary and genital ducts, the *uterus,* walls of *blood vessels,* the capsule of the *spleen,* the iris of the eye, and the *hair follicles* of the skin. See *meat, cardiac muscle* and *skeletal muscle.*

snap bean. A variety of the common garden bean, which includes both round, flat green, yellow or wax beans, and the so-called Italian green beans. Snap beans are also called green beans or string beans. Snap beans have small amounts of carotene* (vitamin A), *iron* and *thiamine**. Green beans have more vitamin A than yellow beans. Caloric values which follow are given for an edible portion of 100 gm:

Fresh, green, raw = 32 calories
Fresh, green, boiled and drained = 25 calories
Canned green, regular pack, solids and liquid = 18 calories
Canned green, regular pack, drained solids = 24 calories
Frozen green, cut style, boiled and drained = 25 calories
Frozen green, French style, boiled and drained = 26 calories
Fresh yellow or wax, raw = 27 calories
Fresh yellow or wax, boiled and drained = 22 calories
Canned yellow or wax, regular pack, solids and liquid = 19 calories
Canned yellow or wax, regular pack, drained solids = 24 calories
Frozen, yellow or wax, boiled and drained = 27 calories

soap. A salt of a long-chain fatty acid. Hard soaps are sodium salts and soft soaps are potassium salts. The soaps emulsify and have a detergent activity. The carboxylate group ($-COO^-$), the anion, is balanced by ionic bond with sodium ion (Na^+) or potassium ion (K^+). It is these parts of the soap that interact with water. The hydrocarbon chain dissolves oily material. The same principles apply to *emulsifiers.*

soda. Chemically soda is a sodium compound of any one of many varieties. In reference to food it is most often sodium bicarbonate or sodium acid bicarbonate, a crystalline salt used in the manufacture of baking powder, carbonated beverages, and effervescent salts.

soda water (carbonated water). A beverage charged with carbon dioxide under pressure, a process which produces a liquid which bubbles, fizzes, or sparkles when opened. The term does not include beverages in which the gas is produced within the beverage by the natural process of fermentation. The carbon dioxide in soda water is produced from sodium bicarbonate by the action of sulphuric or other acid. Soda water is used in combination with various flavorings to produce soft drinks, and combined with liquor for high balls and other alcoholic drinks.

sodium (Na). Elements No. 11. Atom. Wt. 23. It is one of the two important alkali metals, *potassium* is the other. Sodium ions (Na^+) are chiefly in the

Sodium content of some common food:

Food	gm/100gm
Bacon, raw	0.76–1.20
Beef, corned	1.31–1.70
Beef, pork, mutton, raw	0.05–0.11
Biscuits, assorted	0.25–0.39
Bread, all extractions	0.39–0.67
Butter, fresh and salted	0.21–0.99
Cheese, cream	0.12–0.35
Cheese, hard (cheddar, etc)	0.51–1.50
Cornflakes	0.67–1.01
Cornflour	0.05
Egg, fresh, whole	0.14
Fruit, dried, uncooked	0.03–0.08
Ham, boiled, lean	2.0
Ice cream	0.05
Margarine	0.32
Milk, fresh, whole	0.05
Oatmeal	0.03
Sausage, raw	0.74–1.31
Shellfish, fresh and canned	0.07–0.30
Vegetables, canned	0.23–0.60
Vegetables, root and green, cooked and raw	0.01–0.14
Wines, ales, and stout	0.01–0.04

See *potassium, sodium chloride* *.

fluids that circulate outside the cells, and only a small amount of it is inside the cells. Potassium ions (K^+) are mostly inside the cells. Sodium and potassium are vital in keeping a normal balance of water between the cells and the fluids. Sodium and potassium ions are essential for nerves to respond to stimulation, for the nerve impulses to travel to the muscles and for the muscles to contract. All types of muscles including the heart muscle, are influenced by sodium and potassium. Sodium and potassium also work with proteins, phosphates and carbonates to keep a proper balance between the amount of acid and alkali in the blood. The body normally conserves its supply of sodium and potassium ions when the intake is low by reabsorption in the kidneys, which reduces the amount that is filtered in the urine. Excessive sweating can cause a major loss of sodium from the body and muscle cramps. Table salt, sodium chloride (NaC1) is the main source of sodium in a diet and taste and habit determines the amount eaten. Foods from animal sources, including meat, fish, poultry, milk, and cheese, contain more sodium than do foods from plant sources. Most fresh and frozen vegetables contain only small amounts of sodium unless salt is added. Beets, carrots, celery, chard, kale, beet and dandelion greens, and spinach are exceptions; they contain several times more sodium than other vegetables. Foods contain the most sodium when salt has been added to them directly or by brining or pickling, or by curing.

sodium benzoate. Mol. Wt. 144. The sodium salt of benzoic acid. Sodium benzoate is a food preservative which can prevent the growth of almost all microorganisms, (bacteria, fungi, and yeast), but effective only under acidic conditions. Limited to such foods as fruit juices, carbonated drinks, pickles, salad dressing, and preserves. Used at levels of 0.05 to 0.1 percent. Occurs naturally in many fruit and vegetables, notably cranberries (0.05 to 0.09 percent) and prunes.

sodium chloride (table salt). Mol. Wt. 58. The usual intake of sodium chloride is 7 to 15 gm daily. This includes sodium chloride contained in foods, as well as that added as table salt. Deficiency of sodium chloride occurs mainly during hot weather or as a result of heavy work in a hot climate when excessive sweating takes place. The simple provision of extra salt in food or in salt tablets will prevent or correct the condition. Dehydration is generally associated with salt depletion. The blood volume is decreased, the veins collapse, the blood pressure decreases and the pulse rate becomes rapid. Salt depletion can occur without water depletion. The condition is called water intoxication. Large water intakes without salt causes a decreased concentration of salt in the blood that can cause *anorexia,* weakness, and mental apathy. In extreme conditions, convulsions and coma may occur. Reduced salt (sodium chloride) intake is often a recommendation in cases of severe hypertension (diastolic pressure over 120). If the sodium content is significantly lowered there is usually a decrease in blood pressure. The table below gives the approximate daily sodium chloride intakes for various sodium restricted diets.

Diet	gm NaCl/Day
Normal	9
Restricted	6
Low Salt	2

NACl

sodium erythorbate. A close but nonnutritive relative of *ascorbic acid* * (vitamin C). Its most important use is to brighten the pink color of frankfurters, bologna, sliced pastrami, and other cured meats to prevent that color from fading. Occasionally used as an antioxidant in beverages, baked goods, pimento salad, and potato salad.

sodium nitrate. Mol. Wt. 85. $NaNO_3$. The sodium salt of nitric acid (HNO_3). The potassium nitrate salt (KNO_3) is known as saltpeter. Nitrates are used as fertilizers and also as an additive in cured meats such as frankfurters and bologna. Under some conditions nitrates in food can be reduced to potentially toxic nitrites through the action of microorganisms. See *sodium nitrite.*

sodium nitrite. Mol. Wt. 69. $NaNO_2$ Sodium nitrate and *sodium nitrate* * are used in cured meats as coloring, flavoring, and preservatives. They are present in ham, bacon, corned beef, most frankfurters, salami, liverwurst, bologna, and smoked fish. Nitrites can react with secondary amines under certain conditions, such as heat and in the intestines, to form a class of compounds called nitrosamines ($R_2N-N=O$). Dimethylnitrosamine has been shown to cause cancer in experimental animals. There is no evidence that nitrosamines cause cancer in humans, but the addition of nitrites to foods such as bacon has been questioned.

sodium propionate. See *calcium proprionate* and *proprionic acid.*

solute. Any solid particle that dissolves or goes into a liquid solution, usually water. Any particle that dissolves in water does in fact react with water. For example, when a solid particle of *sodium chloride* * (table salt) dissolves, it interacts with water to form a sodium ion and chloride ions which become independent in solution. Each ion is surrounded by a water molecule, that is to say, each ion is hydrated.

solution. A liquid containing dissolved particles or other liquids in a homogeneous single liquid phase.

solvent. The liquid into which solids (*solutes*) dissolves.

sorbic acid. Mol. Wt. 112. Sorbic acid and its sodium and potassium salts are food additives that act as mold and yeast inhibitors. They are often added to cheeses.

$$CH_3-\underset{\underset{H}{|}}{C}=C-C=C-COOH$$

sorbitan monostearate (mono oleate). Polyoxyethylene ether of *stearic acid* * (oleic acid) esters of *sorbitol* * anhydrides. Serves as an emulsifier in cakes, cake icings, whipped vegetable oil toppings, frozen pudding, coconut spread, and many other foods. Used at levels up to 1 percent, often in combination with one of the polysorbate emulsifiers.

sorbitol (glucitol). Mol. Wt. 182. A polyalcohol made commercially by the hydrogenation (reduction) of glucose. Sorbitol is also found naturally in some fruit (such as rowanberries). It is about 60 percent as sweet as *sucrose* (table sugar). Sorbitol is used in the manufacture of diabetic jams, marmalade, canned fruits, fruit drinks and chocolate. Contains 4 calories per gram. Sorbitol is absorbed into the bloodstream and converted to sugar, thereby providing calories. Because sorbitol is absorbed very slowly, blood sugar levels rise only slowly. Foods sweetened with sorbitol instead of sugar provide diabetics with a relatively safe source of sweetness and energy and allow them to decrease their intake of fats.

$$HO-CH_2-\overset{\overset{OH}{|}}{\underset{\underset{H}{|}}{C}}-\overset{\overset{H}{|}}{\underset{\underset{HO}{|}}{C}}-\overset{\overset{OH}{|}}{\underset{\underset{H}{|}}{C}}-\overset{\overset{OH}{|}}{\underset{\underset{H}{|}}{C}}-CH_2OH$$

Sorbitol

sorghum. A genus of grasses with a large number of species, cultivated throughout the world for food, forage, and syrup. They are tall annuals, resembling maize. The grains are smaller and rounder than most of the true cereals such as wheat. The sorghums, although less nutritious than maize, require very little water and can be grown in regions where maize will not flourish. There are four main types of sorghums: grass, grain, broomcorn, and sugar. Grass sorghums are used entirely for hay and pasturage. The grain sorghums grown in the United States include Durra, Milo, Shallu, Kaoliang (Chinese sorghums), Feterita, and Hegari. The grain or seed is used for livestock food and the plants for foliage. Commercial uses include alcohol, beer, oil, and starch. In Asia, India and Africa grain sorghums are a staple human food. Broomcorns, grown in the United States have a panicle with long branches, known as the "brush." These branches are used for carpet and whisk brooms. The sugar sorghums are tall and leafy and their canelike stalk contains a sweet juice which can be boiled down into a syrup. This syrup has been used as a molasses substitute. In sorghum, the syrup is not crystallized into sugar, but rather used in a pure concentrated form. 100 gm = 257 calories.

sorrel (dock) (*Rumex*). A hardy perennial herb with several varieties which differ in shape of leaves and strength of flavor. All varieties are acid to some degrees. The mildest variety is dock (*R. patientia*), also called spinach dock and herb patience dock. A tall plant, growing over 5 feet tall, its foot-long mild leaves are used in the spring as a salad green or potherb. French sorrel (*R. scutatus*) has shield-shape leaves. It has an acid sour flavor, and is used in salads. Very high in *retinol** (vitamin A), with small amounts of calcium and phosphorus and some *ascorbic acid** (vitamin C). Raw, 100 gm = 28 calories; cooked and drained, 100 gm = 19 calories.

sour cream. In its simplest form, sour cream is unpasteurized heavy sweet cream that has been allowed to stand in a warm place until it has become sour. It varies in texture and flavor. Commercial dairy sour cream is made from sweet cream chemically treated with lactic-acid bacteria to produce a thick cream with a mild tangy flavor. The cream is pasteurized and homogenized to distribute the fat evenly throughout. The lactic-acid bacteria is then added and the cream is held at the proper temperature for a specific length of time. When the cream is ready, it is chilled to stop the action of the bacteria and then packaged. Sour cream contains sodium, calcium, phosphorus, potassium, *thiamine**, and *riboflavin**. Good source of *carotene** (vitamin A activity) with some *vitamin D**. 100 gm = 180 calories.

soybean (*Glycine max*). Also called soya, soy pea, soja, and soi, is found in the hairy pods of an erect bushy legume, native to Asia. Soybeans contain a large proportion of assimilable protein, have a considerable fat content, and are low in carbohydrates, having no starch at all. Soybeans have been used as food in China for thousands of years. The whole dry grain contains about 40 percent fat. The protein of soy bean has a high quality with a *net protein utilization* (NPU) value of 65. Soy bean is also a good source of B-complex vitamin. Per 100 grams of soybean the approximate vitamin contents are as follows: *carotene** (vitamin A), 110 I.U.; *thiamine** 1 mg; *riboflavin** 0.3 mg; *niacin** 2 mg; and only a trace of *ascorbic acid**. The food energy is 350 cal/100 gm. The major proteins in soybean are glycinin, phaseolin, and legumelin. The major carbohydrates are *sucrose, raffinose, stachyose,* and *pentosans*. Soybean is now an important raw material, as animal feed, as an oil in margarine, and as a flour in human foods. Soy flour is present in cereal products, sausages, bisquits, infant foods, milk substitutes, and in artificial meat.

Soybean flour, full fat, 100 gm = 421 calories
Soybean flour, high-fat, 100 gm = 380 calories
Soybean flour, low-fat, 100 gm = 356 calories
Soybean flour, 100 gm, defatted = 326 calories
Canned soybeans, solids and liquid, 100 gm = 75 calories
Canned soybeans, drained solids, 100 gm = 103 calories
Dried soybeans, cooked, 100 gm = 130 calories
Soy sauce, 100 gm = 68 calories
Soybean oil, 100 gm = 880 calories.

soybean oil. An oil extracted from the soy bean, which contains about 18 percent oil by weight. Soybean oil is used in the manufacture of margarine shortening, candy and soap. The oil is rich in *unsaturated fatty acids;* 25 percent *oleic acid**, 49 percent *linoleic acid** (an *essential fatty acid*), and 11 percent linolenic acid. About 11 percent of the fatty acids are saturated.

soy sauce. Soy sauce is a mixture of amino acids, polypeptides, simple proteins, carbohydrates and other degradation products obtained by a combination of mold fermentation and acid hydrolysis. More than half of the vitamins in soybeans are destroyed in the process.

spaghetti. One of the most popular members of the pasta family, spaghetti is made from a mixture of semolina, the flour that is milled from durum wheat, and water. The dough is passed through metal discs full of holes to emerge as slender solid rods. The name spaghetti is Italian from the plural form of spaghetto, "string." Spaghetti is a fair source of *iron* and *thiamine**.

Cooked al dente, 100 gm = 148 calories
Cooked tender, 100 gm = 111 calories

Spaghetti in tomato sauce with cheese, home recipe, cooked, 100 gm = about 100 calories

Spaghetti in tomato sauce with cheese, canned, 100 gm = 76 calories

spareribs. A cut of meat consisting of the lower portion of the ribs and breast-bone removed from a fresh side of pig or hog. The ribs have only a small amount of meat but the succulence of the meat and fat makes them good eating. Spare ribs are high in protein, with small amounts of calcium and iron and some phosphorus, *thiamine* *, *riboflavin* *, and *niacin* *. Braised, medium fat, 100 gm = 440 calories; roasted, meat only cut from ribs, 100 gm = 273 calories.

spearmint (Mentha spicata, *var. viridis***).** A strong scented perennial herb, grown for home and culinary use. The word mint and spearmint are often used synonymously. Spearmint has dark green lance-shape leaves and red-tinged stems. Its long pointed flower stalks bear pale purple flowers. Either fresh or dried, the leaves add a pleasant and distinctive flavor to cranberry juice, fruit cup, and some soups; they give delicate flavor to meat ragouts or fish. Mint sauce, chopped mint, and vinegar is a popular accompaniment to roast lamb, as in mint jelly. Fruit compotes, ice cream, fruit beverages, and jellies all use mint.

specific activity (enzymes). Units of enzyme activity per milligram of protein.

specific dynamic action (SDA). When food is ingested, the metabolic rate (energy expenditure) increases above that of the fasting level. The total increase due to SDA of food is about 10 percent per day. Each food type has a different SDA value. The SDA for protein is about 30 percent, carbohydrate 6 percent, and fat 4 percent of increase above the energy value of the food type ingested. The cause of metabolic rate increase is not known.

spices. The oldest of the food additives. Spices are some part of an aromatic plant, e.g., seeds, roots, stems, barks, depending upon the plant. Herbs generally involve the entire plant. Spices were originally used to mask the odors of decaying foods in times before refrigeration. The essential oil of some spices have preservative effects, e.g., clove and cinnamon, but are used now primarily as flavoring agents. Spices are used in quantities too small to provide any nutritional value. Today the word spice tends to be confined to the following group of products made from various parts (most often other than the seeds or leaves) of plants grown in the tropics: allspice, red pepper, and whole chili peppers, from dried fruits; cayenne pepper, from a ground whole plant; cinnamon from bark; cloves, from dried flower buds; mace from the dried aril of the nutmeg, which itself is the kernel of a fruit; paprika, from dried pods; pepper, from a dried berry; and saffron, from the dried stigmas of a flower. See *herbs*.

spinach (*Spinacia oleracea*). An annual potherb which originated in southwestern Asia and is grown for its leafy green leaves. An excellent source of *retinol* * (vitamin A), a very good source of *ascorbic acid* * (vitamin C) and *iron,* and a fair source of *riboflavin* *. It is low in calories. Spinach is a good source of *vitamin K* * which aids in the formation of the blood substance required for clotting of blood.

Fresh, raw, 100 gm = 26 calories
Fresh and frozen, chopped, boiled and drained, 100 gm = 23 calories
Canned, regular pack, solids and liquid, 100 gm = 19 calories
Canned, regular pack, drained solids, 100 gm = 24 calories
Canned, dietary pack, solids and liquid, 100 gm = 21 calories
Canned, dietary pack, drained solids, 100 gm = 26 calories
Frozen, leaf, boiled and drained, 100 gm = 24 calories

sphingomyelin. A phospholipid found in the brain, spinal cord, and kidney. Occurs in large amounts in the myelin sheath of nerve tissue and derives its name from this structure. The sphingomyelins contain phosphorylcholine attached to the terminal carbon atom of sphinogosine and a fatty acid attached in amide linkage to the nitrogen. See *sphingolipids*.

spingolipids. A class of phospholipids that have in common a sphingosine component. The sphingolipids include *ceramides, spingomyelins,* and *glycosphinolipids* (cerebrosides and gangliosides).

$$\underset{\text{Sphingosine (4-sphingenine)}}{CH_3(CH_2)_{12}-CH\!\!=\!\!CH-\overset{\overset{\displaystyle OH}{|}}{CH}-\overset{\overset{\displaystyle NH_2}{|}}{CH_2OH}}$$

spleen. The largest collection of lymphoid tissue in the body, the spleen is located high in the abdominal cavity on the left side, below the diaphragm and behind the stomach. It is somewhat long and ovoid (egg shaped). Although it can be removed (splenectomy) without noticeable harmful effects, the spleen has useful functions, such as serving as a reservoir for blood and red blood cells.

sprat (*Clupea sprattus*). One of the smallest of the herrings, 5 inches is its normal maximum length. Sprats are caught in abundance in many parts of

Europe and extensively eaten there fresh and smoked. A sprat is also called a Norwegian sardine or anchovy. In the United States the term sprat is applied to the young of the common herring and to many other small fishes.

squab. Any young pigeon which has not been allowed to fly. Squabs weigh about 1 pound. Good source of protein, with some phosphorus and a small amount of calcium. Raw, 100 gm = 279 calories.

squash (*Cucurbita*). A gourd fruit native to the Western Hemisphere. The two main types of squash are summer and winter squash. There are many varieties within each group, each differing in shape, size, and color.

squash, summer. Small, quick growing, with thin skins and light-colored flesh. The most common varieties eaten are (1) Scallop, Cymling or Pattypan, disk shape with a scalloped edge. The skin is smooth or slight worted, pale green when young, and turns white as it matures. (2) Cocozelle, cylindrical, with smooth skin, slightly ribbed with alternate stripes of dark green and yellow. Similar to zucchini. (3) Caserta, also cylindrical but thicker than cocozelle at the tip. The skin has alternate stripes of light and dark green. (4) Chayote, pear-shape squash about the size of an acorn squash, light green in color. It has one soft seed in the center. (5) Yellow crookneck, a squash with a curved neck, larger at the top than the base. The worted skin is light yellow in young squash, turning to a deep yellow when mature. (6) Yellow straightneck, similar to the Crookneck except that the neck is straight and it grows to be much larger, 20 inches long and 4 inches thick when mature. (7) Zucchini, sometimes called Marrow or Italian Marrow. It is cylincrical but larger at the base. The skin has a lacy pattern of green and yellow that concentrates to give the appearance of stripes.

squash, winter. Winter squash has a hard, coarse rough rind that is dark green or orange in color. There are many types of winter squash. The most common varieties are: (1) Acorn grows to be 5 to 8 inches long and 4 to 5 inches wide. It has a thin, smooth, hard shell which is widely ribbed, and is dark green, but changes to orange during storage. The flesh is pale orange and there is a large seed cavity. (2) Buttercup has a turbanlike formation at the blossom end. The hard skin is dark green with faint gray pockmarks and stripes and the turban is light gray. The dry sweet flesh is orange in color. (3) Butternut is cylindrical in shape with a bulblike base. The skin is smooth and hard and is a light brown or dark yellow color. (4) Warren Turban is drumshape with a turbanlike formation at the blossom end. The hard worted skin is bright orange, the blossom end slightly striped, and the turban a bluish color. (5) Hubbard globe-shape with a thick tapered neck that is somewhat smaller at the blossom end. The skin may be bronze-green, blue-gray, or orange-red in color; it is hard, worted, and ridged. The flesh is yellowish orange and has a sweet taste. (6) Sugar green or orange rind with ridges round or oval-shape, with stem at the top. The flesh is bright orange with many seeds in the center of the pumpkin. Summer squash provides *ascorbic acid* * (vitamin C), *carotene* * (vitamin A activity), and *niacin* *. Since summer squash is low in calories and sodium it may be used frequently in a sodium-restricted diet, reducing or other special diets. Winter squash is an excellent source of vitamin A, and has a fair *ascorbic acid* * (vitamin C), *riboflavin* * and *iron*.

Summer squash, crookneck and straightneck, boiled and drained, 100 gm = 15 calories

Summer squash, scallop, boiled and drained, 100 gm = 16 calories

Summer squash, cocozelle and zucchini, boiled and drained, 100 gm = 12 calories

Summer squash, other varieties, boiled and drained, 100 gm = 14 calories

Winter squash, acorn, boiled, 100 gm = 34 calories

Winter squash, acorn, baked, 100 gm = 55 calories

Winter squash, butternut, boiled, 100 gm = 41 calories

Winter squash, butternut, baked, 100 gm = 68 calories

Winter squash, hubbard, baked, 100 gm = 50 calories

Winter squash, hubbard, boiled, 100 gm = 30 calories

Winter squash, other varieties, boiled, 100 gm = 38 calories

Winter squash, other varieties, baked, 100 gm = 63 calories

stabilizers and thickeners. Stabilizing substances are added to many foods to impart smooth texture and to help maintain flavor. In chocolate milk and instant breakfasts made basically of skim milk, stabilizers thicken the milk and prevent separation of the chocolate. Carageenin, a seaweed derivative, is widely used in diet milk products. In commercial ice cream and other frozen desserts, stabilizers often are used to increase viscosity and to help prevent the water in the product from freezing into crystals. Flavor oils used in some cake mixes, gelatins, and pudding mixes are highly volatile and stabilizers are used to prevent flavor evaporation and deterioration. Among the thickeners often used commercially to process foods are *pectin* and *gelatins*.

stachyose. An indigestible tetrasaccharide containing *galactose* *, present in beans. There is evidence that the flatulence after consumption of large amounts of beans is due to stachyose and *raffinose* *, a trisaccharide containing *galactose, glucose* *, and *fructose* *, which are not digested by the enzymes in the small intestine but pass to the colon where they are fermented by resident microflora. See *raffinose* *.

Staphylococcus. A common type of bacteria responsible for food poisoning. Food handlers with cutaneous (skin) infections are a major source of this contamination of foods. Staphyloccoci grow in cream fillings, custards, puddings, hollandaise sauce and other starch, eggs, and milk containing mixtures (meat and meat combinations will also support their growth). Rapidly growing staphylococci may spread their enterotoxin within a few hours in fertile media like cream puffs and custard pies if growth is not deterred by proper refrigeration. Warm foods or foods permitted to stand for prolonged periods at room temperatures in summer months are an open invitation for this type of food poisoning. The toxin of staphylococcus acts primarily on the gastrointestinal tract. Since a preformed poisonous substance, the enterotoxin, is involved, onset of symptoms after ingestion is rapid and occurs usually within about 3 hours. Symptoms are acute and include nausea, vomiting, diarrhea, intestinal cramps, headache, and an occasional fever. The attack does not last more than one day and frequently terminates within 6 hours or less.

starch. A high molecular weight polymers of glucose ranging in molecular weights from 50 thousand to several million. Starch occurs in two types of molecules, one type, amylase, consisting of long unbranched chains that form a three-dimensional spiral. The connections between glucose units is α 1$\longrightarrow$4.

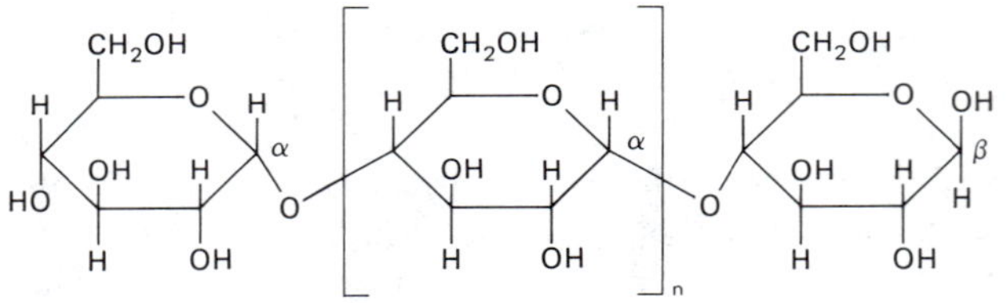

Amylose

The other type, amylopectin, is high branched chains, and very similar to *glycogen,* animal starch. The branching in amylopectin is less than that in glycogen. The branching is α 1$\longrightarrow$6 and the linear backbone is + 1$\longrightarrow$4, as in glycogen.
In amylopectin branching occurs at every 24–30 glucose units (M = 24–30), in glycogen n = 8–12, in the diagram above. Starch in plants is laid down in "granules" coated with a celluloselike substance. When subjected to moist heat, starch granules absorb water, swell, and are ruptured. After treatment, starch forms a colloidal dispersion in water and is more easily digested in this state. Starch is found stored in seeds, roots, tubers, bulbs, and to some extent in the stems and leaves of plants. It is of great importance as a constituent of many natural foods and as a source of *dextrins, maltose**, and *glucose**. It

Amylopectin and glycogen

constitutes one-half to three-fourths of the solid matter of the ordinary cereal grain and at least three-fourths of the solids of mature potatoes. Unripe apples and bananas contain much starch which is to a large extent changed into sugars as these fruit ripen; while on the other hand, young tender corn (maize) kernels and peas contain sugar which is tranformed into starch as these seeds mature. Starch is the most important source of carbohydrate intake in the American diet. The cooking of starch not only improves flavor, but also softens and ruptures the starch cells which facilitate enzymatic digestive processes. The digestion of starch begins in the mouth, where salivary *amylase,* an enzyme, is secreted. Under its influence the chain of glucose units are split into smaller fragments. Hydrolysis continues in the stomach after the food is swallowed until the stomach contents become too acid. The starch fragments and undigested starch and sugars then pass into the small intestine. There the acid is neutralized, more amylase is secreted into the intestine from the pancreas, and the starch is eventually broken down to maltose and *isomaltose *,* disaccharides that consist of two glocuse units. Maltose and isomatltose are hydrolyzed to glucose by their specific maltases.

steapsin. An enzyme in *pancreatic juice* that hydrolyzes fat. It is a *lipase.*

stearic acid. Mol. Wt. 284 ($CH_3(CH_2)_{16}COOH$. A saturated fatty acid. The difference in consistency of various fats at room temperature is due to differences in the kinds and amounts of fatty acids that enter into their composition. *Palmitic ** and stearic acids, which enter largely into the composition of solid fats, have a type formula of $C_nH_{2n}O_2$; they are said to be saturated because they cannot take up any more hydrogen.

$$H-H-H-H-H-H-H-H-H-H-H-H-H-H-H-H-H-H$$
$$H-C-C-C-C-C-C-C-C-C-C-C-C-C-C-C-C-C-C$$
$$H-H-H-H-H-H-H-H-H-H-H-H-H-H-H-H-H-H$$

Stearic acid

stearyl citrate. An ester of stearyl alcohol, $CH_3(CH_2)_{16}CH_2OH$ and citric acid. Stearyl citrate and isopropyl citrate, protect oils by trapping metal (chelates) ions that might otherwise catalyze oxidation reactions and cause rancidity. It is a chelating agent or *sequestrant*. Stearyl citrate is used in margarine, isopropyl citrate is used in vegetable oil and other fat containing foods. It has been found that the body converts these additives to citrate and stearyl or isopropyl alcohol, which are digestible and harmless.

steroids. Complex molecules containing atoms arranged in four interlocking rings, three of which contain six carbon atoms each and the fourth of which contains five. The basic ring structure is a cyclopentanophenanthrene.

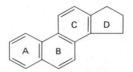

The cyclopentaphenanthrene

Some steroids of biological importance are vitamin D, the male and female sex hormones, the adrenal cortical hormones, *bile salts,* and *cholesterol.* Cholesterol is an important structural component of nervous tissue and other tissues, and the steroid hormones are of prime importance in regulating certain phases of metabolism.

sterols. *Steroids* which possess an alcohol (OH) group. Cholesterol is the most prominent member of this group found in the body, while *ergosterol* and *sitosterol* are common sterols found in plants. Sterols are widely distributed in small amounts in foods and are normal constituents of body tissues. They are concentrated especially in the liver and in lesser amounts in the blood and other tissues. Certain hormones formed in the adrenal cortex and sex glands are also sterols.

stimulants (drugs). Drugs which cause an increase in the activity of an organ or a system. Caffeine, a central nervous system stimulant, decreases drowsiness and fatigue. Digitalis, a heart stimulant, strengthens heart muscle contraction.

stock. A liquid food made by cooking ingredients slowly for a long time so that all the essential flavor and nutrients of the ingredients are dissolved in the liquid. The solid particles remaining are discarded and the liquid may be further concentrated or clarified according to the way it is to be used.

stomach. A baglike structure about 1 foot long and 6 inches wide that can hold about 1.2 liters. It has layers of muscles that contract in different directions. As a result, the stomach can squeeze, twist, and churn food to break it up mechanically and to mix it with digestive secretions. The stomach's thick mucous lining acts like a chemical factory. It produces *hydrochloric acid* * to help in the digestion of proteins and various enzymes to split fats and other food substances. When the stomach is filled, the pyloric sphincter closes and retains the contents until the food has been mixed with certain digestive juices collectively called gastric juice. Gastric juice has two main components, hydrochloric acid, produced by the parietal cells, and pepsin, produced by *chief cells*. The hydrochloric acid in the stomach juice has three important functions: (1) It softens the connective tissues of meat. (2) It kills bacteria destroying many potential disease-producing agents. (3) It activates at least one of the stomach enzymes, which are chemicals that convert food into soluble and absorbable substances.

strawberry (*Fragaria*). A juicy edible fruit belonging to a member of the Rose family, *Rosacae*. The fruits vary in size and color; there are whitish or yellowish fruits as well as the much more common red ones. An excellent source of *ascorbic acid* * (vitamin C). They also contain iron and other minerals.

    Fresh, raw and unsweetened, 100 gm = 37 calories
    Canned, water pack, 100 gm = 22 calories
    Frozen, whole, syrup pack, 100 gm = 92 calories
    Frozen, sliced, syrup pack, 100 gm = 190 calories

stricture. A narrowing of the esophagus resulting from acute or chronic esophagitis or secondary to a tumor. Difficult, painful swallowing, especially when coarse foods are swallowed, is the chief symptom.

stroke. The specific damage to the brain that results from injury to an artery either in the brain or leading to it. The artery damage deprives some of the brain of vital oxygen and other nutrients. In most cases of stroke, blood flow to part of the brain is blocked by a clot in an artery (thrombosis); another problem lies with a leaking or burst artery; or the flow is blocked by a clot coming from another area of the body and lodging in the brain (embolism). In almost every instance of blood clot blockage, the underlying cause is atherosclerosis or disease of the artery wall; and in hemorrhage, the underlying cause is atherosclerosis or a combination of atherosclerosis and high blood pressure.

strontium (Sr.) Element No. 38. Atom. Wt. 88. Like calcium and magnesium, strontium is a divalent alkaline earth metal and its biological behavior is in many ways similar to that of calcium. In general strontium is present in foods which are rich in calcium, especially milk and to a lesser extent fresh vegetables; it is also stored in bone.

sturgeon (*Acipenser*). Various species of fish are known as sturgeon. They are distributed throughout the coastal waters and rivers of the north temperate zone. One related genus, Scaphirhynchus, is recognized as a sturgeon; this is the shovelhead or shovelnosed, freshwater sturgeon found in the Mississippi and other North American rivers. Fresh sturgeon steaks are considered a delicacy, the flavor being so distinct that it requires little seasoning. Another product of the sturgeon is isinglass, made from the swim bladder of the fish. It is used as a clarifying agent and in making jellies and glues. Sturgeon is high in protein. Smoked sturgeon, 100 gm = 149 calories; caviar, granular, 100 gm = 262 calories; caviar, pressed, 100 gm = 316 calories.

subclinical disease. A disease course usually so mild that no definite symptoms that can be recognized by the usual or clinical means.

subcutaneous fat. A layer of fatty tissue, directly under the skin, normally present in well-nourished individuals. The extent and thickness of this layer of subcutaneous fat vary considerably in different individuals, according to sex, general build, and dietary habits. Fat is a very poor conductor of heat, or a good insulator, so that persons with a well-developed layer of fat under the skin lose heat to the exterior much less readily than do those who have little subcutaneous fat.

substrate. A general term for a compound that is chemically altered by the action of an *enzyme*.

succinic acid. Mol. Wt. 118. HOOC CH$_2$CH$_2$ COOH. A four-carbon dicarboxylic acid that is an intermediate in the *Krebs cycle** (tricarboxylic acid cycle, citric acid cycle).

succistearin. An emulsifier used to a limited extent in shortening to help make more tender baked goods. The body converts the additive to *succinic acid**, *stearic acid**, and *propylene glycol**, which may be used as a source of energy.

sucrose. Mol. Wt. 342. Sucrose is commonly known as table sugar. A disaccharide that yields *glucose** and *fructose** when hydrolyzed. Produced by squeezing the juice from sugar cane or sugar beets. This raw juice is neutralized with lime, filtered, and then subjected to vacuum evaporation to remove the excess water. After vacuum evaporation, crystals of raw sugar remain mixed with the mother liquor. The mother liquor, blackstrap molasses, is removed by centrifuging. The raw sugar is dissolved in water and decolorized by filtration through boneblack. Recrystallization is accomplished by vacuum evaporation followed by centrifuging. Sucrose includes no free formyl or carbonyl groups therefore it is not a reducing sugar. The average consumption is about 100 pounds of sugar per year or about 125 frams per day. Large consumption of sugar (sucrose) over many years has been implicated as a cause of dental caries, heart disease, and diabetes, but no firm associations have been established. The diet distribution of food consumed over the last century has varied little with respect to fat, protein, and carbohydrate. However, within the carbohydrate group, sugar has replaced starches to a large extent and represents a major dietary change. With sucrose as a base for comparison given a value of 100, the general relative sweetness of the common sugars have been evaluated as follows:

Fructose	110–175
Sucrose	100
Glucose	75
Galactose	35–70
Lactose	15–30

α-D-glucosyl-(1→2)β-fructoside

Sucrose

suet. The hard fat around the kidneys and loins in beef, mutton, and other carcasses, which yields tallow. In cookery, unless the word is otherwise qualified, the reference is always to beef suet which has a bland taste. Suet is sold in meat markets by the pounds in large pieces, or sold by weight and sliced and ready to be used for barding meats. Suet (beef, kidney fat), raw, 100 gm = 854 calories.

sugar. A polyhydric alcohol containing three or more carbons and an aldehyde of ketone group. A sweet taste is characteristic of polyhydric alcohols. A sweet substance, capable of being crystallized, which is colorless or white when pure. It occurs in many plant juices and forms an important element of human food. Sugar as we usually think of it is, more specifically, cane sugar, which may also be called sucrose or saccharose. By extension, sugar also means any of a class of sweet, soluble compounds comprising the simpler carbohydrates. In addition to cane sugar these carbohydrates or natural sugars are: dextrose or grape sugar, levulose or fruit sugar, lactose or milk sugar, and matose or malt sugar. The chief sources of sugar are the sugar cane and the sugar beet. Cane sugar is made by expressing the juice from the sugar cane. It is then treated with lime to remove impurities, filtered, and evaporated to crystallization. In the case of beet sugar, the sugar is removed by extraction with water and carried to the refined state in one operation. There are various types of sugars: (1) *Granulated sugar* is the product for general use. (2) *Superfine* or *powdered sugar* is a very fine granulated sugar for use in cold drinks, for fruits and cereals, and for special cake baking. (3) *Confectioners' sugar* is granulated sugar that is crushed very fine and mixed with cornstarch to prevent caking. (4) *Brown sugar* is also called soft sugar and consists of extremely fine crystals that are covered with a film or coating of molasses. This coating gives the sugar the characteristic color and taste. (5) *Maple sugar* is made from the sap of the sugar maple, concentrated and crystallized into sugar. Sugar is almost 100 percent carbohydrate and is the most efficient source of energy that can be used by the human body. Brown, 100 gm = 375 calories; white, granulated or powdered, 100 gm = 385 calories. See *sucrose*, glucose*,* and *fructose*.*

sulfitting. Treatment of foods with sulfur dioxide or certain related compounds, sulfites. The sulfur combines with enzymes in the food and prevents them from causing quality deterioration.

sulfonamides (drugs). Drugs which inhibit the growth of or destroy bacteria, particularly the occus worm. One example is sulfisoxazole.

sulfur (S). Element No. 16. Atom. Wt. 32. Occurs principally as a constituent of the amino acids, *cysteine*, cystine*,* and *methionine*,* and is intimately associated with protein metabolism. It is present in all cells of the body but is most prevalent in the epidermal structure, keratin and hair. Sulfur also occurs united to the carbohydrates in some instances. Food proteins contain about 1 percent sulfur, this amount varying with the amount of sulfur-containing animo acids. Sulfur is largely oxidized to sulfate in the liver and is excreted as inorganic and etheral sulfates in the urine. Foods that are good sources of organic sulfur include bluefish, chicken, dried beans, liver, peanuts and turkey, but sulfur is so widespread in foods, especially protein foods, that if the protein in the diet is adequate there is little likelihood of dietary deficiencies of this element occurring.

sulfur dioxide O=S=O (SO$_2$). Mol. Wt. 64. A chemical compound of sulfur and oxygen having antioxidant properties. It is sometimes used in food technology for control of discoloration.

supplement, nutritional. A general term which usually refers to a concentrated source of nutrients, prescribed in addition to the daily diet to increase nutrient intake. A supplement may be a food such as yeast or wheat germ, a concentrate such as cod liver oil, or a pharmaceutical preparation of vitamins or minerals.

surface active agents (surfactants). Similar to *stabilizers* and thickeners in their chemical action. They cause two or more normally incompatible (nonpolar and polar) substances to mix. If the substances are liquids, the surface active agent is called an *emulsifier*. If the surface agent has a sufficient supply of hydroxyl groups, such as the *bile acid* or *cholic acid**, the groups form hydrogen bonds to water. Some surface active agents have hydroxyl groups and a relatively long nonpolar hydrocarbon end. Examples are diglycerides of fatty acids, monopalmitate and sorbitan monostearate. The hydroxyl group on one end of the molecule anchor via hydrogen bonds in the water, and the nonpolar end is held by the nonpolar oils or other substances in the food. This provides tiny islands of water held to oil. These islands are distributed evenly throughout the food.

surfactant. See *emulsifiers*.

sweet basil. See *basil*.

sweet breads. The thymus glands of lamb, veal, or young beef (under 1 year; the thymus disappears in mature beef). Sweetbreads consist of two parts; the heart sweetbread and the throat sweetbread. Lamb and veal sweetbreads are white and tender; beef sweetbreads are redder in color and a little less tender. A good source of protein.

Young beef, raw, 100 gm = 207 calories
Young beef, cooked, 100 gm = 320 calories
Veal, raw, 100 gm = 94 calories
Veal, cooked, 100 gm = 168 calories
Lamb, raw, 100 gm = 94 calories
Lamb, cooked, 100 gm = 175 calories

sweet cicley (*Myrrhis odorata*). A perennial plant with aromatic leaves which are finely chopped in salads and stews. The leaves have a mild aniselike flavor. The seeds can be eaten fresh. The herb is said to improve the flavor of all other herbs with which it is combined. The seeds are especially good in beverages and cordials, fruit salads, and fruit cups.

sweet potato (*Ipomoea batatas*). The enlarged or swollen roots of a perennial vine of the morning glory family. There are hundreds of varieties, with the skins of many colors although yellow tones predominate. They may be slender or globular, forked or beet-shape. The flesh is usually yellow-red, but some sweet potatoes are white. The majority are sweet. Some sweet potatoes have a jellylike consistency, while others are so dry that they have to be moistened with butter or a lubricant before they can be swallowed. The sweet potato, is often confused with the *yam* which it resembles. Yams, however, belong to the completely different botanical genus *Pioscorea*. Excellent source of *ascorbic acid* * (vitamin C) and *carotene* * (vitamin A activity).

Baked in skin, 100 gm = 141 calories
Boiled in skin, 100 gm = 114 calories
Candied, 100 gm = 168 calories
Canned, syrup pack, 100 gm = 114 calories
Dehydrated, reconstituted with water, 100 gm = 95 calories

sweeteners (non-nutritive, artificial). Artificial sweetening ingredients are *saccharin,* sodium saccharin, sodium cyclamates, potassium cyclamate, calcium cyclamate, or any combination of these.

swordfish (*Xiphias gladius*). An oceanic food and sport fish, which may weigh between 200 and 600 pounds. The swordfish is a fish of the Atlantic and Mediterranean. Occasionally it is found in the Pacific. The flesh is red, meaty, and rich. Good source of protein and vitamin A. Fresh, broiled, 100 gm = 174 calories; canned solids and liquid, 100 gm = 102 calories. See *fish* for nutrient content.

sympathetic nervous system. The cell bodies of the connector neurons of the sympathetic nervous system lie in the gray matter of the spinal cord from the levels of the eighth cervical to the second lumbar segments. The nerve fibers from these cells leave the central nervous system in the anterior nerve roots, but they split off from them to end in 22 paired sympathetic ganglia (collection of nerve cells), which are linked together to form the two sympathetic nerve chains running down the back wall of the cavity. These primary efferent nerve fibers are called preganglionic fibers and they end in close approximation to numerous secondary nerve cell bodies in the sympathetic ganglia. The secondary cell bodies give rise to the secondary efferent or postganglionic nerve fibers.

syndrome. A set of symptoms occurring together. The outward signs or symptoms of a disease; e.g., sneezing for hay fever, skin eruption, high fever.

synergism. The joint action of separate agents in which the total effect of their combined action is greater than the sum of their separate actions. Each agent potentiates the action of the other.

synovium. A synovial membrane, lubricated by synovial fluid or mucin. See *membranes*.

synthetases (synthases). A general class or group of enzymes that synthesizes a specific compound. For example, fatty acid synthase is a complex of several enzymes that leads to the synthesis of *fatty acid*. Glycogen synthetase is a single enzyme involved in one of several steps in the synthesis of *glycogen* * (animal starch).

systemic. Pertaining to the body as a whole.

systole. The contraction of the *heart;* the interval between the first and second heart sounds during which blood is forced into the aorta and pulmonary arteries. See *heart*.

systolic hypertension. May be caused either by increase in the amount of blood pumped by the *heart* or by the loss of elasticity of the large arterial walls, most often due to *arteriosclerosis*. May be encountered by many apparently healthy people as they grow older.

T

tachycardia. Rapid beating of the heart.

tamarind (*Tamarindus indica*). A tall tropical shade tree native to the upper Nile region of tropical Africa and possibly southern Asia as well. Its name is derived from the Arabic tamr hindi, "Indian date." Tamarind pulp is used in preparing chutney, curries, and preserves. The juice is used in pickling fish and in making a syrup. This syrup, when diluted with water, makes a cold drink with a milk laxative quality. Raw, 100 = 239 calories.

tangelo (*Citrus*). A member of the citrus family which is a hybrid of the tangerine and grapefruit. They were crossed in 1897 to produce the new fruit. The name is derived from the words "tangerine" and "pomelo," another name by which the grapefruit is known. Tangelos have an orange rind and pale yellow flesh with a pronounced acid flavor. Their size is medium to large. Two of the most successful varieties differ considerably in shape (pear or round) and in peel (thin and smooth or rough and thick). Tangelos are eaten out-of-hand or used in salads. They are also squeezed for juice. Caloric value: juice, 100 gm = 41 calories.

tangerine (*Citrus*). A citrus fruit that is a descendant of the mandarin orange. Tangerines are smaller than oranges. Like all mandarins, tangerines have thin skins which peel off readily and segments that can be easily separated from the pulp. The color of the skin is a rather intense orangy-yellow, and the flavor of the fruit delicate, yet a little spicy and tart. They are named after the North African city of Tangiers, although their original home is China. Tangerines are eaten raw and are used in salads. Peeled and segmented, they can be served with a cheese tray; combined with Tokay grapes or blueberries and sprinkled with coconut; or used in a gelatin. The rind can be used grated as a flavoring. Nutritive food values. A good source of *ascorbic acid* (vitamin C).

Fresh, 100 gm = 46 calories
Juice, fresh;. and canned, unsweetened, 100 gm = 43 calories

Juice, canned, sweetened, 100 gm = 50 calories
Frozen concentrate, unsweetened, undiluted, 100 gm = 162 calories
Frozen concentrate, unsweetened, diluted, 100 gm = 46 calories
See *fruits* and *appendix 9* for nutrient content.

tapeworm. The beef tapeworm *Taenia saginata,* and the pork tapeworm, *Taenia solium* are transmitted by the fecal-oral route, usually in the form of mature eggs in segments of the worm. These cysts are eaten by cattle in sewage-polluted pastures or by hogs in polluted garbage. The larva develop in the animal's intestine, then encyst in the muscle. If man eats the infected meat raw or rare, the adult tapeworm matures in the intestine and continues its reproductive cycles.

tapioca. A valuable farinaceous food made by heating the starch obtained from the roots of the *manioc,* one of the chief tropical food plants. Under the action of the heat the starch grains burst and are converted into small irregular masses. This product, after baking to remove all moisture, is flake tapioca. The pellet form of pearl tapioca is obtained by forcing the moist starch through sieves of various sizes. Granulated tapioca is also marketed in several sizes (made by grinding flake tapioca). An example of this is the quick-cooking tapioca sold in packages in food stores. Nutritive food value is as a carbohydrate food, very easily digested. See *manioc.* Pearl or quick-cooking, raw 100 gm = 352 calories; cream pudding 100 gm = 134 calories.

taro (*Colocasia esculenta*). The plant of the subtropics and tropics, grown for its large underground tuber which has a high starch content and is very easily digested. Its large "elephant ear" leaves can be eaten as greens when young. The large starchy corm or bulb and tuber are boiled, fried, baked or used in soup. However, they have an acrid taste when raw. Poi, a staple food of the Pacific, particularly Hawaii, is made from the taro root.

tarragon (*Artemisia dracunculus*). A perennial shrublike herb, often called French tarragon grows over 18 inches tall. Its dark-green leaves are long, narrow, pointed, and they are one of the most distinctive of the culinary leaf herbs. Fresh or dried, they add a slightly aniselike flavor to chicken livers, vegetable juices, chowders and consommes, tongue, veal, chicken or turkey dishes; broiled fish, shellfish; scrambled eggs or omelets, mustards and mayonnaises. Tarragon's botanical name, *dracunculus,* as well as French name estragon, means "little dragon." It is said that this was chosen because of the way the roots twist about like serpents.

tartar or calculus. Light-yellow to dark-brown deposits on teeth along the gum line which are not true stains. Tartar properly called calculus, is made up of water, inorganic material, and organic material. It collects in layers, and as it forms it mixes with microorganisms, dead cells and other debris in the mouth. It is made mainly of calcium. Tartar collects on bridges, or partial dentures as well as around natural teeth. At first it is soft and may be removed by proper brushing, but as additional layers are formed it becomes hard and difficult to remove from either the natural teeth or bridges and dentures. As tartar forms it pushes the gums away from the teeth, forming pockets in which more tartar forms. Germs and pus accumulate in the pockets, because of irritation of the gums, and infection becomes more difficult to control. Tartar usually is yellowish when it begins to accumulate, above the gum line. It darkens toward black (from blood pigments) as it progresses and slowly pushes the gum away from the tooth.

tartaric acid. Mol. Wt. 150. Occurs naturally in grapes and other fruits and made commercially from waste products of wine productions. Tartaric acid is a constituent of grape and other artificial flavors that are used in beverages, candy, ice cream, baked goods, yogurt, and gelatin desserts. It also serves as the acid in some baking powders. Most of the tartaric acid ingested is destroyed in the intestines by bacteria.

$$
\begin{array}{cc}
\text{COOH} & \text{COOH} \\
| & | \\
\text{H}-\text{C}-\text{OH} & \text{HO}-\text{C}-\text{H} \\
| & | \\
\text{HO}-\text{C}-\text{H} & \text{H}-\text{C}-\text{OH} \\
| & | \\
\text{COOH} & \text{COOH} \\
\text{L-Tartaric acid} & \text{D-Tartaric acid}
\end{array}
$$

taste. Sense organs for taste are taste buds located in the surface of the tongue. The primary taste (gustatory) sensations are sweet, sour, salty, and bitter. The actual sensations of taste, particularly for distinctive flavors, is influenced by the sense of smell. Taste sensation is usually dulled when nasal membranes are congested or when the nostrils are pinched shut while eating foods. Taste depends upon smell to a large extent. Impulses from taste receptors are transmitted by nerve fibers from two cranial nerves, facial and glossopharyngeal, to the temporal lobe. See *tongue* and *smell*.

taste buds. Ovoid bodies, with an external layer of supporting cells, which end in hairlike processes that project through the central taste pore. These cells are the sense cells and the hairlike processes probably are the parts stimulated by the dissolved substances. The taste buds are found on the surface of the tongue, though some are scattered over the soft-palate, fauces, and *epiglottis*. Taste sensitivity is caused largely by receptors on the tongue in adult man. Sensitivity is also found on the palate (for sour and bitter) and the larynx. Strictly speaking, taste receptors give rise only to sensations of sweet, salt, sour and bitter; the complex of the subtle sensations called "taste" in everyday speech, includes smell, chemical common sensitivity, and some esthesis (feeling). A food is said to taste bland when "stinging" common chemical sensations are not present. Food tastes flat when one has a head cold because it is then impossible to smell food.

tea (*Thea sinenis*). The name given to an evergreen shrub or small tree, the leaves of this shrub; the drink made from these leaves. The tea plant is related to the magnolia and, like its relative, would produce blossoms and grow to a great height if it were not pruned. This plant is kept to the size of a bush so the leaves may be easily plucked off as they grow. The principal difference in teas comes from the treatment of the leaves once they are picked. Black tea, by far the most popular, is made by allowing the dried and rolled tea leaves to ferment before they are fired. Green tea, produced in China, Japan, India and Indonesia, is dried, rolled, steamed, and fired, without being allowed to ferment. The leaves retain their greenish color and the resulting beverage is a greenish-yellow color and rather bitter. Oolong tea, from China, Formosa, and Japan has leaves which are partially fermented, giving the beverage the aroma of black tea and "bite" of green tea. Besides these three main types of tea there are special teas which are scented and spiced. The leaves are combined with jasmine, gardenia, mint, orange, or spices. Tea has no nutritive value except when sugar, milk, or cream are added. Tea contains a stimulant called theine which is identical with caffeine in coffee.

teeth. Arise as outgrowths of the primitive mouth (buccal) epithelium and the surrounding connective tissue. A child has a first set of 20, the deciduous teeth, which are shed and replaced by 32 permanent teeth. The fibroelastic periodontal membrane holds the teeth solidly in the sockets of the jawbones. A tooth consists of an exposed crown and one or more buried roots. The junction of the crown and root, the necks, is surrounded by the gingival margins, as shown in the diagram. Enamel covers the crown, while cementum, a hardened type of bone, covers the roots. Beneath the enamel is a thick layer of dentine, another hard, calcified substance much like enamel, but very sensitive. Beneath the cementum is a thinner layer of dentine. The dentine surrounds a central cavity of the tooth which is filled with pulp. Pulp is connective tissue laced with nerves and blood vessels which supply the tooth. Dentine is the main substance of the tooth. Page 456 shows a vertical section of a tooth. Certain antibiotics taken during pregnancy will also show their mark on a child's teeth. Specifically,

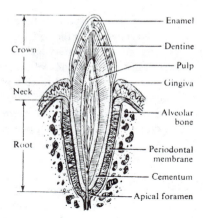

these are the three types of tetracycline (tetracycline, chlortetracycline, and ox-ytetracycline). These drugs travel through the mother's bloodstream. Small amounts are transferred to the unborn baby's blood and are deposited in its developing bones and teeth. The result is a yellow-gray brownish stain on the baby's first teeth. Tetracycline can also stain the teeth of children who receive the antibiotic after birth. The discoloration, however, is not a health hazard.

teeth, nutrition. Dental caries is the most widespread of all chronic diseases. Dental decay results when oral bacteria act on the teeth that are susceptible to decay. Certain microorganisms are prevalent in tooth surface areas protected from cleansing procedures. Carbohydrates, especially table sugar (*sucrose*) accumulate on the teeth and are acted upon by the organisms, readily ferment, and the acid generated by this action penetrates the tooth enamel, thus causing tooth decay. Dental decay in susceptible teeth occurs in direct proportion to the quantity of fermentable carbohydrate in the diet, but frequency of intake and consistency (form) of the food are especially important in the decaying process. Carbohydrates that are sticky and adhere to the teeth are more destructive than those in liquid form. If they are eaten at continuous short intervals the decay process can be practically continuous.

telophase. The stage in mitosis in which the doubled chromosomes have divided and moved apart into newly forming cells.

tendons (sinews). White glistening cords or bands which serve to attach the muscle to the bone. The major substance in tendon is the protein *collagen*.

terminal respiratory chain. The system responsible for the final stage of the oxidation of foodstuffs, fats, carbohydrates, and proteins. It is contained in the membranes of mitochondria and composed of an ordered array of cytochromes. The *cytochromes* (cyto) pass the electrons removed from the foodstuffs by oxidation reactions in a sequential manner to oxygen, the cytochromes themselves undergoing *reduction* and *oxidation* in sequence. Cytochrome oxidase terminates the respiratory chain and transfers the electrons to (reduces) oxygen to form water. The sequence of electron flow is as follows:

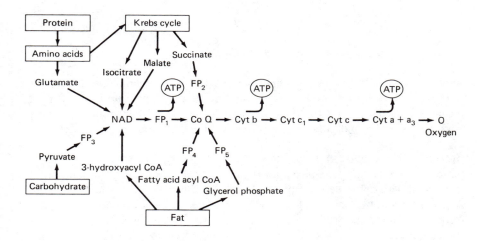

During the process of electron flow through the terminal respiratory chain, about 40 percent of the energy of oxidation is conserved as chemical energy, *adenosine triphosphate* * (ATP), which can be used for the energy needs of cells. The remaining energy, about 60 percent, is converted to heat. See *oxidative phosphorylation* and *Kreb's cycle* *.

Terramycin. A proprietary brand of oxytetracycline, an antibiotic and antiprotozoan.

terpenoids. Very large, important group of compounds which is made up of a simple repeating unit, the isoprenoid unit. This unit, by condensation, gives rise to such compounds as rubber, carotenoids, steroids, and many simpler terpenes. Isoprene, which does not occur in nature, has as its actual biologically active counterpart isopentenyl pyrophosphate, which is formed by a series of enzymically catalyzed steps from mevalonic acid. Isopentenyl pyrophosphate undergoes further reactions to form squalene, which in turn condenses with itself to form *cholesterol* *.

testosterone. Mol. Wt. 288. Testicular steroid hormone synthesized from *cholesterol* *, responsible for male secondary sex characteristics. *Progesterone* * is also a precursor of testosterone. See *steroid*.

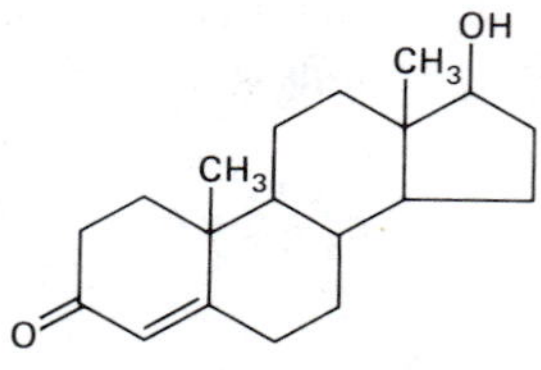

Testosterone

tetany. A disorder caused by abnormal calcium metabolism, fever, intermittent, tonic contractions of the extremities and muscular pain occur, which are usually caused by lowered blood calcium levels. A characteristic diagnostic sign is the inward muscular spasm of the wrist called Trousseau's sign.

tetrahydrofolic acid. Mol. Wt. 445. One of the *B-complex vitamins* and a specific vitamin of the general class of vitamins called *folacin* *. In addition to folic acid with only one glutamic acid group in the molecule, at least two conjugated forms of folacin exist in foods with either three or seven glutamic acid groups per molecule (folic acid glutamates). These conjugated forms serve as the major precursors of the vitamin in the diet. The coenzyme form, tetrahydrofolic acid, the most common form in the body, is also widely distributed in foods. Tetrahydrofolic acid functions prominently in one carbon metabolism, that is to say, it is this vitamin that is directly involved in the transfer of methyl (CH_3), methylene (—CH_2) and hydroxyl methyl (—CH_2OH) groups to several intermediates in metabolic processes. Free, unsubstituted tetrahydrofolic acid appear to be necessary for the production of new *erythrocytes,* and in this important activity, tetrahydrofolic acid is functionally associated with vitamin B_{12} (*cobalamin*) *. Vitamin B_{12} is able to remove the methyl (CH_3) group from methyl-tetrahydrofolic acid to form free tetrahydrofolic acid, in sufficient quan-

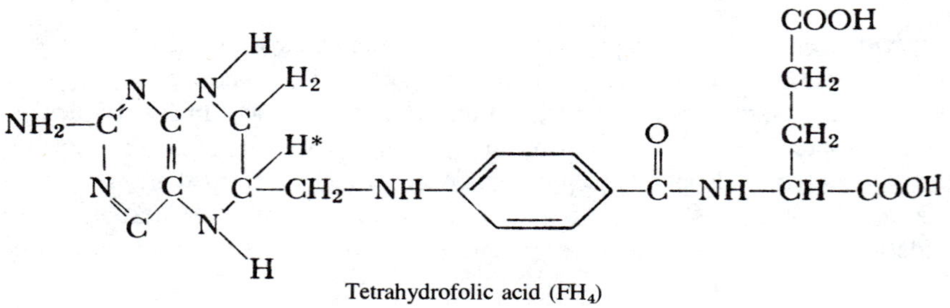

Tetrahydrofolic acid (FH_4)

tity to produce new erythrocytes. In the absence of vitamin B_{12} an anemia develops known as *pernicious anemia*. See *folacin* and *folic acid deficiency*.

thiamine (vitamin B₁). Mol. Wt. 460. One of the B-complex vitamins. It is readily soluble in water, slightly soluble in alcohol, and insoluble in fat solvents. Thiamine may be destroyed during storage or by heating in neutral or alkaline solutions. It is quite stable in the dry state. Synthetic thiamine is usually prepared in the form of one of its salts such as thiamine hydrochloride or thiamine mononitrate, which are more stable than the free vitamin. Thiamine plays a part in promoting appetite and better functioning of the digestive tract, effects that have an indirect influence on promoting growth. After thiamine is absorbed it is distributed widely by the blood throughout the body in all tissues and in somewhat high concentrations in such organs as the heart, liver, and kidneys. The body has limited ability to store thiamine. Tissues are depleted of their normal content of the vitamin in a relatively short period if the diet is deficient, so fresh supplies are needed regularly. The amount of thiamine required by adults varies according to size, degree of activity, dietary habits, and individual differences in how food is utilized. Daily allowances for adults according to the Food and Nutrition Board are calculated on the basis of individual calorie requirements, allowing 0.5 mg per 1000 kcal (minimum requirement is approximately 0.33 mg per 1000 kcal). The thiamine content of most fruits and vegetables, eggs, milk, and cheese does not generally exceed 0.1 mg per 100 gm. The best sources of thiamine, whole grains, organ meats, pork, and legumes are not used in quantity in most American diets. Most thiamine comes from bread and cereals, meat, fish, poultry, eggs, nuts, milk, dairy products, vegetables and fruits.

Function: Especially involved in a *carbohydrate* metabolism. The vitamin is found in the body both in the free form and combined with phosphate as the coenzyme thiamine pyrophosphate (TPP). The coenzyme TPP combines with magnesium and specific proteins to form active enzymes, the decarboxylases. Thus, thiamine aids in the complete breakdown of carbohydrates into carbon dioxide and *acetyl coenzyme A* * releasing energy for the body use. Several of the B-complex vitamins are involved. The coenzyme TPP, which contains thiamine, acts with *nicotinamide adenine dinucleotide* *, which contains the vitamin *niacin* *, coenzyme A, which contains the vitamin *pantothenic acid*, and *lipoic acid* *. Thiamine is the active part of the coenzyme thiamine pyrophosphate shown in the diagram, made in tissue cells by the combining of thiamine with two phosphate groups. This important coenzyme is known to be necessary for at least three different enzyme systems in mammals that are needed for the complete oxidation of carbohydrates. Two of these enzymes function by splitting off carbon dioxide from *pyruvate* * and *alpha(α)-ketoglutarate* * in the course of oxidation in the body. Thiamine pyrophosphate is also necessary for reactions leading to production of ribose, the important pentose sugar needed by all cells in the body for the production of *nucleic acids*.

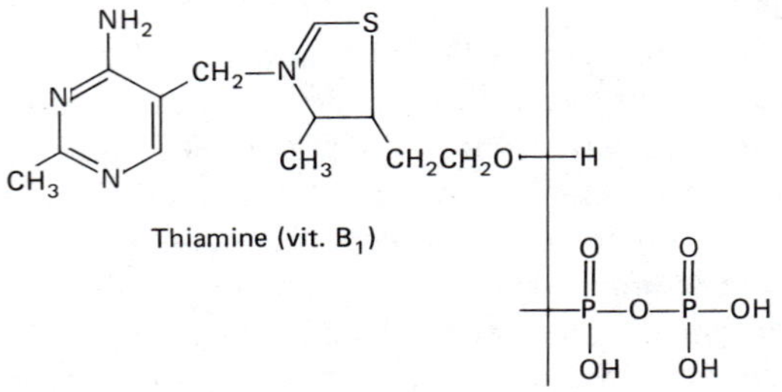

Thiamine (vit. B₁)

Thiamine pyrophosphate (TPP)

Sources of Thiamine

	Thiamine mg/100 gm
Bacon, Canadian	0.83
Beans, pinto	0.84
Buckwheat, flour (dark)	0.58
Cornflakes	0.43
Heart, beef	0.53
Kidneys, hog	0.58
Lentils	0.37
Liver, lamb	0.40
Oatmeal, (dry)	0.60
Peanuts	1.14
Milk chocolate with peanuts	0.25
Peas	0.35
Pecans	0.86
Piñon nuts	1.28
Pork	0.50
Rice, polished	1.84
Rye, whole grain	0.43
Sesame seeds	0.98
Soybeans	1.10
Sunflower seed	1.96
Whole wheat flour	0.55
Wheat germ	2.01
Yeast, Brewer's	15.61

thiaminase. Certain raw fish and seafood, particularly carp, herring, clams, and shrimp, contain the enzyme thiaminase, which is capable of splitting the thiamine molecule into its two major chemical groups, thus making it inactive. The enzyme is also thought to be present in the intestinal flora of man.

thickening agent. Manufacturers use thickening agents to "improve" the texture and consistency of ice cream, pudding, soft drinks, salad dressing, yogurt, soups, baby food and formula, and other foods. These chemicals control the formation of ice crystals in ice cream and other frozen foods. The thickness they create in salad dressing prevents the oil and vinegar from separating out into two layers. These additives are used to stabilize factory made foods, that is, to keep the complex mixture of oils, acids, colors, salts, and nutrients dissolved and at the proper consistency and texture. Most thickening agents are natural carbohydrates (agar, carrageenin, pectin, starch, etc.) or chemically modified carbohydrates (cellulose gum, modified starch, etc.). They work by absorbing part of the water that is present in a food, thereby making the food thicker. See *stabilizers*.

thiocyanic acid or thiocyanate. Mol. Wt. 59. Thiocyanic acid salts (thiocyanates) are goitogenic. They contribute to the formation of a goiter by decreasing *thyroxine* * synthesis in the *thyroid* gland. The mechanism appears to be an inhibition in the synthesis of thyroxine from the thyroglobulin. The *sulfonamides* and 2-thiouracil appear to inhibit thyroxine synthesis by mechanisms similar to the thiocynates. Certain aminobenzenes also inhibit thyroxine synthesis, but the mechanism appears to be related to the formation of stable iodine derivative in the thyroid gland, thus removing the iodine normally used for thyroglobulin formation. Thiocyanates and *thiourea* * another goitogenic compound are found naturally in turnips and cabbages. See *thiourea* * and *food toxins*.

$$HS—C≡N.$$

thiodipropionic acid. A food additive occasionally used in foods to prevent fats and oils from going rancid. It functions by reacting with oxygen which otherwise reacts with fat.

thiourea. Mol. Wt. 60. A goitogenic compound that is found naturally in turnips and cabbages. Thiourea, a thiocarbamide, sulfonamides, and 2-thiouracil inhibit the synthesis of *thyroxine* * in the *thyroid gland*. See *thiocyanic acid* and *food toxins*.

$$H_2N—C—NH_2$$
$$\|$$
$$S$$

thoracic cavity. In the thoracic cavity there are two pleural cavities, each containing a lung. In the space between the pleural cavities is the pericardial cavity, which contains the heart and the mediastinal region, in which are contained the trachea, esophagus, thymus gland, large blood, and lymphatic vessels, lymph nodes, and nerves.

threadworm (*Stronglyoides*). A parasite that produces a chronic intestinal infection with manifestations similar to hookworm infection. In heavy infections there is usually abdominal pain, watery diarrhea, loss of appetite, anemia, nausea, vomiting, and emaciation. Dithiazanine has been used for treatment.

threonine. Mol. Wt. 119. One of the *essential amino acids* found in proteins.

$$CH_3-\underset{\underset{OH}{|}}{CH}-\underset{\overset{|}{NH_2}}{CH}-COOH$$

thrombin. An enzyme in blood that facilitates blood clotting. *Vitamin K** is required for the production of thrombin from *prothrombin*. See *vitamin K**.

thrombus. A clot in a blood vessel formed by coagulation of blood.

thrush. Also called moniliases, these pearly white or bluish-white patches that look like curds in the mouth are the results of infection of the fungus *Candida albicans,* a yeast. Because this same fungus can grow in the vagina, many newborn infants become infected at birth. Thrush also occurs after antibiotic therapy. This is because the antibiotic kills off, along with the disease-causing bacteria, certain useful bacteria in the mouth which normally serve to keep any fungus there under control. When these useful bacteria are killed off, the fungus thrives. Diabetics too, are especially susceptible to thrush as part of their generally poor ability to handle any infection. The white patches also resemble leukopladia and cheek-biting, but with thrush there are usually cracks in the corners of the mouth.

thyme (*Thymus vulgaris*). There are a number of varieties of the herb. Garden and English thyme, are small, bushy perennials, with gray-green leaves; garden thyme's leaves are broad, while the wild or creeping thyme, *T. serpyllum* is a firmly matted ground cover. The wild thyme's leaves may be many colors other than green. The pungent and sweetly fragrant leaves are widely used in cooking. Fresh or dried thyme flavors vegetable juices, soups, meat and poultry dishes, fish, cheese, stuffings, sauces, vegetables, cream and custard desserts, and jellies. It is a relatively powerful herb with a distinctive flavor.

thymine. A pyrimidine found in *deoxyribonucleic acid*.

thyrocalcitonin. A thyroid hormone which prohibits release of calcium from bone. See *calcitonin*.

thyroglobulin. The iodine-containing protein which is synthesized in the *thyroid gland* and can be broken down to *thyroxin* * and small amounts of *triiodothyronine.* *

thyroid gland. The thyroid gland is located in front of the neck and has two lobes, one on either side of the larynx. The hormone produced by the thyroid is *thyroxin* *. This hormone is associated with the rate of metabolism, regulating heat and energy production in the body cells. Thyroid gland cells need a mineral, *iodine,* to manufacture thyroxin. Iodine is ordinarily obtained from foods included in normal diet. Disorders of thyroid function include *hyperthyroidism,* which, when severe, causes a dangerous increase in the metabolic rate; and *hypothyroidism,* an opposite condition, which causes physical and mental sluggishness. An enlargement of the thyroid gland is called a *goiter*. When the enlargement is a modular tumor, it is called an adenoma. The function of the thyroxin regulates the metabolic and oxidative rates in tissue cells of the body, including the liver. It increases the rate of glucose absorption from the intestine and increases the rate of *glucose* * utilization by cells, and stimulates the growth and differentiation of tissues. In the liver it influences conversion of glycogen from noncarbohydrate sources, and conversion of glycogen to glucose, thus raising blood sugar. It increases osteoclastic and osteoblastic activity of bone; it influences the rate of metabolism of lipids, proteins, carbohydrates, water, vitamins, and minerals. The most characteristic function of the thyroid gland is its ability to take up and concentrate *iodine*. The active transport of iodide is under control of *thyroid stimulating hormone* which regulates thyroid function. Iodide exists in food in many forms, and is readily absorbed from the intestinal lumen into the blood. In the thyroid gland iodide is oxidized to elemental iodine, which combines with the amino acid tyrosine in thyroglobulin to form monoiodotyrosine and diiodotyrosine. The thyroid gland also secretes thyroglobulin into the follicles.

thyroid hormones. Several amino acids are release from *thyroglobulin*. The most important is *thyroxine* *. It normally appears in the blood and is considered to be the major hormone of the thyroid gland. Another amino acid, *triio-*

dothyronine * is found in the blood in extremely small amounts. It is physiologically active and considered to be a true product of the thyroid gland and one of the thyroid hormones. Thyroxine is generally referred to as T_4, and triiodothyronine is called T_3. The major function of the thyroid hormones is to control the metabolic rate. The thyroid hormones are also an important factor in growth. Nervous system activity is also influenced by the thyroid hormones.

thyroid stimulating hormone (Thyrotropin, TSH). A hormone secreted by the anterior *pituitary gland* which regulates uptake of *iodine* and synthesis of *thyroxin* by the *thyroid gland*. TSH is a polypeptide with a molecular weight of about 10,000. The major function of TSH is to stimulate the thyroid gland. TSH is thought to increase the amount of cyclic *3', 5 adenosine monophosphate* (c-AMP) in the thyroid cell. The secretion of TSH is regulated in part by thyrotropin releasing factors (TRF).

thyrotropin. See *thyroid stimulating hormone.*

thyroxine (T_4 and triiodothyronine (T_3). These two hormones T_4 and T_3 which are extremely similar chemically, and have exactly the same physiological effect on tissues. The only difference is the speed at which the two hormones act. The most obvious effect that thyroxine has on the body is to increase the rate at which cells burn their fuel, *glucose* *. As well as working in concert with *cortisol* * in defending the body against stress resulting from extreme cold, thyroxine is also involved in other antistress responses. Emotional stress and severe hunger also provide an elevated thyroxine output. In general, thyroxine comes into play when there is an extra demand for energy. Thyroxine also increases the heart rate. The output of the two hormones is controlled directly by *thyroid stimulating hormone* (TSH) secreted by the anterior *pituitary.*

Thyroxine (T_4) Mol. wt. 777

Triiodothyronine (T_3) Mol. wt. 651

Under normal conditions the thyroid secretes about three times as much thyroxine as triiodothyronine. When they are synthesized within the cells of the thyroid the two hormones become a part of a protein (*thyroglobulin*) until they are needed. When needed a complex reaction involving the proteolysis (hyrolysis) of thyroglobulin and the synthesis of thyroxin takes place.

tin. (Sn). Element No. 50. Atomic weight 119. A normal intake is probably in the range of 1.5 to 5 mg a day, depending on the amount of canned foods eaten. Tin is not very toxic. Tin has no known nutritional function.

tissues. The organs can be analyzed into component tissues. For example, the stomach is composed of columnar *epithelial tissue*, smooth muscle tissue, connective tissue, nerves, blood, and lymph. Microscopic study of tissues reveals that tissues are made up of smaller units or cells. Each tissue is a group of cells with more or less intercellular material. The intercellular material varies in amount and in composition and in many cases determines the nature of the tissue. *Connective tissue* is distributed throughout the body to form the supporting framework of the body and to bind together and support other tissues. It binds organs to other organs, muscles to bones, and bones to other bones. The five principle types of connective tissues are adipose, areolar, cartilage, elastic, and reticulur described below.

(1) *Adipose tissue.* A fatty connective tissue which is found under the skin and in many regions of the body. It serves as a padding around and between organs. It insulates the body, reducing heat loss, and serves as a food reserve in emergencies.

(2) *Areolar tissue.* A fibrous connective tissue which forms subcutaneous layers of tissue. It fills many of the small spaces of the body and helps to hold the organs in place.

(3) *Cartilage tissue.* A tough resilient connective tissue found at the ends of the bone, between the bones, and in the nose, throat, and ears.

(4) *Elastic tissue.* A fibrous connective tissue composed of elastic fibers and found in the walls of blood vessels, in the lungs, and in certain ligaments.

(5) *Reticular tissue.* A fibrous connective tissue which forms the supporting framework of lymph glands, liver, spleen, bone marrow, and lungs.

Epithelial tissue forms the outer layer of skin for the protection of the body. It is also a lining tissue. As mucous membrane, it lines the nasal cavity, mouth, larynx, pharynx, trachea, stomach and intestines. As serous membrane, it lines the abdominal, chest, and heart cavities and covers the organs that lie in these cavities. As endothelium it lines the heart and blood vessels. It lines respiratory and digestive organs for the function of protection and absorption. It helps form organs concerned with the excretion of body wastes, certain glands for the purpose of secretion, and certain sensory organs for the reception of stimuli.

tissue fluid. The body fluid that lies outside blood vessels and outside cells, called extravascular (outside blood vessels), or extracellular (outside cells) fluid. Living body cells contain large amounts of water and must be bathed continuously in a watery solution in order to survive and carry on their functions. The colorless and slightly salty tissue fluid is derived from the circulating blood.

tocopherol or vitamin E. Mol. Wt. 432. There are six forms of vitamin E, the alpha (α), beta (β), gamma (γ), delta (δ), eta (η) and zeta (ζ). α-Tocopherol has the widest distribution and greatest biological activity. It is one of the *fat soluble vitamins*. The tocopherols are sensitive to oxidation and to ultraviolet light. As antioxidants, the tocopherols retard oxidation of other fat soluble vitamins and lipoperoxidation in adipose tissue associated with a high intake of polyunsaturated fatty acids. They may also be involved in cell respiration and in nucleoprotein synthesis. Richest sources are the vegetable oils, whole grains, and eggs; the average daily intake has been estimated at 24 mg. Human needs are related to the intake of polyunsaturated fatty acids and may vary between 10 and 30 mg per day for adults. Many claims have been made for vitamin E ranging from specific aid to cardiovascular problems, to a more general aid for fertility. No frank clinical condition due to a lack of vitamin E is known to man. It has sometimes been described as a vitamin in search of a disease (nutritional). Vitamin E deficiencies can be demonstrated in animals, but become complicated by the fact that the symptoms differ in different animals and that the symptoms can sometimes be made to disappear by the addition of selenium or the sulfur amino acids. Vitamin E is not toxic.

Vitamin E (α-tocopherol).

The table on p. 467 shows the tocopherol content in a variety of foods. For the *Recommended Daily Allowance* see Appendix 8.

tofu. Curdlike product made from soybeans or soy flour, used widely in the Orient and prized by health food devotees for its relatively high protein quality.

tomato (*Lycopersicon*). The fruit of a plant which grows on vines. Tomatoes come in many shapes and colors. They may be yellow, green, or whitish, or even varicolored, as well as the best known red. They may be ribbed, round, pearshape, or cherryshape. The small green varieties are often used in pickles,

Food	Mg, per 100 gm of food (tocopherol)
Fats and Oils	
Butter	1
Coconut oil	8
Corn oil, hydrogenated	105
Corn oil, unhydrogenated	100
Cottonseed oil, hydrogenated	80
Cottonseed oil, unhydrogenated	91
Margarine (made with corn oil)	47
Mayonnaise	50
Soybean oil, hydrogenated	73
Soybean oil, unhydrogenated	101
Fruits and Vegetables	
Bananas	0.42
Carrots	0.21
Green peas, frozen	0.65
Orange juice, fresh	0.20
Potatoes, baked	0.085
Tomatoes, fresh	0.85
Cereal Grains	
White bread	0.23
Whole-wheat bread	2.2
Yellow cornmeal	3.4
Meat, Fish, Poultry and Eggs	
Beef liver, broiled	1.62
Egg	1.43
Fillet of haddock, broiled	1.20
Ground beef	0.63
Pork chops, pan-fried	0.60

while the large ripe red ones are most popular in sauces. The deep-red pear-shape tomato is a specialty of Italian tomato pastes. A good source of vitamins and minerals, especially *carotene** (vitamin A activity), and *ascorbic acid** (vitamin C). Tomatoes are low in calories.

Fresh, raw, 100 gm = 22 calories
Fresh, boiled, 100 gm = 26 calories
Canned, regular pack, solids and liquid, 100 gm = 21 calories
Canned, dietary pack, solids and liquid, 100 gm = 20 calories
Ketcup, 100 gm = 106 calories
Chili sauce, 100 gm = 104 calories
Canned tomato juice, 100 gm = 19 calories
Canned tomato juice cocktail, 100 gm = 21 calories
Canned tomato paste, 100 gm = 82 calories
Canned tomato puree, 100 gm = 39 calories

tongue. A fibromuscular organ located partially in the oral cavity and partially in the pharynx. The root of the tongue is anchored to the hyoid bone. In addition to subserving taste functions, the tongue assists in speech, mastication, and swallowing. In mastication the tongue functions to push food between the teeth. Once the food has been broken up by the teeth, the tongue forms a *bolus,* or ball of food, which it propels into the oropharynx. The dorsum of the tongue is covered by numerous minute projections, the papillae, which vary in shape and distribution. Taste buds may be present on any of the papillae but are most numerous at the base of the pallate. See *taste.*

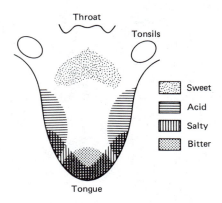

The tongue of beef, veal, lamb, or pork is eaten as meat. Tongue is a nourishing and appetizing food, good hot or cold. A good source of protein, high in fat content, with a good amount of *iron,* fair *niacin** and *riboflavin*.*
Beef, fresh, braised, 100 gm = 244 calories
Veal, braised, 100 gm = 160 calories
Pork, braised, 100 gm = 253 calories
Lamb, braised, 100 gm = 267 calories
Corned, 100 gm = 290 calories
Smoked, 100 gm = 290 calories

tooth. See *teeth.*

Torulopsis. Round to oval fermentative yeasts with multilateral budding cause trouble in breweries and spoil various foods. *T. sphaerica* ferments *lactose** and may spoil milk products. Other species can spoil sweetened condensed milk, fruit-juice concentrates and acid foods.

toxic. Poisonous. Mutations, cancer, blindness, liver damage, are typical of effects that can be caused by toxic materials. See *toxins* and *food poisoning.*

toxicity. The quality of a substance that makes it poisonous or toxic. Toxicity sometimes refers to the degree of severity of the poison or the possibility of being poisonous.

toxicity tests. (a) Acute toxicity tests reveal the effects of mammoth single doses of a chemical. Short-term toxicity tests reveal the effects of 30- to 180-day exposure to a substance with special attention usually given to liver and kidney function and blood composition. (c) Long-term toxicity tests last the lifetime of an animal (2 years in rats or mice and 7 years in dogs). These experiments are the only kind that can reveal whether a chemical causes cancer or chronic effects. (d) Other special tests are designed to detect interference with reproduction and causation of birth defects or mutations.

toxins. Poisonous material produced by plants or microorganisms. See *food poisoning* and *food toxins*.

trace elements. Those elements necessary in the diet in trace amounts, less than 100 mg per day in man. Among the trace elements the range of requirements runs from milligram quantities for iron, zinc, and manganese down to microgram quantities for some of the newly discovered micronutrient elements such as *selenium, chromium,* and *vandium.* A combination total of only about 25 to 30 gm of all trace elements (about 1 ounce) exists in the human body. There is no convenient single way to classify trace elements in nutrition because they vary so much in function, distribution, level of need, and chemical properties. The trace elements found in foods and nature are *iron, iodine, copper, manganese, zinc, fluorine, cobalt, molybdenum, selenium, chromium, nickel, tin, vanadium, silicon.* Except for cobalt, all the trace elements are absorbed (or can be) in the inorganic form before being utilized by the body. Minerals present in organic forms in the food, in general, must be split off to the free inorganic form before absorption. Trace elements have no common biological role other than that they function in the body at the cellular levels, often as constituents of enzymes or an enzyme activator. Some of the trace elements have no known functions. See *minerals*.

trachea. The trachea or windpipe, is a tube held open by cartilaginous tissue. It carries air from the larynx to the bronchi. The trachea is lined with cilia and numerous glands whose secretions provide a sticky film to keep dust and dirt out of the lungs.

tragacanth gum. A vegetable gum stabilizer, that exhibits a resistance to acids which is unexcelled among vegetable gums. This property makes it the ideal thickening agent for foods such as vinegar-containing salad dressing.

tranquilizers (drugs). Drugs that have a sedative effect that is characterized by relief of neuromuscular tension and anxiety without producing sleep. An example is chlorpromazine hydrochloride. See *tyramine* and *food-drug interactions*.

transaminase. A class of enzymes that transfer amino ($-NH_2$) groups from one compound to another. The general reaction is as follows:

$$R_1-\overset{\overset{\text{O}}{\|}}{C}-COOH + R_2-\overset{\overset{NH_2}{|}}{CH}-COOH \overset{(B_6)}{\rightleftharpoons} R_1CH-\overset{\overset{NH_2}{|}}{COOH} + R_2-\overset{\overset{\text{O}}{\|}}{C}-COOH$$

The keto acids acceptors are transformed into the corresponding α-amino acids and the amino group donors become α-keto acids. Essential for these reactions is *pyridoxal phosphate** or *pyridoxamine phosphates,** the *coenzyme* forms of vitamin B_6. These reactions occur with all of the amino acids and their α-keto acid counterparts with exception of the two essential amino acids lysine and threonine. The transaminases are specific for the amino acids and the α-keto acids. In certain diseases or abnormal conditions the level of the transminase activity in the blood increases and the level of certain transaminase activity is used as an aid in diagnosis, particularly in heart and liver pathologies. See *pyridoxine** (vitamin B_6), and *transamination*.

transamination. The act of transferring of an amino group to another molecule, e.g., transfer to a keto acid, thus forming another amino group. Amino acids produced by the digestion of a protein are absorbed through the intestinal wall into the blood and are transported to the liver. Certain of the amino acids are required by the cells for the synthesis of proteins, enzymes, certain hormones and other nitrogen-containing substances. Body tissues are capable of synthesizing some amino acids (nonessential) by removing the required amino groups from other amino acids. The amino group taken from one acid is transferred to an α-keto analogue of the amino acid to be synthesized. The transfer is called transamination. The enzymes that catalyze these reactions are called *transaminases*. The vitamin B_6 (*pyridoxine**) is a part of the coenzyme *pyridoxal phosphate** or *pyridoxamine phosphate** and is required for the transaminases to be active.

transferase. An enzyme that transfers a chemical grouping from one compound to another, for example, *transaminases* transfer amino ($-NH_2$) groups and transphosphorylases transfer phosphate ($-H_2PO_4$) groups.

transferrin or siderophilin. An iron-binding protein that transports iron through the blood. It is a beta (β) pseudoglobulin and occurs in blood at 0.4 mg per 100 ml of blood. Under normal conditions about 3 mg of iron is in the blood which represents about 30 percent of the total transport capability of transferrin. The iron bound to transferrin must be in the oxidized or ferric (Fe^{+3}) state. Ferrous (Fe^{+2}) iron will not bind. Within the cells, the iron is bound by another protein called *ferritin* which also binds only Fe^{+3}. Iron is also stored as an iron-protein complex called *hemosiderin*. The total iron in an adult male is about 700 milligrams.

trans-form. The configuration of substituents around an unsaturated double bond of carbon. The opposite of the *cis-form*.

| Trans-form | Cis-form |

transketolase. An enzyme that transfers two carbon units to other sugar inter-mediates. It requires the coenzyme *thiamine pyrophosphate* * (TPP) which con-tains one of the B-complex vitamins, *thiamine* * (vitamin B₁). Transketolase is necessary for the synthesis of *ribose* * from *glucose* *. Ribose is a five-carbon sugar required for the synthesis of the *nucleic acids, deoxyribonucleic acid* * (DNA) and *ribonucleic acid* * (RNA).

trehalose. A disaccharide composed of two *glucose* * molecules joined at the *anomeric carbons*. It is therefore a nonreducing sugar. It is the principal sugar in insect blood (chemolymph). Trehalose is also present in some molds, fungi, and bacteria and is also known as mushroom sugar. Normally only small amounts are ingested in the diet.

trichinosis (lockjaw). Illness caused by eating raw, improperly cooked pork that is infested by *Trichinella spiralis* a parasitic worm. Most human trichinosis results from the consumption of raw or incompletely cooked pork containing the encysted larvae. The larvae are released into the intestinal tract during digestion and invade the mucous membranes of the first part of the small intes-tine. Symptoms may resemble food poisoning and be followed by muscular pains, weakness, fever, and puffiness of tissues around the eyes and forehead.

trichosporon (*Torula*). Yeasts which bud and form arthrospores. They grow best at low temperatures and are found in breweries and on chilled beef. *T. pullulans* is a common species. They are contaminants.

triglyceride (fat, neutral fat, oil). A compound in which three *fatty acids* are esterified to a molecule of glycerol. The difference between a fat and an oil is that the oils contain a higher number of unsaturated double bonds in the fatty acids. Most natural triglycerides contain mixtures of fatty acids. If a triglyceride contains only one type of fatty acid, it is named after the fatty acid, for example, triolein (an oil) contains only *oleic acid* and tristearin (a *fat*) contains only *stearic acid* *.

triiodothyronine. See *thyroxine* *.

tripe. The inner lining of the stomach of beef. There are three kinds; honeycomb, pocket, and plain or smooth. Honeycomb is considered the most desirable. A good source of protein. Fresh, 100 gm = 100 calories; pickled 100 gm = 62 calories.

triplet code. A trinucleotide. A sequence of three nucleotides in *deoxyribonucleic acid* (DNA) or *messenger* or *ribonucleic acid* (m-RNA) that encodes an amino acid into proteins. Since there are four different nucleotides in DNA and in m-RNA, there are 64 different triplet codes. This means that several of the 20 amino acids are coded for by more than one triplet. The message contained in a sequence of bases in a DNA molecule is transmitted in terms of three bases at a time, a "triplet." Each triplet calls for a particular amino acid to be incorporated into the protein for the message coded. Four different bases made up DNA molecules, and each base in each triplet can be any one of the four.

trout *(Salmo)*. The name given to a large group of fishes of the family Salmonidae. Although most varieties are freshwater fish, a few such as the sea trout and some of the rainbow trout, live in the sea and ascend rivers to breed. Trout vary greatly in size and coloration according to their environment. Among the most widely known are the rainbow trout, *Salmo gairdnerii*, the brook or speckled trout, *Salvelinus fontenalis*, the steelhead, or salmon-trout, which is a variety of the rainbow trout; the cutthroat trout, *Salmo clarkii*, and the Dolly Varden, *Salvelinus malma*. Brook trout, raw, 100 gm = 101 calories; rainbow trout, raw, 100 gm = 195 calories.

trypsin. One of the first enzymes to be discovered. It has a molecular weight of about 24,000 daltons. It digests protein, e.g., meat, in the small intestine. Trypsin is formed initially in the pancreas in an inactive form, trypsinogen. Trypsin is believed to hydrolyze proteins in much the same way as chymotrypsin, another digestive enzyme, because both compounds contain many of the same amino acids in their active sites, including histidine and serine. Trypsin is highly specified and will hydrolyze the peptide bonds at the amino acids *ly-*

sine * and *arginine* *, the basic amino acid. The specificity of chymostrypsin is for *phenylalanine* * and *tyrosine,* * the aromatic amino acids. Trypsin also has the important function of activating chymotrypsinogen to chymotrypsin and of activating all other *zymogen* forms of the proteolytic enzymes of digestion. Trypsin itself is activated from trypsinogen by the intestinal enzyme *enterokinase*. See *trypsinogen* and *zymogen*.

trypsinogen. An inactive form, a zymogen, of trypsin synthesized in the pancreas. During the digestive process, an enzyme *enterokinase* is released by the intestinal mucosa. Enterokinase removes a hexapeptide (six amino acids) from trypsinogen and it becomes active trypsin. See *trypsin* and *zymogen*.

tryptophan. Mol. Wt. 204. An *essential amino acid*. A constituent of body proteins, a precursor of the vitamin *niacin* * and of the vasoconstrictor *serotonin*. Animal protein contains approximately 1.4 percent and vegetable protein 1 percent tryptophan. An average daily diet may provide 500–1000 mg tryptophan. The dietary tryptophan available over the above the body's requirement may be converted to niacin in a proportion of 60 mg Tryptophan to 1 mg niacin.

$$CH_2-CH-COOH$$
$$NH_2$$

Tryptophan

tubules. See *nephron* and *glomerulus*.

Tularemia (tick fever, rabbit fever). Disease is contacted by hunting and killing infected animals, which are cleaned and not cooked properly; by being bitten by a blood-sucking fly or by a tick; or by drinking contaminated water. There are several types. Skin lesions such as red spots, little boils, and red lumps may appear anywhere on the body. The disease may be superficial with a small lump at the site of the cut, or an enlargement of lymph nodes regional to the cut and possible suppuration of nodes. Commonly begins suddenly with a headache, chills, fever, and prostration. Streptomycin, chloramphenicol, and the tetracyline antibiotics have been found effective in treatment.

tuna (*Thunnus*). A saltwater game fish belonging to the *mackerel* family. Tuna is found in almost all the seas of the temperate and warm zones of Asia, Africa, and America. In some parts of the world it can reach weights up to 1500 pounds. There are several varieties, including the albacore, bluefin, skipjack, and yellow-fin. A good source of protein. Fresh, raw, 100 gm = 145 calories; canned in oil, solids and liquid, 100 gm = 288 calories, canned in water, solids and liquid, 100 gm = 127 calories; See *fish* and *Appendix 9* for nutrient content.

turkey. A native American game bird which is related to the pheasant. A good source of protein. Raw, 100 gm = 218 calories; roasted, 100 gm = 263 calories. See *poultry* and *Appendix 9* for nutrient content.

tumeric. The irregularly shaped root of a tropical plant which is related to ginger. When washed, cooked, and then dried, the turmeric root has a mild aroma and a mustardlike bitter taste. One of its characteristics is the brilliant gold color it adds to the dishes in which it is used. Turmeric is used in prepared mustards and is always present in curry powder. Turmeric flavors and colors curried meat, poultry, fish, and shellfish, deviled and creamed eggs, chicken, fish, shellfish; egg, chicken or potato salads.

turnip (*Brassica*). A root vegetable. There are several varieties. The flesh varies in texture; the finer-fleshed turnips are eaten as a vegetable and the coarser ones are fed to livestock. Turnips are white-fleshed. Some varieties have purple tops. Turnip tops are eaten as greens and are used for forage. The greens are an excellent source of *ascorbic acid** (vitamin C) and *carotene** (vitamin A activity), and a good source of calcium, iron, and riboflavin.

Turnip, cooked, 100 gm = 23 calories
Fresh turnip greens, 100 gm = 20 calories
Canned turnip greens, solids and liquid, 100 gm = 18 calories
Frozen turnip greens, cooked and drained, 100 gm = 23 calories.

tyramine. Mol. Wt. 137. Tyramine is formed by the decarboxylation of tyrosine and is found in significant concentration in some foods. Its specific function is not known. Tyramine is a powerful vasopressor normally inactivated by the action of the enzyme *monoamine oxidase* (MAO).

$$HO-\langle \rangle-CH_2-CH_2-NH_2$$

Tyramine

tyramine toxicity. Certain antidepressants such as isocarboxazid and phenelzine sulfate are enzyme inhibitors of mondamine oxidases (MAO) and therefore can be responsible for adverse *food-drug interactions*. Since some antidepressants inhibit MAO, they interfere with the metabolism of tyramine and the ingestion of foods high in tyramine may lead to headaches, nausea, and hypertension. A glass of chianti or an ounce of cheese have sufficient tyramine to cause the toxic effects. Below is a list of foods that have significantly high concentrations of tyramine. See *food toxins* and *food-drug interactions*.

Food	Tyramine mg/100 gms
Cheeses [a]	
Brie	18
Camembert	9
Cheddar	141
Ermanthaler	23
Gruyère	52
Alcoholic beverages	
Beer [a]	0.3
Chianti	2.5
Sherry	0.4
Meats	
Beef livers	0.5
Chicken livers	0.05
Pickled herring	303
Other Possible Agents [b]	
Banana	
Cola	
Coffee	
Pineapples	
Yeast extracts	
Yogurt	

a—Actual content will vary with various brands.
b—Although the content is considered significant definitive data is not available.

tyrosine. Mol. Wt. 181. A nonessential *amino acid* found in proteins that can be formed from the essential *amino acid phenylalanine* *. Tyrosine has a "sparing" effect on phenylalanine since the presence of tyrosine in the diet decreases the amount of phenylalanine required, but can never totally replace it. Tyrosine (and therefore phenylalanine) is a precursor to the pigment *melanin, ubiquinone* *, and *tyramine* *.

$$HO \!-\!\!\bigcirc\!\!-\! CH_2\!-\!\underset{\underset{NH_2}{|}}{CH}\!-\!COOH$$

Tyrosine

U

ubiquinone (coenzyme Q). An electron carrier in the *terminal respiratory chain*. It functions as one of a series of electron carries in a sequential arrangement that transports electrons from foodstuffs to oxygen to form water. Ubiquinone has an isoprene side chain, similar to *retinol* * (vitamin A), *tocopherol* (vitamin E), and *vitamin K* *. Ubiquinone occurs in the mitochondria and in the microsomes.

$$n = 1 \text{ to } 10$$

Ubiquinone

ulcerative colitis. A digestive disease characterized by an inflammation, with the formation of ulcers in the mucosa of the colon. A digestive disorder of unknown cause which produces severe, bloody diarrhea, accompanied by fever and weight loss. Treatment consists of a bland diet, sedatives, sulfa drugs to reduce the number of bacteria in the large bowel, and drugs to reduce diarrhea.

ulcers. A peptic ulcer is an open lesion on the mucosa of the stomach or small intestine. When the ulcer is located in the stomach it is called a gastric ulcer; if it is located in the upper third of the small intestine, it is called a duodenal ulcer. The ulcerated area is thought to be the result of digestion of the membranous lining of the stomach or small intestine by the *gastric juices*.

unit, international vitamin. See *international unit*.

unit pattern (functional pattern). Defined as the smallest aggregate of cells which, when repeated many times, composes an organ. If the liver is studied in this way, it will be seen that the lobules (smallest macroscopic units) are composed of chains of cells with their definite supply paths of blood and lymph and bile capillaries.

unsaturated fatty acid. A *fatty acid* that has a double bond between the two carbon atoms at one or more places in the carbon chain. Examples are *oleic acid**, *linoleic acid**, and *arachidonic acid**. An unsaturated fat is one that contains an unsaturated fatty acid. A saturated fatty acid has no double bonds. See, *oleic acid*1*, and *saturated fatty acid*.

urea. Mol. Wt. 60. Urea is the major nitrogenous constituent of urine, representing between 60 to 90 percent of the total nitrogen excreted in a 24-hour period. The amount of urea excreted is proportional to the protein ingested. Protein is not completely oxidized to CO_2, water, and energy, and the urea represents an end product of that incomplete oxidation. The two nitrogen atoms derive from aspartic acid and ammonia in reactions of the *urea cycle*. Measure of the amount of the urea nitrogen (gm) in a 24-hour collection when multiplied by the factor 6.25 gm of protein/gram of nitrogen yields the amount of protein oxidized for that time period. See *urine*.

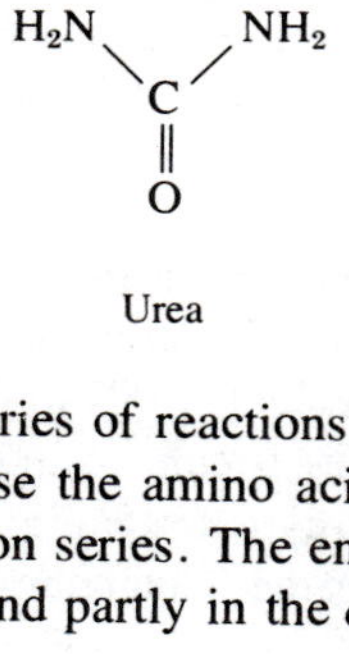

Urea

urea cycle. The biochemical series of reactions that leads to the production of urea. It is called a cycle because the amino acid *ornithine** is continually regenerated to continue the reaction series. The enzymes that constitute the cycle are partly in the *mitochondria* and partly in the *cytosol*. The series of reactions of the urea cycle are as follows.

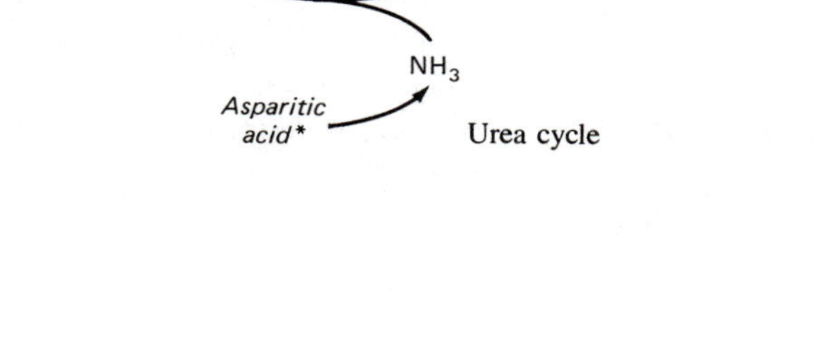

Urea cycle

urease. The first enzyme to be crystallized. It converts *urea** into ammonia and carbon dioxide.

$$H_2O + H_2N-\underset{\underset{\text{urea}}{}}{\overset{\overset{O}{\|}}{C}}-NH_2 \xrightarrow{\text{urease}} 2NH_3 + CO_2$$

water　　urea　　　　ammonia　carbon dioxide

uremia. Progressive degenerative changes in renal tissue bringing marked depression of a kidney function. Few functioning *nephrons* remain, and these gradually deteriorate. Uremia is the term given the symptom complex of adrenal renal insufficiency. Although the name derives from the common finding of elevated blood *urea** levels, the symptoms result not so much from urea concentrations as from disturbances in acid-base balance and in fluid and electrolyte metabolism and from accumulation of other obscure toxic substances not clearly defined.

ureters. The pelvis of each *kidney* is drained by a ureter, a muscular tube extending from the hilus to the posterior portion of the urinary bladder. Ureters are smooth muscles and structures and urine is passed through each ureter by *peristalsis*. Drop by drop, urine passes into the urinary bladder. Ureters are about 15 to 18 inches in length and about $^1/s$ inch in diameter. See *urinary system*.

uric acid. Mol. Wt. 168. An acid found in urine, derived from the metabolism of *purines*. A chemical compound that contains nitrogen and is present in small amounts in the urine, the equivalent of 80 to 200 mg of urinary nitrogen in a 24-hour period. Uric acid stones occurs in individuals who have an increased level of uric acid in the blood (hyperuricemia) and increased urinary excretion of uric acid. It may or may not be accompanied by symptoms of *gout*. Since uric acid is an end-product of purine metabolism, foods with a high purine content are voided. The precipitation of uric acid crystals in the urinary tract occurs most readily at a low urinary pH. See *urine*.

Uric acid

uridine diphosphate (UDP). See *uridine triphosphate*.

uridine monophosphate (UMP). See *uridine triphosphate*.

uridine triphosphate (UTP). Mol. Wt. 484. A high-energy phosphate compound. It is a pyrimidine nucleotide which is energetically equivalent to *adenosine triphosphate* (ATP). The synthesis of animal starch (*glycogen*) depends upon the formation of sugar derivatives of UDP. For example, the reaction that adds a *glucose* molecule to glycogen [(glucose)$_n$] is as follows:

$$\text{UDP-Glucose} + (\text{glucose})_n \xrightarrow[\text{synthetase}]{\text{glycogen}} (\text{glucose})_{n+1} + \text{UDP}.$$

urinary bladder. The urinary bladder, a muscular sac located in the lowest part of the abdominal cavity, stores urine. Normally it holds 300 to 511 ml. The bladder is emptied by contraction of muscles in its walls which force urine out through the *urethra*.

urinary system. The system involving the *kidneys*, the *ureters*, the *urinary bladder*, arteries, veins, and the *urethra*. The purpose of the urinary system is to maintain a constant composition and volume of blood and to maintain its acid-base balance. About 1200 ml of blood flow through the kidneys in a minute. The urinary system is a glomerular filtration of the blood that also involves secretion and absorption of specific materials in the blood. About 125 ml per minute of filtrate (urine) produces through reabsorption, a total of about 1800 milliters of urine concentrate in 24 hours. The composition of urine is similar to plasma except that it contains no proteins or large colloidal particles or glucose under normal conditions. The control of the absorption and secretions of salts and others is a complex matter involving their concentrations and hormonal influences. The resorption of water is directly controlled by the antidiuretic hormone (ADH). The diagram shows the urinary system. See *urine, glomerulus, and nephron.*

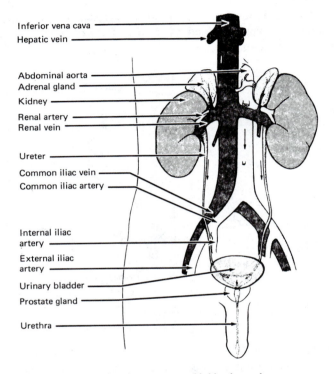

Inferior vena cava
Hepatic vein

Abdominal aorta
Adrenal gland
Kidney
Renal artery
Renal vein

Ureter

Common iliac vein
Common iliac artery

Internal iliac artery

External iliac artery

Urinary bladder
Prostate gland

Urethra

The male urinary system with blood vessels.

urine. The filtrate of the urinary system is urine. It amounts to about 1800 milliliters per day. The composition of urine varies depending upon composition of the diet. The table below shows the composition of urine and their normal ranges. *Uric acid** is an end product of purine metabolism; *urea** is the result of protein (amino acid) oxidation; and *creatinine** is the end product of *creatine phosphate**, a form of chemical energy in the muscles. See *urinary system* and *kidneys.*

United States Recommended Daily Allowances (U.S. RDA, FDA). The U.S. RDA were developed by the Food and Drug Administration (FDA) based on the recommendations of the Food and Nutrition Board. The table given in Appendix 8 contains mandatory nutrients and optional nutrients. The mandatory

	Component	Amount		U/P*
Composition	Sodium	2–4 gm	100–200 meq	0.8–1.5
of average	Potassium	1.5–2.0 gm	35–50 meq	10–15
24-hr urine	Magnesium	0.1–0.2 gm	3–16 meq	
of a normal	Calcium	0.1–0.3 gm	2.5–7.5 meq	
adult	Iron	0.2 mg		
	Ammonia	0.4–1.0 gm N	30–75 meq	
	H^4	0.4–1.0 gm N	4×10^{-8}–4×10^{-6} meq/1	1–100
	Uric acid	0.03–0.2 gm N		20
	Amino acids	0.08–0.15 gm N		
	Hippuric acid	0.04–0.05 gm N		
	Chloride		100–250 meq	0.3–2
	Bicarbonate		0–50 meq	0–2
	Phosphate	0.7–1.6 gm P	20–50 moles	25
	Inorganic sulfate	0.6–1.8 gm S	20–120 meq	50
	Organic sulfates	0.06–0.2 gm S		
	Urea	6–18 gm N		60
	Creatinine	0.3–0.8 gm N		70
	Peptides	0.3–0.7 gm N		

*U/P = ratio of concentration in urine (U) to that in plasma (P).

nutrients are protein, vitamin A (*retinol* *), vitamin C (*ascorbic acid* *), vitamin B$_1$ (*thiamine* *), vitamin B$_2$ (riboflavin*), *niacin* *, *calcium,* and *iron* and are based upon the fact that human nutritional diseases are specifically associated with deficiencies. Optional nutrients are *vitamin D* *, vitamin E (*α-tocopherol* *), vitamin B$_6$ (pyridoxine*), vitamin B$_{12}$ (*cobalamin*), *phosphorous, iodine, magnesium, zinc, copper,* biotin, and *pantothenic acid* *. See *Appendix 8*.

uterus. The uterus, shaped somewhat like a pear, is suspended in the pelvic cavity, supported between the bladder and the rectum by its system of eight ligaments. The normal position of the body of the uterus is anteflexion (bent forward over the bladder). The uterus is about 3 inches long and 3 inches thick at its widest part. It has a thick wall of smooth muscle and a relatively small inner cavity. During pregnancy it can increase about 20 times in size. The upper dome-shaped portion of the uterus is the fundus, the main part is the body, and the lower neck portion is the cervix. The cervix is a canal opening into the vagina. The inner lining of the uterus, the endometrium, undergoes periodic changes during the regular menstrual cycle, to make the uterus ready to receive a fertilized ovum. If the ovum is not fertilized the endometrium gets a message from hormone influences and sheds its surface cells and built-up secretion. Some of the extra blood supply, the surface cells and uterine secretions are eliminated as menstrual flow.

V

vacuoles. Membranous sacs within the cytoplasm that contain water and dissolves substances. The cells of higher animals usually lack vacuoles.

valence. The power of an element or a radical to combine with (or to replace) other elements or radicals. Atoms of various elements combine in definite proportions. The valance number of an element is the number of atoms of hydrogen with which one atom of the element can combine or is equivalent.

valine. Mol. Wt. 117. An essential amino acid. One of the amino acids found in proteins. It is classified as an aliphatic or neutral amino acid.

$$CH_3 \diagdown CH-CH-COOH$$
$$CH_3 \diagup \qquad | \atop NH_2$$

Valine

vanadium (V). Element No. 23. Atom. Wt. 51. It has been reported that vanadium reduces cholesterol production in man. While vanadium is not yet known as an essential micronutrient for man, it is essential in animals. It does have functions in the body, namely as a catalyst for activating enzymes that have to do with fat metabolism and certain nerve hormones, called catecholamines. Vanadium is plentiful in certain foods like seafood, soybeans, corn oil, and many vegetables.

varietal. Differences between varieties of the same plants. Groups of plants within the same species may differ in certain characteristics. For example, different varieties of potatoes may contain widely differing levels of ascorbic acid. Such differences between varieties are known as varietal differences.

vascular. Full of vessels that contain a fluid. In physiology, the blood and lymph vessels in the body. Pertaining to or consisting of vessels.

vasoconstriction. The closing or decreased circumference of blood vessels. Blood pressure is usually increased.

vasodilation. The opening up or increased circumference of blood vessels. Blood pressure is usually reduced.

vassopressin. See *antidiuretic hormone.*

veal. Young beef 4 to 14 weeks of age. An excellent source of protein, iron and *niacin*;* a fair source of riboflavin.

Arm steak, cooked, 100 gm = 298 calories
Blade steak, cooked, 100 gm = 276 calories
Breast, stewed with gravy 100 gm = 346 calories
Cutlet, cooked, 100 gm = 277 calories
Loin chop, cooked, 100 gm = 421 calories
Rib chop, cooked, 100 gm = 318 calories
Rump chop, cooked, 100 gm = 232 calories
Rump, roasted, 100 gm = 174 calories
Sirloin, roasted, 100 gm = 175 calories

vegetables. Plants cultivated for food. Some plants classified as vegetables are botanically classified under other names. For example, the tomato is really a fruit; peas and beans are seeds and are also classified as legumes; and mushrooms are fungi. Normally vegetables include the leafy vegetables such as spinach, lettuce, and cabbage; the stem vegetables, such as celery and asparagus; the roots and tubers of which beets, turnips, carrots, ane potatoes are examples; flower vegetables such as broccoli and cauliflower; seeds and seed pods, which include beans and peas (which are also classified under other names). Vegetables commonly include almost every part of the plant, including leaves, stems, roots, bulbs, tubers, flowers, and seeds. Mature seeds of the grasses make up the cereal group, and those of the leguminous plants make up the peas and beans. The amounts commonly consumed are not important energy-yielding foods; however, their less digestible carbohydrates (hemicellulosis and cellulose fiber) provide sufficient roughage for a normal diet. Their protein is generally of high quality though not abundant in quantity. The value of leafy vegetables lies primarily in their vitamin and mineral content. Most vegetable leaves are rich sources of *carotene** (vitamin A activity), and good sources of iron, calcium, *riboflavin*,* and *folacin*.* The greener the leaf, the higher the carotene content. Carotene (provitamin A) from leafy green vegetables is more readily absorbed and utilized than that from yellow ones. Fresh vegetable leaves are also good sources of *ascorbic acid** (vitamin C). The table

Food, Approximate Measure, and Weight (in grams)		Grams	Water Per- cent	Food Energy Calo- ries	Protein Grams	Fat Grams
Vegetables and Vegetable Products						
Asparagus, green:						
Cooked, drained:						
Spears, ½-in. diam. at base	4 spears	60	94	10	1	Trace
Pieces, 1½ to 2-in. lengths	1 cup	145	94	30	3	Trace
Canned, solids and liquid	1 cup	244	94	45	5	1
Beans:						
Lima, immature seeds, cooked, drained	1 cup	170	71	190	13	1
Snap:						
Green:						
Cooked, drained	1 cup	125	92	30	2	Trace
Canned, solids and liquid	1 cup	239	94	45	2	Trace
Yellow or wax:						
Cooked, drained	1 cup	125	93	30	2	Trace
Canned, solids and liquid	1 cup	239	94	45	2	1
Sprouted mung beans, cooked, drained	1 cup	125	91	35	4	Trace
Beets:						
Cooked, drained, peeled:						
Whole beets, 2-in. diam.	2 beets	100	91	30	1	Trace
Diced or sliced	1 cup	170	91	55	2	Trace
Canned, solids and liquid	1 cup	246	90	85	2	Trace
Beet greens, leaves and stems, cooked, drained	1 cup	145	94	25	3	Trace
Blackeye peas. See Cowpeas						
Broccoli, cooked, drained:						
Whole stalks, medium size	1 stalk	180	91	45	6	1
Stalks cut into ½-in. pieces	1 cup	155	91	40	5	1
Chopped, yield from 10-oz. frozen pkg.	1⅜ cups	250	92	65	7	1
Brussels sprouts, 7–8 sprouts (1¼ to 1½ in. diam.) per cup, cooked	1 cup	155	88	55	7	1
Cabbage:						
Common varieties:						
Raw:						
Coarsely shredded or sliced	1 cup	70	92	15	1	Trace
Finely shredded or chopped	1 cup	90	92	20	1	Trace
Cooked	1 cup	145	94	30	2	Trace
Red raw, coarsely shredded	1 cup	70	90	20	1	Trace

	Fatty Acids									
	Unsaturated									
Satu-rated (total)	Oleic	Lin-oleic	Carbo-hy-drate	Cal-cium	Iron	Vita-min A Value	Thia-mine	Ribo-flavin	Niacin	Ascor-bic Acid
Grams	Grams	Grams	Grams	Milli-grams	Milli-grams	Inter-national units	Milli-grams	Milli-grams	Milli-grams	Milli-grams
—	—	—	2	13	0.4	540	0.10	0.11	0.8	16
—	—	—	5	30	0.9	1,310	0.23	0.26	2.0	38
—	—	—	7	44	4.1	1,240	0.15	0.22	2.0	37
—	—	—	34	80	4.3	480	0.31	0.17	2.2	29
—	—	—	7	63	0.8	680	0.09	0.11	0.6	15
—	—	—	10	81	2.9	690	0.07	0.10	0.7	10
—	—	—	6	63	0.8	290	0.09	0.11	0.6	16
—	—	—	10	81	2.9	140	0.07	0.10	0.7	12
—	—	—	7	21	1.1	30	0.11	0.13	0.9	8
—	—	—	7	14	0.5	20	0.03	0.04	0.3	6
—	—	—	12	24	0.9	30	0.05	0.07	0.5	10
—	—	—	19	34	1.5	20	0.02	0.05	0.2	7
—	—	—	5	144	2.8	7,400	0.10	0.22	0.4	22
—	—	—	8	158	1.4	4,500	0.16	0.36	1.4	162
—	—	—	7	136	1.2	3,880	0.14	0.31	1.2	140
—	—	—	12	135	1.8	6,500	0.15	0.30	1.3	143
—	—	—	10	50	1.7	810	0.12	0.22	1.2	135
—	—	—	4	34	0.3	90	0.04	0.04	0.2	33
—	—	—	5	44	0.4	120	0.05	0.05	0.3	42
—	—	—	6	64	0.4	190	0.06	0.06	0.4	48
—	—	—	5	29	0.6	30	0.06	0.04	0.3	43

Food, Approximate Measure, and Weight (in grams)		Grams	Water Per-cent	Food Energy Calo-ries	Protein Grams	Fat Grams
Savoy, raw, coarsely shredded	1 cup	70	92	15	2	Trace
Cabbage, celery or Chinese raw,	1 cup	75	95	10	1	Trace
Cabbage, spoon (or pakchoy), cooked	1 cup	170	95	25	2	Trace
Carrots:						
Raw:						
Whole, 5½ by 1 inch, (25 thin strips)	1 carrot	50	88	20	1	Trace
Grated	1 cup	110	88	45	1	Trace
Cooked, diced	1 cup	145	91	45	1	Trace
Canned, strained or chopped (baby food)	1 ounce	28	92	10	Trace	Trace
Cauliflower, cooked, flowerbuds	1 cup	120	93	25	3	Trace
Celery, raw:						
Stalk, large outer, 8 by about 1½ inches, at root end	1 stalk	40	94	5	Trace	Trace
Pieces, diced	1 cup	100	94	15	1	Trace
Collards, cooked	1 cup	190	91	55	5	1
Corn sweet:						
Cooked, ear 5 by 1¾ inches	1 ear	140	74	70	3	1
Canned, solids and liquid	1 cup	256	81	170	5	2
Cowpeas, cooked immature seeds	1 cup	160	72	175	13	1
Cucumbers, 10-ounce; 7½ by about 2 inches:						
Raw, pared	1 cucumber	207	96	30	1	Trace
Raw, pared, center slice ⅛-inch thick	6 slices	50	96	5	Trace	Trace
Dandelion greens, cooked	1 cup	180	90	60	4	1
Endive, curly (including escarole)	2 ounces	57	93	10	1	Trace
Kale, leaves including stems, cooked	1 cup	110	91	30	4	1
Lettuce, raw:						
Butterhead, as Boston types: head, 4-inch diameter	1 head	220	95	30	3	Trace
Crisphead, as Iceberg; head, 4¾ inch diameter	1 head	454	96	60	4	Trace
Looseleaf, or bunching varieties, leaves	2 large	50	94	10	1	Trace
Mushrooms, canned, solids and liquid	1 cup	244	93	40	5	Trace
Mustard greens, cooked	1 cup	140	93	35	3	1
Okra, cooked, pod 3 by ⅝ inch	8 pods	85	91	25	2	Trace

Fatty Acids										
Saturated (total)	Unsaturated		Carbo-hy-drate	Cal-cium	Iron	Vita-min A Value	Thia-mine	Ribo-flavin	Niacin	Ascor-bic Acid
	Oleic	Lin-oleic								
Grams	Grams	Grams	Grams	Milli-grams	Milli-grams	Inter-national units	Milli-grams	Milli-grams	Milli-grams	Milli-grams
—	—	—	3	47	0.6	140	0.04	0.06	0.2	39
—	—	—	2	32	0.5	110	0.04	0.03	0.5	19
—	—	—	4	252	1.0	5,270	0.07	0.14	1.2	26
—	—	—	5	18	0.4	5,500	0.03	0.03	0.3	4
—	—	—	11	41	0.8	12,100	0.06	0.06	0.7	9
—	—	—	10	48	0.9	15,220	0.08	0.07	0.7	9
—	—	—	2	7	0.1	3,690	0.01	0.01	0.1	1
—	—	—	5	25	0.8	70	0.11	0.10	0.7	66
—	—	—	2	16	0.1	100	0.01	0.01	0.1	4
—	—	—	4	39	0.3	240	0.03	0.03	0.3	9
—	—	—	9	289	1.1	10,260	0.27	0.37	2.4	87
—	—	—	16	2	0.5	[6]310	0.09	0.08	1.0	7
—	—	—	40	10	1.0	[6]690	0.07	0.12	2.3	13
—	—	—	29	38	3.4	560	0.49	0.18	2.3	28
—	—	—	7	35	0.6	Trace	0.07	0.09	0.4	23
—	—	—	2	8	0.2	Trace	0.02	0.02	0.1	6
—	—	—	12	252	3.2	21,060	0.24	0.29	—	32
—	—	—	2	46	1.0	1,870	0.04	0.08	0.3	6
—	—	—	4	147	1.3	8,140	—	—	—	68
—	—	—	6	77	4.4	2,130	0.14	0.13	0.6	18
—	—	—	13	91	2.3	1,500	0.29	0.27	1.3	29
—	—	—	2	34	0.7	950	0.03	0.04	0.2	9
—	—	—	6	15	1.2	Trace	0.04	0.60	4.8	4
—	—	—	6	193	2.5	8,120	0.11	0.19	0.9	68
—	—	—	5	78	0.4	420	0.11	0.15	0.8	17

Food, Approximate Measure, and Weight (in grams)		Water	Food Energy	Protein	Fat
	Grams	*Per-cent*	*Calo-ries*	*Grams*	*Grams*
Onions:					
Mature:					
Raw, onion 2½-inch diameter 1 onion	110	89	40	2	Trace
Cooked 1 cup	210	92	60	3	Trace
Young green, small, without tops 6 onions	50	88	20	1	Trace
Parsley, raw, chopped 1 tablespoon	4	85	Trace	Trace	Trace
Parsnips, cooked 1 cup	155	82	100	2	1
Peas, green:					
Cooked 1 cup	160	82	115	9	1
Canned, solids and liquid 1 cup	249	83	165	9	1
Canned, strained (baby food) 1 ounce	28	86	15	1	Trace
Peppers, hot, red, without seeds, dried (ground chili powder, added seasonings) 1 tablespoon	15	8	50	2	2
Peppers, sweet:					
Raw, about 5 per pound:					
Green pod without stem and seeds 1 pod	74	93	15	1	Trace
Cooked, boiled, drained 1 pod	73	95	15	1	Trace
Potatoes, medium (about 3 per pound raw):					
Baked, peeled after baking 1 potato	99	75	90	3	Trace
Boiled:					
Peeled after boiling 1 potato	136	80	105	3	Trace
Peeled before boiling 1 potato	122	83	80	2	Trace
French-fried, piece 2 by ½ by ½ inch:					
Cooked in deep fat 10 pieces	57	45	155	2	7
Frozen, heated 10 pieces	57	53	125	2	5
Mashed:					
Milk added 1 cup	195	83	125	4	1
Milk and butter added 1 cup	195	80	185	4	8
Potato chips, medium, 2-inch diameter 10 chips	20	2	115	1	8
Pumpkin, canned 1 cup	228	90	75	2	1
Radishes, raw, small, without tops 4 radishes	40	94	5	Trace	Trace
Sauerkraut, canned, solids and liquid 1 cup	235	93	45	2	Trace
Spinach:					
Cooked 1 cup	180	92	40	5	1
Canned, drained solids 1 cup	180	91	45	5	1

Fatty Acids										
	Unsaturated									
Satu-rated (total)	Oleic	Lin-oleic	Carbo-hy-drate	Cal-cium	Iron	Vita-min A Value	Thia-mine	Ribo-flavin	Niacin	Ascor-bic Acid
Grams	Grams	Grams	Grams	Milli-grams	Milli-grams	Inter-national units	Milli-grams	Milli-grams	Milli-grams	Milli-grams
—	—	—	10	30	0.6	40	0.04	0.04	0.2	11
—	—	—	14	50	0.8	80	0.06	0.06	0.4	14
—	—	—	5	20	0.3	Trace	0.02	0.02	0.2	12
—	—	—	Trace	8	0.2	340	Trace	0.01	Trace	7
—	—	—	23	70	0.9	50	0.11	0.12	0.2	16
—	—	—	19	37	2.9	860	0.44	0.17	3.7	33
—	—	—	31	50	4.2	1,120	0.23	0.13	2.2	22
—	—	—	3	3	0.4	140	0.02	0.02	0.4	3
—	—	—	8	40	2.3	9,750	0.03	0.17	1.3	2
—	—	—	4	7	0.5	310	0.06	0.06	0.4	94
—	—	—	3	7	0.4	310	0.05	0.05	0.4	70
—	—	—	21	9	0.7	Trace	0.10	0.04	1.7	20
—	—	—	23	10	0.8	Trace	0.13	0.05	2.0	22
—	—	—	18	7	0.6	Trace	0.11	0.04	1.4	20
2	2	4	20	9	0.7	Trace	0.07	0.04	1.8	12
1	1	2	19	5	1.0	Trace	0.08	0.01	1.5	12
—	—	—	25	47	0.8	50	0.16	0.10	2.0	19
4	3	Trace	24	47	0.8	330	0.16	0.10	1.9	18
2	2	4	10	8	0.4	Trace	0.04	0.01	1.0	3
—	—	—	18	57	0.9	14,590	0.07	0.12	1.3	12
—	—	—	1	12	0.4	Trace	0.01	0.01	0.1	10
—	—	—	9	85	1.2	120	0.07	0.09	0.4	33
—	—	—	6	167	4.0	14,580	0.13	0.25	1.0	50
—	—	—	6	212	4.7	14,400	0.03	0.21	0.6	24

Food, Approximate Measure, and Weight (in grams)		Water	Food Energy	Protein	Fat
		Grams	*Per-cent*	*Calo-ries*	*Grams*	*Grams*

Food, Approximate Measure, and Weight (in grams)		Grams	Per-cent	Calo-ries	Grams	Grams
Squash:						
Cooked:						
Summer, diced	1 cup	210	96	30	2	Trace
Winter, baked, mashed	1 cup	205	81	130	4	1
Sweetpotatoes:						
Cooked, medium, 5 by 2 inches, weight raw about 6 ounces:						
Baked, peeled after baking	1 sweet-potato	110	64	155	2	1
Boiled, peeled after boiling	1 sweet-potato	147	71	170	2	1
Candied, 3½ by 2¼ inches	1 sweet-potato	175	60	295	2	6
Canned, vacuum or solid pack	1 cup	218	72	235	4	Trace
Tomatoes:						
Raw, approx. 3-in. diam. 2⅛ in. high; wt., 7 oz.	1 tomato	200	94	40	2	Trace
Canned, solids and liquid	1 cup	241	94	50	2	1
Tomato catsup:						
Cup	1 cup	273	69	290	6	1
Tablespoon	1 tbsp.	15	69	15	Trace	Trace
Tomato juice, canned:						
Cup	1 cup	243	94	45	2	Trace
Glass (6 fl oz)	1 glass	182	94	35	2	Trace
Turnips, cooked, diced	1 cup	155	94	35	1	Trace
Turnips greens, cooked	1 cup	145	94	30	3	Trace

Dashes in the columns for nutrients show that no suitable value could be found although there is reason to believe that a measurable amount of the nutrient may be present.

[1] Value applies to unfortified product; value for fortified low-density product would be 1500 I.U., and the fortified high-density product would be 2290 I.U.

lists the nutrient content of some common vegetables. See *Appendix 9* for nutrient contents.

vegeterian. A vegetarian may be generally described as a person who omits one or more of the following food groups from the diet; meat, poultry; fish; milk; eggs. Pure vegetarians include only plant foods in the diet. Fruitarians limit their food intake to raw and dried fruits, nuts, honey and oils. Those who

Fatty Acids										
Satu-rated (total)	Unsaturated		Carbo-hy-drate	Cal-cium	Iron	Vita-min A Value	Thia-mine	Ribo-flavin	Niacin	Ascor-bic Acid
	Oleic	Lin-oleic								
Grams	Grams	Grams	Grams	Milli-grams	Milli-grams	Inter-national units	Milli-grams	Milli-grams	Milli-grams	Milli-grams
—	—	—	7	52	0.8	820	0.10	0.16	1.6	21
—	—	—	32	57	1.6	8,610	0.10	0.27	1.4	27
—	—	—	36	44	1.0	8,910	0.10	0.07	0.7	24
—	—	—	39	47	1.0	11,610	0.13	0.09	0.9	25
2	3	1	60	65	1.6	11,030	0.10	0.08	0.8	17
—	—	—	54	54	1.7	17,000	0.10	0.10	1.4	30
—	—	—	9	24	0.9	1,640	0.11	0.07	1.3	[7]42
—	—	—	10	14	1.2	2,170	0.12	0.07	1.7	41
—	—	—	69	60	2.2	3,820	0.25	0.19	4.4	41
—	—	—	4	3	0.1	210	0.01	0.01	0.2	2
—	—	—	10	17	2.2	1,940	0.12	0.07	1.9	39
—	—	—	8	13	1.6	1,460	0.09	0.05	1.5	29
—	—	—	8	54	0.6	Trace	0.06	0.08	0.5	34
—	—	—	5	252	1.5	8,270	0.15	0.33	0.7	68

*Table 1, Nutritive Values of the Edible Parts of Foods, in *Nutritive Value of Foods*, Home and Garden Bulletin No. 72. United States Department of Agriculture, United States Government Printing Office, Washington, D.C., 1971.

[2]Contributed largely from beta-carotene used for coloring.

include plant foods and milk in their diet, but eliminate meat, poultry or eggs are called lactovegetarians. Those who abstain from poultry, fish and meat, but include eggs, milk and plant foods in their diets are called lacto-ovo-vege-tarians. Strict or pure vegetarians have two areas of possible concern where malnutrition problems may develop. The omission of milk or milk products in a vegetarian diet may lead to inadequate intakes of calcium. Large amounts of dark green vegetables can provide appreciable amounts of calcium. The deficiency of *cobalamin** (vitamin B_{12}) is a serious deficiency that may develop in pure or strict vegetarian diets. Only animal products supply cobalamin and the deficiency symptoms are insidious because they may not occur until years after the vegetarian diet was adopted. Pregnant females who are strict vegetarians should be mindful that it is possible for a child to be born with cobalamin deficiency symptoms although they are not evident in the mother. See cobalamin* (vitamin B_{12})

verbena (*Lippia citriodora*). A perennial shrub varying greatly according to the conditions under which it is grown. The long, narrow pointed leaves are yellow-green. Dried or fresh, the leaves have a lemony flavor and smell. They may be used to garnish fruit cups or fruit salads, or put into jellies. Lemon verbena tea is a popular herb tea.

vescicles. A small bladder or bladderlike structure.

villikinin. A hormone produced by glands in the upper intestinal mucosa in response to pressure of *chyme* entering the intestine. Villikinin stimulates alternating contractions and extensions of the villi (*villus*). This motion of the villii constantly agitates the mucosal surface, which stirs and mixes the chyme, and exposes additional nutrient material for absorption.

villus. A finger like structure that is a part of the mucous membrane of the small *intestine* which serves to increase the efficiency of absorption of nutrients and excretion of mucous. Villi also occur in the placenta.

viosterol. A solution of irradiated *ergosterol** in oil, in which the active agent is *calciferol** (vitamin D_2).

vinegar. Produced by the oxidation of *ethanol** to *acetic acid** by acetic acid bacteria. Any material that has undergone alcoholic fermentation can be used to produce vinegar, wine, fermented potatoes, or malt and cider. In vinegar strength is considered as well as flavor. Vinegar's bite and sourness is in direct proportion to the amount of acetic acid in it, and a 4 percent vinegar will be far less pungent than one with 5 percent or higher. The term "40- or 50-grain strength" is used by some manufacturers instead, "grain" standing for 10 times the percent acetic-acid content. The strength has no effect on the calorie count. One of the most universal of all foods, vinegar is an essential of characteristic dishes of many nations.

visual purple. See *rhodopsin**. Photosensitive pigment found in the rods of the retina. Rhodopsin requires *retinol** (vitamin A) to be formed.

vitamins. Vitamins are low molecular weight *organic* compounds required in the diet for the maintenance of good health or growth. Some dietary requirements fit this general description, but are not classified as vitamins. The *essential fatty acids,* for example, were called vitamin F at one time, but the designation is no longer used, nor are they considered vitamins. Vitamins are not considered to be incorporated into the structure of the cell in general. However, since neither all of the functions, nor all of the forms of all of the vitamins are presently known, some now designated as vitamins now may have a structural function. Indeed the designation of a compound as a vitamin is more of a historical classification than a highly selective category. In 1906, J. Gowland Hopkins of England showed that laboratory animals could not live on purified proteins, fats, and carbohydrates and concluded that small quantities of a vital substance was required in the diet. The vital substances or accessory factors were thought to be amines. In 1911, C. Funk called these vital amines vitamines. Later, the "e" was dropped. The vitamins are generally classified according to their solubility, the "fat soluble" and "water soluble" vitamin. The use of the alphabet to designate the vitamins derives from work of McCollum and Davis at the University of Wisconsin, and Osborne and Mendel at Yale who were isolating the factor that prevented the nutritional disease beri-beri. It was recognized there were two factors in different fractions of separation procedures. A fat-soluble "fraction A" that prevented a nutritional eye disease, and a water-soluble "fraction B" that prevented beri-beri. The water-soluble *antiscorbutic* factor, vitamin C (*ascorbic acid* *) was recognized as distinct from the "fraction B" or vitamin B. It was soon determined that the fat-soluble A fraction contained two factors, one that prevented nutritional eye disease, vitamin A (*retinol* *) and another (antirachitic) factor that prevented the nutritional disease *rickets, vitamin D* *. The vitamin B fraction was found to be a complex of various substances and as their structures were discovered they were given subscripts, for example, vitamin B_1 (*thiamine* *), vitamin B_2 (*riboflavin* *), vitamin B_6 (*pyridoxine* *), and vitamin B_{12} (*cobalamin* *). The determination that these substances were vitamins occurred in laboratory animals. In man, the avitaminosis of the water-soluble vitamins manifest themselves as beri-beri, due to lack of thiamine; *pellagra* due to lack of niacin; *pernicious anemia,* due to lack of *cobalamin* *; and *scurvy* due to lack of ascorbic acid. The avitaminosis of the fat-soluble vitamin manifests themselves as *nyctalopia* (night blindness) due to a lack of vitamin A (*retinol* *); rickets due to a lack of vitamin D; and hemorrhage due to lack of *vitamin K* *. No specific diseases or set of clinical symptoms in man are associated with a lack of any of the other vitamins outside of experimental conditions. The division of the vitamins into the fat-soluble and water-soluble vitamins has more than historical significance. Certain generalities derive from the differences in solubility. In general, the fat-soluble vitamins are stored in the lipid deposits of the body, particularly in the liver. Because of their lack of solubility in water, the daily requirements for the fat-soluble vitamins is generally less stringent than for the water-soluble vitamins. In some instances, vitamins A and D, dosages can last up to several months. By the same token, in vitamin toxicity (hypervitaminosis) of the fat-soluble vitamins, the removal of the overload runs its course very slowly. The water-soluble vitamins must be replenished frequently because their solubility permits their excretion in *urine*.

Exactly what is and what is not a vitamin is a source of confusion. Retinol, thiamine, pyridoxine, ascorbic acid, vitamin D, and vitamin K are definitely established vitamins in man, and their lack in the diet leads to the associated diseases given above. All other vitamins have been demonstrated as necessary for the health of man under experimental conditions only, or have been demonstrated as necessary for the health of experimental animals. The extrapolations of the results in animals to man must be done with caution. For example, vitamin C (*ascorbic acid* *) is a dietary requirement for primates (man), guinea pig, and one species of fruit bat. All other animals are capable of the biosynthesis of ascorbic acid from *glucose* *. An additional source of confusion related to the vitamins was the frequent reporting of vitamins that later proved to be combinations of known vitamins or were not determined to be vitamins in more than one species of animals. More than 50 vitamins have been reported. The trend is to designate vitamins by their chemical or generic name in order to circumvent the multiplicity and confusion of designations by alphabet and subscripts. See *fat soluble vitamins* and *water soluble vitamins*

vitamin A: See *retinol* *. A group of related vitamins.

vitamin B₁: See *thiamine* *.

vitamin B₂: See *riboflavin* *. An obsolete term.

vitamin B₃: Necessary for growth in pigeons. It is probably the same as *pantothenic acid* *.

vitamin B₄: Required in rats and chicks. Possibly a mixture of *arginine* *, *glycine* *, *pryidoxine* *, and *riboflavin* *.

vitamin B₅: Needed for growth in pigeons. Possibly *niacin* *.

vitamin B₆: See *pyridoxine* *.

vitamin B₇ (vitamin I): A factor that prevents disturbances in digestion in pigeons.

vitamin B$_8$: *Adenylic acid* * (AMP). This is not classified as a vitamin.

vitamin B$_{10}$: A factor for feather growth in chicks.

vitamin B$_{12}$ (*cobalamin* *): See *folacin* *.

vitamin B$_{11}$: A growth factor in chicks. Probably vitamin B$_{12}$ (*cobalamin* *) and *folacin.* *

vitamin B$_{13}$: An uncharacterized growth factor in rats.

vitamin B$_{14}$: No confirmations that vitamin B$_{14}$ exists.

vitamin B$_{15}$ (pangamic acid): Reported to facilitate oxygen uptake in rabbits.

vitamin B$_{17}$ (amygdalin, laetrile): See *amygdalin* *.

vitamin B$_c$: Identical with *folacin*.

vitamin B$_p$: Replaceable by manganese and *choline* *, in chicks.

vitamin B$_t$ (*carnitine*): A growth factor in insects.

vitamin B$_w$: Identical with *biotin* *.

vitamin B$_x$: Both *pantothenic acid* * and *para-amino benozic acid* * have been given this designation.

vitamin B complex: As originally used, this term referred to the water-soluble vitamins occurring in yeast, liver, meats, and whole-grain cereals, but some of the newer B-complex vitamins, for example, *folacin* * and vitamin B$_{12}$ (*cobalamin* *) do not correspond to this distribution; includes a number of compounds which have been identified, isolated and synthesized; *thiamine* *, *riboflavin* *, *niacin* *, *pyridoxine* *, *pantothenic acid* *, *bitoin* *, *folic acid* (*folacin*), *inositol* * and *choline* *.

vitamin C: See *ascorbic acid* *.

vitamin C$_2$ (vitamin J): A postulated antipneumonia factor.

vitamin D: Vitamin D comprises a group of vitamin derivatives of calciferol which prevent rickets (antirachitic factors). The forms of vitamin D that are of therapeutic or nutritional importance are vitamin D_2 or ergocalciferol; vitamin D_3 or cholecalciferol; 25-hydrocholecalciferol (25 HCC); 1,25-dihydrocholecalciferol (DHCC); and 1,24,25-trihydroxycholecalciferol (THCC). All are structurally related to *cholesterol* *. In addition to dietary sources for vitamin D, humans are able to biosynthesize the provitamin 7-dehydrocholesterol. Vitamin D_2 and D_3 are derived from their respective protovitamins ergosterol, from yeast, and 7-dehydrocholesterol, in the skin, by ultraviolet irradiation. The structures are as follows:

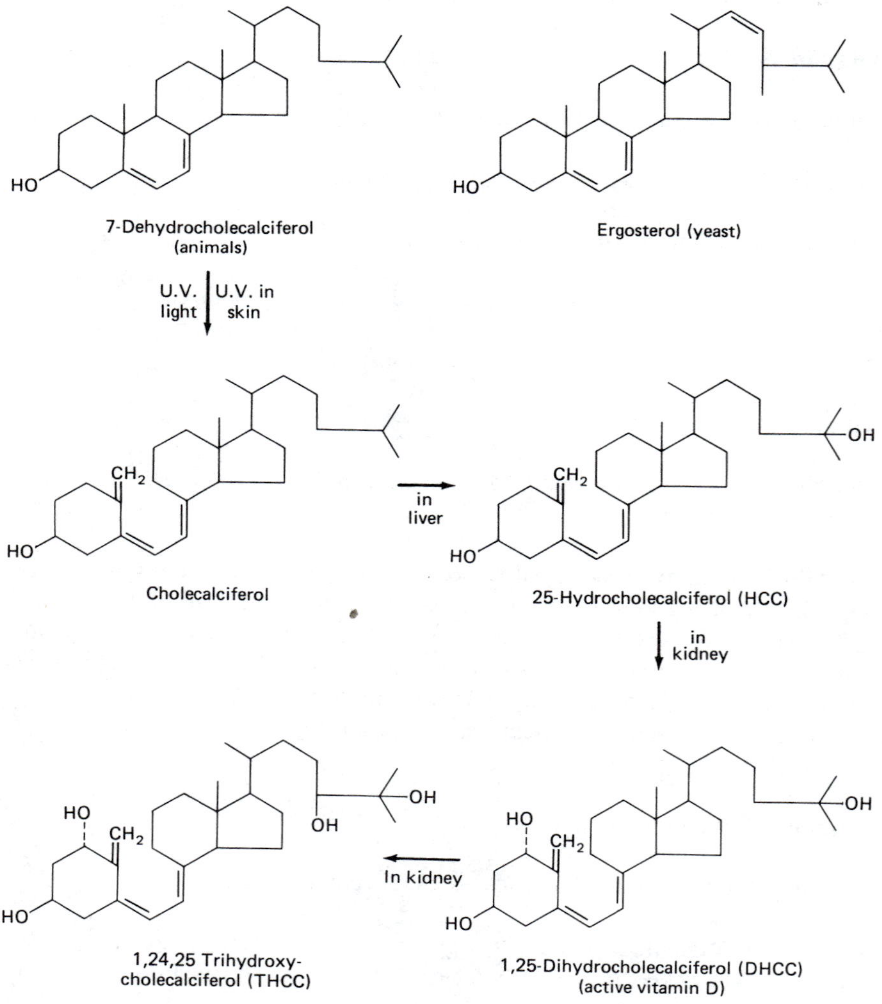

7-Dehydrocholecalciferol
(animals)

Ergosterol (yeast)

U.V. | U.V. in
light | skin

Cholecalciferol

in
liver

25-Hydrocholecalciferol (HCC)

in
kidney

1,24,25 Trihydroxy-
cholecalciferol (THCC)

In kidney

1,25-Dihydrocholecalciferol (DHCC)
(active vitamin D)

The active form of the vitamin is considered to be the 1,25-HCC with respect to intestinal *calcium* transport and bone mineral mobilization.

Vitamin D increases the availability, retention, and utilization of calcium and phosphorus for proper mineralization of the skeleton. Deficiency of vitamin D is a major cause of *rickets* in the infant, and one of the causes of *osteomalacia* in the adult. The requirements of infants are generally met through the use of vitamin D milk. The needs of most adults are probably supplied by the average diet and casual exposure to sunshine. Vitamin D is absorbed in the presence of *bile,* primarily from the *jejunum* (small intestine) and is transported to the liver and then to the kidney for conversion to the active form, 1,25 dihydrocholecalciferol (1,25 DHCC). The 1,25 DHCC is carried by the bloodstream by a specific binding protein to the intestinal wall and to the bone. Reserves of vitamin D are stored as such in the liver and kidneys. After the absorption of calcium and phosphorus through the intestinal wall, vitamin D continues to work in partnership with calcium and phosphorus in the calcification aspect of bone formation. Tracer studies with radioactive isotopes have shown that 1,25-DHCC directly increases the role of mineral accretion and resorption in bone by which the tissue is built and maintained.

The 1,25-DHCC activates the production of a specific protein in the intestinal wall which carries the calcium from the small intestine into the blood, thereby increasing the availability of calcium for bone deposition. In vitamin D deficiency, not only is calcium absorption from the small intestine decreased, but the mobilization of calcium from the bone is depressed resulting in *hypocalcemia*. In addition there is an increase in the urinary losses of phosphorus and amino acids. See *calcitonin* and *parathyroid hormone.*

Sunshine is an important source of vitamin D. In the skin, a form of cholesterol, the provitamin 7-dehydrocholecalciferol, is activated to vitamin D_3 when exposed to sunlight. The natural distribution of vitamin D in common foods is limited to small, often insignificant amounts in cream, butter, eggs, and liver. For this reason it is necessary to depend upon fortified foods, fish-liver oils or concentrates for preventative and therapeutic use. Vitamin D_3 milk is produced by adding a vitamin D_3 concentrate to homogenized milk. All brands of evaporated milk also have vitamin D_3 added. Fish liver oils have a wide range of potency. The chart on p. 498 shows some natural sources of vitamin D (1 μg is equal to 40 of the old international units).

Vitamin D_2, ergocalciferol, is manufactured by exposing ergosterol, a sterol found in fungi and yeasts to ultraviolet (u.v.) light. Although ergocalciferol, vitamin D_2, is widely used in therapeutics, it occurs very rarely in nature. It is absent in almost all plants and animal tissues except for small amounts in certain fish-liver oils. Ergosterol, from which it is derived, occurs only in plants. The fat-soluble antirachitic factor vitamin D_2 is obtained by ultraviolet-ray activation of 7-dehydrocholesterol. It occurs in fish-liver oils and in irradiated foods of animal origin; termed "natural" vitamin D. Vitamin D in milk may be produced by three different methods: (1) "Fortified" milk, which is more generally distributed than other types, is that to which a vitamin D concentrate has been added: (2) "Metabolized" milk is produced by feeding cows irradiated yeast; and (3) "Irradiated" milk has been exposed directly to ultraviolet rays. The standard amount used for fortification is 400 I.U. vitamin D per quart of fresh or reconstituted milk.

Source	Range (μg/100 g)
Fatty fish and their oils	
Cod-liver oil	200–750
Halibut-liver oil	500–10,000
Swordfish-liver oil	25,000
Shark-liver oil	30–125
Fat fish (fresh or canned, e.g., herring, salmon, sardine, pilchard)	5–45
Dairy produce	
Eggs, whole	1.25–1.5
Eggs, yolk	4–10
Margarine, vitamised	2–9
Butter	0.25–2.5
Cheese	about 0.3
Milk	less than 0.1

vitamin deficiency. The absence or an inadequacy of vitamins in the diet of man results in signs of poor health. Since a deficiency in a single specific vitamin is difficult to achieve even under experimental conditions, such an achievement in any diet is unlikely. For example, for the most part, the B-complex vitamins occur in the same foods. Therefore it is difficult to provide a diet deficient in *pyridoxine* * (vitamin B_6) that would not also be deficient in *thiamine* * (vitamin B_1) and *riboflavin* *. The clinical symptoms of vitamin deficiencies are not always clear or specific, partly because of problems of multiple deficiencies and partly because of the fact that many of the symptoms of the individual vitamin deficiencies overlap with one another. For example, a dermatitis manifests itself in five different vitamin deficiencies. The known vitamin deficiencies in man (Table, p. 499,) represent the clinical symptoms and the specific names given to the avitaminosis. In general, experimentally induced avitaminoses are not considered in the table. More information is given under the listing of the vitamin.

vitamin E: See *tocopherols* *.

Vitamin	Symptoms
*Ascorbic acid***** (vitamin C)	Scurvy: red, swollen, bleeding gums, perifolliculosis, poor wound healing, subcutaneous hemorrhage, swelling of joints.
*Cobalamin***** (vitamin B₁₂)	Pernicious anemia. Generally due to genetic lack of *intrinsic factor*. Weakness, numbness, and dementia. Some of the symptoms (anemia) related to an induced free *folic acid* (folacin) deficiency. Dietary deficiency occasionally seen in strict vegetarians.
*Folacin***** (folic acid)	Glossitis, gastrointestinal disturbances, diarrhea and megaloblastic anemia. The anemia is related to the type seen in *cobalamin***** (vitamin B₁₂) deficiency.
*Niacin***** (Nicotinic acid, nicotin-amides)	Pellagra: bilateral dermatitis particularly in areas exposed to sunlight, glossitis, diarrhea, irritability, mental confusion, eventually delirium or psychotic symptoms.
*Pyridoxine***** (vitamin B₆)	Convulsions have been observed in infants. Experimental deficiency in man: seborrheic dermatitis, glossitis, angular stomatitis, abnormal electroence-phalogram
*Retinol***** (vitamin A)	Night blindness (nyctalopia), hyperkeratinization of epithelial tissues, xe-ophthalmia.
*Riboflavin*****	Ariboflavinosis: chelosis, angular stomatitis, labial dermatitis, photophobia, corneal vascularization.
*Thiamine***** (vitamin B₁)	Beriberi; chiefly nervous and cardiovascular systems affected; mental confusion, muscular weakness, loss of ankle and knee jerks, painful calf muscles, peripheral paralysis, edema (wet beri-beri), muscle wasting (dry beri-beri), enlarged heart.
*Vitamin D*****	Rickets in the young. Osteomalacia in adults.
*Vitamin K*****	"Hemorrhagic disease of the newborn." Hemorrhage or slowed blood-clot times. The deficiency is sometimes associated with steatorrhea (fatty stools), diarrhea, or high antibiotic therapy.

vitamin F: An obsolete designation for the essential fatty acids, *linolenic*, linoleic*,* and *arachidonic** acids. It was also once used for vitamin B₁ (*thiamine**).

vitamin G: An obsolete name for *riboflavin**.

vitamin H: An obsolete name for *biotin**.

vitamin I (vitamin B₇): A factor that prevents disturbances in digestion in pigeons.

vitamin J (vitamin C₂): A postulated antipneumonia factor.

vitamin K (phyloquinone, farnoquinone): A group of fat-soluble, light-sensitive vitamins possessing a common naphthoquinone structure; natural forms include vitamin K_1 occurring in green leaves, and vitamin K_2 produced by intestinal bacteria; synthetic forms such as *menadione* * are available as water-soluble esters. The major function of vitamin K is to catalyze the synthesis of normal *prothrombin* by the liver. Normal prothrombin has a terminal amino acid, gamma (γ)-carboxyglutamic acid. Vitamin K is necessary to carboxylate (add CO_2) to this terminal amino acid. In the absence of vitamin K, the terminal *glutamic acid* * residue in the protein is not converted to a γ-carboxyglutamyl residue and normal prothrombin is not formed. Only normal prothrombin can be converted to thrombin by the proteolytic enzyme proaccelerin or factor V. Without vitamin K the whole vital process of blood clotting cannot be initiated. Vitamin K function is therefore essential in blood coagulation for the maintenance of normal prothrombin time through its effect on prothrombin and other clotting factors. Prothrombin levels regulate the rate of blood coagulation; when they are low, the coagulation is depressed. Coumarin drugs, such as *dicumarol* * are anticoagulants and act as vitamin K antagonists (*antivitamins*). They are used in anticoagulation therapy. Vitamin K deficiency, which is characterized by hemorrhagic tendencies, may result from reduced synthesis by intestinal bacteria or poor intestinal absorption; prophylaxis is achieved with 1–2 mg. vitamin K per day administered orally. It can be synthesized in the lower gastrointestinal tract by the bacterial flora. Because vitamin K is absorbed mainly from the upper section of the tract, only limited amounts are probably absorbed. Medication such as antibiotics which reduce intestinal flora decrease the synthesis of vitamin K.

Dietary sources of vitamin K are absorbed in the small intestine where fats are absorbed. Bile salts are necessary for effective absorption. The vitamin passes

Vitamin K_1 Mol. Wt. 450

Vitamin K_2 Mol. Wt. 580

into the lacteals, through the thoracic duct, and into the liver. Here it functions in synthesis of the proteins, prothrombin, proconvertin factors, and the Steward factor. All these are necessary for blood clotting.

Vitamin K is fairly wide distributed in foods. It appears abundantly in cauliflower, cabbage, spinach, pork liver, and soybeans and to a lesser extent in wheat and oats.

Major Sources of Vitamin K

Sources	Vitamin K (gm/100 grams edible portion)
Alfalfa	425–850
Cabbage	250
Cauliflower	275
Liver, pork	115–230
Soybeans	190
Spinach	334
Wheat, whole	36
Wheat bran	80
Wheat germ	37

The dietary vitamin K requirement is unknown and there is no *United States Recommended Daily Allowance* (U.S. RDA).

vitamin L₁: Reported to be needed for lactation in rats.

vitamin L₂: Reported to be related to adenosine and necessary for lactation in rats.

vitamin M: An obsolete name for *folacin* *.

vitamin N: A name given to extracts from the stomach and brain of animals that were reported to inhibit cancer. It is obsolete.

vitamin P (citrin): A group of bioflavinoids shown to prevent capillary fragility in animals under experimental conditions. The flavinoids were extracted from lemon peel. The bioflavinoids are not considered as vitamins.

vitamin R: A bacterial growth factor. Probably a derivative of the *folacin* * group.

vitamin S: A bacterial growth factor. It is probably identical with *biotin* *.

vitamin T: Reported to promote excessive growth in insects (termite factor) and to improve protein uptake in rats.

vitamin toxicity: *Hypervitaminosis.* The water-soluble vitamins are not toxic in general. Of the fat-soluble vitamins, *retinol** and *vitamin D** can produce severe toxic symptoms. The guide below gives the ratio of the *Recommended Daily Allowance* (RDA) to a toxic level in humans. The toxic level is broadly defined as a level that produces some physiological change no matter how transient. For example, hypervitamin therapy with pyridoxine causes a flushing, itching and warm sensation that lasts about 30 seconds. It should be borne in mind that toxicity levels vary greatly from individual to individual. In vitamin D toxicity for example, the variations in toxic levels among individuals may be greater than 10-fold.

Vitamin	Ratio of RDA/Toxic Level
Retinol* (vitamin A)	1 : 7,500
Vitamin D*	1 : 2,000
Cobalamin* (vitamin B_{12})	1 : 100,000
Niacin*	1 : 5,000
Pyridoxine* (vitamin B_6)	1 : 60,000
Thiamine* (vitamin B_1)	1 : 25,000

vitamin U: A bacterial growth factor. Probably a derivative of the *folacin**.

vitamin V: A bacterial growth factor. Probably a derivative of *niacin**, *nicotinamide adenine dinucleotide** (NAD).

vitamin W: A bacterial growth factor. Probably *biotin**.

vitamin X: A bacterial growth factor. Probably *biotin**.

vitamin Y: Appears to be identical with *pyridoxine**.

W

walnut (*Juglans regia*). The edible nut of the fruit of the walnut tree. The most commonly known walnut is the English, or Persian, walnut. This hard-shelled nut has a wrinkled white kernel with two very irregularly shaped halves covered with a light-brown skin. The shell is thin and light tan; it is made up of two distinct halves. Walnuts have some protein, iron, and B vitamins. Walnuts are high in fat. English, shelled, 100 gm = 651 calories; black, shelled, 100 gm = 628 calories.

water. Mol. Wt. 18. H—O—H (H_2O). Water is the medium for transporting the food materials to be used in the body. In a state of solution or suspension, simple sugars, amino acids, fats, minerals, and vitamins are passed through the intestinal walls and are then carried to the cells by blood and lymph, the two most fluid tissues of the body. Waste products are carried and excreted in a similar manner. Oxygen and carbon dioxide are also transported by the bloodstream. After absorption much fluid reenters the alimentary tract, where it serves as a carrier of digestive enzymes. Large quantities of digestive juices are secreted daily by the body. It has been estimated that the 24-hour secretion of *saliva,* expressed in milliliters, is from 500 to 1500; of *gastric juice,* 1000 to 2500; of *bile,* 100 to 400; and of intestinal secretions 700 to 300. Water is an efficient heat conductor and serves to maintain the uniform body temperature essential for health. As a protector of internal organs, water is indispensible; it serves as a cushion and prevents the transmission of shock from the outside. By means of the synovial fluid present in all joints, these surfaces are kept lubricated and moist; the central nervous system is bathed by the cerebospinal fluid. In terms of life need, water is second only to oxygen. The body can be deprived of oxygen for up to about 20 minutes, in rare instances can survive water deprivation for only a few days, and can live without food for weeks. When the body water loss exceeds 20 percent, death is likely.

Water is found in all parts of the body. The water within the cells (intercellular fluid) comprises the largest part of the total amount and furnishes an aqueous medium for the chemical reactions which constantly occur. When considered in relation to total body weight, water may vary from about 40 percent in very obese to 70 percent in the very lean person. The different parts of the body vary markedly in their water content. Muscle has about 75 percent water, and bone about 25 percent. Blood plasma and red blood cells have about 92 and 60 percent. *Adipose* (fat) *tissue* may vary from 10 to 30 percent.

In addition to direct ingestion, water is obtained from food as a part of its content and is obtained also as a result of its metabolism. In the oxidation of foodstuffs to obtain energy, the process results in carbon dioxide, water, and energy. The table below shows the water content of some common classes of food. Except for fat, pure sugars and dry cereals, water is the major constituent of most foods.

Food	Approximate Percent Water
Bread	35
Cooked cereals	80–90
Dry cereal	3
Eggs	75
Fruits and vegetables	70–95
Meat (cooked rare)	75
Meat (well done)	40
Milk	85

The table that follows shows the amount of water that is produced by the oxidation of the foodstuff. The oxidation of the sugar glucose is given as an example of how the water arises in the balance chemical equation:

$$C_6H_{12}O_6 + 6O_2 \longrightarrow 6CO_2 + 6H_2O + 686,000 \text{ calories}$$
Glucose + Oxygen⟶carbon dioxide + water + energy.

Food (100 gm)	ml or gms of H_2O Formed
Fat	107
Carbohydrate	56
Protein	41

See *water balance* and *water regulation*

water balance. The total blood flow through the kidneys is about 1200 ml per minute and the total extracellular fluid amounts to about 15 liters, about 3 liters of that total is *plasma*. The blood plasma and the extracellular fluid are in equilibrium with each other and therefore an amount of blood equivalent to all the extracellular fluid can pass through the kidney once every 15 minutes. The water and electrolyte content of the blood plasma, and therefore, indirectly, of the extracellular fluid are closely controlled by the kidney. Any increase of water content of the body, such as a water load by drinking, leads to the prompt production of a corresponding amount of *urine*, with a low specific gravity. Water absorption in the tubules is controlled by the *antidiuretic hormone* (ADH) of the pituitary gland, which modifies the amount of water taken up in the distal part of the renal tubule. An increase in the amount of water in the body lowers the osmotic pressure of the carotid body and reduces the production of ADH which causes an increased production of urine. The diagram below shows the relationships among the various water compartments of the body and the outside world.

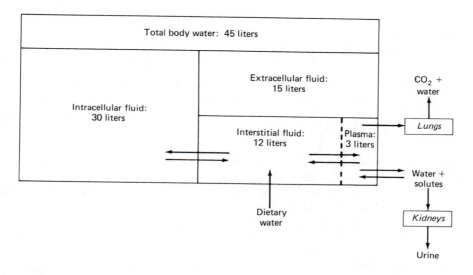

The typical water balance for an adult over a 24-hour period during light activity is approximately as follows:

Water Intake	ml	Water Output	ml
Water	1200	Urine	1300
Foods	900	Feces	200
Water of oxidation	300	Perspiration	500
		Lungs	400

water chestnut (*Trapa*). The fruit of a water plant with floating leaves and small white flowers. The nutlike fruit kernel resembles a true chestnut in shape and color, but is crunchy in texture. Water chestnuts can be used in poultry, meat, seafood, and egg dishes, and adds a pleasant crispness when combined with soft foods. Raw, 100 gm = 79 calories.

watercress (*Nasturtium officinale*). The most popular and widely eaten of the cresses, plants of the mustard family which includes peppergrass or garden cress, winter cress or rocket, and spring or Belle Isle cress. All have crisp green leaves and a pungent, rather bitter taste, each variety with its own characteristics. Peppergrass is sometimes sprinkled over such dishes as beet soup. All the cresses may be boiled as *potherbs*. Watercress gets its name because it grows in cold running water. The word "cress" is perhaps related to the Latin word for grass, and even further back to the Sanskrit verb meaning "to eat," especially gnawing or nibbling. Watercress is a good source of *ascorbic acid* * (vitamin C) and *carotene* * (vitamin A activity), and supplies a variety of minerals including iron if eaten in large amounts. 100 gm = 19 calories.

water extract. Whatever can be removed or dissolved out of a substance with water. A substance like sugar is completely soluble in water, whereas when yeast is shaken up with water only a small portion of it goes into solution. What remains is insoluble and does not pass into the water-extract.

water regulation. The *water balance* is regulated by several complex mechanisms. *Antidiuretic hormone* (ADH) from the posterior *pituitary* causes an increase in water absorption by the kidney and therefore a decreased urine output. A high *osmotic pressure* (a high concentration of solutes in the blood) signals the release of ADH. Diuretics and alcohol inhibit the release of ADH from the pituitary and increased urine output is the result. Increased urine output (diuresis) generally accompanies an increased excretion of solutes into the urine because the solutes carry the water of hydration along with them. The diuresis due to the disease *diabetes mellitus* (sugar diabetes) is due to the high blood sugar which "spills over" into the urine and carries large amounts of water of hydration. The large water loss is in turn accompanied by increased water intake (thirst or polydipsia) and the water balance is maintained. Water regulation is also intimately associated with salt (electrolyte) balance and some steroids, *aldosterone* * in particular. Aldosterone and deoxycorticosterone promote the reabsorption sodium ion (Na^+) and retention of the water. The release of aldosterone by the adrenal glands is controlled indirectly by the Na^+ plasma concentration. When the Na^+ in plasma is low, the kidneys release renin which causes the liver angiotensinogen to be active angiotensin which stimulates the adrenal glands to release aldosterone. Aldosterone can also be released by stimulation of the adrenal glands by *adrenocorticotrophic hormone* (ACTH) from the pituitary. Stress can cause the release ACTH by the pituitary. The diagram below shows these relationships.

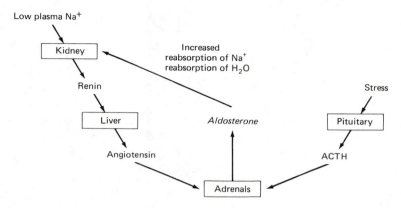

The female hormone, *progesterone* promotes the retention of salt and water and accounts for the retention of water at certain stages of the menstral cycle.

A change in the diet can cause a temporary retention or loss of water until a new water balance is reached. The carbohydrate content of the diet has a pronounced influence on water retention. In general, a decrease in dietary carbohydrate is accompanied by an increased loss of water. All of the diets that promise rapid weight loss are low in carbohydrates, and take full advantage of the weight loss due to increased water excretion. Conversely, if the shift is to a high carbohydrate intake, the rapid increase in weight is due largely to water retention. There are several different theories as to why carbohydrates have an effect on water retention but the mechanism is not understood clearly.

watermelon (*Citrullus vulgaris*). A member of the gourd family, most commonly a spherical fruit with pink or red flesh and many seeds. There are many varieties among which are yellow and white watermelons as well as the red. Seeds may be white, red, brown, black, green, or speckled. The rind is usually dark green. Watermelons average 24 to 40 pounds, although there are some small 2- to 10-pound varieties. The flesh is sweet with a high water content. Watermelons are a good source of vitamin A activity and a fair source of *ascorbic acid* * (vitamin C). 100 gm = 26 calories. See *fruits* and Appendix 8 for nutrient content.

water-soluble vitamins. The water-soluble vitamins make up a large group, and all but one belong to the B complex. The remaining water-soluble vitamin is *ascorbic acid* (vitamin C). For the most part, water-soluble vitamins are not

Summary of Water-Soluble Vitamins

Nomenclature	Important Sources	Physiology and Function	Effects of Deficiency	Recommended Allowances
Ascorbic acid Vitamin C	Citrus fruits; tomatoes; melons; cabbage; broccoli; strawberries; fresh potatoes; green leafy vegetables	Very little storage in body. Formation of intercellular cement substance; synthesis of collagen. Absorption and use of iron. Prevents oxidation of folacin	Weakened cartilages and capillary walls. Cutaneous hemorrhage; sore, bleeding gums, anemia. Poor wound healing. Poor bone and tooth development. Scurvy	Men 45 mg. Women: 45 mg. Pregnancy: 60 mg. Lactation: 60 mg. Infants: 35 mg. Children under 10: 40 mg. Boys and girls: 45 mg
Thiamin Vitamin B$_1$	Whole-grain and enriched breads, cereals, flours; organ meats, pork; other meats, poultry, fish; legumes, nuts; milk; green vegetables	Limited body storage. Thiamin pyrophosphate (TPP) is coenzyme for decarboxylation and transketolation; chiefly involved in carbohydrate metabolism	Poor appetite; atony of gastrointestinal tract, constipation. Mental depression, apathy, polyneuritis. Cachexia, edema. Cardiac failure. Beriberi	Men: 1.4 mg. Women: 1.0 mg. Pregnancy: 1.3 mg. Lactation: 1.3 mg. Infants: 0.3–0.5 mg. Children under 10: 0.7–1.2 mg. Boys and girls: 1.1–1.5 mg
Riboflavin Vitamin B$_2$	Milk; organ meats; eggs; green leafy vegetables	Limited body stores, but reserves retained carefully. Coenzymes for removal and transfer of hydrogen; flavin mononucleotide (FMN) and flavin adenine dinucleotide (FAD)	Cheilosis (cracks at corners of lips). Scaly desquamation around nose, ears. Sore tongue and mouth. Burning and itching of eyes. Photophobia	Men: 1.6 mg. Women: 1.2 mg. Pregnancy: 1.5 mg. Lactation: 1.7 mg. Infants: 0.4–0.6 mg. Children under 10: 0.8–1.2 mg. Boys and girls: 1.3–1.8 mg

Vitamin	Food sources	Functions	Deficiency	Requirements
Niacin Nicotinic acid Nicotinamide	Meat, poultry, fish; whole-grain and enriched breads, flours, cereals; nuts, legumes Tryptophan as a precursor	Coenzyme for glycolysis, fat synthesis, tissue respiration. Coenzymes NAD and NADP accept hydrogen and transfer it	Anorexia, glossitis, diarrhea Dermatitis Neurologic degeneration Pellagra	Men: 18 mg Women: 13 mg Pregnancy: 15 mg Lactation: 17 mg Infants: 5–8 mg Children under 10: 9–16 mg Boys and girls: 14–20 mg
Vitamin B$_6$ Three active forms: pyridoxine, pyridoxal, pyridoxamine	Meat, poultry, fish; potatoes, sweet potatoes, vegetables	Pyridoxal phosphate is coenzyme for transamination, decarboxylation, transulfuration Conversion of tryptophan to niacin; conversion of glycogen to glucose	Nervous irritability, convulsions Weakness, ataxia, abdominal pain Dermatitis; anemia	Adults: 2.0 mg Pregnancy: 2.5 mg Lactation: 2.5 mg Infants: 0.3–0.4 mg Children under 10: 0.6–1.2 mg Boys and girls: 1.6–2.0 mg
Pantothenic acid	Meat, poultry, fish; whole-grain cereals; legumes Smaller amounts in fruits, vegetables, milk	Constituent of coenzyme A: oxidation of pyruvic acid, α-ketoglutarate, fatty acids; synthesis of fatty acids, sterols, and porphyrin	Deficiency seen only with severe multiple B-complex deficits; then, gastrointestinal disturbances, neuritis, burning sensations of feet	Not known; probably about 5–10 mg
Biotin	Organ meats, egg yolks, nuts, legumes	*Avidin*, a protein in raw egg white, blocks absorption; large amounts of raw eggs must be eaten Coenzyme for deamination, carboxylation, and decarboxylation	Deficiency only when many raw egg whites are consumed for long periods of time Dermatitis, anorexia, hyperesthesia, anemia	Not known; probably about 5–10 mg
Vitamin B$_{12}$ Cyanocobalamin Hydroxycobalamin	In animal foods only: organ meats, muscle meats, fish, poultry; eggs; milk	Requires intrinsic factor for absorption Biosynthesis of methyl groups Synthesis of DNA and RNA Formation of mature red blood cells	Lack of intrinsic factor leads to deficiency; pernicious anemia, following gastrectomy Macrocytic anemia Neurologic degeneration	Adults: 3 mcg Pregnancy: 4 mcg Lactation: 4 mcg Infants: 1–2 mcg Boys and girls: 3 mcg

Summary of Water-Soluble Vitamins

Nomenclature	Important Sources	Physiology and Function	Effects of Deficiency	Recommended Allowances
Folacin Folic acid Tetrahydrofolic acid	Organ meats, deep-green leafy vegetables; muscle meats, poultry, fish, eggs; whole-grain cereals	Active form is folinic acid; requires ascorbic acid for conversion Coenzyme for transmethylation; synthesis of nucleoproteins; maturation of red blood cells Interrelated with vitamin B$_{12}$	Megaloblastic anemia of infancy, pregnancy, tropical sprue	Adults: 400 mcg Pregnancy: 800 mcg Lactation: 600 mcg Infants: 50 mcg Children under 10: 100–300 mcg Boys and girls: 400 mcg
Choline	Egg yolk, meat, poultry, fish, milk, whole grains	Probably not a true vitamin Donor of methyl groups: lipotropic action Component of acetylcholine	Has not been observed in humans	Not known; typical diet supplies 200–600 mg
Lipoic acid Thioctic acid Protogen		Probably not a true vitamin Coenzyme for decarboxylation of keto acids		Not known
Inositol	Widely distributed in all foods	Lipotropic agent Vitamin nature not established	Has not been observed in humans	Not known

510

stored in the body. Excesses are largely excreted, thus eliminating the possibilities for toxicity that exist with overdoses of *fat-soluble vitamins*. At least 11 vitamins compose the B complex. Seven of them are essential in human nutrition; six are included in the allowance table of the Food and Nutrition Board. These are *thiamine* * (vitamin B_1), *riboflavin* *, *niacin* *, *folacin, pyridoxine* (vitamin B_6), and *cobalamin* * (vitamin B_{12}). All are concerned with converting the end products of carbohydrate, fat and protein digestion into a form of energy the body can use. They serve basically as coenzymes. Pages 508–510 contain a summary of some water soluble vitamins.

waxes. Defined chemically as fatty acid esters of higher alcohols. Occur widely in the cuticles of leaves and fruit and in the secretions of insects, and may be mixed with very long chain hydrocarbons (C_{21435}). The structure of myricyl palmitate, a major constituent of beeswax is given below. They replace the *triglycerides* to some extent in the tissues of aquatic animals, e.g., crustaceans. So far waxes have not been shown to be an important constituent of any of the higher land animals, nor do they contribute importantly to normal human diet.

$$CH_3(CH_2)_{14} \overset{\overset{\displaystyle O}{\|}}{C} - O(CH_2)_{29}CH_3$$

Palmitic acid   Myricyl alcohol

waxy flour. A flour prepared from certain varieties of rice or corn that contain a type of starch that has waxy adhesive qualities. The flour acts as a stabilizer when it is used as an ingredient in sauces or gravies and binds the mixture together so there is no separation when the mixture is frozen.

Wernicke's encephalopathy. A syndrome related to *thiamin* * deficiency characterized by anorexia, nystagmus, double vision, opthalmoplegia, ataxia, loss of memory, confusion, confabulations, and hallucinations, which may progress to stupor and coma. Thiamine deficiency is largely responsible for the condition, though associated insufficiencies of other water-soluble vitamins may be involved. See *thiamine* *.

whale liver oil. Oil is extracted from the liver of whales caught in the Antarctic and is used for the production of commercial vitamin concentrates employed in the fortification of margarines, with the fat-soluble vitamins. The vitamin of the oil differs from that of other sources.

wheat (*Triticum*). The grain of a grass most widely grown of the cereal grains. The little wheat kernels grow in beads at the top of stalks or straw. The flour made by grinding wheat grain is the best of all fours for breadmaking because of the presence of gluten, a form of protein that makes a soft and spongy dough. A grain of wheat has three main parts. The outer covering is the bran, the inner part the endosperm, and the tiny nucleus within the endosperm is the germ. If the entire kernel is ground, the result is whole-wheat flour, graham flour, or entire wheat flour. If just the endosperm is used, the result is flour, wheat flour, and plain flour. Below is a cross-section of a grain of whole wheat. The Bran. The brown outer layers. This part contains: (1) Bulk-forming carbohydrates, (2) B vitamins, (3) Minerals, especially iron. The Aleurone Layers: The layers located right under the bran. They are rich in: (1) Proteins, (2) Phosphorus, a mineral. The Endosperm. The white center. This consists mainly of: (1) Carbohydrates (starches and sugars), (2) Protein.

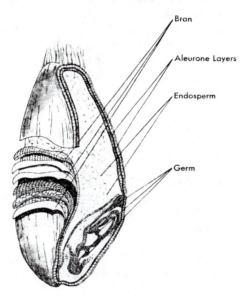

The wheat proteins occupy a unique position among the cereal grains. *Gluten* or wheat protein is composed of two major proteins, gliadin (a *prolamine*) and glutenin (a *glutelin*). The combination in wheat flour gives a characteristic stickiness when mixed with water which enables the molecules to bond together under heat. This allows the wheat flour dough to bake to form bread. Rye contains a small amount of gluten and it too can be made into bread. However, oats, barley, corn, rice, and millets cannot be made into rising breads. These grains or their flours can be boiled into porridges or tortillas. Wheat has a nutritive value similar to that of the other cereals.

Most of the flour used today is highly refined. Milling in general consists of grinding and sifting through fine sieves in order to obtain fine, white wheat flour. The table below shows the nutritive content of wheat flour relative to the percent of the whole wheat flour in the finely milled flour. Most fine flours contain less than 70 percent of the whole wheat flour.

Values Per 100 gm of flour	Percent of Whole-wheat Flour			
	100	80	70	45
Fiber (gm)	2.2	0.1	trace	trace
Fat (gm)	2.5	1.4	1.2	0.9
Protein (g)	13.6	13.2	12.8	11.8
Biotin (μg)	5	1.4	1.2	0.7
Folacin (μg)	35	13	—	8
Niacin (mg)	5.0	2.0	1.6	0.7
Pyridoxine (μg)	400	108	64	—
Riboflavin (mg)	160	83	53	50
Thiamine (mg)	0.4	0.3	0.1	0.03

The limiting amino acid in wheat protein is lysine, and typical of the cereal grains it contains only a trace of the *carotene* and no *ascorbic acid*. In white flour, starch is present in greater proportion and is more digestible than it is in whole-wheat flour. Therefore, it is higher in caloric value. If enriched, white flour contains added *thiamine, riboflavin, niacin* and *iron. Calcium* and *vitamin D** may also be added. Wholewheat flour, which contains all the nutrients available in the whole grain, is high in phosphorus, potassium, and has moderate amounts of protein, niacin, thiamine, and riboflavin. The caloric values of 100 gm of the most commonly available wheat flours and other foods are:

Whole-wheat flour = 333 calories
Flour, enriched or unenriched = 364 calories
Self-rising, enriched = 352 calories
Bulgur, dry = 357 calories
Wheat germ = 363 calories
Whole-wheat crackers = 403 calories
Graham crackers, plain = 384 calories
Graham crackers, sugar-honey-coated = 411 calories
Cereal, rolled wheat, cooked = 75 calories
Cereal, wheat and malted barley, quick-cooking = 65 calories
Cereal, wheat-flakes, ready-to-eat = 354 calories
Cereal, wheat germ, ready-to-eat = 391 calories
Cereal, puffed wheat, ready-to-eat = 363 calories
Cereal, puffed wheat with sugar and honey, ready-to-eat = 354 calories
Cereal, shredded wheat, ready-to-eat = 354 calories

Cereal, bran with sugar and malt, ready-to-eat = 240 calories
Cereal, bran with sugar and wheat germ, ready-to-eat = 238 calories
Cereal, bran flakes, ready-to-eat = 303 calories
Cereal, bran flakes with raisins, ready to eat = 287 calories
See *cereal grains* and *appendix 8* for nutrient content.

whey. The liquid part of milk which remains after the thicker part, or curd is removed. The curd is used in making cheese. Whey contains sugar, minerals, and lactalbumin. See *milk*.

whiskey or whisky. A spirit distilled from such grains as barley, rye, and corn, and subsequently refined, colored, and flavored by various processes. Each country produces a distinctive type of whiskey. The Latin term used to describe distilled spirits was aquavitae, "water of life." The Scotch and Irish translated it to usquebaugh in Galeic. The name was later contracted to uisge and still later anglicized to whiskey. The four steps of whiskey production are malting, fermenting, distilling, and aging. Whiskey, strictly defined by the United States Federal standards is a grain spirit, distilled at less than 190° proof and 1 day old. Thirty-three whiskey variations are listed among the United States Standards, but general usage divides whiskey into two major subdivisions, straight whiskey and blended whiskey. Straight whiskey is whiskey which is unmixed with other liquors or substances, such as straight bourbon whiskey and straight rye whiskey. Federal law requires that straight whiskey be aged in new charred oak barrels for at least 2 years. A blended whiskey is a balanced blending of straight whiskeys and neutral grain spirits (a high distillate, at least 190 proof, of any fermented mash), containing at least 20 percent straight whiskeys and bottled at not less than 80 proof. The word proof applied to distilled spirits indicates the amount of alcohol in a liquor. Proof is twice the percentage of alcohol. A bonded whiskey is straight whiskey produced and bottled in accordance with the Federal Bottling-in-Bond Act. It must be at least 4 years old, must be bottled at 100° proof, must have been produced in a single distillery, by the same distiller, and be the product of a single season or year. Caloric value: Bourbon 86 proof, 43 ml (1½ ounces), = about 125 calories; Irish, 43 ml (1½ ounces), 86 proof = about 125 calories; Rye, 43 ml (1½ ounces), 86 proof = about 125 calories; Scotch, 86 proof 43 ml (1½ ounces), = about 110 calories.

white blood cells. See *blood cells, white*.

whitefish (*Coregonus*). A fatty freshwater fish caught in North America lakes, belonging to the salmon family. Whitefish are prepared in almost any way that fish can be prepared: broiled, panfried, baked, or poached. Whitefish are very high in protein and *retinol** (vitamin A), phosphorus and potassium; has some *thiamine**, *riboflavin**, and *niacin**. Fresh, raw, 100 gm = 155 calories; fresh, baked and stuffed 100 gm = 215 calories; smoked, 100 gm = 155 calories.

whiting (*Merluccius, Merlangus, or Menticirrhus*). Small gray and white salt-water fish sometimes called kingfish or silver hake. Whiting grow to an average length of 12 inches and weigh from 1 to 4 pounds. The fish has tender white flesh, fine in texture, flaky, with a delicate flavor. It can be broiled, panfried, baked, or poached. A good source of protein. Fresh, raw, 100 gm = 105 calories.

wild rice (*Zizania aquatica*). A native American grass, that bears a grain used for food. It is a tall plant that grows in water in the western Great Lakes area and has never been domesticated. Wild rice is high in protein, phosphorus, and potassium, with some *riboflavin**, *thiamine**, and *niacin**. Uncooked 100 gm = 353 calories.

wine. Wine is the product of the natural fermentation of the juice of the grape. The term is also used to describe beverages made from other fruit juices or vegetable juices by adding sugar and yeast and fermenting the mixture—examples are dandelion wine and elderberry wine. But strictly speaking wine is the product of the vine, for grapes contain naturally all the ingredients needed for a normal fermentation of the juice. No sugar nor yeast need be added. The true wine yeast is *Saccharomyces cerevisiae* var. *ellipsoideus*. The raw grape juice or "must" is high in sugar and strongly acid. An unsuitable medium for the growth of bacteria but highly suitable for yeast and molds. Fermentation is either allowed to proceed spontaneously or it is started with a must from a previously successful fermentation. The must is aerated slightly until yeast growth is vigorous and then stopped. The carbon dioxide produced by the yeast is sufficient to keep conditions anaerobic, inhibiting the growth of molds and bacteria. The ageing process ensues after sufficient sugar has been utilized and sufficient alcohol produced. See *saccharomyces, yeast, alcohol* and *ethanol*.

woodruff, sweet (*Asperula adorata*). A spreading plant with small white flowers whose slim yellow leaves are used to flavor beverages. The characteristic odor of its leaves is released when they are somewhat dried; they then smell like new-mown hay. The leaves may be used to flavor cold fruit drinks and wine cups.

work. The result of the utilization of energy to produce a change. In this sense, the use of chemical energy to produce a new compound (a synthesis) would be chemical "work." Work also has a technical definition in physics restricted to linear displacement.

X

xanthoproteic test. A yellow color reaction produced when a protein is treated with concentrated nitric acid. The test is simply a nitration of the aromatic ring of certain amino acids (*tyrosine* *, *phenylalanine* *, and *tryptophan* *). Recognized as the familiar nitric acid stain. The test is done on urine and the presence of protein in urine usually indicates a dysfunction or pathology of the kidney.

xanthelasma. Common form of xanthoma (yellow tumor). The condition occurs when there is a high level of *cholesterol* * and cholesterol esters in the blood. The lesion occurs on the eyelids. The tumors are flat, soft, yellow-colored plaques of varying size. May be a forerunner of angina or high blood pressure.

xanthine. A purine intermediate in the metabolism of purines. It is related to *uric acid* *.

xanthomatosis. Accumulation of lipids in the form of tumors in various parts of the body.

xeroderma. Means dryness of the skin. Instead of the normal smooth, moist, velvet texture, the skin feels dry and often rough. On uncovering the legs, a cloud of fine, branny dandruff is often seen. Xeroderma is commonly but not constantly associated with follicular keratosis and "crackled skin."

xerophthalmia. An extreme dryness of the conjunctiva of the eye condition caused by lack of *retinol* * (vitamin A). See *retinol* *.

xylitol Mol. Wt. 152. A five-carbon polyhydric alcohol used as a sugar substitute. Xylitol is a natural product and is metabolized and enters the five-carbon sugar metabolism by its oxidation to D-xylulose and then to D-xylulose phosphate. It is a part of the series of reaction that produces *ribose* in the pentose shunt or hexose monophosphate shunt. See *sorbitol*.

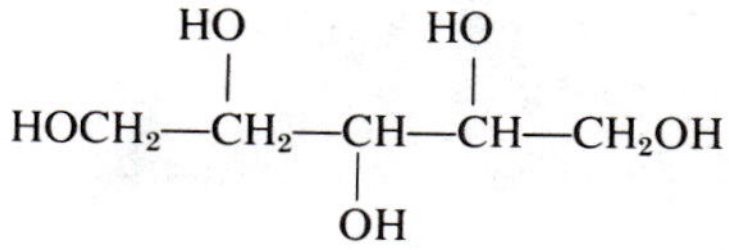

$$\underset{\overset{|}{OH}}{HOCH_2-CH_2-\overset{\overset{HO}{|}}{CH}-\overset{\overset{HO}{|}}{CH}-CH_2OH}$$

xylose (wood sugar). Mol. Wt. 150. A five-carbon sugar that is not metabolized by the body. It occurs in wood nuts and other vegetables as a polymer class called the xylans which occur in the cell walls of plants.

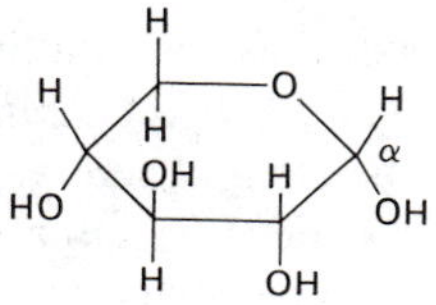

α D-xylose
(α D-xylopyranose)

xylulose. Mol. Wt. 150. A five-carbon sugar intermediate in the pentose cycle (hexose monophosphate shunt) that leads to the biosynthesis of *ribose*.

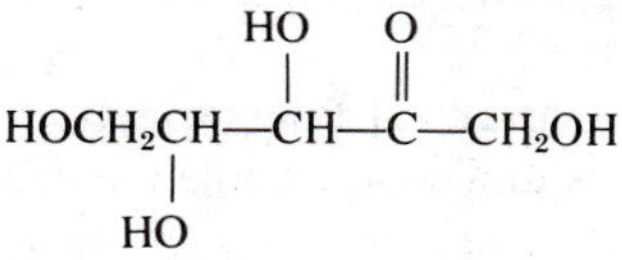

$$\underset{\overset{|}{HO}}{HOCH_2CH-\overset{\overset{HO}{|}}{CH}-\overset{\overset{O}{\|}}{C}-CH_2OH}$$

D-xylulose

Y

yams (*Disocorea*). The two most important cultivated varieties are the greater yam (*D. alata*) and the lesser yams (*D. esculentia*). The yam is a thick tuber which develops at the base of the stem. There are more than 150 species, with some varieties growing up to 100 pounds; some are no larger than a small potato. The consistency varies from coarse and mealy to tender and mushy, with some crisp varieties. Like potatoes, the yam tubers are rich in starch, but also contain significant amounts of protein. Yams are often confused with *sweet potatoes (Ipomoea batatas)*, which they resemble, but they belong to different botanical genera. Both yams and sweet potatoes are not sweet until cooked. The warming process of cooking activates the amylases and these enzymes hydrolize the starches to sugars. Raw, 100 gm = 101 calories.

yeast (*Sacchromycetes*). One-celled fungi widely distributed in nature. Some convert sugar in fruit juices to alcohol. Some are used to produce carbon dioxide for a leavening agent in breadmaking. From an industrial and technical view the yeast are easily the most important single group of microorganism. There are many varieties of yeast, but the most commonly used by man are *S. cerevisiae* and its variety *ellipsoideus*. Man has used yeast in processing his food, drink, and textiles since prehistoric times. Yeast are used in the preparation of beer, wine, cheese, butter, and flax. Yeast is an excellent source of protein and the B-complex vitamins. The table below gives the nutritive value of yeast.

Nutrient Value of Yeast Per 100 Grams			
Protein	38 g	Thiamin*	16 mg
Carbohydrate	38 g	Riboflavin*	4 mg
Fat	trace	Niacin*	38 mg
Carotene* (vitamin A)	trace	Ascorbic acid*	trace

Baker's compressed, 100 gm = 86 calories
Baker's dry, active, 100 gm = 282 calories

Brewer's dry, 100 gm = 283 calories
Torula, 100 gm = 277 calories

yogurt. A semisolid milk product that has been made acid by the addition of bacterial cultures which have much greater acidfying power than natural ferments. A good source of the B-vitamins and calcium. Plain, made from whole milk 100 gm = 62 calories; plain, made from partially skimmed milk, 100 gm = 50 calories. See *milk* and *milk products*.

Z

zein. A major protein in *corn*. It has a low biologic value, with an *net protein utilization* (NPU) value of about 40. Zein is relatively poor in the *essential amino acids lysine* and *tryptophan*.

zinc. (Zn) Element No. 30. Atom. Wt. 65.38 The adult human body contains about 2–3 gm zinc. Zinc is present in most tissues of the animal body. Extraordinarily high concentrations occur in choroid of the eye and in male reproductive organs. Liver, voluntary muscle, and bone contain considerably less, but more than other tissues. Most of the zinc in blood is present in the erythrocytes; almost all of the zinc occurs associated with carbonic anhydrase. Zinc is a component of a number of metaloenzymes including the pancreatic peptidases, carbonic anhydrase, alcohol dehydrogenation, and other dehydrogenases. Zinc has

Food	mg per 100-gm Edible Portion	Food	mg per 100-gm Edible Portion
Applesauce, canned	1.2–1.4	Liver, pork	3–15
Barley	2.7	Milk, cow	0.4–3.0
Beef	2–5	Milk, dry skim	4.5
Beets	2.8	Oatmeal	14.0
Bread, whole wheat	2.4–3.5	Oranges	0.1
Bread, rye	2.2	Oysters	160
Butter	0.3	Peanut butter	2.0
Cabbage	0.2–1.5	Pears, canned	1.5–1.8
Carrots	0.5–3.6	Peas	3–5
Cherries, canned	1.6–2.2	Potatoes	0.2
Clams	2.0	Rice	1.5
Corn, whole	2.5	Spinach	0.3–0.9
Eggs, dry whole	5.5	Syrup, maple	5.2–10.5
Egg yolk	2.6–4.0	Wheat	2.5–8.5
Herring	70–120	Wheat bran	14
Lettuce	0.1–0.7	Yeast, dry	8
Liver, beef	3.0–8.5		

been found to accelerate wound healing, and is necessary in man for growth, sexual maturation, the body syntheses of collagen tissue, in the metabolism of the all-important *nucleic acids,* and as a vital component of many enzymes which are the key to a variety of functions in human health. Many enzymes in man have zinc as a component or it activates them. Precisely how zinc works with enzymes is not known, but it is known that in almost 20 enzyme systems, functions are disturbed in zinc deficiency. Many foods are comparatively rich in zinc such as seafood (especially oysters), liver, wheat germ, wheat bran, dried green split peas, lima beans, yeast, nuts, and milk. The table on p. 520 gives the zinc content of some common foods.

zucchini (*Cucurbita*). A variety of summer squash developed in Italy. It is also known as vegetable marrow or Italian marrow. Zucchini is cylindrical in shape but larger at its base than at its top. The skin has a lacy pattern of green and yellow that concentrates to give the appearance of stripes. It grows to be 10 to 12 inches long and 2 to 3 inches thick, and has pale-green flesh and a delicate flavor. Zucchini provides fair quantities of *carotene** (vitamin A activity), *ascorbic acid** (vitamin C), and small amounts of other vitamins. Cooked and drained, 100 gm = 12 calories. See summer squash under *squash*.

zwieback. A sweet biscuit or rusk which is first baked and then sliced and toasted in the oven to make it into a kind of dry toast. The word comes from the German, and means "baked twice." 100 gm = 423 calories.

zwitterion. Dipolar ions that carry both a positive and negative charge in aqueous solution and are internally neutralized. The neutral amino acids are examples of zwitterions, because they have an *acid* group, the carboxyl group (—COOH) and a basic group, the amino group (—NH$_2$). As shown below, with near neutral pH's the zwitterion is internally neutralized.

$$H_2-\overset{\overset{\displaystyle H}{|}}{\underset{\underset{\displaystyle NH_3^+}{|}}{C}}-COO^-$$

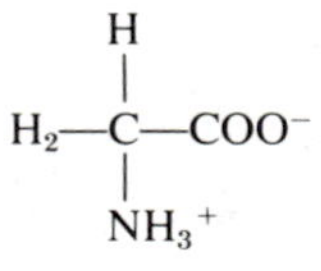

Glycine

zygosaccharomyces. Yeasts notable for their ability to grow in high concentrates of sugar (hence are termed osmophilic), and are involved in the spoilage of honey, syrups, and molasses and in the fermentation of soy sauce and some wines. *Z. nussbaumer* grows in honey.

zygote. The fertilized egg or the individual, resulting from the union of a sperm with an unfertilized egg.

zymogen. A general term for an inactive enzyme precursor that can be activated by hydrolysis, e.g., pepsinogen. Most of the proteases, digestive enzymes, are zymogens. They become activated by hydrolysis of specific *peptide* bonds in the protein chain. The hydrolysis of the peptide bonds is by the acid HCl, in the case of the pepsinogen to *pepsin* activation in the stomach. In the small intestine, most of the activations proceed by enzymic hydrolysis. For example, *trypsinogen* is activated to *trypsin* by the proteolytic enzyme *enterokinase*.

Appendix

1. Common Abbreviations
2. Prefixes
3. Table of Atomic Weights
4. Weights and Measures: Conversion Tables
   a. Temperature
   b. Weights
   c. Length
   d. Area and volume
   e. Relative sizes of microbial forms and the red blood cell
5. Greek Alphabet
6. Weight Ranges for Heights of Men and Women
7. Normal Constituents of Human Blood
8. Recommended Daily Allowances (RDA)
9. Mineral and Vitamin Content of Foods
10. Numerical Factors: Protein, Fat and Carbohydrate Metabolism
11. Nomograms for Estimation of Heat Production (Metabolic Rate)

APPENDIX 1: COMMON ABBREVIATIONS

AcCoA: acetyl coenzyme A
ACTH: adrenocorticotropic hormone
ADH: antidiuretic hormone
ADP: adenosine-5'-diphosphate
AMP: adenosine-5'-phosphate
ATP: adenosine-5'-triphosphate
ATPase: adenosine triphosphatase
BMR: basal metabolic rate
BUN: blood urea nitrogen
cal: calorie
cc: cubic centimeter
Co I: coenzyme I (NAD)
Co II: coenzyme II (NADP)
DNA: deoxyribonucleic acid
Dopa: dioxy-or dihydroxyphenylalanine
EAA: essential amino acid
EF: extrinsic factor
EFA: essential fatty acid
FAD: flavin adenine dinucleotide, oxidized form
FADH$_2$: flavin adenine dinucleotide, reduced form
FAO: Food and Agriculture Organization
FDA: Food and Drug Administration
FFA: free fatty acid
FMN: flavin mononucleotide
FSH: follicle-stimulating hormone
GFR: glomerular filtration rate
gm: gram(s)
GOT: glutamate oxalacetate transaminase
GTF: glucose tolerance factor
Hb: hemoglobin
HbO$_2$: oxyhemoglobin
HMP shunt: hexose monophosphate shunt
IF: intrinsic factor
INH: isonicotinic acid hydrazide
I.U.: international unit
J: joule
kcal: kilocalorie(s)
kg: kilogram
kJ: kilojoule
L: liter

lb: pound
LCT: long-chain triglyceride
LH: luteinizing hormone
μg: microgram(s)
MCT: medium-chain triglyceride
mEq: milliequivalent(s)
mg: milligram(s)
ml: milliliter(s)
mm: millimeter(s)
mRNA: messenger ribonucleic acid
NAD: nicotinamide adenine dinucleotide
NADP: nicotinamide adenine dinucleotide phosphate
NEFA: nonesterified fatty acid
ng: nanogram(s)
NPN: nonprotein nitrogen
NRC: National Research Council
oz: ounce
PABA: para-amino benzoic acid
PBI: protein-bound iodine
PCBs: polychlorinated biphenyls
pg: picogram(s)
pH: hydrogen ion concentration
PKU: phenylketonuria
ppm: parts per million
PTH: parathyroid hormone
RDA: Recommended Dietary Allowances
RNA: ribonucleic acid
RNAse: ribonuclease
RQ: respiratory quotient
SH: sulfhydryl
TCA: tricarboxylic acid cycle
TPP: thiamin pyrophosphate
tRNA: transfer ribonucleic acid
TSH: thyroid-stimulating hormone
UNESCO: United Nations Educational, Scientific, and Cultural Organization
UNICEF: United Nations Children's Fund
USDA: United States Department of Agriculture
USP: United States Pharmacopeia
WHO: World Health Organization

APPENDIX 2: PREFIXES AND SUFFIXES

The list below is not intended to be complete. Many of the prefixes and suffixes are used in medicine and a medical dictionary is advised for a more comprehensive list. In the ists below, the examples given arein this text or are of common usage.

Prefix	Meaning	Example
A, AN	without, lack of	
A used before consonants		aphasia
AN used before vowels		anemia
AB	away from	abnormal
AD	toward, to, at	additive
ADEN, ADENO	relating to a gland	adenoid
ANA	again, back, building up	anabolism
ANTE, ANTERO	before, in front of	anterior
ANTI	against, opposed to	antigen
ARTHRO	pertaining to joints	arthritis
AUTO	self	autotrophic
BIO	pertaining to life	biochemical
BLAST, BLASTO	cell, germ	megaloblastic
CARDIO	pertaining to the heart	cardiovascular
CHOLE	pertaining to bile	cholecystokinin
CO, COM, CON	with, together	complication
CONTRA	against, opposite	contracture
CYSTO	pertaining to urinary bladder	cystitis
CYTO	pertaining to a cell	cytoplasm
DE	down, away from	deglutition
DERM, DERMATO	pertaining to the skin	dermatitis
DI	two, twice, double	disulfide
DIA	through	dialysis
DIS	reversal, separation	discharge
DYS	difficult, painful	dyspepsia
E, EC, ECTO, EX, EXO	out, outside, away from	extract
EM, EN	in	emphysema
ENDO	within	endogenous
ENTERO	relation to the intestine	enterokinase
EPI	upon, above	epidermis
EXTRA	outside of, beyond, in addition	extracellular

Prefix	Meaning	Example
GLYCO	sweetness (sugar)	glycogen
HEM, HEMO, HAEMO	some relation to the blood	hemoglobin
HETERO	other, other than, different from	heterogeneous
HISTO	some relation to tissues	histogenesis
HOMO	similarity	homeostatis
HYDRO	relation to water or hydrogen	hydrolysis
HYPER	above, over, excessive	hyperglycemia
HYPO	lack, deficiency	hypoglycemia
INFRA	below	inframandibular
INTER	between	intercellular
INTRA, INTRO	within	intracellular
LAC, LACTO	pertaining to milk	lactose
LEUCO, LEUKO	pertaining to anything white	leukocyte
MACRO	pertaining to anything large	macrocytic
MEGA, MEGALO	pertaining to anything great	megaloblastic
META	between, after, beyond- indicates changes, transformation into a succeeding stage, exchange	metabolism
MICRO	pertaining to anything small	microscopic
NEO	new, recent, young	neonatal
NEPHRO	pertaining to kidneys	nephron
NEURO	pertaining to nerves	neuralgia
ODONTO	pertaining or some relation to teeth	odontocele
OSSEO, OSSI, OSTEO	pertaining to bone	osteomalacia
PARA	beside, beyond, accessory to	parasympathetic
PATHO	pertaining to disease	pathogen
PERI	around	peristalsis
PHOTO	pertaining to light	photosynthesis
POLY	many	polysaccharide
POST	after, behind	postprandial
PRE	before	precursor
PYO	pertaining to pus	pyorrhea
SEPTI	pertaining to poison	septicemia
SUB	under, almost	subclinical
SYN	union	synthesize
THERMO	relating to heat	thermometer
TOX, TOXI, TOXICO	relating to poison	toxic
TRANS	across, through	transplant
VASO	pertaining to vessel	vasodilation

Suffix	Meaning	Example
-AC	pertaining to	hemophiliac
-AEMIA, -EMIA	denoting a condition of the blood	leukemia
-ALGIA, -ALGY	a painful condition	neuralgia
-ASE	enzyme	sucrase

Suffix	Meaning	Example
-BLAST	germ, cell	myeloblast
-COCCUS	round bacterium	streptococcus
-CYTE	hollow vessels, used to denote a cell	lymphocyte
-ECTOMY	excision of	appendectomy
-ITIS	inflammation	gastritis
-LOGY, -OLOGY	the science of	bacteriology
-LYSIS	a loosening, a dissolving	hemolysis
-OMA	morbid condition, especially a tumor	carcinoma
-OREXIA	appetite, desire	anorexia
-OSE	carbohydrate	glucose
-OSIS	a condition or process, particularly a disease condition or morbid process	xanthomatosis
OSTOMY, -STOMY	the making of a mouth	colostomy
-OUS	full of, having, possessing	fibrous
-PHAGIA	eating	polyphagia
-PHASIA	speech	aphasia
-RRHAGIA, -RRHAGE	excessive flow	hemorrhage
-URIA	urine	polyuria

APPENDIX 3

TABLE OF INTERNATIONAL ATOMIC WEIGHTS

Element	Symbol	Atomic No.	Atomic Weight	Element	Symbol	Atomic No.	Atomic Weight
Actinium	Ac	89		Germanium	Ge	32	72.59
Aluminum	Al	13	26.9815	Gold	Au	79	196.967
Americium	Am	95		Hafnium	Hf	72	178.49
Antimony	Sb	51	121.75	Helium	He	2	4.0026
Argon	Ar	18	39.948	Holmium	Ho	67	164.930
Arsenic	As	33	74.9216	Hydrogen	H	1	1.00797[a]
Astatine	At	85		Indium	In	49	114.82
Barium	Ba	56	137.34	Iodine	I	53	126.9044
Berkelium	Bk	97		Iridium	Ir	77	192.2
Beryllium	Be	4	9.0122	Iron	Fe	26	55.847[b]
Bismuth	Bi	83	208.980	Krypton	Kr	36	83.80
Boron	B	5	10.811[a]	Lanthanum	La	57	138.91
Bromine	Br	35	79.909[b]	Lead	Pb	82	207.19
Cadmium	Cd	48	112.40	Lithium	Li	3	6.939
Calcium	Ca	20	40.08	Lutetium	Lu	71	174.97
Californium	Cf	98		Magnesium	Mg	12	24.312
Carbon	C	6	12.01115[a]	Manganese	Mn	25	54.9380
Cerium	Ce	58	140.12	Mendelevium	Md	101	
Cesium	Cs	55	132.905	Mercury	Hg	80	200.59
Chlorine	Cl	17	35.453[b]	Molybdenum	Mo	42	95.94
Chromium	Cr	24	51.996[b]	Neodymium	Nd	60	144.24
Cobalt	Co	27	58.9332	Neon	Ne	10	20.183
Copper	Cu	29	63.54	Neptunium	Np	93	
Curium	Cm	96		Nickel	Ni	28	58.71
Dysprosium	Dy	66	162.50	Niobium	Nb	41	92.906
Einsteinium	Es	99		Nitrogen	N	7	14.0067
Erbium	Er	68	167.26	Nobelium	No	102	
Europium	Eu	63	151.96	Osmium	Os	76	190.2
Fermium	Fm	100		Oxygen	O	8	15.9994[a]
Fluorine	F	9	18.9984	Palladium	Pd	46	106.4
Francium	Fr	87		Phosphorus	P	15	30.9738
Gadolinium	Gd	64	157.25	Platinum	Pt	78	195.09
Gallium	Ga	31	69.72	Plutonium	Pu	94	

Element	Symbol	Atomic No.	Atomic Weight	Element	Symbol	Atomic No.	Atomic Weight
Polonium	Po	84		Sulfur	S	16	32.064[a]
Potassium	K	19	39.102	Tantalum	Ta	73	180.948
Praseodymium	Pr	59	140.907	Technetium	Tc	43	
Promethium	Pm	61		Tellurium	Te	52	127.60
Protactinum	Pa	91		Terbium	Tb	65	158.924
Radium	Ra	88		Thallium	Tl	81	204.37
Radon	Rn	86		Thorium	Th	90	232.038
Rhenium	Re	75	186.2	Thulium	Tm	69	168.934
Rhodium	Rh	45	102.905	Tin	Sn	50	118.69
Rubidium	Rb	37	85.47	Titanium	Ti	22	47.90
Ruthenium	Ru	44	101.07	Tungsten	W	74	183.85
Samarium	Sm	62	150.35	Uranium	U	92	238.03
Scandium	Sc	21	44.956	Vanadium	V	23	50.942
Selenium	Se	34	78.96	Xenon	Xe	54	131.30
Silicon	Si	14	28.086[a]	Ytterbium	Yb	70	173.04
Silver	Ag	47	107.870[b]	Yttrium	Y	39	88.905
Sodium	Na	11	22.9898	Zinc	Zn	30	65.37
Strontium	Sr	38	87.62	Zirconium	Zr	40	91.22

[a] The atomic weight varies because of natural variations in the isotopic composition of the element. The observed ranges are boron, ± 0.003; carbon, ± 0.00005; hydrogen, ± 0.00001; oxygen, ± 0.0001; silicon, ± 0.001; sulfur, ± 0.003.

[b] The atomic weight is believed to have an experimental uncertainty of the following magnitude; bromine, ± 0.002; chlorine, ± 0.001; chromium, ± 0.001; iron, ± 0.003; silver, ± 0.003. For other elements the last digit given is believed to be reliable to ± 0.5.

APPENDIX 4: WEIGHTS AND MEASURES: CONVERSION TABLES

The formula for the conversion of °Celsius (°Centrigrade) to °Fahrenheit (°F)

$$°F = (20 °C \times \frac{9}{5}) + 32°$$

The formula for the conversion of °Fahrenheit (°F) to °Celsius (°Centrigrade).

$$°C = \frac{5}{9}(°F - 32°)$$

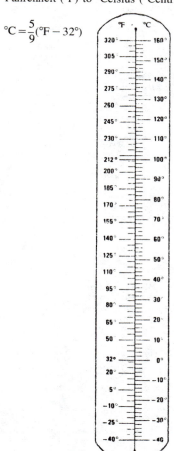

32° Fahrenheit = 0° Centigrade
0° Fahrenheit = −17.8° Centigrade

Conversion to and from Metric Measures:

If measure is in	Multiply by	To find
Length		
inches	25.4	millimeters
inches	2.54	centimeters
feet	30.48	centimeters
feet	0.305	meters
centimeters	0.394	inches
meters	3.281	feet
Weight		
grains	64.799	milligrams
ounces (Av.)	28.35	grams
pounds (Av.)	454	grams
pounds	0.454	kilograms
grams	15.432	grains
grams	0.035	ounces (Av.)
grams	0.0022	pounds (Av.)
kilograms	2.205	pounds
Capacity (liquid)		
teaspoons	4.7	milliliters
tablespoons	14.1	milliliters
fluid ounces	29.573	milliliters
cups (8 ounces)	238	milliliters
pints	0.473	liters
quarts	0.946	liters
milliliters	0.034	fluid ounces
liters	1.057	quarts
Energy units		
kilocalories	4.184	kilojoules
kilojoules	0.239	kilocalories
Temperature		
Fahrenheit	subtract 32; then multiply by $\frac{5}{9}$	Celsius (Centigrade)
Celsius	multiply by $\frac{9}{5}$; then add 32	Fahrenheit

Metric equivalents
  1 kilogram (kg) = 1000 grams
  1 gram (gm) = 1000 milligrams
  1 milligram (mg) = 1000 micrograms
  1 microgram (mcg, μg, γ) = 1000 nanograms
  1 nanogram (ng) = 1000 picograms (pg)
Multiples
  deca- 10
  hecto- 10^2 (100)
  kilo- 10^3 (1000)
  mega- 10^6 (1,000,000)
Submultiples
  deci- = one tenth 10^{-1} (0.1)
  centi- = one hundredth 10^{-2} (0.01)
  milli- = one thousandth 10^{-3} (0.001)
  micro- = one millionth 10^{-6} (0.000,001)
  nano- = one billionth 10^{-9} (0.000,000,001)
  pico- = one trillionth 10^{-12} (0.000,000,000,001)

b. Weight Conversions

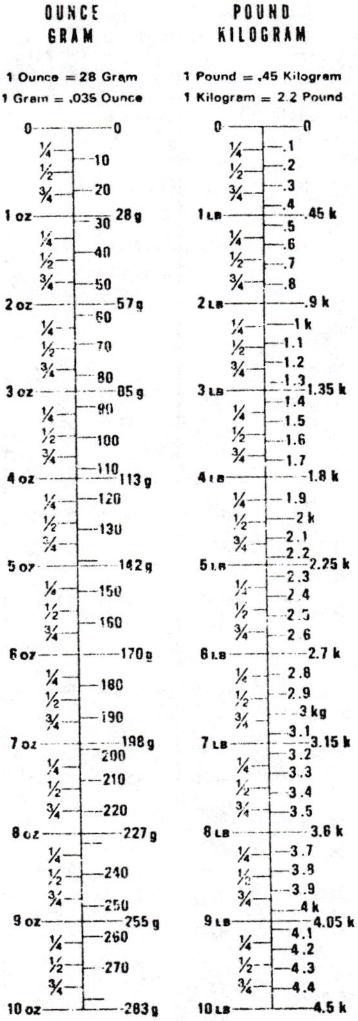
OUNCE
GRAM
1 Ounce = 28 Gram
1 Gram = .035 Ounce
0 ¼ ½ ¾ 1 oz ¼ ½ ¾ 2 oz ¼ ½ ¾ 3 oz ¼ ½ ¾ 4 oz ¼ ½ ¾ 5 oz ¼ ½ ¾ 6 oz ¼ ½ ¾ 7 oz ¼ ½ ¾ 8 oz ¼ ½ ¾ 9 oz ¼ ½ ¾ 10 oz
0 10 20 30 28 g 40 50 57 g 60 70 80 85 g 90 100 110 113 g 120 130 142 g 150 160 170 g 180 190 198 g 200 210 220 227 g 240 250 255 g 260 270 283 g
POUND
KILOGRAM
1 Pound = .45 Kilogram
1 Kilogram = 2.2 Pound
0 ¼ ½ ¾ 1 LB ¼ ½ ¾ 2 LB ¼ ½ ¾ 3 LB ¼ ½ ¾ 4 LB ¼ ½ ¾ 5 LB ¼ ½ ¾ 6 LB ¼ ½ ¾ 7 LB ¼ ½ ¾ 8 LB ¼ ½ ¾ 9 LB ¼ ½ ¾ 10 LB
0 .1 .2 .3 .4 .45 k .5 .6 .7 .8 .9 k 1 k 1.1 1.2 1.3 1.35 k 1.4 1.5 1.6 1.7 1.8 k 1.9 2 k 2.1 2.2 2.25 k 2.3 2.4 2.5 2.6 2.7 k 2.8 2.9 3 kg 3.1 3.15 k 3.2 3.3 3.4 3.5 3.6 k 3.7 3.8 3.9 4 k 4.05 k 4.1 4.2 4.3 4.4 4.5 k

c. Length Conversions

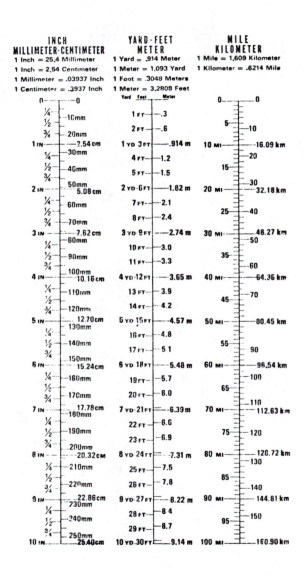

INCH MILLIMETER-CENTIMETER	YARD-FEET METER	MILE KILOMETER
1 Inch = 25.4 Millimeter	1 Yard = .914 Meter	1 Mile = 1,609 Kilometer
1 Inch = 2.54 Centimeter	1 Meter = 1,093 Yard	1 Kilometer = .6214 Mile
1 Millimeter = .03937 Inch	1 Foot = .3048 Meters	
1 Centimeter = .3937 Inch	1 Meter = 3.2808 Feet	

d. Area And Volume Conversions

Area

1 Sq Ft = 144 Sq In = 929.03 Sq Cm
1 Sq In = 6.4516 Sq Cm
1 Sq Cm = .155 Sq In

Square Foot	Square Inch	Square Centimeter
	0	0
	4	31
	12	93
	20	155
	28	217
	36	
48 sq in	44	279
	52	309 sq cm
		341
	60	403
	68	465
	76	527
	84	
96 sq in	92	589
	100	619 sq cm / 651
	108	713
	116	775
	124	837
	132	
	140	899
1 SQ FT	144 SQ IN	929 sq cm

1 Sq Yd = 9 Sq Ft = .82 Sq M
1 Sq Ft = .092 Sq M
1 Sq M = 10.8 Sq Ft

Square Yard	Square Foot	Square Meter
	0	0
	1 sq ft	
	3 sq ft	.25
	5 sq ft	.50
	7 sq ft	.75
1 SQ YD	9 sq ft	.82 m²
	11 sq ft	1 sq m
	13 sq ft	1.25 sq m
	15 sq ft	1.50 sq m
	17 sq ft	1.65 m
2 SQ YD	19 sq ft	1.75 sq m
	21 sq ft	2 sq m
	23 sq ft	2.25 sq m
	25 sq ft	
3 SQ YD	27 sq ft	2.48 sq m

Volume

Unit	U.S. Fluid Ounce	U.S. Liquid Pint	U.S. Liquid Quart	Cubic Inch	Cubic Centimeter	Deci-liter	Liter
1 U.S. FL OZ =	1	.0625	.03125	1.8047	29.574	.2957	.0296
1 U.S. LIQ PT =	16	1	.5	28.875	473.18	4.7316	.4732
1 U.S. LIQ QT =	32	2	1	57.75	946.35	9.4633	.9463
1 Cubic Inch =	0.5541	.03463	.01732	1	16.387	.1639	.0164
1 Cubic Centimeter =							
1 Milliliter =	0.0338	.00211	.00106	.06102	1	.01	.001
1 Deciliter =	3.3815	.2113	.1057	6.1025	100	1	.1
1 Liter =	33.815	2.1134	1.0567	61.025	1000	10	1

The Figures shown above have been rounded where full extension was impossible

Quarts Pints	Fluid Ounces	Cubic Inches	Cubic Centimeters	Milliliters	Deciliters	Liters
			1 cc = 1 ml			
		2	50	50		
	2	4				
		6	100	100	1	
	4	8				
		10 ci	164cc	150		
	6	12	200	200	2	
		14	250	250		
	8	16				
		18	300	300	3	
	10	20 ci	328cc			
	12	22	350	350		
		24	400	400	4	
	14	26				
½ QT·1 PT	16	28	450	450		
		30 ci	492cc	500	5	
	18	32	550	550		
		34				
	20	36	600	600	6	
		38				
	22	40 ci	655cc	650		
	24	42	700	700	7	
		44				
	26	46	750	750		
		48	800	800	8	
	28	50 ci	819cc			
		52	850	850		
	30	54	900	900	9	
		56				
1 QT·2 PT	32	58	950	950		
	34	60 ci	983cc / 1000	1000	10	1 ltr.

e. Relative Sizes of Microbial Forms and the Red Blood Cell

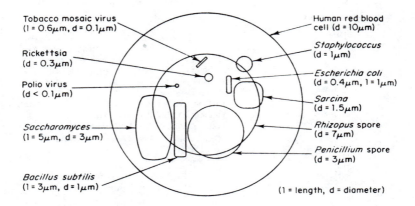

From: *Food Microbiology* by R. V. Lechovich in "Food Science and Nutrition Current Issues and Answers" Fergus Clydesdale (Ed.) Prentice-Hall Inc, 1979.

APPENDIX 5:GREEK ALPHABET

The letters of the Greek alphabet are frequently employed by chemists. Many of the metabolic intermediate carry the Greek alphabet as part of the name, e.g., alpha (α) amino acid and beta (β) carotene, usually to denote the position of some substituent in the molecule. *Ortho, para,* and *meta* are also used to designate positions in aromatic ring compounds. Ortho means straight, para means along side of, and meta means in the midst of or between.

Name of Letter	Capital	Small
alpha	A	α
beta	B	β
gamma	Γ	γ
delta	Δ	δ
epsilon	E	ϵ
zeta	Z	ζ
eta	H	η
theta	Θ	θ
iota	I	ι
kappa	K	κ
lambda	Λ	λ
mu	M	μ
nu	N	ν
xi	Ξ	ξ
omicron	O	o
pi	Π	π
rho	P	ρ
sigma	Σ	σ
tau	T	τ
upsilon	Υ	υ
phi	Φ	ϕ
chi	X	χ
psi	Ψ	ψ
omega	Ω	ω

APPENDIX 6: WEIGHT RANGES FOR HEIGHTS OF MEN AND WOMEN

Height (without shoes) inches	Weight (without clothing) Low	Median pounds	High	Height centimeters	Low	Weight Median kilograms	High
Men							
63	118	129	141	160	54	59	64
64	122	133	145	163	55	60	66
65	126	137	149	165	57	62	68
66	130	142	155	167	59	65	70
67	134	147	161	170	61	67	73
68	139	151	166	173	63	69	75
69	143	155	170	175	65	70	77
70	147	159	174	178	67	72	80
71	150	163	178	180	68	74	81
72	154	167	183	183	70	76	83
73	158	171	188	185	72	77	85
74	162	175	192	188	74	80	87
75	165	178	195	191	75	81	89
Women							
60	100	109	118	152	45	50	54
61	104	112	121	155	47	51	55
62	107	115	125	157	49	52	57
63	110	118	128	160	50	54	58
64	113	122	132	163	51	55	60
65	116	125	135	165	53	57	61
66	120	129	139	167	55	59	63
67	123	132	142	170	56	60	65
68	126	136	146	173	57	62	66
69	130	140	151	175	59	64	69
70	133	144	156	178	60	65	71
71	137	148	161	180	62	67	73
72	141	152	166	183	64	69	75

* Data for heights in inches and weights in pounds taken from: Hathaway, M. L., and Foard, E. D.: *Heights and Weights of Adults in the United States*. Home Economics Research Report No. 10, U.S. Department of Agriculture, Washington, D.C.

Conversions to centimeters and kilograms were rounded off to the nearest whole number.

APPENDIX 7: NORMAL CONSTITUENTS OF HUMAN BLOOD
(B = WHOLE BLOOD: P = PLASMA: S = SERUM)

Constituent	Normal Range		Examples of Deviations
Physical Measurements			
Specific gravity (S)	1.025–1.029		
Bleeding time, capillary	1–3	min	
Prothrombin time (Quick, P)	10–20	sec	
Sedimentation rate (Wintrobe)			
Men	0–9	mm/hr	
Women	0–20	mm/hr	
Viscosity (water as unity) (b)	4.5–5.5		
Acid-Base Constituents			
Base, total fixed cations (Na + K + Ca + Mg) (S)	143–150	mEq/L	Low in alkali deficit; diabetic acidosis
Sodium (S)	320–335	mg/100 ml	Low in alkali deficit, diabetic acidosis,
	139–146	mEq/L	excessive fluid administration
Potassium (S)	16–22	mg/100 ml	High in acute infections, pneumonia,
	4.1–5.6	mEq/L	Addison's disease; low in diarrhea, vomiting, correction of diabetic acidosis
Calcium (S)	9–11	mg/100 ml	High with excessive vitamin D, hyper-
	4.5–5.5	mEq/L	parathyroidism; low in infantile tetany, steatorrhea, severe nephritis, defective vitamin D absorption
Calcium, ionized (S)	50–60	percent	
Magnesium (S)	2–3	mg/100 ml	High in chronic nephritis, liver disease;
	1.65–2.5	mEq/L	low in uremia, tetany, severe diarrhea
Chloride (S)	340–372	mg/100 ml	High in congestive heart failure,
	96–105	mEq/L	eclampsia, nephritis
As NaCl (S)	560–614	mg/100 ml	
	96–105	mEq/L	
Phosphorus, inorganic as P (S)			
Child	4.0–6.5	mg/100 ml	High in chronic nephritis, hypopara- thyroidism; low during treatment of
Adult	2.5–4.5	mg/100 ml	diabetic coma, hyperparathyroidism
Sulfates as SO$_4$—(S)	2.5–5.0	mg/100 ml	
	0.5–1.0	mEq/L	
Bicarbonate cation-binding power (S)	19–30	mEq/L	
Serum protein cation-binding power (S)	15.5–18.0	mEq/L	
Lactic acid (S)	10–20	mg/100 ml	
	1.1–2.2	mEq/L	
pH at 38°C (B, P, or S)	7.30–7.45		High in uncompensated alkalosis; low in uncompensated acidosis

Constituent	Normal Range		Examples of Deviations
Blood Gases			
CO_2 content (venous S)	45–70	vol %	Low in primary alkali deficit, diarrhea;
	20.3–31.5	mM/L	high in hypoventilation
CO_2 content (venous B)	40–60	vol %	
	18–27	mM/L	
CO_2 tension (pCO_2) arterial blood	35–45	mm Hg	pCO_2 in venous blood is about 6 mm higher than arterial or capillary blood
Oxygen content (arterial B)	15–22	vol %	High in polycythemia; low in emphysema
Oxygen content (venous B)	11–16	vol %	
Oxygen capacity (B)	16–24	vol %	
Oxygen tension (pO_2)	85–100	mm Hg	
Carbohydrates			
Glucose			
Reducing substances (B)	90–120	mg/100 ml	High in diabetes mellitus; low in hyperinsulinism
"True"	60–85	mg/100 ml	
Glucose tolerance			
Fasting sugar	90–120	mg/100 ml	
Highest value	130–140	mg/100 ml	
Highest value reached in	45–60	minutes	
Return to fasting in	1.5–2.5	hr	
Lactose tolerance			
Fasting blood glucose (B)	90–120	mg/100 ml	In lactase deficiency the rise in blood
Increase in blood glucose after test dose lactose	20	mg/100 ml	glucose after test dose of lactose is less than 20 mg in 1 hour
Citric acid (B)	1.3–2.3	mg/100 ml	
(P)	1.6–2.7	mg/100 ml	
Lactic acid (see acid-base constituents)			
Pyruvic acid, fasting (B)	0.7–1.2	mg/100 ml	
Enzymes			
Amylase (Somogyi) (S)	60–180	units/100 ml	High in acute pancreatitis, acute appendicitis
Lactic dehydrogenase (S)	25–100	units/ml	High in myocardial infarction
Lipase (S)	0.2–1.5	units/ml	High in pancreatitis
Leucine-aminopeptidase (S)	1–3.5	units/ml	High in hemolytic anemias
Phosphatase, alkaline			
(Bodansky) (S) Child	4–14	units/100 ml	High in rickets, bone cancer, Paget's
Adult	1–4		disease, hyperparathyroidism, vitamin D inadequacy; indicates rapid bone growth in young
Transaminases			
Glutamic-oxalacetic (SGOT) (Karmen) (S)	10–40	units/ml	Increased within 24 hours in myocardial infarction; normal after 6 to 7 days
Glutamic-pyruvic (SGPT) (Karmen) (S)	5–35	units/ml	High in hepatic disease, and trauma after surgery

Constituent	Normal Range		Examples of Deviations
Hematologic Studies			
Cell volume	39–50	percent	High in polycythemia; low in anemia, prolonged iron deficiency
Red blood cells	4.25–5.25	million per cu mm	High in polycythemia, dehydration; low in anemia, hemorrhage
White blood cells	5000–9000	per cu mm	Increased in acute infections, leukemias
Lymphocytes	25–30	percent	
Neutrophils	60–65	percent	
Monocytes	4–8	percent	
Eosinophils	0.5–4	percent	
Basophils	0–1.5	percent	
Platelets	125,000–300,000	per cu mm	
Lipids			
Acetone (S)	0.3–2.0	mg/100 ml	High in uncontrolled diabetes and starvation
Cholesterol, total (S)	125–225	mg/100 ml	High in uncontrolled diabetes mellitus,
esters	50–67	percent	nephrosis, hypothyroidism,
free	33–50	per cent	hyperlipidemias
Fatty acids, unesterified (P)	8–31	mg/100 ml	
17-Hydroxycorticosteroids (P)	10–13.5	μg/100 ml	
Lipids, total (P)	570–820	mg/100 ml	
Phospholipid (S)	150–300	mg/100 ml	
Triglycerides (S)	30–140	mg/100 ml	Increased in hyperlipidemias
Nitrogenous Constituents			
Alpha-amino acid nitrogen (S)	3.5–5.5	mg/100 ml	High in severe liver disease; low in nephrosis
Ammonia (B)	40–70	μg/100 ml	High in liver disease
Creatinine (S)	0.5–1.2	mg/100 ml	Increased in renal insufficiency
Creatinine clearance endogenous (B)	120 ± 20	ml	Blood cleared per min by kidney; measure of glomerular filtration
Nonprotein N (NPN) (B)	25–35	mg/100 ml	High in acute glomerulonephritis, dehydration, metallic poisoning, intestinal obstruction, renal failure
Phenylalanine (S)	0.7–4	mg/100 ml	Increased in phenylketonuria
Urea nitrogen (BUN) (B)	8–18	mg/100 ml	High in renal failure, acute glomerulonephritis, mercury poisoning, dehydration; low in hepatic failure
Urea clearance (B)	75	ml/min C_m	C_m = maximal clearance
	54	ml/min C_s	C_s = standard clearance
Uric acid (S)	2–6	mg/100 ml	High in gout, nephritis, arthritis
Proteins			
Total protein (S)	6.5–7.5	gm/100 ml	High in dehydration; low in liver disease, nephrosis
Albumin (S)	3.9–4.5	gm/100 ml	Low in starvation, cirrhosis, proteinuria
Globulin (S)	2.3–3.5	gm/100 ml	High in infections, liver disease, multiple myeloma
Albumin globulin ratio	1.2–1.9		Low in liver disease, nephrosis
Fibrinogen (P)	0.2–0.5	gm/100 ml	High in infections; low in severe liver disease

Constituent	Normal Range		Examples of Deviations
Ceruloplasmin (S)	16–33	mg/100 ml	
Gamma globulin (S)	0.7–1.2	gm/100 ml	
Hemoglobin (B)			High in polycythemia; low in prolonged
Males	14–17	gm/100 ml	dietary deficiency, anemia
Females	12–16	gm/100 ml	
Vitamins			
Ascorbic acid (S)	0.3–1.4	mg/100 ml	
Folic acid (*L. casei*) (S)	6–10	ng/ml	
(*L. casei*) (B)	100–220	ng/ml	
Niacin (S)	30–150	μg/100 ml	
Riboflavin (S)	2.3–3.7	μg/100 ml	
Thiamine (B)	5.5–9.5	μg/100 ml	
Tocopherol (S)	0.6–2.0	mg/100 ml	
Vitamin A (S)	25–90	μg/100 ml	
Carotene (S)	40–125	μg/100 ml	
Vitamin B_6 (B)	1–18	μg/100 ml	
Vitamin B_{12} (S)	10–90	μg/100 ml	
Miscellaneous			
Bilirubin (S)	0–1.5	mg/100 ml	High in red cell destruction, liver disease
Icterus index	4–6	units	High in jaundice
Copper (S)	80–240	μg/100 ml	Low in anemia, Wilson's disease
Iron (S)			
Men	80–165	μg/100 ml	High in hemochromatosis, liver disease,
Women	65–130	μg/100 ml	transfusion hemosiderosis; low in
			iron-deficiency anemia
Iron-binding capacity (S)			
Men	250–430	μg/100 ml	High in anemia
Women	220–415	μg/100 ml	
Lead (S)	1–3	μg/100 ml	
Manganese (S)	2–5	μg/100 ml	
Protein-bound iodine (PBI) (S)	3–8	μg/100 ml	High in hyperthyroidism; low in hypothy-
			roidism
Zinc (S)	100–140	μg/100 ml	

ml = milliliters   gm = grams
mg = milligrams   cu mm = cubic millimeters
μg = micrograms
mEq = milliequivalents

$$mEq \text{ per liter} = \frac{mg \text{ per liter}}{\text{equivalent weight}} \quad mM \text{ (millimoles) per liter} = \frac{mg \text{ per liter}}{\text{molecular weight}}$$

$$\text{equivalent weight} = \frac{\text{atomic weight}}{\text{valence of element}} \quad \text{volumes per cent} = mM \text{ per liter} \times 2.24$$

Sources of Data:

Oser, B. L., ed.: *Hawk's Physiological Chemistry,* 14th ed. McGraw-Hill Book Company, New York, 1965, pp. 977–79.

Robinson, H. W.: "Biochemistry," in *Rypins' Medical Licensure Examinations,* 11th ed., A. W. Wright, ed. J. B. Lippincott Company, Philadelphia, 1970, pp. 202–5.

APPENDIX 8: RECOMMENDED DAILY ALLOWANCES (RDA)

Table B–1. Food and Nutrition Board, National Academy of Sciences —National Research Council Recommended Daily Dietary Allowances,[a] Revised 1974* Designed for the maintenance of good nutrition of practically all healthy people in the USA

	Age	Weight		Height		Energy	Protein	Vitamin A Activity RE[c]	I.U.	Vitamin D I.U.	Vitamin E Activity[e] I.U.
	yrs	kg	lbs	cm	in.	Cal[b]	g				
Infants	0.0–0.5	6	14	60	24	kg × 117	kg × 2.2	420[d]	1400	400	4
	0.5–1.0	9	20	71	28	kg × 108	kg × 2.0	400	2000	400	5
Children	1–3	13	28	86	34	1300	23	400	2000	400	7
	4–6	20	44	110	44	1800	30	500	2500	400	9
	7–10	30	66	135	54	2400	36	700	3300	400	10
Males	11–14	44	97	158	63	2800	44	1000	5000	400	12
	15–18	61	134	172	69	3000	54	1000	5000	400	15
	19–22	67	147	172	69	3000	54	1000	5000	400	15
	23–50	70	154	172	69	2700	56	1000	5000		15
	51+	70	154	172	69	2400	56	1000	5000		15
Females	11–14	44	97	155	62	2400	44	800	4000	400	12
	15–18	54	119	162	65	2100	48	800	4000	400	12
	19–22	58	128	162	65	2100	46	800	4000	400	12
	23–50	58	128	162	65	2000	46	800	4000		12
	51+	58	128	162	65	1800	46	800	4000		12
Pregnant						+300	+30	1000	5000	400	15
Lactating						+500	+20	1200	6000	400	15

*Recommended Dietary Allowances, 8th ed. National Academy of Sciences, 1974, p 128. Reproduced with permission of the National Academy of Sciences

[a]The allowances are intended to provide for individual variations among most normal persons as they live in the United States under usual environmental stresses. Diets should be based on a variety of common foods in order to provide other nutrients for which human requirements have been less well defined. See text for more detailed discussion of allowances and of nutrients not tabulated

[b]Kilojoules (kJ) = 4.2 × Cal

[c]Retinol equivalents

[d]Assumed to be all as retinol in milk during the first 6 months of life. All subsequent intakes are assumed to be half as retinol and half as β-carotene when calculated from international units. As retinol equivalents, three-fourths are as retinol and one-fourth as β-carotene

| | Water-soluble Vitamins | | | | | | | Minerals | | | | | |
Ascorbid Acid μg	Folacin[f] μg	Niacin[g] μg	Riboflavin μg	Thiamin μg	Vitamin B6 μg	Vitamin B12 μg	Calcium μg	Phosphorus μg	Iodine μg	Iron μg	Magnesium μg	Zinc μg
35	50	5	0.4	0.3	0.3	0.3	360	240	35	10	60	3
35	50	8	0.6	0.5	0.4	0.3	540	400	45	15	70	5
40	100	9	0.8	0.7	0.6	1.0	800	800	60	15	150	10
40	200	12	1.1	0.9	0.9	1.5	800	800	80	10	200	10
40	300	16	1.2	1.2	1.2	2.0	800	800	110	10	250	10
45	400	18	1.5	1.4	1.6	3.0	1200	1200	130	18	350	15
45	400	20	1.8	1.5	2.0	3.0	1200	1200	150	18	400	15
45	400	20	1.8	1.5	2.0	3.0	800	800	140	10	350	15
45	400	18	1.6	1.4	2.0	3.0	800	800	130	10	350	15
45	400	16	1.5	1.2	2.0	3.0	800	800	110	10	350	15
45	400	16	1.3	1.2	1.6	3.0	1200	1200	115	18	300	15
45	400	14	1.4	1.1	2.0	3.0	1200	1200	115	18	300	15
45	400	14	1.4	1.1	2.0	3.0	800	800	100	18	300	15
45	400	13	1.2	1.0	2.0	3.0	800	800	100	18	300	15
45	400	12	1.1	1.0	2.0	3.0	800	800	80	10	300	15
60	800	+2	+0.3	+0.3	2.5	4.0	1200	1200	125	18[h]	450	20
80	600	+4	+0.5	+0.3	2.5	4.0	1200	1200	150	18	450	25

[e] Total vitamin E activity, estimated to be 80% as α-tocopherol and 20% other tocopherols

[f] The folacin allowances refer to dietary sources as determined by *Lactobacillus casei* assay. Pure forms of folacin may be effective in doses less than one-fourth of the recommended dietary allowance

[g] Although allowances are expressed as niacin, it is recognized that on the average 1 μg niacin is derived from each 60 μg dietary tryptophan

[h] This increased requirement cannot be met by ordinary diets; therefore, the use of supplemental iron is recommended

Mineral and Vitamin Content of Foods: Sodium, Potassium, Phosphorus, Magnesium, and Zinc: Folacin, Pantothenic Acid, Vitamin B6, Vitamin B12, and Vitamin E (Values for 100 g, edible portion).

Item No.	Food	Sodium mg	Potassium mg	Phosphorus mg	Magnesium mg	Zinc mg	Folacin μg	Pantothenic Acid μg	Vitamin B6 μg	Vitamin B12 μg	Vitamin E mg
1	Almonds, dried	4	773	504	270		45	470	100	0	
2	Roasted, salted	198	773	504	—[1]			250	95	0	
3	Apples, raw, not peeled	1	110	10	8	0.05	2	105	30	0	0.31
4	Apple brown Betty	153	100	22	—						
5	Apple juice, bottled	1	101	9	4		trace	—	30	0	
6	Applesauce, sweetened	2	65	5	5	0.1		85	30	0	
7	Apricots, raw	1	281	23	12		3	240	70	0	
8	Canned	1	234	15	7		1	92	54	0	
9	Dried, sulfured, uncooked	26	979	108	62		5[2]	753[2]	169[2]	0	
10	Cooked, sweetened	7	278	31	20						
11	Apricot nectar	trace	151	12	—						
12	Asparagus, green, cooked	1	183	50	20 (raw)		109				
13	Canned, regular pack	236	166	53	—		27	195	55	0	
14	Low sodium	3	166	53	—						
15	Frozen, spears, cooked	1	238	67	14		109	410	155		
16	Avocado	4	604	42	45		30	1,070	420	0	
17	Bacon, cooked, drained	1,021	236	224	25		—	330 (raw)	125 (raw)	0.70 (raw)	0.53
18	Canadian, cooked	2,555	432	218	24						
	Baking powder, home use:										
19	Sodium aluminum sulfate	10,953	150	2,904							
20	Straight phosphate	8,220	170	9,438							
21	Tartrate	7,300	3,800	0							
22	Low sodium, commercial	6	10,948								
23	Low sodium, noncommercial formula		20,729								
24	Banana	1	370	26	33	0.2	10	260	510	0	0.22

25	Barley, pearled, light	3	160	189	37			503	224	0	
26	Bass, sea, raw	68	256	—	—			512	—	—	0.47
	Beans, common, mature:										
27	White, dry	19	1,196	425	170	2.8	125	725	560	0	
28	Cooked	7	416	148	—	1.0					
29	Canned with pork and tomato sauce	463	210	92	37			92	—	0	
30	Red, dry	10	984	406	163		180[1]	500	441	0	
31	Cooked	3	340	140	—						
	Beans, Lima, immature:										
32	Cooked	1	422	121	67 (raw)		34				
33	Canned, regular pack	236	222	70	—		13	130	90	0	
34	Low sodium	4	222	70	—					0	
35	Frozen, Fordhook, cooked	101	426	90	48		34	240	150	0	
36	Mature seeds, dry	4	1,529	385	180 (raw)	2.8	103	975	580	0	
37	Cooked	2	612	154	—	0.9	128				
38	Beans, Mung, sprouts, cooked	4	156	48	32	0.3	145	190 (raw)	80	0	
39	Beans, snap, green, cooked	4	151	37	— (raw)		28				
40	Canned, regular pack	236	95	25	14	0.3	12	75	40 (raw)	0	0.03
41	Low sodium	2	95	25	—						
42	Frozen, cooked	1	152	32	21		28	135	70	0	0.11
43	Yellow, cooked	3	151	37	— (raw)		32	250 (raw)		0	
44	Canned, regular pack	236	95	25	—			—	42 (raw)	0	
45	Low sodium	2	95	25	—						
	Beef:										
46	All cuts, lean, broiled or roasted average	60	370	246	29	5.8	11	620 (raw)	435 (raw)	1.8 (raw)	0.13
47	Simmered, average	60	370	194	18	6.2			(raw)	(raw)	
48	Hamburger, regular, cooked	47	450	194	21		7			0	0.37

Item No. Food	Sodium mg	Potassium mg	Phosphorus mg	Magnesium mg	Zinc mg	Folacin μg	Pantothenic Acid μg	Vitamin B6 μg	Vitamin B12 μg	Vitamin E mg
49 Beef, canned, roast beef	—	259	116	—						
50 Beef, corned, cooked	1,740	150	93	—					1.84 (canned)	
51 Hash, canned	540	200	67	—				75 (with potato)	—	
52 Beef, dried	4,300	200	404	—				—	1.84	
53 Beef potpie, commercial	366	93	48	—						
54 Home recipe	284	159	71	—						
55 Beef and vegetable stew, canned	411	174	45	—				—	0.65	
56 Home recipe	37	250	75	—						
57 Beets, cooked	43	208	23	25 (raw)		14	150 (raw)	55 (raw)	0	
58 Canned, regular pack	236	167	18	15		3	100	50	0	
59 Low sodium	46	167	18	—						
60 Beet greens, cooked	76	332	25	106 (raw)		60	250 (raw)	100 (raw)	0	
Beverages, alcoholic										
61 Beer	7	25	30				80	60	0	
62 Gin	1	2								
63 Wine, table	5	92	10	10			30	40	0	
Biscuits, baking powder:										
64 Enriched	626	117	175	—						
65 Self-rising flour	660[3]	64	317[3]	—						
66 Biscuit dough, commercial in cans	868	65	497							
67 Blackberries, raw	1	170	19	30		14	240	50	0	
68 Blueberries, raw	1	81	13	6		8	156	67	0	
69 Frozen, sweetened	1	66	11	4		8	121	54	0	
70 Bluefish, baked or broiled, prepared with butter	104	—	287	—						

71 Bouillon cube	24,000	100	—	—						
72 Bran, with sugar and malt extract	1,060	1,070	1,176	—						
73 Bran flakes (40 per cent bran)	925	—	495	—	3.6		875	384	0	
74 Bran flakes with raisins	800	—	396	—						
75 Brazil nuts	1	715	693	225		5	231	170	0	
Breads:										
76 Boston brown	251	292	160	—						
77 Cracked wheat	529	134	128	35		25	607	92	0	
78 French or Vienna	580	90	85	22		9	378	53	0	
79 Italian	585	74	77	—		—				
80 Raisin	365	233	87	24						
81 Rye, American	557	145	147	42	1.6	16	450	100	0	
82 Pumpernickel	569	454	229	71			500	160	0	
83 White, 3–4 per cent nonfat milk solids	507	105	97	22	0.6	15	430	40	trace	0.10
84 Whole-wheat bread, 2 per cent nonfat milk solids	527	273	228	78	1.8	30	760	180	0	0.45
85 Broccoli spears, cooked	10	267	62	24 (raw)		54				
86 Frozen, cooked	12	220	58	21		54	525	170	0	
87 Brownies with nuts	251	190	148	—						
88 Brussels sprouts, cooked	10	273	72	29 (raw)		49	420 (frozen)	175 (frozen)	0	
89 Butter, salted	987	23	16	2	0.1	—	—	3	trace	1.00
90 Unsalted	under 10									
91 Buttermilk	130	140	95	14	0.4	11	307	36	0.22	
92 Cabbage, raw	20	233	29	13	0.4	32[2]	205	160	0	
93 Cooked, small amount of water	14	163	20	—						
94 Cabbage, celery or Chinese	23	253	40	14						
Cakes (home recipe)[4]										
95 Angel food	283	88	22	—						
96 Chocolate with icing	235	154	131	—			200 (commercial)	—	—	

Item No.	Food	Sodium mg	Potassium mg	Phosphorus mg	Magnesium mg	Zinc mg	Folacin µg	Pantothenic Acid µg	Vitamin B6 µg	Vitamin B12 µg	Vitamin E mg
97	Fruitcake, dark	158	496	113	—						
98	Gingerbread	237	454	65	—						
99	Plain with icing	229	114	104	—						
100	Plain without icing	300	79	102	—	0.2		—	40[5]	—	
101	Poundcake, old fashioned	110	60	79	—						1.10
102	Sponge	167	87	112	—						
	Candy:										
103	Caramels	226	192	122	—						
104	Chocolate, milk, plain	94	384	231	58						1.10
105	Fudge, plain	190	147	84	—						
106	Hard	32	4	7	trace						
107	Marshmallows	39	6	6	—						
108	Peanut brittle	31	151	95	—						
109	Cantaloupe	12	251	16	16		7	250	86	0	0.14
110	Carrots, raw	47	341	36	23	0.4	8	280	150	0	0.11[2]
111	Cooked	33	222	31	—	0.3					
112	Canned, regular pack	236	120	22	—	0.3	3	130	30	0	0.11
113	Low sodium	39	120	22	—						
114	Cashew nuts, unsalted	15	464	373	267		—	1,300	—	0	
115	Cauliflower, raw	13	295	56	24		22[2]	1,000	210	0	
116	Cooked	9	206	42	—						
117	Frozen, cooked	10	207	38	13			540	190	0	
118	Celery, raw	126	341	28	22 (raw)						
119	Cooked	88	239	22	—		7	429	60	0	
120	Chard, Swiss, cooked	86	321	24	65 (raw)		42	172 (raw)	—	0	
	Cheese:										
121	Cheddar or American	700	82	478	45	4.0	16	500	80	1	0.38
122	Cheddar, process	1,136[6]	80	771[6]	—		11	400	80	0.80	

123	Cottage, creamed	229	85	152	—		31,	220	40	1	0.37
124	Uncreamed	290	72	175	—					
125	Cream	250	74	95	—			270	55	0.22
126	Parmesan	734	149	781	48			530	96	—
127	Swiss	710	104	563	—			370	75	1.80
128	Cherries, raw, sweet	2	191	19	14		6	261	32	0
129	Canned, syrup pack	1	124	12	9		3		30	0
130	Frozen, sweetened	2	130	15	8			83	58	0
	Chicken, broiled:									
131	Light without skin	64	411	265	19	0.9	3	800	683	0.45
132	Dark without skin	86	321	229	—	2.8	3	1,000	325	0.40
133	Chicken, canned, boneless	—	138	247	—			850	300	0.79
134	Chicken potpie, frozen, commercial	411	153	50	13					
135	Chicory	7	182	21			28	140	45	0
136	Chili con carne, canned with beans	531	233	126	—				103	—
137	Chili powder with seasonings	1,574	1,000	204	169					
138	Chocolate, bitter	4	830	384	292			190	35	0
139	Chocolate syrup, thin	52	282	92	63	0.9				
140	Clams, raw, soft, meat only	36	235	183	—	1.5		300	80	98
141	Hard, round, meat only	205	311	151	—	1.5				
142	• Canned	—	140	137	—	1.2	2		83	—
143	Cocoa, breakfast, dry powder	6	1,522	648	420	5.6				
144	Processed with alkali	717	651	648	46					
145	Coconut, fresh, shredded	23	256	95	77		28	200	44	0
146	Dried, sweetened	—	353	112	456					
147	Coffee, instant, dry powder	72	3,256	383		0.6		400	32	0
148	Beverage	1	36	4		0.03		4	trace	0
149	Collards, cooked	25	234	39	57 (raw)	0.4	102	450 (frozen)	195 (frozen)	0
150	Cookies, plain and assorted	365	67	163	15	0.3				
151	Fig bars	252	198	60	—					
152	Corn, sweet, cooked	trace	165	89	48	0.4	28[2]	540 (raw)	161 (raw)	0
153	Canned, whole kernel, regular pack	236	97	49	19 (raw)	0.4	8	220	200	0
154	Low-sodium pack	2	97	49	—					0.5

Item No.	Food	Sodium mg	Potassium mg	Phosphorus mg	Magnesium mg	Zinc mg	Folacin µg	Pantothenic Acid µg	Vitamin B_6 µg	Vitamin B_{12} µg	Vitamin E mg
	Corn cereals, ready to eat:										
155	Cornflakes	1,005	120	45	16	0.3	6	185	65	0	0.12
156	Cornflakes, sugar coated	775	—	24	—						
157	Corn, puffed	1,060	—	90	—			288	—	0	
158	Corn, shredded	988	—	39	—						
159	Corn, rice, and wheat flakes	950	—	120	—						
160	Corn grits, dry	1	80	73	20	0.4		—	147	0	0.31
161	Cooked	—	11	10	3						
162	Cornbread, southern style, degermed cornmeal	591	157	156	—						
	Cornmeal, white or yellow, dry:										
163	Whole ground	(1)	(284)	256	106	1.8	7	580[5]	250[5]	0	
164	Degermed, dry	1	120	99	47	0.8	9				
165	Cooked	—	16	14	7	0.1			•		0.64[5]
166	Cowpeas, immature, cooked	1	379	146	55		41		95 (frozen)		
167	Canned, regular pack	236	352	112	—		26	162	53	0	
168	Cowpeas, dry seeds, cooked	8	229	95	230	1.2	439	1,050	562	0	
169	Crabmeat, canned	1,000	110	182	34		trace	600	300	10	
170	Crackers, graham, plain	670	384	149	51	1.1					
171	Saltines	(1,100)	(120)	90	—	0.5		—	68	0	
172	Soda	1,100	120	89	29						
173	Cranberry juice	1	10	3	—						
174	Cranberry sauce	1	30	4	2			—	22	0	
175	Cream, half-and-half	46	129	85	—						
176	Light, coffee	43	122	80	11			321	33	0.25	
177	Whipping, light	36	102	67	9			—	29	0.20	
178	Cream substitute (cream, skim milk, lactose)	575	—	—	—						

179	Cucumbers, not peeled	6	160	27	11		7	250[5]	42[5]	0
180	Custard, baked	79	146	117	—					
181	Dandelion greens, cooked	44	232	42	36 (raw)					0.46 (cooked)
182	Dates, domestic	1	648	63	58		25	780	153	0
183	Doughnuts, cake type	501	90	190	—	0.5		387[5]	—	—
184	Duck, flesh only, raw	74	285	(203)	—					
185	Eggplant, cooked	1	150	21	16 (raw)		10	220 (raw)	81 (raw)	0
186	Eggs, whole	122	129	205	11 (raw)	1.0	5	1,600 (raw)	110 (raw)	2.0 (raw)
187	White	146	139	15	9	0.02	1	200 (raw)	2 (raw)	0.10 (raw)
188	Yolk	52	98	569	16	3.0	13	4,400	300	6
189	Endive, curly	14	294	54	10		47	90 (canned)	20 (canned)	0
190	Farina, regular, dry	2	83	107	25	0.5	13	515	67	0
191	Cooked, salted	144	9	12	3	0.06				
192	Instant cooking, cooked	188	13	60	4					
193	Fats, vegetable	0	0	0	0					
194	Figs, raw	2	194	22	20		14	300	113	0
195	Canned	2	149	13	—			69	—	0
196	Dried, uncooked	34	640	77	71		32	435	175	0
197	Flounder, raw	78	342	195	—	0.7		850	170	1.2 (raw)
198	Fruit cocktail	5	161	12	7			—	33	0
199	Gelatin, dry	—	—	—	33			—	7	—
200	Sweetened, ready to eat	51	—	—	—					
201	Goose, flesh only, raw	86	420	203	—		3			
202	Grapefruit, raw	1	135	16	12			283	34	0
203	Canned, sweetened	1	135	14	11			120	20	0
204	Grapefruit juice, canned	1	162	14	—		2	130	11	0.04
205	Frozen, diluted	1	170	17	9		1	162	14	0
206	Grapes, American	3	158	12	13		5	75[5]	80[5]	0

Item No.	Food	Sodium mg	Potassium mg	Phosphorus mg	Magnesium mg	Zinc mg	Folacin μg	Pantothenic Acid μg	Vitamin B_6 μg	Vitamin B_{12} μg	Vitamin E mg
207	European	3	173	20	6						
208	Grape juice, bottled	2	116	12	12						
209	Haddock, raw	61	304	197	24	0.7		130	180	1.3	0.60 (broiled)
210	Fried (dipped in egg, milk, bread crumbs)	177	348	247	24						
211	Heart, beef, lean, raw	86	193	195	18			2,500	250	11	
212	Cooked, braised	104	232	181							
213	Herring, raw, Pacific	74	420	225	—			—	—		
214	Smoked, hard	6,231	157	—	—			500	200	2	
215	Honey, strained	5	51	6	3		3	200	20	7	
216	Honeydew melon	12	251	16	—		5	207	56	0	
217	Ice cream, no added salt, approximately 12% fat	40	112	99	14	0.5		492	—	—	0.06
218	Ice milk, no added salt	68	195	124	—						
219	Jams and preserves	12	88	9	5			—	25	0	
220	Jellies	17	75	7	4						
221	Kale, cooked, leaves with stems	43	221	46	37		70	376 (frozen)	185 (frozen)	0	
222	Lamb, average of lean cuts, cooked	70	290	223	21 (raw)	4.3	3	550 (raw)	275 (raw)	2.15 (raw)	0.16
223	Lard	0	0	0	0	0.2					
224	Lemon juice, fresh	1	141	10	8		—	—	20	0	
225	Lemonade, frozen, diluted	trace	16	1	1		1	103	46	0	
226	Lettuce, butterhead	9	264	26			25	11	5		
227	Crisphead	9	175	22	11	0.4	21[5]	200[5]	55[5]	0	0.06
228	Looseleaf	9	264	25		0.4	44				
229	Lime juice, fresh or canned	1	104	11	—			314 (sweet)	— (sweet)	0	

No.	Item	A	B	C	D	E	F	G	H	I	J
230	Limeade, frozen, diluted	trace	13	1	—						
	Liver, cooked, fried:										
231	Beef	184	380	476	18	5.1	294 (raw)	7,700 (raw)	840 (raw)	80 (raw)	0.63 (broiled)
232	Calf	118	453	537	26	6.1		8,000 (raw)	670 (raw)	60 (raw)	
233	Pork	111	395	539	24		221	6,400 (raw)	650 (raw)	32 (raw)	
234	Lobster, canned or cooked	210	180	192	22 (raw)	2.2		1,500 (raw)	—	0.5 (raw)	
235	Macaroni, dry	2	197	162	48	1.5			64	0	
236	Cooked, firm	1	79	65	20						
237	Tender	1	61	50	18	0.5					
238	Macaroni and cheese, baked	543	120	161	—						
239	Margarine, salted	987	23	16		0.2	—				
240	Unsalted	under 10									
241	Milk, whole	50	144	93	13	0.4	1	340	40	0.4	0.04
242	Skim	52	145	95	14	0.4	trace	370	42	0.4	
243	Dry, nonfat, instant	526	1,725	1,005	143	4.5		3,600	380	3.2	
244	Evaporated, undiluted	118	303	205	25	0.8	1	640	50	0.16	
245	Milk, goat's	34	180	106	17			320	45	0.08	
246	Milk, human	16	51	14	4			220	10	0.04	
	Milk beverages:										
247	Chocolate flavored, with skim milk	46	142	91	—						
248	Malted, with whole milk	91	200	122	—						
249	Molasses, light	15	917	45	46		10[5]				
250	Blackstrap	96	2,927	84	258						
251	Muffins, corn, enriched degermed cornmeal	481	135	169	—			350[5]	200[5]	0[5]	
252	Plain	441	125	151	—						
253	Mushrooms, raw	15	414	116			24	2,200	125	0	
254	Canned	400	197	68	8		4	1,000	60	0	
255	Mustard, prepared, yellow	1,252	130	73	48						1.75

Item No. / Food	Sodium mg	Potassium mg	Phosphorus mg	Magnesium mg	Zinc mg	Folacin μg	Pantothenic Acid μg	Vitamin B6 μg	Vitamin B12 μg	Vitamin E mg
256 Mustard greens, cooked	18	220	32	27 (raw)		60	164 (frozen)	133 (frozen)	0 (frozen)	1.75 (raw)
257 Nectarine	6	294	24	13		20	—	17	0	
258 Noodles, enriched, dry	5	136	183	—			—	88	trace	
259 Cooked	2	44	59	—						
260 Oatmeal, dry	2	352	405	144	3.4	30	1,500	140	0	2.27[2]
261 Cooked, salted	218	61	57	21	0.5	33				
262 Oil, vegetable	0	0	0	0	0.2	—				36.0 (corn)[7]
263 Okra, cooked	2	174	41	41 (raw)		24	215 (frozen)	45 (frozen)	0 (frozen)	
264 Olives, green	2,400	55	17	22			18	—	0	
265 Ripe	813	34	16	—		1	15	14	0	
266 Onions, mature, raw	10	157	36	12	0.3	11	130	130	0	
267 Cooked	7	110	29	—		10				
268 Onions, young green	5	231	39	—	0.3	14	144	—	0	
269 Oranges, peeled	1	200	20	11	0.2	5	250	60	0	
270 Orange juice, fresh	1	200	17	11	0.02	2	190	40	0	0.04
271 Canned	1	199	18	—	0.07	2	150	35	0	
272 Frozen, diluted	1	186	16	10	0.02	2	164	28	0	
273 Oysters, eastern, raw	73	121	143	32	74.7	11 (canned)	250	50	18	
274 Pancakes, buckwheat, from mix	464	245	337	—			218			
275 Wheat, home recipe	425	123	139	—						
276 Papayas, raw	3	234	16	—				—	0	
277 Parsley	45	727	63	41		38	300	164	0	
278 Parsnips, cooked	8	379	62	32		23	600[2]	90[2]	0[2]	
279 Peaches, raw	1	202	19	10 (raw)	0.2	4	170	24	0	

280	Canned	2	130	12	6	0.1	1	50	19	0	
281	Dried, sulfured, uncooked	16	950	117	48		5	—	100[2]	0[2]	
282	Cooked with sugar	4	261	32	15			132	18	0	
283	Frozen	2	124	13	6		4				
284	Peach nectar	1	78	11	—						
285	Peanuts, roasted	5	701	407	175	3.0	57	2,100	400	0	7.70 (dry)
286	Salted	418	674	401	175		57	—	330	0	
287	Peanut butter	607	670	407	173	2.9	2	70	17	0	
288	Pears, raw	2	130	11	7			70	14	0	
289	Canned	1	84	7	5			22			
290	Pear nectar	1	39	5	—						
291	Peas, green, cooked	1	196	99	35 (raw)	0.7	25				0.55
292	Canned, regular pack	236	96	76	20	0.8	10	150	50	0	0.02
293	Low-sodium pack	3	96	76	—						
294	Frozen, not thawed[8]	129[8]	150	90	24		25	315	130	0	0.25
295	Peas, dry, split, raw	40	895	268	180	3.2	51[2]	2,000	130	0	
296	Cooked	13	296	89	—	1.1		220 (canned)	20 (canned)	(canned)	
297	Pecans	Trace	603	289	142		27	1,707	183	0	
298	Peppers, sweet, green, raw	13	213	22	18		7	230	260	0	
299	Perch, ocean, Atlantic, raw	79	269	207	8						
300	Persimmons, Japanese	6	174	26	12				7[5]	0[5]	
301	Pickles, dill	1,428	200	21	—						
302	Relish, sweet	712	—	14	—						
	Pies, home recipe:										
303	Apple	301	80	22				110	—	0	2.50
304	Cherry	304	105	25					—	0	
305	Custard	287	137	113				946		0	
306	Lemon meringue	282	50	49				—			
307	Mince	448	178	38					—		
308	Pumpkin	214	160	69				519	—	—	

Item No.	Food	Sodium mg	Potassium mg	Phosphorus mg	Magnesium mg	Zinc mg	Folacin μg	Pantothenic Acid μg	Vitamin B$_6$ μg	Vitamin B$_{12}$ μg	Vitamin E mg
309	Piecrust, baked	611	50	50	—			—	115	—	
310	Pike, walleye, raw	51	319	214	—			160	88	0	
311	Pineapple, raw	1	146	8	13		6	100	74	0	
312	Canned	1	96	5	8		1	100	96	0	
313	Pineapple juice, canned	1	149	9	12		1				
314	Pizza, cheese, home recipe	702	130	195							
315	Plums, raw	2	299	17	9			186	52	0	
316	Canned, purple	1	142	10	5		1	72	27	0	
317	Popcorn, salted	1,940	—	216	—	3.0		—	204	0	
	Pork, fresh:										
318	Ham, lean, roasted	65	390	308	29	3.1	2 (loin)	790 (raw)	450 (raw)	0.70 (raw)	0.16 (chops, fried)
319	Picnic ham, lean, simmered	65	390	176	18	4.0					
	Pork, cured:										
320	Ham, light cure, lean, cooked	930	326	200	20	4.0	11	675 (raw)	400 (raw)	0.60 (raw)	0.28 (fried)
321	Canned, spiced or unspiced	(1,100)	(340)	156	— (raw)			(raw)	360	—	
322	Potatoes, baked	4	503	65	22			—	233[5]		0.03
323	Boiled, unsalted	2	285	42	—	0.3		540 (frozen)	174 (frozen)	0	0.04
324	French fried	6	853	111	—		7		180		0.28
325	Mashed, with milk, table fat, salted	331	250	48	—						
326	Potato chips	variable to 1,000	1,130	139	—			— (frozen)	180 (frozen)	0	6.40
327	Pretzels	1,680[9]	130	131	40						
328	Prunes, dried, uncooked	118	694	79	40		5	540	19	trace	0.15
329	Cooked, without sugar	4	327	37	20			460[2]	240[2]	0[2]	

330	Prune juice, canned	2	235	20	10					
	Pudding, home recipe:									
331	Bread with raisins	201	215	114	—					
332	Chocolate	56	171	98	—					
333	Cornstarch (blanc mange)	65	138	91	—					
334	Rennin, using mix	46	128	92	—					
335	Rice with raisins	71	177	94	—					
336	Tapioca cream	156	135	109	—					
337	Pumpkin, canned, unsalted	2	240	26	12		8	400	56	0
					(raw)					
338	Radishes, raw	18	322	31	15		7	184	75	0
339	Raisins, dried	27	763	101	35		10	45	240	0
340	Raspberries, red, raw	1	168	22	20		5	240	60	0
341	Frozen	1	100	17	—		5	270	38	0
342	Rhubarb, cooked	2	203	15	13		4[5]	70	25	0
343	Rice, white, dry	5	92	94	28	1.3		550 (frozen)	170 (frozen)	0
344	Cooked, salted	374	28	28	8	0.4	16			0.18
	Rice cereals:									
345	Flakes	987	180	132	—	1.4	8	340	125	0.04
346	Puffed, without salt	2	100	92	—	1.4		378	75	0
347	Rolls, commercial, plain	506	95	85	—	0.6		310	35	—
348	Sweet	389	124	107	—					
349	Whole wheat	564	292	281	—					
350	Rutabagas, cooked	4	167	31	15		5	160[2]	100[2]	0[2]
					(raw)					
351	Rye flour, light	1	156	185	73					
352	Rye wafers	882	600	388	—		16	720	90	0
	Salad dressings:[10]									
353	Blue cheese	1,094	37	74						
354	Commercial, mayonnaise type	586	9	26						
355	French	1,370	79	14	10	0.2				
356	Home cooked	728	116	93	2					
357	Mayonnaise	597	34	28		0.2				

Item No.	Food	Sodium mg	Potassium mg	Phosphorus mg	Magnesium mg	Zinc mg	Folacin µg	Pantothenic Acid µg	Vitamin B6 µg	Vitamin B12 µg	Vitamin E mg
358	Thousand island	700	113	17							
359	Salmon, pink, raw	64	306	—	—			300	700	4	1.35 (broiled)
360	Canned	387[11]	361	286	30	0.9	1	550	300	6.89	
361	Sardines, Pacific, canned in tomato sauce	400	320	478	24		1	700	160	10	
362	Sauerkraut	747[12]	140	18	—			93	130	0	
	Sausage:										
363	Bologna	1,300	230	128	—	1.8	—	—	100	—	0.06
364	Frankfurters, raw	1,100	220	133	—	2.0	—	430	140	1.30	
365	Pork links, cooked	958	269	162	16		12	682	165	0.54	0.16 (fried)
366	Scallops, bay steamed	265	476	338	—			132 (raw)	—	1.20 (raw)	0.60 (frozen, deep fried)
367	Shad, raw	54	330	260	—						
368	Baked, with butter or margarine	79	377	313	—			608	—	—	
369	Sherbet, orange	10	22	13	—						
370	Shrimp, raw	140	220	166	42	1.5		280	100	0.90	0.60 (fried)
371	Canned, dry pack	—	122	263	51	2.1	2	210	60	—	
	Soup, canned, diluted with equal part water:										
372	Bean with pork	403	158	51	—						
373	Beef bouillon	326	54	13	—						
374	Beef noodle	382	32	20	—						
375	Chicken noodle	408	23	15	—						
376	Clam chowder, Manhattan type	383	75	19	—						

377 Cream soup (mushroom), prepared with milk	424	114	69	—						
378 Minestrone	406	128	24	—						
379 Pea, green	367	80	46	—						
380 Tomato	396	94	14	9						
381 Vegetable with beef broth	345	98	16	—			140		0	
382 Spaghetti, dry	2	197	162	—			—	64	0	
383 Cooked, tender	1	61	50	—						
384 Spaghetti with meatballs, canned	488	98	45	—						
385 Spaghetti in tomato sauce with cheese, home recipe	(382)	163	54	—						
386 Spinach, raw	71	470	51	88	0.8	77	300	280	0	
387 Cooked	50	324	38	—	0.7	75	75	130	0	
388 Canned, regular pack	236	250	26	63	0.8	49	65 (frozen)	70 (frozen)	0	0.02
389 Low sodium	32	250	26	—						
390 Squash, summer, cooked	1	141	25	16		11	173	63	0	
391 Winter, cooked	1	258	32	17 (raw)		12	282 (frozen)	91 (frozen)	0	
392 Strawberries, raw	1	164	21	12		9	340	55	0	0.13
393 Frozen	1	112	17	9		9	135	43	0	0.21
394 Sugar, brown	30	344	19	—						
395 Granulated	1	3	0	trace	0.06					
396 Sweet potatoes, baked	12	300	58	31 (raw)		12[5]	820 (raw)	218 (raw)	0	
397 Boiled	10	243	47	(raw)						
398 Candied	42	190	43	—						
399 Syrup, table blend	68	4	16	—						
400 Tangerines, raw	2	126	18	—		7	200	67	0	
401 Tangerine juice, canned	1	178	14	—			—	32	0	
402 Tapioca, dry	3	18	18	3		6				
403 Tea, instant, dry powder	—	4,530	—	395						

Item No. Food	Sodium mg	Potassium mg	Phosphorus mg	Magnesium mg	Zinc mg	Folacin µg	Pantothenic Acid µg	Vitamin B6 µg	Vitamin B12 µg	Vitamin E mg
404 Beverage	—	25		22	0.02					
405 Tomatoes, raw	3	244	27	14		8	330	100	0	
406 Canned, regular pack	130	217	19	12	0.2	4	230	90	0	0.40
407 Low sodium	3	217	19	—	0.2					
408 Tomato catsup, regular pack	1,042	363	50	21			—	107		
409 Tomato juice, canned, regular pack	200	227	18	10		7	250	192	0	
410 Canned, low sodium	3	227	18	—					0	0.22
411 Tongue, beef, braised	61	164	117	16						
412 Tuna, canned in oil, solids and liquid	800	301	294	(raw)		2	320	425		
413 Turkey, light, roasted	82	411	(251)	28	1.0	8[5]	591	—	2.20	
414 Dark, roasted	99	398	(251)	—	2.1		1,128	—	—	
415 Turnips, cooked, diced	34	188	24	20	4.4	4	200	90	—	
416 Turnip greens, canned, regular pack	236	243	30	(raw)			(raw)	(raw)	0	
417 Frozen, not thawed	23	188	41	58		42	68			
418 Veal, lean, stewed	80	500	140	(raw)	4.2	5	1,060	100	1.75	
419 Roasted	80	500	235	19	4.1		(raw)	400	0 (raw)	0.05 (fried)
420 Vinegar, cider	1	100	9	1				(raw)	(raw)	
421 Waffles, home recipe	475	145	173	—			650	1[5]	0	
422 Walnuts, black	3	460	570	190		77	900		—	
423 English	2	450	380	131			300			
424 Watermelon	1	100	10	8		1		730	0	
425 Wheat bran, crude	9	1,121	1,276	490	9.8	195		68	0	
Wheat cereals, cooked:										
426 Wheat and malted barley, dry	1	—	350	168	3.6	33				

No.											
427	Cooked	72	trace	59	31	0.5					0.61[2]
428	Wheat, rolled, cooked	trace	84	76	—		49				
	Wheat cereals, ready to eat:										
429	Wheat flakes	1,032	—	309	—	2.3	47	469	292	0	
430	Wheat, puffed, without salt	4	340	322	—	2.6		—	170	0	
431	Wheat, shredded, plain	3	348	388	133	2.8	55	706	244	0	
	Wheat flours:										
432	All purpose or family	2	95	87	25	0.7	8	465	60	0	
433	Cake	2	95	73		0.3	5	320	45	0	
434	Self-rising	1,079	90[13]	466	—						
435	Whole wheat	3	370	372	113	2.4	38	1,100	340	0	
436	Wheat germ	3	827	1,118	336	14.3	305	1,200	1,150	0	
437	White sauce, medium	379	139	93	—						
	Yeast, bakers':										
438	Compressed	16	610	394	59			3,500	600	0	
439	Dry active	(52)	(1,998)	(1,291)	—			11,000	2,000	0	
440	Brewers', dry	121	1,894	1,753	231		2,022	12,000	2,500	0	
441	Yogurt, made from partially skimmed milk	51	143	94	—			313	46	0.11	

[1] Dashes denote lack of reliable data for a constituent believed to be present in measurable amounts.

[2] Source of data does not indicate whether raw or cooked; it is assumed that the values are for the raw food.

[3] Based on use of self-rising flour containing anhydrous monocalcium phosphate.

[4] Based on calculations using sodium aluminum sulfate powder with monocalcium phosphate monohydrate.

[5] Nature of samples not clearly defined.

[6] Values for phosphorus and sodium are based on use of 1.5 percent anhydrous disodium phosphate as the emulsifying agent. If the emulsifying agent does not contain either phosphorus or sodium, the content of these nutrients per 100 gm is sodium, 650 mg; phosphorus, 444 mg.

[7] Vitamin E in other oils as follows: cottonseed, 60.5; olive, 67.0; peanut, 61.0; safflower, 90.0; and soybean, 21.0 mg per 100 gm.

[8] Average weighted in accordance with commercial practices in freezing vegetables.

[9] Sodium content is variable. For example, very thin pretzel sticks contain about twice the average amount listed.

[10] For salad dressing without salt, sodium content is low, ranging from less than 10 mg to 50 mg per 100 gm; the amount is usually indicated on the label.

[11] If canned without salt, the sodium value is about the same as for raw salmon.

[12] Based on salt content of 1.9 percent; may vary significantly from this level.

[13] Ninety milligrams potassium per 100 gm contributed by flour. Small quantities of additional potassium may be contributed by other ingredients.

APPENDIX 10: NUMERICAL FACTORS: PROTEIN, FAT, AND CARBOHYDRATE METABOLISM

The factors below are determined from the metabolism of protein, fat, and carbohydrate. The protein metabolized is determined both as protein weight directly (1 g) and as a 1 g of nitrogen, since urinary nitrogen is the common measure for protein. The values of grams of protein and grams of nitrogen differ by the factor 6.25 grams protein/gram of nitrogen which is based upon a 16 percent nitrogen content in the average protein.

(a) "Water of Oxidation" in the table below shows the amount of water produced by the oxidation of the weight of the foodstuff given. Fat when oxidized to $CO_2 + H_2O +$ energy gives rise to a weight of water greater than the weight of fat, i.e., 1 g fat produces 1.07 g H_2O

(b) "Gas Exchange" gives the amount of oxygen utilized per gram of foodstuff and the amount of CO_2 produced in terms of volume and weight. The "respiratory quotient" is calculated from the volume of CO_2 produced divided by the volume of O_2 metabolized.

(c) "Metabolizable Energy" gives the amount of energy in the protein, fat or carbohydrate as determined after complete metabolism. The "Gross, kcal" is the theoretical value with corrections made for incomplete oxidation. The "Metabolizable, kcal" includes a correction factor for incomplete absorption. Protein, fat, and carbohydrate have an absorption efficiency during digestion of 92 percent, 95 percent, and 97 percent respectively.

The "Caloric Value" of protein, fat, and carbohydrate are very similar. The utilization of 1 liter of O_2 will give rise to 4.60, 4.69, and 5.05 kcal, respectively for the oxidation of that foodstuff. The average of these values, 4.8 kcal is the value used to determine the heat production in indirect calorimetry. The value of 4.8 kcal is called caloric equivalent.

(d) "Specific dynamic action" (SDA) gives the increase in heat production that is associated with the ingestion of each type of foodstuff. Protein has the highest SDA. Some amino acids also exhibit the same effect. The quantitation of the SDA is difficult to measure in man. A value of about 10 percent of the total calories ingested is the usual SDA for the average meal and the SDA is generally not considered as significant in the design of meals or as a strategy for obesity.

Numerical Factors for Protein, Fat, and Carbohydrate
Metabolized in the Human Body*

Item and Units	Protein		Fat, 1 g	Carbo-hydrate, 1 g
	As Protein, 1 g	As Nitrogen, 1 g		
a. Water of oxidation, gm	0.41	2.56	1.07	0.60
b. Gas exchange				
Oxygen, ml	966	6,030	2,019	829
Oxygen, gm	1.38	8.61	2.88	1.185
Carbon dioxide, ml	782	4,880	1,427	829
Carbon dioxide, gm	1.53	9.57	2.80	1.63
Respiratory quotient	0.81	0.81	0.71	1.00
c. Metabolizable energy				
Gross, kcal	4.4	27.5	9.5	4.2
Metabolizable, kcal	4.1	25.6	9.0	4.1
Caloric values				
Oxygen, 1 liter	4.60	28.7	4.69	5.05
Oxygen, 1 gm	6.07	38.0	6.70	7.21
Carbon dioxide, 1 liter	5.68	35.6	6.63	5.05
Carbon dioxide, 1 gm	11.15	69.7	13.01	9.93
d. Specific dynamic action, kcal/100 kcal	30	30	4	6

Weights of oxygen and carbon dioxide
$$1 \text{ liter } O_2 = 1.4290 \text{ gm} \qquad 1 \text{ gm } O_2 = 0.6998 \text{ liter}$$
$$1 \text{ liter } CO_2 = 1.9769 \text{ gm} \qquad 1 \text{ gm } CO_2 = 0.5158 \text{ liter}$$
* A. Magnus-Levy (1907).

APPENDIX 11: NOMOGRAPHS FOR ESTIMATION OF HEAT PRODUCTION (METABOLIC RATE)

The heat production per squared meter (M²) of body surface is very similar for all mammals. For example, the kcal/M²/24 hr for man is about 1042, 1185 for the mouse, and 1142 for the average mammal. All values are with 10 percent of one another. There is no explanation for the universal nature of these values. There is also a relationship between the height (H) and weight (W) of man and the surface area. The relationship can only be determined empirically, i.e., there is no theoretical development for an equation.

Nomogram 1 was developed from direct measurements of surface areas, heights, and weights, the approach being the empirical determination of the exponents of W and H and the factor, 71.84. The measurements and information required to determine the heat production (metabolic rate) or kcal/M²/hr are the height, weight, oxygen consumption per hour, sex, and age. As an example, the heat production of the individual below will be calculated.

Data: Sex: Female
       Height: 5 ft 3 in (160 cm)
       Weight: 111 lbs (50 kg)
       Age: 25 yrs
       Oxygen consumption: 0.20 liters/min
       Conditions: At rest, 18 hrs postprandial (basal conditions)

Step 1: Using Nomogram 1, the height and the body weight (shown as dots on those scales), the line joining these values intersects the center scale at 1.5 M², the body surface area.

Step 2: Using Nomogram 2, the surface body area (1.t M²) and the oxygen consumption (0.20 liters/min (a determined value), the line joining these values intersects the center scale at 38 kcal/M²/hr. This is the heat production. It is sometimes referred to as the basal metabolic rate (BMR) when measured under basal conditions, but as will be shown in Nomogram 3, the BMR is truely expressed as a percent above or below normal value (0).

Step 3: Using Nomogram 3, the heat production (38 kcal/M²/hr, the sex (female, and age 25), the line joining the values intersects the center scale +9. This means that this individual has a basal metabolic rate (BMR) of 9 percent above the normal, and she is within the accepted normal range of ±20 percent. The normal (zero percent)) is a value obtained by averaging the heat productions of a large number of clinically normal individuals of a given age and sex. The normal heat production for any age and sex can be determined by pivoting a straight edge around the 0 (zero) of the center scale. It can be observed, for example, that heat production kcal/M²/hr declines with age.

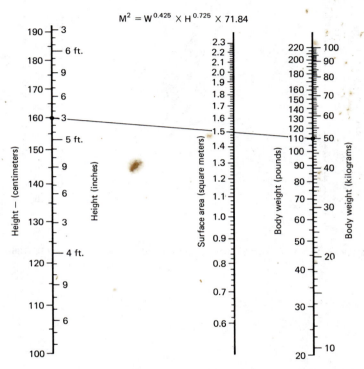

Surface area from height and weight. Nomogram constructed from the DuBois-Mech formula for surface area.

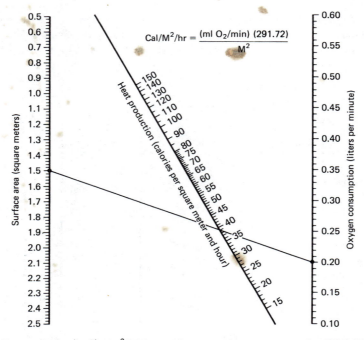

Heat production (kcal/meter^2/hr) from surface area and oxygen consumption (RQ 0.85)

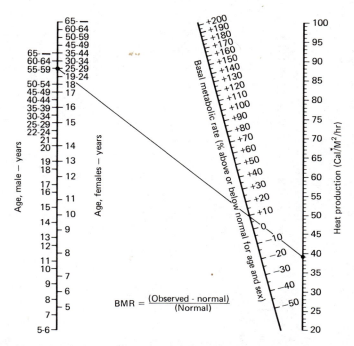

Metabolic rate from heat production, age, and sex. The Mayo Clinic standards were employed. [*Boothby, Berkson,* and *Dunn* (1936)].